Dermal Absorption and Toxicity Assessment

DRUGS AND THE PHARMACEUTICAL SCIENCES
A Series of Textbooks and Monographs

Executive Editor

James Swarbrick
PharmaceuTech, Inc.
Pinehurst, North Carolina

Dermal Absorption and Toxicity Assessment
Second Edition

Edited by

Michael S. Roberts
School of Medicine, University of Queensland
Princess Alexandra Hospital
Buranda, Australia

Kenneth A. Walters
An-eX Analytical Services Ltd.
Cardiff, United Kingdom

informa
healthcare

New York London

Informa Healthcare USA, Inc.
52 Vanderbilt Avenue
New York, NY 10017

© 2008 by Informa Healthcare USA, Inc.
Informa Healthcare is an Informa business

No claim to original U.S. Government works
Printed in the United States of America on acid-free paper
10 9 8 7 6 5 4 3 2 1

International Standard Book Number-10: 0-8493-7591-6 (Hardcover)
International Standard Book Number-13: 978-0-8493-7591-0 (Hardcover)

Library of Congress Cataloging-in-Publication Data

Dermal absorption and toxicity assessment/edited by Michael S. Roberts, Kenneth A. Walters – 2nd ed.
    p. ; cm. – (Drugs and the pharmaceutical sciences ; v. 177)
Includes bibliographical references and index.
ISBN-13: 978-0-8493-7591-0 (hb : alk. paper)
ISBN-10: 0-8493-7591-6 (hb : alk. paper)
    1. Dermatotoxicology. 2. Dermatologic agents–Toxicology. 3. Cosmetics–Toxicology. 4. Skin absorption. 5. Health risk assessment. I. Roberts, Michael S., 1949– II. Walters, Kenneth A., 1949– III. Series.
    [DNLM: 1. Skin Absorption–physiology. 2. Cosmetics–adverse effects. 3. Cosmetics–pharmacokinetics. 4. Environmental Exposure. 5. Pharmaceutical Preparations–adverse effects. 6. Risk Assessment. W1 DR893B v.117 2007/WR 102 D434 2007]
    RL803.D44 2007
    615'.778–dc22   2007031873

For Corporate Sales and Reprint Permissions call 212-520-2700 or write to: Sales Department, 52 Vanderbilt, 16th floor, New York, NY 10017.

Visit the Informa Web site at
www.informa.com

and the Informa Healthcare Web site at
www.informahealthcare.com

Preface to the Second Edition

Since this book was first published in 1998, there have been significant advances in our understanding of the morphology of the skin and the properties that govern the transport of molecules into and across the three major strata. The multitude of data that has been generated has allowed the development of predictive models for both the rate and extent of dermal absorption and has increased our ability to predict the likelihood of local toxic events subsequent to solute penetration and permeation. In this second edition we have completely revised and updated many of the chapters that appeared in the earlier version and we have expanded the scope of the volume to include coverage of the more recent exciting and innovative areas of research. Those chapters concerned with dermatological and cosmeceutical therapy have been moved to a companion publication, *Dermatologic, Cosmeceutic, and Cosmetic Development: Therapeutic and Novel Approaches*.

This second edition has been divided into six parts covering skin structure and absorption, measurement of absorption, modeling of dermal absorption and risk assessment, skin toxicity and its prevention, regulatory issues, and specific examples of the absorption of environmental materials. As in the first edition, this book provides an overview of the dermal absorption process, with particular emphasis on the determinants for toxicity arising from dermal exposure. A general introduction, covering the structure of human and animal skin and its relationship to dermal absorption, is followed by Part I, which expands on the specific barrier properties of the skin, such as its physical structure, biosensor properties, cutaneous metabolism, skin lipid morphology, and dermal blood and lymphatic flow. The range of methods used to assess skin absorption is fully discussed in Part II. There, the use of standard established laboratory methods, such as diffusion cell technology, are covered together with some of the newer techniques, such as the use of cultured skin equivalents. Many of the techniques used for measurement and modeling of dermal absorption and risk assessment are discussed in Part III. This section also includes the use of mathematical models, many of which have been refined to provide more realistic predictions, together with structure-penetration relationships as principles for estimating dermal risk assessment. In addition, this part covers the estimation of systemic exposure subsequent to dermal absorption, pharmacodynamics and the pharmacokinetics of skin delivery, and the use of various real life exposure scenarios in dermal risk assessment.

The next two parts of the book focus on local toxicity and its prevention and regulatory initiatives. Within the local toxicity section, issues such as skin damage, irritation, sensitisation, phototoxicity, and the prevention of toxicity are covered. The regulatory section provides information on the various governmental and industrial programs concerning the issues surrounding skin permeation and toxicity, including alternative in silico, in vitro, and in vivo strategies to conduct studies for regulatory approval.

The final section provides some examples of substances absorbed through the skin, giving particular emphasis to environmental contaminants and cosmetic ingredients. This section includes the U.S. Environmental Protection Agency's defined common environmental substances, together with discussions on the percutaneous absorption of compounds from soil and bathing water, and the permeation of pesticides, metals, fragrances, and other cosmetic ingredients.

This book is intended for scientists involved in dermal absorption and for those concerned with the marketing of products that may be absorbed through the skin intentionally or unintentionally. To this end, we have been fortunate in obtaining the agreement of many internationally recognized experts in the field of dermal absorption and toxicity assessment to provide coverage of their specific fields of expertise. To all of our authors we extend our sincere thanks for their unreserved efforts and time.

Michael S. Roberts
Kenneth A. Walters

Preface from the First Edition

The development and use of chemicals, especially those in the pharmaceutical, general chemical, and cosmetic fields, are associated with hazards arising from human exposure. For these compounds, absorption into the skin may represent a major route of entry into the body. In addition, a number of such substances are applied to the skin for therapeutic or cosmetic purposes. The rate and extent of penetration into and absorption through the skin are defined by a number of variables, including environmental conditions, skin physiology, permeant structure, method of application, and species differences.

This volume provides and overview of the dermal absorption process, with particular emphasis on the determinants for toxicity arising from dermal exposure. Part I is concerned with the structure of the skin and the underlying principles defining percutaneous absorption and toxicity. In Part II, the concept of dermal risk assessment, predicted from epidemiological factors, physiological models, in vitro/in vivo experimentation, and chemical structures, is examined by experts in these areas. This section also describes the use of mathematical models together with structure-penetration relationships as principles for estimating dermal risk assessment.

Parts III and IV are concerned with dermal absorption and risk assessment as applied to specific product types: pharmaceuticals and cosmetics. The individual chapters discuss specific product classes such as drugs used for pain and inflammation, fragrances, sunscreens, and hair dyes. The final section, Part V, provides information on skin permeation following environmental exposure and includes discussions on the percutaneous absorption of compounds from soil and bathing water. Throughout this volume, pharmacokinetic data and models often used in dermal risk assessment are fully described.

The book has been written for scientists interested in dermal absorption and those concerned with the marketing of products that may be absorbed through the skin either intentionally or unintentionally. We hope that this book will prove useful to those involved in research and development in the pharmaceutical, cosmetic, agrochemical, household, and general chemical industries.

Michael S. Roberts
Kenneth A. Walters

Contents

Contributors

Yuri G. Anissimov   School of Biomolecular and Physical Sciences, Griffith University, Nathan, Queensland, Australia

Martin D. Barratt   Marlin Consultancy, Carlton, Bedford, U.K.

Andrew Bartholomaeus   Drug Safety and Evaluation Branch, Therapeutic Goods Administration, Woden, Australia

Edward D. Bashaw   Division III, Office of Clinical Pharmacology, U.S. Food and Drug Administration, Rockville, Maryland, U.S.A.

Ronald E. Baynes   Center for Chemical Toxicology Research and Pharmacokinetics, College of Veterinary Medicine, North Carolina State University, Raleigh, North Carolina, U.S.A.

Eva Benfeldt   Department of Dermatology, Gentofte Hospital, University of Copenhagen, Hellerup, Denmark

Keith R. Brain   An-eX Analytical Services, Ltd., and Cardiff University, Cardiff, U.K.

Robert L. Bronaugh   Office of Cosmetics and Colors, Food and Drug Administration, College Park, Maryland, U.S.A.

Annette L. Bunge   Department of Chemical Engineering, Colorado School of Mines, Golden, Colorado, U.S.A.

Heidi P. Chan   Department of Dermatology, School of Medicine, University of California San Francisco, San Francisco, California, U.S.A.

John Corish   School of Chemistry, Trinity College, University of Dublin, Dublin, Ireland

Mark T. D. Cronin   School of Pharmacy and Chemistry, Liverpool John Moores University, Liverpool, U.K.

Yuri Dancik   Department of Medicine, Princess Alexandra Hospital, University of Queensland, Woolloongabba, Queensland, Australia

Michael Dellarco   U.S. Environmental Protection Agency, National Center for Environmental Assessment, Washington, D.C., U.S.A.

Mitsuhiro Denda   Shiseido Research Center, Yokohama, Japan

William E. Dressler   Independent Consultant, Huntington, Connecticut, U.S.A.

Peter M. Elias   Dermatology and Medical (Metabolism) Services, Veterans Affairs Medical Center, and Departments of Dermatology and Medicine, University of California, San Francisco, California, U.S.A.

Steven J. Enoch   School of Pharmacy and Chemistry, Liverpool John Moores University, Liverpool, U.K.

David J. Esdaile   LAB International Research Centre, Szabadságpuszta, Veszprém, Hungary

Kenneth R. Feingold   Dermatology and Medical (Metabolism) Services, Veterans Affairs Medical Center, and Departments of Dermatology and Medicine, University of California, San Francisco, California, U.S.A.

Dara Fitzpatrick   Department of Chemistry, University College Cork, Cork, Ireland

Susi Freeman   Department of Dermatology, School of Medicine, University of California San Francisco, San Francisco, California, U.S.A.

Ulrike Günther   Institute of Pharmaceutics and Biopharmaceutics, Martin Luther University of Halle-Wittenberg, Halle, Germany

Ingrid Gerner   Weidenauer Weg, Berlin, Germany

Audrey Gierden   Department of Medicine, Princess Alexandra Hospital, University of Queensland, Woolloongabba, Queensland, Australia

Darach Golden   Centre for High Performance Computing, Trinity College, University of Dublin, Dublin, Ireland

Jonathan Hadgraft   The School of Pharmacy, University of London, London, U.K.

Betty Hakkert   National Institute for Public Health and the Environment, Expertise Centre for Substances, Bilthoven, The Netherlands

Brian Henry   Pfizer Global Research and Development, Sandwich, Kent, U.K.

Matthias Herzler   Federal Institute for Risk Assessment, Safety of Substances and Preparations, Thielallee, Berlin, Germany

Jon R. Heylings   Research and Investigative Toxicology, Syngenta Central Toxicology Laboratory, Macclesfield, Cheshire, U.K.

Jennifer R. Hill   Dows Institute, University of Iowa, Iowa City, Iowa, U.S.A.

Etje Hulzebos   National Institute for Public Health and the Environment, Expertise Centre for Substances, Bilthoven, The Netherlands

Mark Jenner   Scitox Assessment Services, Kambah, Australia

Owen G. Jepps   Department of Medicine, Princess Alexandra Hospital, University of Queensland, Woolloongabba, Queensland, Australia

Gerald B. Kasting,   James L. Winkle College of Pharmacy, University of Cincinnati Academic Health Center, Cincinnati, Ohio, U.S.A.

Janet Kielhorn   Fraunhofer Institute of Toxicology and Experimental Medicine, Hannover, Germany

John C. Kissel   Department of Environmental and Occupational Health Sciences, University of Washington, Seattle, Washington, U.S.A.

Jon Lalko   Research Institute for Fragrance Materials, Woodcliff Lake, New Jersey, U.S.A.

Majella E. Lane   The School of Pharmacy, University of London, London, U.K.

C. S. Leopold   Department of Pharmaceutical Technology, Institute of Pharmacy, University of Hamburg, Hamburg, Germany

Cheryl Y. Levin   Department of Dermatology, School of Medicine, University of California San Francisco, San Francisco, California, U.S.A.

Manfred Liebsch   Federal Institute for Risk Assessment, Centre for Alternative Methods to Animal Experiments—ZEBET, Diedersdorfer Weg, Berlin, Germany

B. C. Lippold   Institute of Pharmaceutics and Biopharmaceutics, Heinrich Heine University, Duesseldorf, Germany

Richard Lyons   Pfizer Global Research and Development, Sandwich, Kent, U.K.

Judith C. Madden   School of Pharmacy and Chemistry, Liverpool John Moores University, Liverpool, U.K.

Howard I. Maibach   Department of Dermatology, School of Medicine, University of California San Francisco, San Francisco, California, U.S.A.

Dawn McCleverty   Pfizer Global Research and Development, Sandwich, Kent, U.K.

James N. McDougal   Department of Pharmacology and Toxicology, Boonschoft School of Medicine, Wright State University, Dayton, Ohio, U.S.A.

Stephanie Melching-Kollmuß   Fraunhofer Institute of Toxicology and Experimental Medicine, Hannover, Germany

Hendrik Metz   Institute of Pharmaceutics and Biopharmaceutics, Martin Luther University of Halle-Wittenberg, Halle, Germany

Wim J. A. Meuling   Business Unit Biosciences, TNO Quality of Life, Zeist, The Netherlands

Nancy A. Monteiro-Riviere Center for Chemical Toxicology Research and Pharmacokinetics, College of Veterinary Medicine, North Carolina State University, Raleigh, North Carolina, U.S.A.

Richard P. Moody Healthy Environments and Consumer Safety Branch, Environmental Health Centre, Ottawa, Canada

Utz Mueller Food Standards Australia New Zealand, Canberra BC, Australia

Reinhard H. H. Neubert Institute of Pharmaceutics and Biopharmaceutics, Martin Luther University of Halle-Wittenberg, Halle, Germany

Johannes M. Nitsche Department of Chemical and Biological Engineering, University at Buffalo, State University of New York, Buffalo, New York, U.S.A.

Lars Norlén Medical Nobel Institute, Department of Cellular and Molecular Biology, Karolinska Institute, Stockholm, Sweden

Jim E. Riviere Center for Chemical Toxicology Research and Pharmacokinetics, College of Veterinary Medicine, North Carolina State University, Raleigh, North Carolina, U.S.A.

Michael S. Roberts Department of Medicine, Princess Alexandra Hospital, University of Queensland, Woolloongabba, Queensland, Australia

Emiel Rorije National Institute for Public Health and the Environment, Expertise Centre for Substances, Bilthoven, The Netherlands

Monika Schäfer-Korting Institut für Pharmazie (Pharmakologie und Toxikologie) der Freien Universität Berlin, Berlin, Germany

U. F. Schaefer Biopharmaceutics and Pharmaceutical Technology, Saarland University, Saarbruecken, Germany

Sylvia Schreiber Institut für Pharmazie (Pharmakologie und Toxikologie) der Freien Universität Berlin, Berlin, Germany

Vinod P. Shah Pharmaceutical Consultant, North Potomac, Maryland, U.S.A.

Jeffry H. Shirai Department of Environmental and Occupational Health Sciences, University of Washington, Seattle, Washington, U.S.A.

Kenneth B. Sloan Department of Medicinal Chemistry, University of Florida, Gainesville, Florida, U.S.A.

Elizabeth W. Spalt Integral Consulting, Inc., Mercer Island, Washington, U.S.A.

Horst Spielmann Federal Institute for Risk Assessment, Centre for Alternative Methods to Animal Experiments—ZEBET, Diedersdorfer Weg, Berlin, Germany

Winfried Steiling   Henkel KGaA, Corporate SHE and Product Safety—Human Safety Assessment, Düsseldorf, Germany

Haw-Yueh Thong   Department of Dermatology, School of Medicine, University of California San Francisco, San Francisco, California, U.S.A.

Johannes J. M. van de Sandt   Business Unit Food and Chemical Risk Analysis, TNO Quality of Life, Zeist, The Netherlands

Joop J. van Hemmen   Business Unit Food and Chemical Risk Analysis, TNO Quality of Life, Zeist, The Netherlands

Hans-Werner Vohr   Department of Toxicology, Bayer HealthCare AG, Wuppertal, Germany

John D. Walker   TSCA Interagency Testing Committee, Office of Pollution Prevention and Toxics, U.S. Environmental Protection Agency, Washington, D.C., U.S.A.

Kenneth A. Walters   An-eX Analytical Services, Ltd., Cardiff, U.K.

Siegfried Wartewig   Institute for Applied Dermatopharmacy, Halle, Germany

Scott C. Wasdo   Department of Medicinal Chemistry, University of Florida, Gainesville, Florida, U.S.A.

Philip W. Wertz   Dows Institute, University of Iowa, Iowa City, Iowa, U.S.A.

Simon C. Wilkinson   Medical Toxicology Research Centre, Newcastle University, Newcastle upon Tyne, U.K.

Faith M. Williams   Medical Toxicology Research Centre and Institute for Research on Environment and Sustainability, Newcastle University, Newcastle upon Tyne, U.K.

Introduction

Human Skin Morphology and Dermal Absorption

Michael S. Roberts
Department of Medicine, Princess Alexandra Hospital, University of Queensland, Woolloongabba, Queensland, Australia

Kenneth A. Walters
An-eX Analytical Services, Ltd., Cardiff, U.K.

INTRODUCTION

The relationship between the structure of human skin and its barrier properties has been the subject of extensive research over the past half century (1,2). There can be little doubt that the stratum corneum, the skin's outermost layer, plays an important role in this respect by providing protection against the ingress of environmental materials and controlling the egress of water. Investigations by many researchers have further refined our understanding of the precise nature of the diffusion-controlling barrier with consensus on the major role of the intercellular lipid lamellae of the stratum corneum (3). There are many excellent and recent reviews covering the structure of skin (4,5), the nature of the epidermis and its many protective functions (6–8), and permeation across the skin (9,10). Although it has been experimentally well established that it is the chemical morphology of the stratum corneum that controls the overall rate at which chemicals can permeate across the skin, other factors can contribute to the extent of such permeation. Figure 1 shows that a number of major secondary factors governing the extent of percutaneous absorption include permeant clearance from the skin (11) and desquamation (12), as well as response and toxicity. It is not the purpose of this chapter to reiterate the information already adequately reviewed elsewhere by colleagues and by us. In this introductory chapter, therefore, we have elected to cover some recent information relevant to the subject matter of the book, dermal absorption and toxicity assessment. Thus we discuss new insights in skin biology and barrier formation including the initiation of keratinocyte migration and differentiation in the basal layer of the epidermis, the constituents and morphology of the intercellular lipids and the process of desquamation (Fig. 2).

INITIATION OF KERATINOCYTE MIGRATION AND DIFFERENTIATION

The cells of the epidermis originate in the basal lamina between the dermis and viable epidermis. In this layer there are melanocytes, Langerhans cells, Merkel cells, and keratinocytes. The keratinocytes of the basal lamina are attached to the basement membrane by hemidesmosomes and focal adhesions that are comprised of several distinct proteins. The hemidesmosome complex contains two bullous pemphigoid antigens (BPAg1 and BPAg2) and several integrins (including integrins

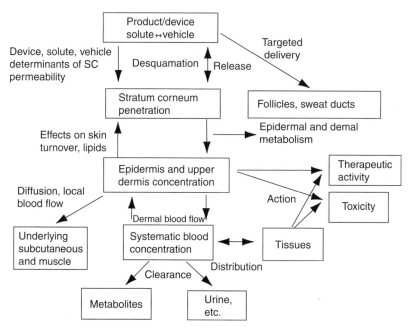

FIGURE 1 Dermal absorption; sites of action and toxicity. *Abbreviation*: SC, stratum corneum.

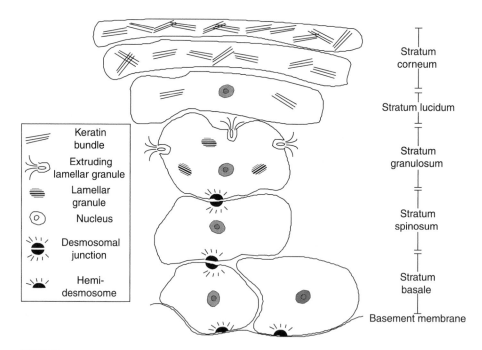

FIGURE 2 Major events in epidermal differentiation.

α6β4 and α3β1), together with multiple laminins (13–16), all of which are involved in securing the cell to the basement membrane. BPAg2 is a collagen that has an amino terminus within the hemidesmosome and a carboxy terminus within the lamina lucida of the basement membrane and may form part of the anchoring filament. The fundamental importance of these basal membrane-anchoring proteins is reflected in the devastating skin disorders associated with inherited and acquired encoding gene mutations such as dystrophic epidermolysis bullosa (type VII collagen) and bullous pemphigoid (integrin α6β4) (14).

In addition to hemidesmosome binding, another site for adhesion of the cells of the epidermal basal layer and the basal membrane is the adherens junction (17). The adherens junction expresses a different protein profile to desmosomes and hemidesmosomes, containing talin, vinculin, and cadherins; whereas, the hemidesmosomes are linked to cytoplasmic keratin, the proteins of the adherens junctions are linked to cytoplasmic actin microfilaments and appear to play an important role in cell migration (18) and may also have a functional role in nuclear signaling (19).

Although a secure link between the basal keratinocytes and the basal matrix is essential for skin integrity, these cells must also be capable of detaching and migrating to begin the process of terminal differentiation that will form the stratum corneum. Among the proteins implicated in detachment is CD151, a transmembrane protein of the tetraspanin family (20). CD151 is localized with integrin α6β4 at cell–matrix interfaces and it is suggested that dissociation of this complex allows remodeling of the cell–matrix attachment and subsequent cell migration. Another important link in the chain is integrin-linked kinase, which connects integrins to actin fibers and is thought to be highly involved in cell–matrix and cell–cell adhesion and migration (21). Similarly a role has been suggested for the calcium/manganese-ATPase, ATP2C1, in cell migration where it may act as a regulator of the integrin-linked basal attachment (22).

The relatively short-lived adherens junctions and the more stable hemidesmosomes regulate cell–matrix adhesion. Both types of adhesion must be disrupted to allow the keratinocyte to detach from the basal membrane. Rear detachment is accompanied by membrane ripping and the loss of cellular material in keratinocytes. Rigort and colleagues (23) showed that migrating keratinocytes leave behind "migration tracks" of cellular remnants that were anchored to a meshwork of extracellular matrix proteins consisting of collagen type IV, fibronectin, laminin, and laminin 5. These tracts were classified on the basis of their size, distribution, and molecular composition. Type I macroaggregates appeared as spherical and tubular structures with a diameter of about 50 to 100 nm. These structures appeared to be derived from fragmentation of long tubular extensions, the retracting fibers, at the cell rear and contained high amounts of α3β1 integrin, a component of fibronectin and laminin receptors in migrating keratinocytes usually found in focal adhesions. Type II macroaggregates were spherical structures with a diameter of about 30 to 50 nm that were arranged in clusters and scattered over the gaps between type I, macroaggregates. Type II macroaggregates contained high amounts of α6β4 integrin and probably derived from former hemidesmosomes. Their observations support the concept that the release of macroaggregates represents a distinct cellular mechanism of rear detachment based on the loss of adhesive receptors embedded in membrane-covered cellular remnants.

The role of the non-neuronal cholinergic system of human epidermis has been reviewed recently (24). The system is known as the keratinocyte acetylcholine axis and is composed of the enzymes mediating acetylcholine synthesis and degradation, and two classes of acetylcholine receptors, the nicotinic and muscarinic receptors. Regulation of keratinocyte cell–cell and cell–matrix adhesion is one of the important biological functions of cutaneous acetylcholine. The targets include both the intercellular adhesion molecules, such as desmosomal cadherins, and the cell–matrix adhesion molecules (integrins). The signaling pathways include activation or inhibition of kinase cascades resulting in either up- or down-regulation of the expression of cell adhesion molecules or changes in their phosphorylation status, or both. For example, it has been proposed that the muscarinic M3 receptor activation is linked to up-regulation of $\alpha2\beta1$-integrin and $\alpha3\beta1$-integrin-mediated cell adhesion, whereas activation of the muscarinic M4 receptor stimulates keratinocyte motility by up-regulating the migratory integrins $\alpha5\beta1$, $\alpha v\beta5$, and $\alpha v\beta6$ (25).

Nguyen and colleagues investigated the role of the non-neuronal acetylcholine axis in the control of cell–cell adhesion of human epidermal keratinocytes (26). Cholinergic effects on the expression of desmoglein 1 and 3 were measured using semiquantitative immunofluorescence and Western blot assays. Keratinocyte mono-layers were treated with the cholinergic agonist carbachol or the acetylcholinesterase inhibitor pyridostigmine bromide. Both compounds increased the relative amounts of desmoglein 1 and 3. The role for cholinergic receptor-mediated phosphorylation of desmoglein molecules in the assembly and disassembly of keratinocyte desmosomes was investigated by evaluating the effects of a cholinergic antagonist, atropine, on keratinocyte adhesion and desmoglein phosphorylation status. Atropine induced a rapid detachment of cells from each other and increased phosphorylation of desmoglein 3. The atropine-dependent phosphorylation of desmoglein 3 was inhibited by carbachol. It was concluded that keratinocyte cholinergic receptors regulate desmosomal adhesion of keratinocytes by altering the level of expression of both desmoglein 1 and 3 and the phosphorylation state of desmoglein 3.

The same group also investigated the roles of the muscarinic M3, the nicotinic $\alpha3$ and the mixed muscarinic–nicotinic $\alpha9$ acetylcholine receptors in the physiologic control of keratinocyte adhesion (27). Both muscarinic and nicotinic antagonists caused keratinocyte detachment and reversibly increased the permeability of keratinocyte monolayers. Phosphorylation of adhesion proteins is known to play an important role in the assembly and disassembly of intercellular junctions. The authors found that the phosphorylation levels of E-cadherin, β-catenin, and γ-catenin increased following pharmacological blockage of muscarinic receptors. Long-term blocking of all three receptor-signaling pathways with antisense oligonucleotides resulted in cell–cell detachment and changes in the expression levels of E-cadherin, β-catenin, and γ-catenin in cultured human keratinocytes. Overall, the data indicated that the three acetylcholine receptors played key synergistic roles in regulating keratinocyte adhesion, most likely by modulating the levels and activities of cadherin and catenin.

The keratinocyte cholinergic axis may prove to be a very interesting biochemical pathway to probe in the search for new therapeutic entities for the treatment of skin adhesion malfunction, such as Hailey–Hailey and Darier's diseases.

THE INTERCELLULAR LIPIDS OF THE STRATUM CORNEUM

The development of the stratum corneum from the keratinocytes of the basal layer involves several steps of cell differentiation that have resulted in a structure based classification of the layers above the basal layer (the stratum basale). Thus the cells progress through the stratum spinosum, the stratum granulosum, the stratum lucidium to the stratum corneum. Cell turnover, from stratum basale to stratum corneum, is about 21 days. The stratum spinosum (prickle cell layer), which lies immediately above the basal layer, consists of several layers of cells that are connected by desmosomes and contain prominent keratin tonofilaments. In the outer cell layers of the stratum spinosum, membrane-coating granules appear and this region forms the border with the overlying stratum granulosum. The most characteristic feature of the stratum granulosum are the many intracellular membrane-coating granules, the assembly of which appears to take place in the endoplasmic reticulum and Golgi regions (28). Lamellar subunits are observed within these granules and these are the precursors of the intercellular lipid lamellae of the stratum corneum. In the outermost layers of the stratum granulosum, the lamellar granules migrate to the apical cell surface where they fuse and eventually extrude their contents into the intercellular space. At this stage, in the differentiation process, the keratinocytes lose their nuclei and other cytoplasmic organelles, become flattened and compacted to form the stratum lucidum, which eventually forms the stratum corneum. The extrusion of the contents of lamellar granules is a fundamental requirement for the formation of the epidermal permeability barrier (29) and disturbances in this process have been implicated in various dermatological disorders (30–32).

There has been some debate on the physical structure and state of the intercellular lipid regions. A structural model of the skin barrier was proposed by Norlen (33), who postulated that the stratum corneum intercellular lipid existed as a single and coherent lamellar gel phase. The proposed intercellular structure was stabilized by the unique mixture of lipids and their chain length distributions and had virtually no phase boundaries. The intact gel phase was suggested to be located mainly in the lower half of stratum corneum. In the outermost regions of the stratum corneum, crystalline segregation and phase separation may be the result of the desquamation process. This single gel phase model differed significantly from earlier models in that it predicted that no phase separation was present in the unperturbed barrier structure. Norlen and colleagues went on to show, using atomic force microscopy on Langmuir–Blodgett films composed of extracted human stratum corneum ceramides, cholesterol, free fatty acids, cholesterol sulfate, and cholesteryl oleate, that the saturated long-chain free fatty acid distribution of human stratum corneum prevented hydrocarbon chain segregation (34). More recently, this group used differential scanning calorimetry, fluorescence spectroscopy, and two-photon excitation and laser scanning confocal fluorescence microscopy to show that, at normal skin temperatures, the phase state of hydrated bilayers made from human stratum corneum lipids corresponded microscopically to a single gel-phase at pH 7. There was coexistence of different gel-phases between pH 5 and 6, and no fluid phase at any pH [(35), see also Chapter 3 of this volume].

It is not surprising that the biologically unique stratum corneum lipid composition, mainly long chain ceramides, free fatty acids and cholesterol [(36), see also Chapter 4 of this volume], results in lipid phase behavior that is different from that of other biological membranes. The extensive work of Bouwstra and her colleagues suggests that crystalline phases are predominantly present in the stratum corneum intercellular lipid, but also that there is probably a subpopulation of lipids that form a liquid phase, probably promoted by the presence of free fatty acids (37). The authors pointed out that mixtures prepared only with ceramides and cholesterol formed a lamellar phase with a 13 nm periodicity. When free fatty acids were present the lattice density of the structure increased. The presence of ceramide 1 is essential to the formation of the 13 nm lamellar phase. Bouwstra's group proposed a molecular model for the structural organization of the 13 nm lamellar phase (the sandwich model), in which crystalline and liquid domains coexisted (38).

The discussion on the precise nature of the stratum corneum intercellular lipid state seems set to continue (34,39,40), but, whatever the actual state is, the possibility of using the collective knowledge of the structure of the skin barrier to formulate vesicles for improved drug delivery across the skin has been the subject of intense investigation. For example, the Leiden group focused on differences between the effects of gel-state vesicles, liquid-state vesicles, and elastic vesicles (41–43). The in vivo and in vitro interactions between elastic-, rigid vesicles and micelles with human skin were investigated (42). Following application of the solutions containing the vesicles and micelles, the stratum corneum was tape-stripped and subsequently visualized by freeze fracture electron microscopy. There were no ultrastructural changes in skin treated with rigid vesicles. Elastic vesicles appeared to rapidly partition intact into the deeper layers of the stratum corneum, where they accumulated in channel-like regions. Since only small amounts of vesicle material was found in the deepest layers of the stratum corneum, it was concluded that partitioning of intact vesicles into the viable epidermis was unlikely. There was excellent in vitro/in vivo correlation. It was concluded that elastic vesicles were superior to rigid vesicles for interaction with skin and drug delivery.

Distribution profiles in the stratum corneum were obtained for the elastic and rigid vesicle material and for the model drug ketorolac (43). As suggested by earlier work (42), the elastic vesicle rapidly entered the deeper layers of the stratum corneum. The rigid vesicle material did not penetrate deeply into the stratum corneum. As expected, the elastic vesicles delivered more ketorolac into the stratum corneum than the rigid vesicles. Distribution of ketorolac in the deeper layers of the stratum corneum was different than that of the vesicle material, suggesting that the ketorolac was released from the vesicles in the skin.

Similarly, deformable or elastic liposomal formulations have proved to be superior to rigid and traditional liposomes in the delivery of many compounds into and across the skin, including estradiol (44), diclofenac (45), and propranolol (46). The use of vesicles such as liposomes to modulate drug delivery into and through the skin has become reasonably accepted but the mechanism(s) of action remains unclear. As recently pointed out by El Maghraby and colleagues (47), vesicles vary considerably with respect to size, lamellarity, charge, membrane fluidity or elasticity, which allows for multiple functions ranging from local to transdermal effects and this may result in multiple modes of action.

DESQUAMATION

During the process of terminal differentiation, keratinocytes migrate from the basal layer toward the stratum corneum where they ultimately detach in the process of desquamation. Since the keratinocytes are linked by desmosomes, it is perhaps not surprising that it is the degradation of these links that signals the initiation of desquamation. The major adhesive molecules in the desmosome are cadherins. These are Ca^{++}-dependent molecules and they cooperate to make up the adhesive core of the desmosome. The adhesion molecules may have differentiation-specific functions over and above their roles in cell adhesion (for review see Ref. 48).

The most important cadherins located in the desmosome are desmoglein 1, desmocollin 1, and corneodesmosin, and it is thought that, while desmoglein 1 promotes the formation of the adhesive link, it is the relative level of desmoglein and desmocollin expressed at the cell surface that regulates the adhesive process (49). For desquamation to occur, it is necessary for the desmosomal link to degrade. Human tissue kallikreins are a family of 15 trypsin- or chymotrypsin-like secreted serine proteases (KLK1–KLK15) that have been identified in normal stratum corneum, and are candidate desquamation-related proteases. Two serine proteases of the kallikrein family have been implicated in this process: the stratum corneum chymotryptic enzyme (SCCE/KLK7/Hk7) and the stratum corneum tryptic enzyme (SCTE/KLK5/Hk5). The capacity of these enzymes to cleave desmoglein 1, desmocollin 1, and corneodesmosin has been investigated (50). At acidic pHs similar to that of the stratum corneum, SCCE cleaved corneodesmosin and desmocollin 1 but was unable to degrade desmoglein 1. On the other hand, incubation with SCTE induced degradation of all three proteins. The data suggested that SCTE was able to activate the proform of SCCE and that both kallikreins were involved in desquamation. More recently, it was found that the epidermal pH gradient regulates the activity of KLK5 with acidic conditions being required for its activation in the superficial layers of the stratum corneum (51).

There are several more serine proteases (apart from KLK5 and KLK7) that are located in the epidermis. Borgono and colleagues (52) investigated the contribution of KLK1, KLK5, KLK6, KLK13, and KLK14 to the desquamation process by examining their interaction with a colocalized serine protease inhibitor lympho-epithelial Kazal-type-related inhibitor (LEKTI) and their ability to digest desmoglein 1. Apart from KLK13, all kallikreins digested the ectodomain of desmoglein 1 within cadherin repeats, Ca^{++}-binding sites, or in the juxtamembrane region suggesting that multiple kallikreins participate in desquamation.

As is quite common in biological systems, evolution has resulted in an extremely complex mechanism for shedding a layer of skin each day. It is a simple matter to accept that this happens for a reason but not so simple to figure out just what that reason (or reasons) is. Why does the stratum corneum keep renewing itself? Milstone (12) puts forward the concept that continuous desquamation might reflect "a first line of defense against a myriad of known as well as unanticipated or novel physical, chemical or toxic assailants." The argument is intriguing, the discussion is continuing.

INTERRELATIONSHIP BETWEEN SKIN PHYSIOLOGY AND KINETICS OF DERMAL ABSORPTION

As some of the key concepts concerning these inter-relationships are covered in the later chapters "Physiologically-based pharmacokinetics and pharmacodynamics of skin" and "Beyond stratum corneum," this section is limited to a summary of the key principles and implications.

Principles of Dermal Absorption

The amount of a compound absorbed (Q) into the body depends on effective flux through the epidermis J_s, the area of application (A), the effective lag time (lag), and the exposure time (T):

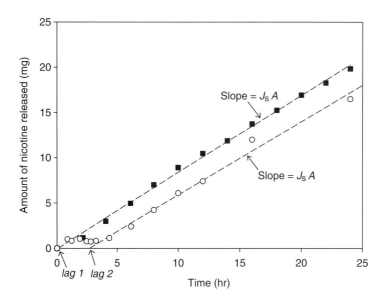

FIGURE 3 Nicotine release from patches in vitro (■) and in vivo (○). *Source*: Adapted from Ref. 63.

$$Q = J_s A(T - \text{lag}) \tag{1}$$

The time required to reach a steady-state flux $J_s A$ is ∼2 times the lag time. Figure 3 shows an illustration of equation (1) for release of nicotine from a patch in vivo and in vitro. It is apparent that in vivo there is an additional pharmacokinetic lag and the $J_s A$ is only slightly less consistent, with release from the patch being the rate-determining step in the absorption process. The effective flux into a target site in the epidermis or dermis in turn is dependent on the first pass availability of the solute through the skin F_s, recognizing that this may be less than one through loss from removal on clothing, evaporation, adsorption to outermost layers in the stratum corneum, vaporization, desquamation or by skin first pass metabolism prior to reaching the site. In general, the in vivo flux:

$$J_{s,\,\text{in vivo}} = F_s J_{s,\,\text{in vitro}} \tag{2}$$

Wester et al. (53) estimated F_s to be 0.57 for nitroglycerin in the monkey using the AUC ratio for unchanged nitroglycerin after transdermal and intravenous administration. A higher F_s of 0.77 was obtained when the AUC of total radioactivity was used implying about 20% of the nitroglycerin had been metabolized during the topical absorption process.

Solute flux through the stratum corneum may occur by a number of pathways and be retarded by various barriers and removal by the cutaneous blood supply, as discussed later. Of practical interest, is the maximum flux J_{max} as this should apply across all vehicles and may be used to estimate J_s for a given vehicle if the fractional solubility in that vehicle is known. The precise determinant of J_{max} is unclear, as shown in Figure 4, although solute size can be shown to be a dominant determinant (54,55). It is evident that the J_{max}, for steroids at approximately the same molecular weight, is similar except for the most polar one for both infinite (55) and finite (56) dosing (Fig. 4). The maximum flux concept does, however, have limitations in that

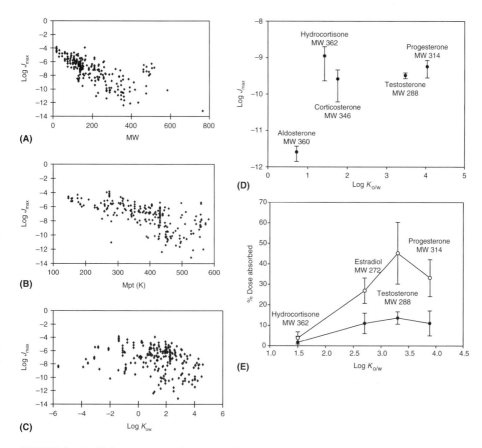

FIGURE 4 (**A–C**) Determinants of maximum flux for a large set of solutes, (**D**) steroids from an infinite dosing situation, and (**E**) steroids from finite dosing for occluded (*open symbols*) and non-occluded (*closed symbols*) conditions. *Abbreviations*: Mpt, melting point; MW, molecular weight. *Source*: From Refs. 54–56.

solutes in high concentrations may exhibit nonlinear concentration dependencies due to effects on the stratum corneum or association in the vehicle. An ideal maximum flux may be estimated as a product of aqueous solubility and permeability coefficient k_p, where k_p may be defined in terms of octanol–water partition coefficients log K_{oct} and molecular weight (MW) by an expression similar to that developed by Potts and Guy (57):

$$\log k_p = 0.71 \log K_{oct} - 0.0061\,\text{MW} - 2.72 \tag{3}$$

Epidermal Reservoir and Dermal Clearance
Lipophilic solutes may also accumulate in the skin to form a so-called skin reservoir (58). Rehydration of the skin may cause such solutes to be released. An example of the historical evidence of this effect is illustrated by the work of Vickers (59) in

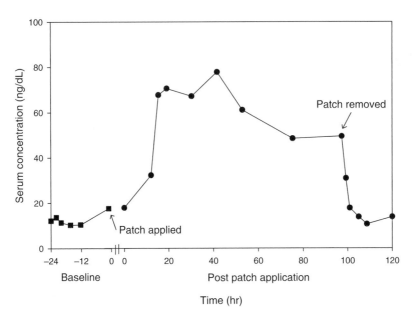

FIGURE 5 Mean total testosterone serum concentrations over time from a single 28 cm^2 patch applied for 96 hours and systemically delivering testosterone ~300 µg/day. *Source*: From Ref. 64.

which vasoconstriction was achieved by occluding an area of skin with plastic film 12 to 14 days after an initial application of steroid under occlusion and a fading of the vasoconstriction on removal of the film at 16 hours. The clearance of a solute from the epidermis is also an important determinant of dermal absorption and toxicity and, if impaired e.g., by vasoconstriction, may lead to higher levels of the solute in the stratum corneum and in the viable epidermis. Altered topical absorption due to changing blood flow can also occur as a consequence of elevated temperature or exercise or coadministration of vasodilating drugs.

Systemic Concentrations of Solutes

Figure 5 shows serum plasma concentrations of testosterone obtained on the application of a patch and on its removal. It is noted that there is a lag prior to reaching maximal levels and on in returning to baseline on patch removal. Further, after reaching a maximum, the serum levels slowly decline with time, consistent with a reduction in flux due to a gradual depletion in the amount of testosterone in the patch. Topical products, especially transdermal patches, often seek to provide constant therapeutically effective plasma concentrations C_{ss}. The release flux J_s ideally needed to reach such concentrations is given by

$$J_s = \frac{C_{ss}Cl_{body}}{F_s} \tag{4}$$

Table 1 shows some estimated transdermal fluxes required for the topical administration of a number of pharmaceuticals which are used in transdermal

TABLE 1 Examples of Solutes on the Market and their Indications, Effective Plasma Levels, Body Clearances (Cl_{body}), Availability (F_s), Elimination Half-Life ($t_{1/2}$), and Physicochemical Data Used to Estimate Required Solute Transdermal Flux (J_s) [from equation (4)] for Passive Topical Delivery Systems

Solute	Indication	Plasma level (µg/L)	Cl_{body} (L/h/70kg)	F_s	Estimated J_s required (µg/hr)	$t_{1/2}$ (hr)	MW	MP (°C)	Log K_{oct}
Buprenorphine	Pain relief	0.1–0.52	76	0.5	15–80	4	468	209	3.44
Clonidine	Hypertension	0.2–2.0	13	0.5–0.95	2.7–28	6–20	230	140	1.77
Estradiol	Estrogen replacement	0.04–0.15			1–4	1	272	176	2.69
Fentanyl	Pain relief	1	25–75	0.3–0.95	25–75	17	337	83	4.37
Isosorbide dinitrate	Angina	22	1.22		28	105	236	68	1.31
Methylphenidate	Attention-deficit hyperactivity disorder (ADHD)	20–46	60 (L/h/30kg in children)		1200–2760	3–5	233	74.5	2.55
Nicotine	Smoking cessation	10–30	72	0.8	900–2630	2	162	~80	1.17
Nitroglycerin	Angina	1.2–11	13.5	0.75	16.2–148.5	0.04	227	13.5	1.62
Oxybutynin	Urinary incontinence	3–4	25–34		75–135	2	357	130	5.19
Rivastigmine	Dementia in Alzheimer and Parkinson disease	2–10	130		260–1300	1–4	250	124 (tartrate)	2.14
Rotigotine	Parkinson disease	0.2–0.6	630		126–378	5–7	315		4.97
Scopolamine	Motion sickness	0.04	67–205		2.68–8.10	1.2–2.9	303	59	1.23
Selegiline	Depression	2		0.25–0.3	250–500	2	187	138	2.95
Testosterone	Hormone replacement	60–100	3–5	—	300	2.3	288	153	3.31
Timolol	Hypertension	5–15	38	0.75	250–750	4.1	316	72	2.46
Triprolidine	Antihistamine	5–15	43.7	1.0	218.5–655.5	2–6	278	60	4.22

Abbreviations: MP, melting point; MW, molecular weight; Log K_{oct}, logarithm of the octanol–water partition coefficient.

- Drug concentrations across human skin in vivo

    ○ Blood and/or urine levels

    ○ Target tissue levels (e.g., biopsy, microdialysis)

    ○ Stratum corneum tape stripping

    ○ Remainder in topically applied product

- Pharmacodynamic response in vivo

    ○ Direct: Clinical trial

    ○ Indirect: Related response (e.g., vasoconstriction, TEWL)

- In vivo animal studies

- In vitro pharmacokinetic studies

    ○ Cadaver skin percutaneous absorption

    ○ Membrane rate of release

SCHEME 1 Strategies used to define percutaneous absorption. *Abbreviation*: TEWL, transepidermal water loss.

systems based on the substitution of desired plasma concentrations and body clearances into equation (4).

Physiological and Pathological Determinants of Barrier Function

Age, gender, race, environment, species, and application site can affect percutaneous absorption (60). The interrelationship between skin pathology and dermal absorption and toxicity assessment is variable and, usually, related to the severity of the pathology. Transepidermal water loss (TEWL) is one measure of skin barrier function that is either unaffected or compromised by the disease process. In general, percutaneous absorption appears to show an association with TEWL (61).

Various strategies to impair and enhance skin permeability are detailed elsewhere in the companion to this book (62). Technologies considered include: chemical enhancement, iontophoresis, ultrasound, microneedles, and pressure waves. Prodrugs are considered later in this volume.

There are also a range of strategies that can be used to assess topical bioavailability and bioequivalence as summarized in Scheme 1.

TOXICITY ASSESSMENT

In general, toxicity after topical exposure may be classified as (*i*) accidental arising from environmental, occupational or recreational exposure or (*ii*) cosmetic or therapeutic related. In this second edition, a greater emphasis has been placed on toxicity issues, with a section devoted specifically to regulatory issues.

CONCLUSION

Dermal absorption and toxicity may be defined by the interrelationship of the anatomy and physiology of the skin with the physicochemical properties of the solutes and the conditions under which they are used. A number of structure–transport/activity relationships and pharmacokinetic models have been developed to be able to predict both absorption and toxicity under a range of conditions. One challenge is to be able to quantify solute concentrations and effects in the lower layers of the epidermis in vivo in dynamic studies.

ACKNOWLEDGMENT

One of us (MSR) thanks the Australian National Health & Medical Research Council for support.

REFERENCES

1. Flesh P, Kligman AM, Baldridge GD. Improved method for the separation of the epidermis of laboratory animals. J Invest Dermatol 1951; 16:86.
2. Kligman AM. A brief history of how the dead stratum corneum became alive. In: Elias PM, Feingold KR, eds. Skin Barrier. New York: Taylor & Francis, 2006:15–24.
3. Madison KC. Barrier function of the skin: "La raison d'etre" of the epidermis. J Invest Dermatol 2003; 121:231–41.
4. Walters KA, Roberts MS. The structure and function of skin. In: Walters KA, ed. Dermatological and Transdermal Formulations. New York: Marcel Dekker, 2002:1–39.
5. Monteiro-Riviere NA. Structure and function of skin. In: Riviere JE, ed. Dermal Absorption Models in Toxicology and Pharmacology. New York: Taylor & Francis, 2006:1–19.
6. Elias PM. Stratum corneum defensive functions: an integrated view. J Invest Dermatol 2005; 125:183–200.
7. Di Nardo A, Gallo RL. Cutaneous barriers in defense against microbial invasion. In: Elias PM, Feingold KR, eds. Skin Barrier. New York: Taylor & Francis, 2006:363–77.
8. Bouwstra JA, Pilgram GSK, Ponec M. Structure of the skin barrier. In: Elias PM, Feingold KR, eds. Skin Barrier. New York: Taylor & Francis, 2006:65–95.
9. Roberts MS, Cross SE, Pellett MA. Skin transport. In: Walters KA, ed. Dermatological and Transdermal Formulations. New York: Marcel Dekker, 2002:89–195.
10. Bronaugh RL, Maibach HI. Percutaneous Absorption. 4th ed. New York: Taylor & Francis, 2005.
11. Cross SE, Roberts MS. Dermal blood flow, lymphatics, and binding as determinants of topical absorption, clearance, and distribution. In: Riviere JE, ed. Dermal Absorption Models in Toxicology and Pharmacology. New York: Taylor & Francis, 2006:251–81.
12. Milstone LM. Epidermal desquamation. J Dermatol Sci 2004; 36:131–40.
13. Borradori L, Sonnenberg A. Structure and function of hemidesmosomes: more than simple adhesion complexes. J Invest Dermatol 1999; 112:411–8.
14. Fassihi H, Wong T, Wessagowit V, et al. Target proteins in inherited and acquired blistering skin disorders. Clin Exp Dermatol 2006; 31:252–9.
15. McMillan JR, Akiyama M, Nakamura H, et al. Colocalization of multiple laminin isoforms predominantly beneath hemidesmosomes in the upper lamina densa of the epidermal basement membrane. J Histochem Cytochem 2006; 54:109–18.
16. Aumailley M, El Khal A, Knoss N, et al. Laminin 5 processing and its integration into the ECM. Matrix Biol 2003; 22:49–54.
17. Kaiser HW, Ness W, Jungblut I, et al. Adherens junctions: demonstration in human epidermis. J Invest Dermatol 1993; 100:180–5.
18. Haftek M, Hansen MU, Kaiser HW, Kreysel HW, Schmitt D. Interkeratinocyte adherens junctions: immunocytochemical visualization of cell–cell junctional structures, distict from desmosomes, in human epidermis. J Invest Dermatol 1996; 106:498–504.

19. Hu P, Berkowitz P, O'Keefe EJ, et al. Keratinocyte adherens junctions initiate nuclear signalling by translocation of plakoglobulin from the membrane to the nucleus. J Invest Dermatol 2003; 121:242–51.
20. Chometon G, Zhang Z-G, Rubinstein E, et al. Dissociation of the complex between CD151 and laminin-binding integrins permits migration of epithelial cells. Exp Cell Res 2006; 312:983–95.
21. Vespa A, D'Souza SJA, Dagnino L. A novel role for integrin-linked kinase in epithelial sheet morphogenesis. Mol Biol Cell 2005; 16:4084–95.
22. Yoshida M, Yamasaki K, Daiho T, et al. ATP2C1 is specifically localized in the basal layer of normal epidermis and its depletion triggers keratinocyte differentiation. J Dermatol Sci 2006; 43:21–33.
23. Rigort A, Grunewald J, Herzog V, et al. Release of integrin macroaggregates as a mechanism of rear detachment during keratinocyte migration. Eur J Cell Biol 2004; 83:725–33.
24. Grando SA. Cholinergic control of epidermal cohesion. Exp Dermatol 2006; 15:265–82.
25. Chernyavsky AI, Arredondo J, Wess J, et al. Novel signalling pathways mediating reciprocal control of keratinocyte migration and wound epithelialization by M3 and M4 muscarinic receptors. J Cell Biol 2004; 166:261–72.
26. Nguyen VT, Arredondo J, Chernyavsky AI, et al. Keratinocyte acetylcholine receptors regulate cell adhesion. Life Sci 2003; 72:2081–5.
27. Nguyen VT, Chernyavsky AI, Arredondo J, et al. Synergistic control of keratinocyte adhesion through muscarinic and nicotinic acetylcholine receptor subtypes. Exp Cell Res 2004; 294:534–49.
28. Madison KC, Howard EJ. Ceramides are transported through the Golgi apparatus in human keratinocytes in vitro. J Invest Dermatol 1996; 106:1030–5.
29. Menon GK, Feingold KR, Elias PM. Lamellar body secretory response to barrier disruption. J Invest Dermatol 1992; 98:279–89.
30. Fartasch M, Bassukas ID, Diepgen TL. Disturbed extruding mechanism of lamellar bodies in dry non-eczematous skin of atopics. Br J Dermatol 1992; 127:221–7.
31. Pilgram GS, Vissers DC, van der Meulen H, et al. Aberrant lipid organization in stratum corneum of patients with atopic dermatitis and lamellar ichthyosis. J Invest Dermatol 2001; 117:710–7.
32. Bouwstra JA, Ponec M. The skin barrier in healthy and diseased state. Biochim Biophys Acta 2006; 1758:2080–95.
33. Norlen L. Skin barrier structure and function: the single gel phase model. J Invest Dermatol 2001; 117:830–6.
34. Norlen L, Gil IP, Simonsen A, et al. Human stratum corneum lipid organization as observed by atomic force microscopy on Langmuir–Blodgett films. J Struct Biol 2007; 158:386–400.
35. Plasencia-Gil MI, Norlen L, Bagatolli LA. Direct visualization of lipid domains in human skin stratum corneum's lipid membranes: effect of pH and temperature. Biophys J 2007; 93:3142–55.
36. Hill J, Paslin D, Wertz PW. A new covalently bound ceramide from human stratum corneum—ω-hydroxyacylphytosphingosine. Int J Cosmet Sci 2006; 28:225–30.
37. Bouwstra JA, Gooris GS, Dubbelaar FE, et al. Phase behavior of lipid mixtures based on human ceramides: coexistence of crystalline and liquid phases. J Lipid Res 2001; 42:1759–70.
38. Bouwstra JA, Dubbelaar FE, Gooris GS, et al. The lipid organisation in the skin barrier. Acta Derm Venereol Suppl (Stockh) 2000; 208:23–30.
39. Moore DJ, Snyder RG, Rerek ME, et al. Kinetics of membrane raft formation: fatty acid domains in stratum corneum lipid models. J Phys Chem B 2006; 110:2378–86.
40. Gooris GS, Bouwstra JA. Infrared spectroscopic study of stratum corneum model membranes prepared from human ceramides, cholesterol, and fatty acids. Biophys J 2007; 92:2785–95.
41. Bouwstra JA, Honeywell-Nguyen PL, Gooris GS, et al. Structure of the skin barrier and its modulation by vesicular formulations. Prog Lipid Res 2003; 42:1–36.

42. Honeywell-Nguyen PL, deGraaff AM, Groenink HW, et al. The in vivo and in vitro interactions of elastic and rigid vesicles with human skin. Biochim Biophys Acta 2002; 1573:130–40.
43. Honeywell-Nguyen PL, Gooris GS, Bouwstra JA. Quantitative assessment of the transport of elastic and rigid vesicle components and a model drug from these vesicle formulations into human skin in vivo. J Invest Dermatol 2004; 123:902–10.
44. El Maghraby GM, Williams AC, Barry BW. Skin delivery of oestradiol from deformable and traditional liposomes: mechanistic studies. J Pharm Pharmacol 1999; 51:1123–34.
45. Jain S, Jain N, Bhadra D, et al. Transdermal delivery of an analgesic agent using elastic liposomes: preparation, characterization and performance evaluation. Curr Drug Deliv 2005; 2:223–33.
46. Mishra D, Garg M, Dubey V, et al. Elastic liposomes mediated transdermal delivery of an anti-hypertensive agent: propranolol hydrochloride. J Pharm Sci 2007; 96:145–55.
47. El Maghraby GM, Williams AC, Barry BW. Can drug-bearing liposomes penetrate intact skin? J Pharm Pharmacol 2006; 58:415–29.
48. Dusek RL, Godsel LM, Green KJ. Discriminating roles of desmosomal cadherins: beyond desmosomal adhesion. J Dermatol Sci 2007; 45:7–21.
49. Getsios S, Amargo EV, Dusek RL, et al. Coordinated expression of desmoglein 1 and desmocollin 1 regulates intercellular adhesion. Differentiation 2004; 72:419–33.
50. Caubet C, Jonca N, Brattsand M, et al. Degradation of corneodesmosome proteins by two serine proteases of the kallikrein family, SCTE/KLK5/hK5 and SCCE/KLK7/hK7. J Invest Dermatol 2004; 122:1235–44.
51. Deraison C, Bonnart C, Lopez F, et al. LEKTI fragments specifically inhibit KLK5, KLK7, and KLK14 and control desquamation through a pH-dependent interaction. Mol Biol Cell 2007; 18:3607–19 .
52. Borgono CA, Michael IP, Komatsu N, et al. A potential role for multiple tissue kallikrein serine proteases in epidermal desquamation. J Biol Chem 2007; 282:3640–52.
53. Wester RC, Noonan PK, Smeach S, Kosoboud L. Pharmacokinetics and bioavailability of intravenous and topical nitroglycerin in the rhesus monkey: estimates of percutaneous first pass metabolism. J Pharm Sci 1983; 72:745–8.
54. Magnusson BM, Anissimov YG, Cross SE, Roberts MS. Molecular size as the main determinant of solute maximum flux across the skin. J Invest Dermatol 2004; 122:993–9.
55. Magnusson BM, Cross SE, Winckle G, Roberts MS. Percutaneous absorption of steroids: determination of in vitro permeability and tissue reservoir characteristics in human skin layers. Skin Pharmacol Physiol 2006; 19:336–42.
56. Bucks D, Maibach H. Occlusion does not uniformly enhance penetration in vivo. In: Bronaugh RL, Maibach HI, eds. Percutaneous Absorption. 4th ed. New York: Marcel Dekker, 2005:81–105.
57. Potts RO, Guy RH. Predicting skin permeability. Pharm Res 1992; 9:663–9.
58. Roberts MS, Anissimov YG, Cross SE. Factors affecting the formation of a skin reservoir for topically applied solutes. Skin Pharmacol Physiol 2004; 17(1):3–16.
59. Vickers CFH. Existence of reservoir in stratum corneum. Experimental proof. Arch Dermatol 1963; 88:21–3.
60. Roberts MS, Walters KA. The relationship between structure and barrier function of skin. In: Roberts MS, Walters KA, eds. Dermal Absorption and Toxicity Assessment. New York: Marcel Dekker, 1998:1–42.
61. Levin J, Maibach H. The correlation between transepidermal water loss and percutaneous absorption: an overview. J Control Release 2005; 103:291–9.
62. Walters KA, Roberts MS, eds. Dermatological, Cosmeceutic, and Cosmetic Development: Therapeutics and Novel Approaches. New York: Informa Healthcare, 2008.
63. Chan KKH, Ross HD, Berner B, Piraino AJ. Pharmacokinetics of a single dose of nicotine in healthy smokers. J Control Rel 1990; 14:145–51.
64. European Medicines Agency. EPARs for authorised medicinal products for human use: scientific discussion. http://www.emea.europa.eu/humandocs/PDFs/EPAR/intrinsa/063406en6.pdf (last accessed 23 October, 2007).

2 Animal Skin Morphology and Dermal Absorption

Nancy A. Monteiro-Riviere, Ronald E. Baynes, and Jim E. Riviere
Center for Chemical Toxicology Research and Pharmacokinetics, College of Veterinary Medicine, North Carolina State University, Raleigh, North Carolina, U.S.A.

INTRODUCTION

There is a flourishing interest in dermal toxicology because of environmental and occupational exposures and the development of novel transdermal drug delivery systems. Skin is one of the largest organs of the body and is the primary barrier to absorption from the environment. Because of its accessibility and continuous exposure to a myriad of chemicals, both accidentally and deliberately (cosmetics), it is a common target for toxic chemicals. This requires that substantial testing occur to assess both the rate and extent of dermal absorption as well as to characterize the dermatotoxic potential of chemicals.

Because of the ethical considerations and inability to conduct such research and testing in humans, animal models have been developed and extensively utilized. The global animal rights movement has had a major impact on the type of testing that is done by researchers. In response, new in vitro testing methods have been developed to study irritation, absorption, corrosion, and toxicity. However, before data from these tests can be interpreted, these surrogate models must be analyzed from the perspective of their capability to mimic the wide range of responses seen with intact skin in both animals and humans.

One of the primary functions of skin is to act as a barrier between the well-regulated *milieu interieur* and the outside environment. However, skin is a complex, integrated, dynamic organ which has several functions that go far beyond its role as a barrier to the environment, some of which are listed in Table 1. Skin is a very nonhomogeneous organ, being anatomically comprised of two principal and distinct components: a stratified, avascular, outer cellular epidermis, and an underlying dermis consisting of connective tissue with numerous cell types and special adnexial structures. The comparative anatomy and physiology of skin, as well as its comparative histology, have been reviewed in depth (1,2).

The two properties of a chemical that relate to its propensity to cause dermatotoxicity are its ability to penetrate the skin and its subsequent interactions with the biological components of skin that could elicit a toxicological response. Species differences may have impacts on how these properties are assessed. Many of the functions of skin (especially temperature regulation) impact on structural differences between species. This chapter reviews the basic anatomical factors that may affect both of these processes (absorption, potential targets for toxicity) relative to how they are expressed in different species. This is followed by specific examples where similarities and differences have been seen.

TABLE 1 Functions of Skin that Impact on Animal Species Differences

Environmental barrier
Diffusion barrier
Metabolic barrier
Temperature regulation
Regulation of blood flow
Hair and fur
Sweating
Immunological affector and effector axis
Mechanical support
Neurosensory reception
Endocrine (e.g., vitamin D)
Apocrine/eccrine/sebaceous glandular secretion
Metabolism
Keratin
Collagen
Melanin
Lipid
Carbohydrate
Respiration
Biotransformation of xenobiotics

Source: Modified from Ref. 1.

RELEVANT ANATOMY AND PHYSIOLOGY

Figure 1 is a "generic" representation of the microstructure of skin across all species depicting features that may modulate chemical absorption or toxicity. Differences in the thickness of epidermal layers and the dermis across nine species are listed in Table 2.

Epidermis

The epidermis consists of a keratinized stratified squamous epithelium that undergoes an orderly pattern of proliferation, differentiation, and keratinization. Various skin appendages, such as hair, sweat and sebaceous glands, digital organs (hoof, claw, nail), feathers, horn, and glandular structures are actually special-izations of the epidermis. Two primary cell types, the keratinocytes (stratum basale, stratum spinosum, stratum granulosum, stratum lucidum, and stratum corneum) and the non-keratinocytes (melanocytes, Merkel cells, and Langerhans cells), both play important roles in determining the dermatotoxic potential of topically applied compounds.

The stratum basale is a single layer of columnar to cuboidal cells attached to the underlying basement membrane by hemidesmosomes and laterally to each other and to the overlying stratum spinosum cells by desmosomes. The basal cells are constantly undergoing mitosis causing the daughter cells to be displaced outward keeping the epidermis replenished as the stratum corneum cells are constantly being sloughed from the surface epidermis. This process of cell turnover and self-replacement in normal human skin is thought to take approximately 45 to 75 days depending on the region of the body, age, disease states, and other modulating factors. It varies greatly between animal species, with rodents having a much more accelerated turnover (4,5). The epidermal kinetics of cell proliferation in pigs and humans are very similar having a 30-day epidermal cell turnover time (6).

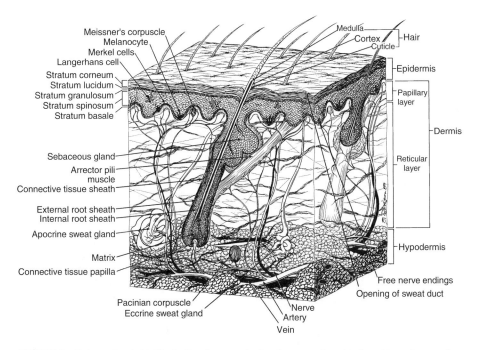

FIGURE 1 Schematic of skin illustrating the complexity of mammalian skin found in various regions of the body. *Source*: From Ref. 1.

TABLE 2 Comparative Epidermal Thickness, Stratum Corneum Thickness, and Number of Cell Layers from the Back and Abdomen of Nine Species

Species	Area	Epidermal thickness (μm)	Stratum corneum thickness (μm)	Number of cell layers
Cat	Back	12.97±0.93	5.84±1.02	1.28±0.13
	Abdomen	23.36±10.17	4.32±0.95	2.06±0.73
Cow	Back	36.76±2.95	8.65±1.17	2.22±0.11
	Abdomen	27.41±2.62	8.07±0.56	2.39±0.13
Dog	Back	21.16±2.55	5.56±0.85	1.89±0.16
	Abdomen	22.47±2.40	8.61±1.92	2.33±0.12
Horse	Back	33.59±2.16	7.26±1.04	2.50±0.25
	Abdomen	29.11±5.03	6.95±1.07	2.89±0.44
Monkey	Back	26.87±3.14	12.05±2.30	2.67±0.24
	Abdomen	17.14±2.22	5.33±0.40	2.08±0.08
Mouse	Back	13.32±1.19	2.90±0.12	1.75±0.08
	Abdomen	9.73±2.28	3.01±0.30	1.75±0.25
Pig	Back	51.89±1.49	12.28±0.72	3.94±0.13
	Abdomen	46.76±2.01	14.90±1.91	4.47±0.37
Rabbit	Back	10.85±1.00	6.56±0.37	1.22±0.11
	Abdomen	15.14±1.42	4.86±0.79	1.50±0.11
Rat	Back	21.66±2.23	5.00±0.85	1.83±0.17
	Abdomen	11.58±1.02	4.56±0.61	1.44±0.19

Paraffin sections stained with hematoxylin and eosin; $n=6$, mean±SE.
Source: Modified from Ref. 3.

Chemicals whose mode of action is related to genotoxicity cause damage to these cells. Carcinogens that transform basal keratinocytes may result in squamous cell carcinomas.

The succeeding outer layer is the stratum spinosum, or "prickle cell layer," which consists of several layers of irregular polyhedral cells that become flattened as they reach the surface. These cells are connected to adjacent stratum spinosum cells and to the stratum basale cells by desmosomes and contain the same complement of organelles as the stratum basale cells, with only the presence of tonofilaments differentiating them morphologically from the other cell layers. The uppermost layers of the stratum spinosum contain small membrane-bound organelles known as lamellar granules.

The third layer is the stratum granulosum, which consists of several layers of flattened cells lying parallel to the epidermal–dermal junction. This layer contains irregularly shaped, nonmembrane-bound, electron-dense keratohyalin granules. These granules are thought to play a role in keratinization and barrier function. Another characteristic feature is the presence of lipid-containing lamellar granules (Odland bodies, lamellated bodies, or membrane-coating granules), which are smaller than mitochondria and are found near the Golgi complex and smooth endoplasmic reticulum. In the upper epidermis, the lamellar granules increase in number and size, move toward the cell membrane, and release their lipid contents by exocytosis into the intercellular space between the stratum granulosum and the stratum corneum, thereby coating the cell membrane of the stratum corneum cells. They are composed primarily of lipids including the ceramides, cholesterol, fatty acids, and small amounts of cholesterol esters, as well as hydrolytic enzymes such as acid phosphates, proteases, lipases, and glycosidases. The content and mixture of lipids can vary between species and are considered to function as the primary component of the permeability barrier. Lipid extraction studies conducted in the abdominal, inguinal, and back regions of pigs demonstrated relative proportions of individual lipids (ceramides 1–6, fatty acids, cholesterol, triglycerides, and cholesterol esters) extractions were similar across all body regions (7). However, a higher concentration of total lipids could be extracted from the back. Chapter 4 covers this area in greater depth. Toxicants that target the formation or function of these granules or alter activity of their constitutive enzymes may be manifested in impaired barrier function.

The stratum lucidum is a thin, translucent, homogeneous layer between the stratum granulosum and the stratum corneum. It is only found in distinct anatomical areas of exceptionally thick skin or hairless regions (e.g., plantar and palmar surfaces). It consists of several layers of fully keratinized, closely compacted, dense cells devoid of nuclei and cytoplasmic organelles. Their cytoplasm contains protein-bound phospholipids and a keratin-like protein, eleidin.

The outermost layer of the epidermis is the stratum corneum consisting of several layers of completely keratinized dead cells that are constantly being shed. The stratum corneum is considered the primary barrier to dermal absorption of compounds. This layer appears clear, enucleated, and lacks cytoplasmic organelles by transmission electron microscopy. The most superficial layers of the stratum corneum that undergo constant desquamation are referred to as the stratum disjunctum. The stratum corneum cell layers vary in thickness in different areas (i.e., abdomen vs. back) of the body and between species (Table 2). The stratum corneum cells are highly organized and stacked upon one another to form vertical interlocking columns having a flattened tetrakaidecahedron shape. This 14-sided polygonal provides a minimum surface-to-volume ratio, which allows for space to be filled by packing without interstices. This spatial arrangement helps facilitate the maintenance of the skin's efficient barrier function. The intercellular lipids derived from the lamellar granules of the stratum granulosum are located between the stratum corneum cells and form the intercellular lipid component of the complex stratum corneum barrier. This prevents both the penetration of substances from the environment and the insensible loss of body water by surface evaporation. These cells are surrounded by a plasma membrane and a thick submembranous layer that contains the protein involucrin. This protein is synthesized in the stratum spinosum and cross-linked in the stratum granulosum by an enzyme that makes it highly stable. Involucrin provides structural support to the cell, allowing the cell to resist invasion by microorganisms and destruction by environmental agents, but does not appear to play a role in barrier permeability. It is partitioning and diffusion through the intercellular lipids which is most closely correlated with chemical and drug penetration. The much higher penetration of compounds across mouse skin is largely secondary to the relative thinness of the stratum corneum compared with other animals (Table 2).

Non-Keratinocytes

Melanocytes are derivatives of the neural crest and are located in the basal layer of the epidermis. These cells have several dendritic processes that extend between adjacent keratinocytes or run parallel to the dermal surface. The cytoplasm is clear except for pigment-containing membrane-bound ovoid granules, referred to as melanosomes, which impart color to skin and hair. Melanosomes are transferred to keratinocytes where they are randomly distributed within the keratinocyte's cytoplasm. They often become localized over the nucleus of the keratinocyte to form a cap-like structure that protects the sensitive genetic material from ultraviolet radiation. Skin color is determined by several factors including the number, size, distribution, and degree of melanization of melanosomes. As expected, this aspect of skin structure is a major variable across animal species. In chemical carcinogenesis, chemicals that transform melanocytes may result in malignant melanomas.

Merkel cells are located in the basal region of the epidermis. These cells contain spherical electron-dense granules, and are connected to adjacent keratinocytes by desmosomes. When these cells are associated with axons, they are referred to as a Merkel cell–neurite complex. Specialized areas containing these complexes are known as Haarscheiben (hair disks, tactile hair disks, or tylotrich pads). The axon associated with a Merkel cell arises from a myelinated nerve, but as it approaches the epidermis it loses its myelin sheath and terminates as a flat meniscus on the basal aspect of the cell. Merkel cells are thought to function as slow adapting mechanoreceptors for touch.

Langerhans cells are most commonly found in the upper spinous layer of the epidermis, yet have been identified in other stratified squamous epithelium. Ultrastructurally, Langerhans cells have an indented nucleus, and contain common organelles, but lack tonofilaments and desmosomes. A unique feature of this cell is the presence of distinctive rod- or racket-shaped granules known as Langerhans, (Birbeck) cell granules. Langerhans cells have long dendritic processes that traverse the intercellular space up to the granular cell layer. Langerhans cells are derived from bone marrow and are functionally and immunologically related to the monocyte–macrophage series. They play a major role in the skin immune response because they are capable of presenting antigen to lymphocytes and transporting them to lymph nodes for lymphocyte activation. They are considered to be the initial receptor for initiating a cutaneous immune response (delayed-type hypersensitivity) to certain contact allergens and thus play an initiating role in some forms of immune-mediated dermatotoxic reactions.

Dermal–Epidermal Junction

All of these cell layers are situated above the basement membrane zone or dermal–epidermal junction, which provides mechanical support to the epidermis. Ultra-structurally, this junction consists of the following four components:

1. The cell membrane of the basal epithelial cell, which includes the hemidesmosomes
2. The lamina lucida (lamina rara)
3. The lamina densa (basal lamina)
4. The subbasal lamina (reticular lamina) that contains a variety of fibrous structures (anchoring fibrils, dermal microfibril bundles, microthread-like filaments)

The basement membrane has a complex molecular architecture with numerous components that play a key role in adhesion of the epidermis to the dermis. The basement membrane components that are ubiquitous components of all basement membranes in the body include type IV collagen, laminin, entactin/nidogen, and heparan sulfate proteoglycans. Other basement membrane components such as bullous pemphigoid antigen (BPA), epidermolysis bullosa acquisita (EBA), fibronectin, GB3, L3d, and 19-DEJ-1 are limited to skin. The basal cell membrane of the epidermal–dermal junction is undulating and irregular, forming finger-like projections into the dermis. Several functions have been attributed to the basement membrane: maintaining epidermal–dermal adhesion, acting as a selective barrier between the epidermis and the dermis by restricting some molecules and permitting the passage of others, influencing cell behavior and wound healing, and serving as a target for both immunological and non-immunological injury. The basement membrane is the target for vesicating chemical agents that cause blister formation after topical exposure. Sulfur mustard is a potent cutaneous vesicant that causes separation within the upper portion of the lamina lucida in pig skin. Characterization of the epidermal–dermal junction in pig skin by indirect immunohistochemistry and immunoelectron microscopy showed the distribution of eight epitopes. Mapping antibodies to laminin, type IV collagen, fibronectin, GB3, BPA, and EBA were similar to human skin but L3d and 19-DEJ-1 were not similar (8). The conservation of human epitopes in the epidermal–dermal junction of the pig further emphasizes the similarities between human and pig skin. In addition, the basement membrane zone contains integrins that are glycoproteins composed of α- and β-subunits. Proper expression of the correct complement of integrins makes it possible for cells to maintain their structural association and functional communication, which is very important in wound healing studies. Zhang and Monteiro-Riviere (9) studied the distribution of these integrins and found that three major integrins in the epidermis, α2β1, α3β1, and α6β4, are also expressed in perfused porcine skin, and their immunostaining pattern was similar to that of human skin. The distribution of α6β4 in sulfur mustard–treated perfused porcine skin was also similar to some of the basement membrane blistering diseases of humans such as bullous pemphigoid and junctional epidermolysis bullosa.

Dermis

The dermis or corium consists of dense irregular connective tissue that extends to the hypodermis or subcutaneous tissue. The matrix of this connective tissue is composed of collagen, elastic, and reticular fibers embedded in an amorphous ground substance of mucopolysaccharides. The cells of the dermis include fibroblasts, mast cells, and macrophages. Plasma cells, chromatophores, fat cells, and extravasated leukocytes are often found along with blood vessels, nerves, and lymphatics. In addition, adnexial appendages such as sweat glands, sebaceous glands, hair follicles, and arrector pili muscles are anchored within the dermis. The dermis can be arbitrarily divided into a superficial papillary layer that blends into a deep reticular layer. The papillary layer is thin and consists of loose connective tissue, which is in contact with the epidermis and conforms to the contour of the basal epithelial ridges and grooves. It can protrude into the epidermis, giving rise to the dermal papilla. When the epidermis invaginates the dermis, epidermal pegs are formed. The reticular layer is thicker and constitutes irregular dense connective tissue with fewer cells and more fibers. A major component of the dermis is the extensive network of capillaries that function to both regulate body temperature and transport topically absorbed chemicals into the systemic circulation. A lymphatic network transports migrating immune cells as well as larger molecules (>60 kDa) into the lymphatic system. Blood flow through skin can vary by a factor of 100-fold depending on environmental conditions, making it one of the most highly perfused organs in the body. There are large species differences in blood flow that could impact on the absorptive properties of many topically applied compounds.

There is considerable variation in skin thickness both between species and within the same species in various regions of the body (3). Over the dorsal and lateral surfaces of limbs, skin is thick and on the ventral and medial surfaces of limbs, the skin is thinner. In hairy areas the epidermis is thin, while in nonhairy skin, such as mucocutaneous junctions, the epidermis is thicker. The stratum corneum is the thickest on the palmar and plantar surfaces, where considerable abrasive action occurs.

Adnexial Appendages

Hair

Hairs are keratinized structures derived from epidermal invaginations and are found almost everywhere on the body surface except for specific body sites including the palms, soles, and mucocutaneous junctions. The variation, in terms of density, structure, and rate of growth of hair is often the primary distinguishing feature between animal species. The hair follicle is embedded at an angle in the dermis, with the bulb sometimes extending as deep as the hypodermis. This fundamental anatomical arrangement is often ignored when dermatomed skin sections or epidermal membranes are employed in in vitro diffusion cell systems. In these preparations, holes appear where the hair shafts once were (10). Similarly, when animal skin is obtained from an abattoir, the dehairing procedure (scalding) often significantly damages the skin. Skin must be obtained immediately after slaughter and before extensive processing begins.

The hair follicle consists of four major components: (1) internal root sheath, (2) external root sheath, (3) dermal papilla, and (4) hair matrix. The cells covering the dermal papilla and composing most of the hair bulb are the hair matrix cells.

These are comparable with stratum basale cells of regular epidermis except that they have less lipid and produce harder keratin than their epidermal counterparts.

Hair growth varies from species to species, body site, and age of an individual. Whereas the process of keratinization is continuous in the epidermis, the matrix cells of the hair follicle undergo periods of quiescence during which no mitotic activity occurs. Cyclic activity of the hair bulb accounts for the seasonal change in the hair coat of domestic animals. The part of the hair cycle in which the cells of the hair bulb are active and growth occurs is called anagen. When the follicles go through a regressive stage and metabolic activity slows down, it is referred to as catagen. In this phase, the base of the follicle migrates upward in the skin toward the epidermal surface. The hair follicle then enters telogen, a resting or quiescent phase, in which growth stops and the base of the bulb is at the level of the sebaceous canal. Following this phase, mitotic activity and keratinization start over again and a new hair is formed. As the new hair grows beneath the telogen follicle, it gradually pushes the old follicle upward toward the surface, where it is eventually shed. This intermittent mitotic activity and keratinization of the hair matrix cells constitutes the hair cycle that is controlled by several factors, including length of daily periods of light, ambient temperature, nutrition, and hormones, particularly estrogen, testosterone, adrenal steroids, and thyroid hormone (2). This is important for considering certain dermatotoxic responses to chemicals whose mechanism of action requires interaction with an active metabolic process. Toxicity may only occur when hair growth is in an active growth phase. Exposure at other times may not elicit any response. Many cytotoxic chemicals (e.g., cancer chemo-therapeutic drugs and immunosuppressants like cyclophosphamide) whose mechanism of action is to kill dividing cells will produce hair loss (alopecia) as an unwanted side effect of nonselective activity, without causing any other damage to the skin.

Bundles of smooth muscle fibers that make up the arrector pili muscle are associated with most hair follicles. This muscle, innervated by autonomic nerve fibers, attaches to the connective tissue sheath of the hair follicle and extends toward the epidermis, where it connects to the papillary layer of the dermis. The arrector pili muscles are especially well developed in humans and when they contract during cold weather they elevate the hairs, forming "goose pimples." Contraction of this muscle may also play a role in emptying the sebaceous glands. Pig skin has single hair follicles that may be grouped into clusters of two to four follicles, with clusters of three most common in young pigs. This is a perceptual effect related to age, since there is a tendency for the grouping to become less obvious as the skin area expands with growth. This basic arrangement of hair follicles occurring in groups of three during the early stages of development is common in a number of species (11).

Sebaceous Glands

Sebaceous glands secrete lipid and consist of a single layer of low cuboidal cells. These cells move inward through mitotic activity and accumulate lipid droplets to release their secretory product, sebum by the holocrine mode of secretion. The major lipids in the human sebaceous gland consist of squalene, cholesterol, cholesterol esters, wax esters, and triglycerides (12). In lower mammals, sebaceous glands can become specialized and are often associated with a pheromone-secreting role, making their exact composition species specific. For more detail on how pig excretory glands compare with those of humans, see Argenzio and Monteiro-Riviere (13).

Human sebum plays a major role during early adolescence in acne vulgaris and thus its production is involved in the evaluation of anti-acne drug candidates. Toxicants that interact with sebaceous gland function can induce an acne-like response and produce comedones, a severe condition of which is termed chloracne. Several chloracnegens, including chloronaphthalenes, polychlorinated biphenyls, tetrachloroazoxybenzene, tetrachloroazobenzene, polychlorinated dibenzodioxins, polychlorinated dibenzofurans, and polychlorinated biphenyls elicit responses in humans. Most of these chloracnegens induce a cytochrome P-450 mediated microsomal monoxygenase response (14).

Eccrine Sweat Gland

Sweat glands can be classified into apocrine or eccrine (merocrine) based on their morphological and functional characteristics. In domestic animals, the apocrine gland is extensively developed and found throughout most of the skin. In humans, the eccrine glands are found over the entire body surface except for the lips, external ear canal, clitoris, and labia minora. They are simple tubular glands that open directly onto the skin surface. Myoepithelial cells are found in the secretory portion and are specialized smooth muscle cells that, upon contraction, aid in moving the secretions toward the duct. The duct of the eccrine sweat glands is comprised of two layers of cuboidal epithelium resting on the basal lamina and opens in a straight path onto the epidermal surface. Some workers postulate that the ducts of these glands provide an alternate pathway for the absorption of polar molecules through the skin.

This exocrine gland, whose principal function is thermoregulation, is one of the major cutaneous appendages and is functionally very active in humans. Sweating in humans refers to a distinct physiological function of excreting body fluids to the surface of the skin, which is necessary for fluid and electrolyte homeostasis. Physiologically stressed individuals can excrete 2 L/hr to support evaporative heat loss. Only the higher primates and horses have a built-in mechanism that can accommodate this large volume loss without circulatory collapse. The secretory portion secretes isotonic fluid that is low in protein and similar to plasma in ionic composition and osmolarity. On passage down the duct portion, it becomes hypotonic and reabsorption of sodium chloride, bicarbonate, lactate, and small amounts of water occurs (15,16). Abnormality in this fluid and electrolyte transport system leads to cystic fibrosis, and analysis of this secretion is a prime diagnostic tool for this disease.

When comparing percutaneous absorption of drugs in human and other species, the presence of sweat on the surface of skin is a major variable. In vivo, drugs dosed topically to humans may become dissolved in sweat, thus allowing sweat to function as a vehicle for drug solubilization. This may not be present in other species. In many cases, when sweat is considered an important factor, "artificial sweat" is often used as a dosing vehicle. In contrast, the solubilizing substance in sheep is lanolin, which has properties significantly different than human eccrine sweat secretions, again illustrating select differences in a species' physiology that could impact their use in dermal absorption and toxicity studies.

Apocrine Sweat Gland
In humans apocrine sweat glands are limited to the axillary, pubic, areolae, and perianal regions. They can be a simple sacular or tubular structure, having a coiled secretory portion and a straight duct. The secretory portion is usually found in the lower reticular dermis and hypodermis. Depending on the stage of secretory activity, the epithelium may be simple columnar or cuboidal. The acini portion of the sweat gland contains two types of secretory cells, a clear cell and a dark seromucous cell. Myoepithelial cells are present between the basal lamina and the secretory cells to aid in cell secretion. The duct has a narrow lumen consisting of two layers of cuboidal cells and is found adjacent to the hair follicle. The duct runs parallel to the follicle, penetrates the epidermis of the follicle, and opens alongside the follicle at the surface. Based on physiological and evolutionary development, the axillary apocrine sweat glands and possibly other apocrine glands function as scent glands in humans (17).

IMPACT OF ANATOMY ON PERCUTANEOUS ABSORPTION AND TOXICOLOGY

There are a number of species-specific factors that may influence the extrapolation of pharmacology and toxicology data across animal species and humans. These include the obvious presence or absence of fur and different types of sweat glands and products. However, it also relates to differences in the thickness and structure of the relevant cellular layers, especially the epidermis and stratum corneum that play a central role in barrier function.

Different cell types may be targets for chemical toxicants. The toxicological response of the primary cells (keratinocytes, melanocytes, Langerhans cells), structures (stratum corneum, basement membrane), or adnexial appendages (hair follicles, sebaceous, and sweat glands) will define the nature of the dermatotoxicity produced. Two of these cells, the keratinocytes and melanocytes, are the target cells that undergo transformation in the process of chemical carcinogenesis and produce the squamous cell carcinomas and melanomas observed in "skin painting" carcinogenicity bioassays. When these epidermal cells are affected by exogenous chemicals, independent of etiology, the dermis often reacts to their damage in a process mediated by cytokines of epidermal origin. The dermis, being primarily a vascular organ, responds by increasing blood flow to remove the offending toxicant and brings in cellular components of the immune system to affect repair. This dermal reaction is macroscopically observed as erythema and edema, the two hallmarks of cutaneous toxicity. If a chemical is capable of interacting with one of these cutaneous cell types, the potential for dermatotoxicity exists. However, the chemical must be able to reach the target cell to affect its action. The barrier properties of the stratum corneum must be overcome for this potential toxicity to be expressed.

Percutaneous Absorption and Penetration
The skin is generally considered to be an efficient barrier preventing absorption (and thus systemic exposure) of most topically administered compounds. It is a membrane that is relatively impermeable to aqueous solutions and most ions. It is, however, permeable in varying degrees to a large number of lipophilic solid, liquid, and gaseous xenobiotics making the concept of barrier inappropriate for these substances. Studies have also demonstrated that the skin may be responsible for metabolizing topically applied compounds by both Phase I and II metabolic

pathways (see chap. 6). For some compounds, the extent of cutaneous metabolism influences the overall fraction of a topically applied compound that is absorbed, making this process function as an alternate absorption pathway. Cutaneous biotransformation is used to promote the absorption of some topical drugs that normally would not penetrate the skin. By modifying these drugs to more lipid-soluble ester analogues, the drug penetrates the stratum corneum and the free drug is liberated through the action of cutaneous esterases. Cutaneous metabolism may also be important for certain aspects of skin toxicology when nontoxic compounds are bioactivated within the epidermis [e.g., benzo(*a*)pyrene]. Species differences in the presence and concentration of dermal metabolizing enzymes would be expected to be very large, as is seen with hepatic drug metabolizing systems. Unfortunately, few systematic studies documenting these differences have been conducted.

The stratum corneum appears to afford the greatest deterrent to absorption. This layer of dead proteinaceous keratinocytes embedded in an extracellular lipid matrix composed primarily of sterols, other neutral lipids, and ceramides was referred to by Elias (18) as a "brick and mortar" model. The intercellular lipids composition is not homogeneous in all layers of the epidermis, making the lipid topography complex. Species differences are also evident. Although highly water retarding, the dead, keratinized cells are highly water absorbent (hydrophilic), a property that keeps the skin supple and soft. A natural oil covering the skin, the sebum, appears to maintain the water-holding capacity of the epidermis but has no appreciable role in retarding the penetration of xenobiotics. This is especially prevalent in some species including sheep.

Compared with most routes of drug absorption, the skin is by far the most diverse across species (e.g., sheep vs. pig) and body sites (e.g., human forearm compared with scalp). The ability of a toxicant to enter skin is a primary determinant of its dermatotoxic potential. The quantitative prediction of the rate and extent of percutaneous penetration (into skin) and absorption (through skin) of topically applied chemicals is complicated by the biological variability inherent in skin across animal species. The many varied biological roles lead to functional and structural adaptations that impact on the skin's barrier properties and thus the rate and extent of percutaneous absorption. This area is becoming of increased importance in veterinary therapeutics where increased use of topical drugs for systemic therapy (pour-on, spot-on, gels, patches) is occurring (19). These differences were clearly illustrated when transdermal fentanyl patches, designed for human use, were first applied for clinical analgesia postoperatively in dogs, cats, and horses. Absorption patterns were different, not only in skin permeability, but also in their transit through the dermis. A database is developing that will see more products, specifically designed for individual veterinary species, be approved by the relevant regulatory authorities. As veterinary transdermal compounds get developed and marketed, additional research conducted in non-laboratory species (dogs, cats, sheep, cattle) may shed light on the importance of differences in skin structure on chemical absorption.

Selection of Animal Model for Human Skin

There is no single animal species that exactly matches the morphology and physiology of human skin. Even the genetically closest primate model is different because of the presence of hair. Rodent models are often used so that data can be compared to other routes of administration, since the predominant species used in routine toxicology testing are rats and mice. Rabbits and guinea pigs have been employed in dermatotoxicology testing often because of immunological consider-ations and comparison with historical databases. On a purely morphological basis, the domestic pig is the closest match to human skin.

Pig Skin as a Model

The integument of the pig is very similar to that of humans (Fig. 2). It has a relatively large surface area that makes it amenable to test transdermal patches designed for human use without further scale-up. Similarly, the absorption of topical formu-lations may be investigated over surface areas as appropriate for applications in humans. The surface characteristics of porcine skin are similar to those of human (relatively hairless, similar texture). Finally, the skin surface area to body weight ratio in the pig compares favorably with that in humans, an attribute not present in smaller laboratory animal species. This, coupled with a similar dosing surface area, makes extrapolation of systemic drug delivery or assessment of the potential for systemic toxicity straightforward without resorting to complex mathematical transformations. In addition, noninvasive techniques such as stratum corneum tape stripping, assessment of transepidermal water loss, laser Doppler velocimetry, and colorimetry may utilize the same techniques and instrumentation used in human clinical settings. Pigs are widely used in developing surgical techniques for humans, as models for UV phototoxicity and are an accepted dermatological model for many diseases (20). All of these similarities single out *Sus scrofa* as an excellent animal model for conducting preclinical trials for drug development and cutaneous toxicology studies targeted at *Homo sapiens*.

The use of a pig as a surrogate for human percutaneous absorption studies has been extensively reviewed and validated over many years. These comparisons hold for both in vitro and in vivo models. For most compounds tested, absorption through pig skin is very similar to human skin (50–150%), especially when compared with rodent models that often differ by orders of magnitude. Table 3 lists some compounds for which absorption in pigs and humans are approximately equivalent (21–26). A few of these compounds are particularly significant. For example, the pesticide paraquat is readily absorbed in most rodent models investigated, but minimally absorbed in human and porcine skin (27). There would be an obvious impact to risk assessment if the incorrect animal model were selected to assess human toxicity.

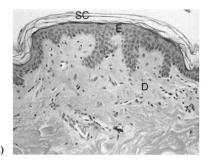 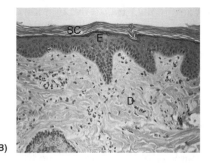

(A)   (B)

FIGURE 2 Microscopic anatomy of (**A**) human skin compared to (**B**) pig skin. Note the relative thickness of the epidermis. *Abbreviations*: D, dermis; E, epidermis; SC, stratum corneum.

TABLE 3 Compounds where Absorption in Pig and in Human Skin is Similar

2,4-Diamine	Hydrocortisone
Benzoic acid	Lindane
Benzopyrene	Malathion
Butter yellow	p-Nitrophenol
Caffeine	Paraquat
Carbaryl	Parathion
Cortisone	Permethrin
Dichlorodiphenyltrichloroethane	Phenol
Diethyl-m-toluamide	Progesterone
Diisopropylfluorophosphate	Salicylic acid
Fluocinolone acetonide	Testosterone
Haloprogin	Theophylline

Ratio of percent absorbed in pigs is 50% to 150% of that in humans.

Comparison of Rodent and Porcine Model Chemical Absorption

Rodent species such as the guinea pig, mouse, and rat are often used in initial dermal absorption and dermatotoxicity studies to determine systemic bioavailability of drugs and potential human toxicants following dermal exposure. The data generated from these studies often overestimate dermal absorption primarily because of the previously described anatomical and biochemical differences between human skin and rodent skin. For example, our laboratory demonstrated that dermal absorption of the insect repellent and insecticide, Diethyl-m-toluamide, and permethrin, was significantly greater in mouse or rat skin than in human and/or pig skin (26). For both chemicals, absorption was significantly greater in mouse skin than in rat or pig skin. In vitro dermal studies also demonstrated that the permeability of the charged herbicide paraquat in various rodent species was 40 to 1600 times greater than that in humans (28), while porcine skin was similar to humans (27). In vivo studies demonstrated more than a 10-fold difference (0.29% vs. 3.5%) in percent dermal absorption between rats and human volunteers over a longer exposure period than the in vitro studies (29,30). Species differences were also observed with the coronary vasodilator, nicorandil when compared using rodent, dog, pig, and human skin in vitro (31). Nicorandil permeability in pig skin was comparable to that in human skin; however, permeability differences were most significant when comparing human skin with rodent skin. Although differences in epidermal microanatomy played a role, permeability differences were also attributed to species-specific lipids on the skin surface.

As previously stated, pig skin is functionally and structurally similar to human skin and should be the ideal model for predicting absorption in human skin. Our laboratory demonstrated that permethrin absorption is indeed very limited in pig skin (0.11–0.68% dose) (32), but this compared favorably with recent human in vivo studies (0.7% to <2%) (33). These comparisons and similarities have been reported for comparisons of pig in vitro and human in vivo dermal absorption of various other drugs, pesticides, and environmental contaminants (21,34). This strong correlation between human and pig skin may not be applicable to more hydrophilic chemicals (35) and in vivo dermal absorption in pig skin does not always reflect in vivo dermal absorption in humans (Fig. 3) (21). These differences become more critical not only in assessing the potential dermal absorption of environmental toxicants, but also when determining the most

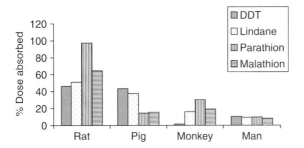

FIGURE 3   In vivo dermal absorption. *Abbreviation*: DDT, dichlorodiphenyltrichloroethane. *Source*: Data obtained from Refs. 21,36,37.

appropriate animal to be used in testing cosmetic and pharmaceutical formulations intended for topical use in humans.

VETERINARY COMPARISONS

Veterinary pharmaceuticals face a greater challenge as the pharmaceutical and pesticide industry have often found that the dermatopharmacokinetics of any one drug or pesticide vary considerably across domestic animal species. There are many topical sprays and pour-ons approved for use in dogs and cats to treat internal and external parasites. Veterinarians also use transdermal patches in clinical situations where steady-state delivery is required for an extended time period and/or when other routes of administration are not practical. A good example of this is the use of human transdermal patches containing an opioid analgesic, fentanyl, to manage pain associated with injury, perioperative procedures, and chronic pain in dogs and cats.

These transdermal patches that are only approved for use in humans can produce therapeutic drug levels (0.6–1.0 ng/mL) within 7 hours in the cat and 24 hours in the dog, but require as long as 40 hours in humans (38–40). Drug depot formation in the stratum corneum is more remarkable in humans and cats than in dogs as evidenced by the more persistent blood concentrations after patch removal. The transdermal bioavailability of fentanyl is 92% in human skin (41), but 63% in the dog and 36% in the cat (40,42,43). These data are not consistent with the previously described physiological and anatomical differences between species, although the patch–skin interface may vary across species and account for these apparent differences (19).

The fentanyl patch is only one of the many transdermal delivery systems that are often used in veterinary medicine. Other popular transdermal systems contain drugs to treat and manage hyperthyroidism (methimazole), diabetes (glipizide), or congestive heart failure (diltiazem) in cats. The literature suggests that many of these transdermal systems, which are primarily gels containing pluronic and lecithin, may not have clinical applications. Some of these gels do not achieve therapeutic plasma concentrations and dermal bioavailability is often difficult to assess (44,45). In contrast to these observations, more recent clinical efficacy studies suggest that methimazole absorption in cats may be significant enough to manage feline hyperthyroidism (46). It should be noted that compared with healthy cats, hyperthyroidism is associated with increased blood flow and thinner skin, which will promote dermal absorption. This may in part explain why efficacy responses vary widely with regard to transdermal application of this drug. It should be noted that none of these transdermal gels or patches are approved for use in veterinary species and are regarded as off-label applications. Therefore, care must be taken as the dermatopharmacokinetics of these delivery systems have demonstrated significant interspecies and intraspecies variability, as shown in humans, and can impact efficacy and toxicity.

Many of the topical insecticides that are widely used in veterinary medicine have a larger margin of safety compared with the drugs described above. Therefore, control of the release of these active ingredients on the skin surface may not be as critical but are still of clinical importance. Some of these formulations result in systemic absorption (e.g., pour-ons) and other formulations (e.g., topicals) are not significantly absorbed into the blood stream, but move laterally across the skin surface of the animal.

The spot-on selamectin product (Revolution®; Pfizer, Inc., New York, New York, U.S.A.) has a completely different pharmacokinetic profile in dogs when compared with cats following topical application (47). Dermal bioavailability in cats (74%) is much greater than that in dogs (4%) (Fig. 4), although self-grooming, which is more common among cats than dogs, may have partially contributed to the differences in bioavailability. This drug is slowly absorbed across the skin in both species and displays flip-flop kinetics. That is, dermal absorption is the rate-limiting step in the kinetics of this drug in both species. However, it is worth noting that selamectin flux is three times greater in cat skin (0.1 µg/cm^2/hr) than in dog skin (0.03 µg/cm^2/hr). The much longer elimination half-life in the cat (69 hours) than in the dog (14 hours) may be due to differences in liver metabolism. These

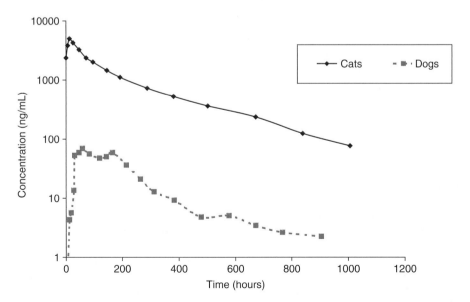

FIGURE 4 Mean plasma concentration of selamectin after topical application of 24 mg/kg to the skin of dogs and cats. *Source*: Kinetic profile obtained from Ref. 47 and plotted from Unscan-it® software (Silk Scientific, Orem, Utah, U.S.A.).

pharmacokinetic features favor more persistent blood drug concentrations, redistribution to targeted areas in the skin, such as the sebaceous glands, and skin regions where ectoparasites reside, and, most importantly, reduce the need for frequent reapplication. In essence, slow release from the topical application resulted in more persistent blood concentrations than oral dosing, suggesting improved therapeutic efficacy with the dermal application. For these and other reasons, selamectin is approved and marketed for topical use only in cats and dogs.

Although avermectins are widely used in several ruminants, pour-on applications are only approved for bovine species and not ovine and caprine species. Recent studies demonstrated that off-label applications by the dermal route in small ruminants may not necessarily result in therapeutic success. Based on the in vivo half-life of absorption (0.36 vs. 0.93 days), eprinomectin is more rapidly absorbed across goat skin than cattle skin (48,49). However, more of the drug was absorbed across cattle skin than goat skin based on significant AUC differences. The reason for the low dermal bioavailability in goats compared with cattle is unclear, although it may be related to greater depot formation in goat skin than cattle skin. This observation together with other efficacy studies (50) suggests that transdermal application in goats may not provide as satisfactory antiparasitic efficacy as demonstrated in cattle at the labeled dose of 0.5 mg/kg. Although a small percentage (0.1% in cattle and 0.3–0.5% in goats) of a topical dose of 0.5 mg/kg appears in the milk, eprinomectin levels in milk were below the tolerance level of 12 ng/mL. From a human health perspective, eprinomectin is safer to give to lactating ruminants than, say, ivermectin whose topical application results in a 5% elimination of the topical dose in the milk.

Our laboratory recently demonstrated differences across ruminant species for the dermal absorption of another avermectin, abamectin (51). We also demonstrated that abamectin deposition into the viable epidermis at eight hours was significantly greater in ruminant species than porcine species, irrespective of the aqueous or oil formulations tested. Although small amounts of abamectin were absorbed (<0.2% dose) during the 8-h study in the ruminant and swine model, this was similar to the extent of absorption in rhesus monkeys over a 10-day study period (52). These avermectins are very lipophilic, and it is not unusual to observe comparable absorption across these species.

CONCLUSION

As can be appreciated from this overview, large differences exist in the morphology of animal and human skin that could impact the properties of the cutaneous barrier and the mechanism of action of cytotoxic agents. Clear species differences exist in the extent of percutaneous absorption. These factors apply equally to the study of effects of exposure to occupational chemicals (solvents, corrosives), environmental pollutants (pesticides and other organics), vesicant agents, cosmetics or dermatologics, or transdermal drugs that are designed to cross the epidermal barrier. To properly study the dermatotoxicity of these chemicals, the ability to penetrate the stratum corneum barrier must be assessed. The target cells or structures in skin must then be defined, the potential cytotoxic response classified, and the ubiquitous cutaneous immune response taken into account. The proper human surrogate in vivo animal models that are capable of characterizing all of these events must be selected to adequately study the nature of the response seen after human exposure. Unfortunately, there is no single universal animal model that is appropriate for predicting both absorption and toxicity of all drugs in humans.

REFERENCES

1. Monteiro-Riviere NA. Comparative anatomy, physiology, and biochemistry of mammalian skin. In: Hobson DW, ed. Dermal and Ocular Toxicology: Fundamentals and Methods. New York: CRC Press Inc., 1991:3–71.
2. Monteiro-Riviere NA. The integument. In: Eurell J, Frappier B, eds. Dellmann's Textbook of Veterinary Histology. Ames, Iowa: Blackwell Publishing, 2006:320–49.
3. Monteiro-Riviere NA, Bristol DG, Manning TO, et al. Interspecies and inter-regional analysis of the comparative histological thickness and laser doppler blood flow measurements at five cutaneous sites in nine species. J Invest Dermatol 1990; 95:582–6.
4. Halprin KM. Epidermal "turnover time" a reexamination. Br J Dermatol 1972; 86:14–9.
5. Bergstresser PR, Taylor JR. Epidermal "turnover time" a new examination. Br J Dermatol 1977; 96:503–9.
6. Weinstein GD. Comparison turnover time of keratinous protein fractions in swine and human epidermis. In: Bustad LK, McClellan RO, Burns MP, eds. Swine in Biomedical Research. Richland, WA: Pacific Northwest Laboratory, 1966:287–97.
7. Monteiro-Riviere NA, Inman AO, Mak V, et al. Effect of selective lipid extraction from different body regions on epidermal barrier function. Pharm Res 2001; 18:992–8.
8. Monteiro-Riviere NA, Inman AO. Indirect immunohistochemistry and immunoelectron microscopy distribution of eight epidermal–dermal junction epitopes in the pig and in isolated perfused skin treated with bis (2-chloroethyl) sulfide. Toxicol Pathol 1995; 23:313–25.
9. Zhang Z, Monteiro-Riviere NA. Comparison of integrins in human skin, pig skin, and perfused skin: an in vitro skin toxicology model. J Appl Toxicol 1997; 17:247–53.
10. Grissom RE, Monteiro-Riviere NA, Guthrie FE. A method for preparing mouse skin for assessing in vitro dermal penetration of xenobiotics. Toxicol Lett 1987; 36:251–8.
11. Monteiro-Riviere NA. The integument. In: Pond WG, Mersmann HJ, eds. The Biology of the Domestic Pig. Ithaca, NY: Cornell University Press, 2001:625–52.
12. Stewart ME. Sebaceous gland lipids. Semin Dermatol 1992; 11:100–5.
13. Argenzio RA, Monteiro-Riviere NA. The excretory system. In: Pond WG, Mersmann HJ, eds. The Biology of the Domestic Pig. Ithaca, NY: Cornell University Press, 2001:585–624.
14. Crow KD, Puhvel M. Chloracne. In: Marzulli FN, Maibach HI, eds. Dermatotoxicology. 3rd ed. Washington: Hemisphere Publishing, 1977:515–34.
15. Bijman J. Transport processes in the eccrine sweat gland. Kidney Int 1987; 32:S109–12.
16. Quinton PM, Reddy MM. Cl^- conductance and acid secretion in the human sweat duct. Ann NY Acad Sci 1989; 574:438–46.
17. Ebling FJG. Aprocine glands in health and disorder. Int J Dermatol 1989; 28:508–11.
18. Elias PM. Epidermal lipids, barrier function, and desquamation. J Invest Dermatol 1983; 80:44–9.
19. Riviere JE, Papich M. Potential and problems of developing transdermal patches for veterinary applications. Adv Drug Deliv Rev 2001; 50:175–203.
20. Monteiro-Riviere NA. Anatomical factors affecting barrier function. In: Marzulli FN, Maibach HI, eds. Dermatotoxicology. 5th ed. Washington: Taylor & Francis, 1996:3–17.
21. Bartek MJ, LaBudde JL, Maibach HI. Skin permeability in vivo: comparison in rat, rabbit, pig and man. J Invest Dermatol 1972; 58:114–23.
22. Hawkins GS, Reifenrath WG. Development of an in vitro model for determining the fate of chemicals applied to the skin. Fundam Appl Toxicol 1984; 4:S133–44.
23. Riviere JE, Monteiro-Riviere NA. The isolated perfused porcine skin flap as an in vitro model for percutaneous absorption and cutaneous toxicology. CRC Crit Rev Toxicol 1991; 21:329–44.
24. Wester RC, Maibach HI. Animal models for percutaneous absorption. In: Wang RGM, Knaak JB, Maibach HI, eds. Health Risk Assessment: Dermal and Inhalation Exposure and Absorption of Toxicants. Boca Raton, FL: CRC Press, 1993:89–104.

25. Riviere JE, Monteiro-Riviere NA, Williams PL. Isolated perfused porcine skin flap as an in vitro model for predicting transdermal pharmacokinetics. Eur J Pharm Biopharm 1995; 41:152–62.

26. Baynes RE, Halling KB, Riviere JE. The influence of diethyl-*m*-toluamide (DEET) on the percutaneous absorption of permethrin and carbaryl. Toxicol Appl Pharmacol 1997; 144:332–9.

27. Srikrishna V, Riviere JE, Monteiro-Riviere NA. Cutaneous toxicity and absorption of paraquat in porcine skin. Toxicol Appl Pharmacol 1992; 115:89–97.

28. Walker M, Dugard PH, Scott RC. In vitro percutaneous absorption studies: a comparison of human and laboratory species. Hum Toxicol 1983; 2:561–8.

29. Wester RC, Maibach HI, Bucks DA, et al. In vivo percutaneous absorption of paraquat from hand, leg, and forearm of humans. J Toxicol Environ Health 1984; 14:759–62.

30. Chui YC, Poon G, Law F. Toxicokinetics and bioavailability of paraquat in rats following different routes of administration. Toxicol Ind Health 1988; 4:203–19.

31. Sato K, Sugibayashi K, Morimoto Y. Species differences in percutaneous absorption of nicorandil. J Pharm Sci 1991; 80:104–7.

32. Baynes RE, Monteiro-Riviere NA, Riviere JE. Pyridostigmine bromide modulates the dermal disposotion of [^{14}C] permethrin. Toxicol Appl Pharmacol 2002; 181:164–73.

33. Franz TJ, Lehman PA, Franz SF, et al. Comparative percutaneous absorption of lindane and permethrin. Arch Dermatol 1996; 132:901–5.

34. Wester RC, Melendres J, Sedik L, et al. Percutaneous absorption of salicylic acid, theophylline, 2,4-dimethylamine, diethyl hexyl phthalic acid, and *p*-aminobenzoic acid in the isolated perfused porcine skin flap compared to man in vivo. Toxicol Appl Pharmacol 1998; 151:159–65.

35. Dick IP, Scott RC. Pig ear skin as an in-vitro model for human skin permeability. J Pharm Pharmacol 1992; 44:640–5.

36. Bartek MJ, LaBudde JA. Percutaneous absorption in vitro. In: Maibach HI, ed. Animal Models in Dermatology. New York: Churchill-Livingstone, 1975:103–20.

37. Feldmann RJ, Maibach HI. Percutaneous penetration of some pesticides and herbicides in man. Toxicol Appl Pharmacol 1974; 28:126–32.

38. Grond S, Radbruch L, Lehmann KA. Clinical pharmacokinetics of transdermal opioids: focus on transdermal fentanyl. Clin Pharmacokinet 2000; 38:59–89.

39. Hofmeister EH, Egger CM. Transdermal fentanyl patches in small animals. J Am Anim Hosp Assoc 2004; 40:468–78.

40. Kyles AE, Papich M, Hardie EM. Disposition of transdermally administered fentanyl in dogs. Am J Vet Res 1996; 57:715–9.

41. Varvel JR, Shafer SL, Hwang SS, et al. Absorption characteristics of transdermally administered fentanyl. Anesthesiology 1989; 70:928–34.

42. Lee DD, Papich MG, Hardie EM. Comparison of pharmacokinetics of fentanyl after intravenous and transdermal administration in cats. Am J Vet Res 2000; 61:672–7.

43. Roy SD, Hou SL, Withman SL, et al. Transdermal delivery of narcotic analgesics: comparative metabolism and permeability of human cadaver skin and hairless mouse skin. J Pharm Sci 1994; 83:1723–8.

44. Hoffman SB, Yoder AR, Trepanier LA. Bioavailability of transdermal methimazole in a pluronic lecithin organogel (PLO) in healthy cats. J Vet Pharmacol Ther 2002; 25:189–93.

45. Bennett N, Papich MG, Hoenig M, et al. Evaluation of transdermal application of glipizide in a pluronic lecithin gel to healthy cats. Am J Vet Res 2005; 66:581–8.

46. Lécuyer M, Prini S, Dunn M, et al. Clinical efficacy and safety of transdermal methimazole in the treatment of feline hyperthyroidism. Can Vet J 2006; 47:131–5.

47. Sarasola P, Jernigan AD, Walker DK, et al. Pharmacokinetics of selamectin following intravenous, oral and topical administration in cats and dogs. Vet Pharmacol Ther 2002; 25:265–72.

48. Alvinerie M, Lacoste E, Sutra JF, et al. Some pharmacokinetic parameters of eprino-mectin in goats following pour-on administration. Vet Res Commun 1999; 23:449–55.

49. Alvinerie M, Sutra JF, Galtier P, et al. Pharmacokinetics of eprinomectin in plasma and milk following topical administration to lactating dairy cattle. Res Vet Sci 1999; 67:229–32.

50. Chartier C, Etter E, Pors I, et al. Activity of eprinomectin in goats against experimental infections with Haemonchus contortus, Teladorsagia circumcincta and Trichostrongylus colubriformis. Vet Rec 1999; 144:99–100.
51. Baynes RE. In vitro dermal disposition of abamectin (avermectin B1) in livestock. Res Vet Sci 2004; 76:235–42.
52. Wislocki PG, Feely WF, White S, et al. Dermal penetration of avermectin B1a in the rhesus monkey. Toxicol Appl Pharmacol 1988; 94:238–45.

3 The Physical Structure of the Skin Barrier

Lars Norlén

Medical Nobel Institute, Department of Cellular and Molecular Biology, Karolinska Institute, Stockholm, Sweden

INTRODUCTION

The main function of skin is to serve as barrier at the interface between body and environment. This is manifested in different ways, e.g., as a barrier to mechanical stress, to UV-light damage, and to the penetration of drugs, allergens, microorganisms, toxic substances, etc. For many dermatological patients, the skin may also represent a strong social barrier. However, from an evolutional point of view, the single most important task of skin is to create a watertight enclosure of the body to prevent water loss. Water homeostasis is a strict requirement for normal body function as an uncontrolled loss of water results in a dramatic increase in ion concentrations with consequent harmful effects on cells and tissues.

It is generally believed that the permeability of the skin is mainly a function of the physical state and the structural organization of the stratum corneum intercellular lipid matrix [cf. (1,2)]. A better understanding of stratum corneum lipid organization may thus aid the development of more rational transdermal drug administration systems. In order to achieve this, several problems of fundamental character must be overcome. These are, e.g., that precise quantitative compositional lipid data are still lacking, which severely handicaps experimental and theoretical model building. Such model building is further complicated by the structural complexity of the stratum corneum and the many gradients (e.g., in water chemical potential, pH, and ion concentrations) through the stratum corneum in the native situation. For example, as the osmotic pressure (i.e., chemical potential) of water is the driving force for both swelling and phase transitions of lipid bilayers (3,4), a transition from a gel into a liquid crystalline structure could occur locally in stratum corneum at a critical chemical potential of water. Thus the physical state of the intercellular lipid compartment may not be identical throughout the stratum corneum (5). These gradients further suggest that the stacked lamellar lipid matrix of the stratum corneum intercellular space, like most other biological system, may not essentially be an equilibrium structure, but rather stabilized by secondary, or higher, minimum energy order steady states [cf. (6)]. Consequently, the pathway followed during the formation of this multilamellar membrane structure may have profound implications for its structural organization and physical characteristics (7).

A fundamental problem for skin barrier research is that it is not known what artifacts are introduced during sample storage and sample preparation procedures, e.g., conventional X-ray diffraction and electron microscopy. Separation of the epidermis with or without heat, trypsination, desiccation, storage in freezer as well as chemical fixation, solvent exposure, dehydration, plastic embedding, and staining are procedures that may have profound effects on the structural organization of lipid membranes and other constituents of the epidermis.

One way to obtain morphological skin barrier data largely unaffected by preparation-induced artifacts may be cryo-electron microscopy of vitreous skin sections (CEMOVIS) (8) and cryo-electron tomography of vitreous skin sections (CETOVIS) (9). Using CEMOVIS it has been shown that the extracellular space of stratum corneum, i.e., the area representing the skin barrier, is dominated by ~44-nm-thick regions interconnected by thinner linker regions. The ~44-nm-thick regions contain eight electron-dense parallel lines with a characteristic, complex non-bilayer pattern. The linker regions are represented by ~9-, ~14-, ~25-, ~33-, ~39-, and ~48-nm-thick spaces containing 1, 2, 4, 6, 8, and 10 parallel electron-dense lines, respectively, forming stacked bilayer-like patterns between adjacent corneocyte plasma membranes (or "lipid envelopes") (10). Further, it has been shown that the extracellular space between viable and cornified epidermis, i.e., the area where the skin barrier is formed, contains transition desmosomes at different stages of reorganization interconnected by areas expressing a rich variety of complex membrane-like structures, resembling cubic-to-lamellar membrane transitions (8,10).

There follows a description of the physical structure of the skin barrier as observed by CEMOVIS together with a discussion of the closely related subjects of skin permeability and skin barrier lipid composition.

SKIN BARRIER STRUCTURE
Cryo-Electron Microscopy of Vitreous Epidermal Sections

Due to limitations imposed by available technology our view of skin ultrastructure has, until recently, mainly been derived from observations made on dehydrated specimens. As water activity represents a major factor governing lipid-phase behavior and structural organization (3,4,11–13) it is not unlikely that dehydration during sample preparation of skin for conventional X-ray diffraction or electron microscopy, may perturb the structural organization of the lipid matrix of the stratum corneum extracellular space. Dehydration during sample preparation for conventional electron microscopy results in inevitable aggregation, and partial loss, of nonaqueous biomaterial (Fig. 1). Further, conventional electron microscopy uses heavy metal staining in order to increase image contrast (to compensate for the strong background noise created by the plastic embedding medium). Consequently, it is not the epidermal biomaterial per se that is observed, but deposits of contrast agents on remaining dehydrated, and consequently heavily aggregated, plastic-embedded biomaterial (14).

Cryo-electron microscopy (15,16) consists in vitrifying (rapid cooling such that ice crystals do not have time to form) a biological sample (typically a suspension of proteins) and observing it in a cryo-electron microscope at a temperature where vitreous water is stable and does not evaporate ($< -140°C$). The native structure of the skin may then be preserved down to atomic resolution. Further, biostructures are often better visualized unstained in their aqueous environment than stained in conventional preparations. This is because the signal-to-noise ratio is optimal in vitreous water where the only source of noise is electron statistic. Recently, the method has been extended to tissues (8,10,14). This requires successful vitrification and subsequent cutting of ultrathin cryo-sections that are then directly observed in the cryo-electron microscope. As a consequence, it is now possible to study the ultrastructure of tissues in their native fully

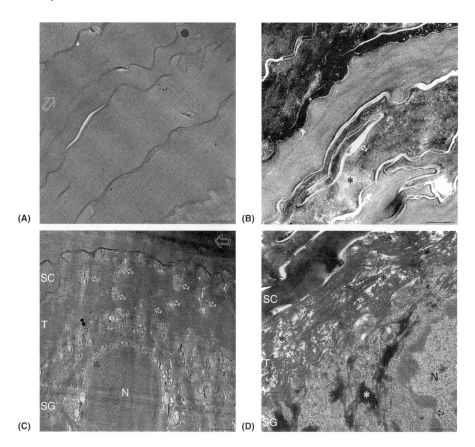

FIGURE 1 Conventional sample preparation for electron microscopy results in important losses of epidermal biomaterial. Low magnification transmission electron micrographs of human epidermis at the interzone between viable and cornified cell layers (**A,B**: lowermost stratum corneum; **C,D**: uppermost stratum granulosum). (**A,C**) Cryo-electron micrographs of vitreous sections of native epidermis. (**B,D**) Conventional electron micrographs of resin-embedded sections. In the vitreous cryo-fixed epidermis (**A,C**) cellular as well as intercellular space appears densely packed with organic material, while in the conventionally fixed epidermis (**B,D**) the distribution of biomaterial is characteristically inhomogeneous. Loss of biomaterial appears to have taken place in (**B,D**), both in the cytoplasmic (*black asterisk*) and intercellular (*white arrow*) space. Large portions of the biomass of the viable cells appear as aggregated, heavily stained clusters, so-called keratohyalin granules (**D**,*white asterisk*). Furthermore, the rich variety of cytoplasmic organelles and multigranular structures presents in the stratum corneum/stratum granulosum transition (T) cells of native epidermis (**C**, *white arrows*) are replaced by empty space in resin-embedded samples (**D**, *black asterisk*). Inner and outer nuclear envelopes and nuclear pores are clearly distinguished in the native, cryo-fixed, non-stained specimen (**C**, *black arrow*), while they are difficult to distinguish in the conventionally fixed stained specimen (**D**, *black arrow*). Electron-dense single spot in (**A**) and double spot in (**C**) correspond to surface ice contamination. *Abbreviations*: N, nucleus; SC, lowermost stratum corneum cell; SG, uppermost stratum granulosum cell; T, transition cell. *Open white double arrow* (**A,C**): section cutting direction. Section thicknesses ~100 nm (**A,C**) and ~50 nm (**B, D**). Scale bars 500 nm (**A–D**). *Source*: Adapted from Ref. 10.

hydrated state, without chemical fixation or staining. Our results have shown that micrographs of human skin obtained by CEMOVIS not only show more detail but also differ dramatically from those obtained by conventional methods (10,14).

Computerized Electron Tomography of Vitreous Epidermal Sections

What limits the amount of information that can be extracted from cryo-electron micrographs of vitreous epidermal sections is mainly superposition of biomaterial in the section thickness dimension (9). This problem can be circumvented by CETOVIS in which a three-dimensional image is reconstructed from a large series of tilted electron micrographs. To maximize preservation of the vitreous tissue specimen, each electron micrograph in the tilt series is recorded with minimum electron dose. This yields a very low electron contrast for the individual micrographs in the tilt series, which consequently become difficult to align during tomographic reconstruction. In fact, tilt series image alignment has represented the main obstacle for the development of molecular resolution CETOVIS. However, we recently developed a method allowing reliable image alignment for electron tomography on vitreous skin sections (9). Quantum dots, which form liquid suspensions in organic solvents at cryo-temperatures, are deposited directly onto vitreous sections and subsequently used as electron-dense markers to align the tilt series. The new method allows for molecular resolution three-dimensional imaging of epidermis in its native hydrated state in situ.

Global Structure of the Stratum Corneum

Based on conventional electron microscopy data, human stratum corneum has been proposed to contain three distinct zones (17). The topmost part, the stratum disjunctum, comprises corneocytes with varying translucency that represents varying degrees of mass loss. In the lowermost part, the stratum compactum, the electron contrast seems more homogeneous. However, in human forearm epidermis prepared by direct vitreous cryo-fixation, the corneocyte density is approximately homogeneous throughout the stratum corneum (Fig. 2) (8,10,14). Given the lack of evidence in cryo-electron micrographs for differences in densities between the upper and lower stratum corneum these earlier reported differences may, to a large extent, have been artifactual.

In conventional electron micrographs of human forearm epidermis, the stratum corneum extracellular space is largely empty looking (Fig. 1B,D). Furthermore, the rich variety of cytoplasmic organelles and multigranular structures present in the stratum corneum/stratum granulosum transition (T) cell cytoplasm of vitreous epidermis (Fig. 1C, white arrows) is partly replaced by empty space in resin-embedded epidermis (Fig. 1D, black asterisk). Consequently, cytoplasmic structures responsible for the formation of the lipid matrix of the stratum corneum extracellular space may largely be absent in conventionally fixed resin-embedded epidermal samples.

Structure of the Interface Between Stratum Granulosum and Stratum Corneum as Observed by CEMOVIS

For a recent theoretical model on skin barrier formation, see Ref. (18). A striking feature of cryo-electron micrographs of vitreous epidermal sections is the usually clearly non-lamellar content of "lamellar bodies" at the stratum granulosum/stratum corneum interface (8). This difference from conventional electron

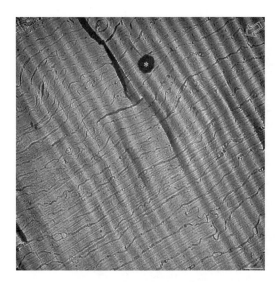

FIGURE 2 The ultrastructure of vitreous native stratum corneum is approximately homogeneous throughout its thickness dimension. Low magnification cryo-transmission electron micrograph of vitreous section of native human stratum corneum. Note the approximately homogeneous corneocyte density, size, and form throughout the stratum corneum, with the exception of the lowermost corneocytes that generally are larger and characterized by a seemingly more highly invaginated cell surface (*lower right corner*). Electron-dense spot corresponds to surface ice contamination (*white asterisk*). Wave-like diagonal pattern in the upper right corner is due to section compression during cutting. *Open white double arrow*: section cutting direction. Section thickness ~50 nm. Scale bar 1.0 μm.

micrographs, where numerous lamellae containing "lamellar bodies" can usually be identified, could be explained by an artifactual dehydration-driven lamellarization of "lamellar body" lipid content taking place during conventional sample preparation for electron microscopy. The absence of lamellae containing "lamellar bodies" in cryo-preserved epidermis suggests that the conventional model for skin barrier formation, based on the concept of coordinated fusion of lamellar body disks in the extracellular space of lowermost stratum corneum (19), may be regarded with skepticism.

In cryo-electron micrographs, the extracellular space between viable and cornified epidermis is characterized by a rich variety of complex features. About half of the length of the extracellular space is occupied by structures reminiscent of desmosomes, referred to as "transition desmosomes" (Fig. 3, solid white arrows). The remaining half is occupied by widened areas, frequently extending as deep cell invaginations (Fig. 3, thin white arrows), containing complex membrane-like structures (10). In our experience, the most frequently observed internal feature of widened areas is a stacked multilamellar electron density pattern associated with a granular pattern (Fig. 4A; white asterisk in Fig. 5A,C). Other patterns observed are check patterns (Fig. 4A, central white box) incorporated in complex arrangements of irregular layers and multilamellar electron densities enclosing a granular structure (Fig. 4B). The region visualized in Fig. 4B is probably a cross section through a large invagination originating at the interface between viable and cornified epidermis (inset box, solid white arrows). The multilamellar "shell"

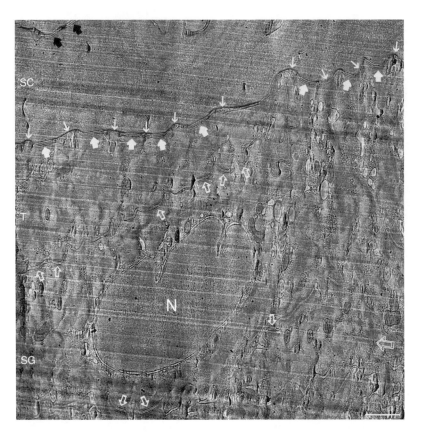

FIGURE 3 Transition desmosomes are exclusively found at the interface between stratum granulosum and stratum corneum. Low magnification cryo-transmission electron micrograph of vitreous section of human epidermis at the interface between viable and cornified cell layers. About 50% of the extracellular space at this location is occupied by transition desmosomes (*solid white arrows*) and the remaining 50% by widened areas (*thin white arrows*) containing complex electron density patterns (cf. Figs. 4 and 5). *Open white arrows*: desmosomes (cf. Fig. 16) and *solid black arrows*: ~44-nm-thick regions of the stratum corneum extracellular space (cf. Fig. 12). *Abbreviations*: N, nucleus; SC, lowermost stratum corneum cell; SG, uppermost stratum granulosum cell; T, transition cell. *Open white double arrow* (**B**): section cutting direction. Section thickness ~50 nm. Scale bar 500 nm. *Source*: Adapted from Ref. 10.

domain is composed of at least 25 electron-dense lines at its thickest part, with an apparent decreasing lamellar repeat distance from ~5 nm in the central part to ~4 nm in the peripheral part. Also, complex stacks of small portions of bent double-layer electron density patterns (Fig. 5B, white box) and stacks of electron-dense double-layer patterns (Fig. 5D, region "1") seemingly extending into the extracellular core domain of transition desmosomes (Fig. 5A, open white arrow) are seen (10).

No widened extracellular areas are usually found above the third stratum corneum cell, although apparently featureless extracellular dilatations can be observed throughout the mature stratum corneum (cf. Fig. 6A,C, black asterisk). In the first to third stratum corneum extracellular space loosely packed extended double-layer patterns (pairs of thin white arrows) are found in remaining widened

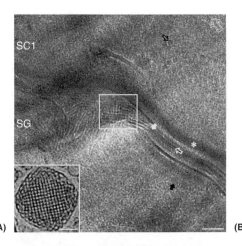 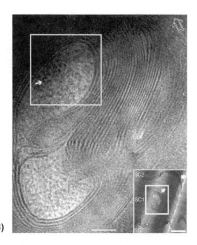

(A)   (B)

FIGURE 4 Check pattern (**A**) and bent multilamellar (**B**) electron density pattern in widened areas. High magnification cryo-electron micrographs (**A**,**B**) of widened areas of the extracellular space between stratum granulosum and stratum corneum of vitreous epidermis. The electron density check pattern in (**A**, *central white box*) resembles, including its dimensions, the cryo-electron density pattern of cubic lipid/water in vitro phases (inset box in **A**). *Open white arrow* (**A**): central electron-dense double-layer pattern of transition desmosome extracellular core domain in possible continuity (*solid white arrow*) with lamellar lipid material of adjacent widened areas (**A**, *central white box*); *solid black arrow* (**A**): remnants of the inner cytoplasmic desmosome plaque; SG (**A**): uppermost stratum granulosum cell; SC1 (**A**): lowermost stratum corneum cell; *white asterisk* (**A**): cornified envelope; *open black arrow* (**A**): keratin intermediate filament cut perpendicularly to its length axis; *thin white arrow* (**B**): sinusoid-like dot pattern. Inset box (**A**): cryo-transmission electron micrograph of a lipid/water in vitro phase with cubic (D-type) symmetry (scale bar 50 nm). *Source*: From Ref. 20. Inset box (**B**): low magnification cryo-electron micrograph of the locality from which (**B**) was obtained (*white box*). *Solid white arrows* (inset box in **B**): extracellular space; *open white double arrow* (**A**,**B**): section cutting direction. Section thickness (**A**,**B**) ~50 nm. Scale bar (A, B) 50 nm and (inset box in **B**) 500 nm. *Source*: Adapted from Ref. 10.

areas (Fig. 7A). The most peripheral double-layer patterns (peripheral-most pairs of thin white arrows) adhere closely to the corneocyte lipid envelope (pair of thin black arrows) giving the corneocyte cell periphery a trilamellar aspect (Fig. 7A,B, small square bracket). The loosely packed extended double-layer patterns are observed to be associated laterally either with the characteristic eight-line pattern of ~44-nm-thick regions (cf. below; Fig. 7B,C) or with the stacked lamellae of linker regions (cf. below; Fig. 13A,C, large white box) (10).

Transition desmosomes are recognized at low magnification by the fact that they lack a cytoplasmic plaque on the upper (corneocyte) side (Fig. 3, solid white arrows). In contrast to normal desmosomes (open white arrows), they therefore appear asymmetric. Transition desmosomes are exclusively found at the interface between stratum granulosum and stratum corneum. High magnification views are shown in Figure 5. The median width of the extracellular core domain of transition desmosomes has been estimated to ~43 nm (Table 1). The single cytoplasmic plaque on the lower (stratum granulosum) side is characterized by a central ~10-nm-thick electron-dense band (solid white arrows in Fig. 5A–D and inset box in Fig. 5C), paralleled on each side by a very weak ~2- to 4-nm-thick electron-dense double-line (thin white arrow in inset box in Fig. 5C; thin black arrows in Fig. 5B,D). The cytoplasmic plaque is situated ~11 nm from the plasma membrane

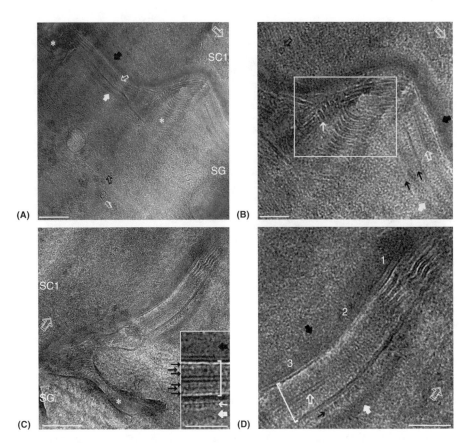

FIGURE 5 Transition desmosomes. High magnification cryo-electron micrographs of the interface between stratum granulosum and stratum corneum of vitreous epidermis (**B,D** represent enlargements of the upper right part of **A,C**, respectively). Transition desmosomes are characterized by a ∼43-nm-thick extracellular core domain (*white square brackets* in **D** and *inset box* in **C**; Table 1) and by a single cornified envelope (*solid black arrows*) situated on the upper cytoplasmic side and a single cytoplasmic plaque (*solid white arrows*) situated on the lower cytoplasmic side. Note that stacked lipid bilayer-like material (**D**, region "1") sometimes appears in the transition desmosome extracellular core domain (**A**, *open white arrow*) already before the desmosome cytoplasmic plaque (**A**, *solid white arrow*) has disappeared. Widened areas (**A,C**, *white asterisk*) between transition desmosomes express a complex electron density pattern (**B**, *white box*; cf. Fig. 4). The flattened circular electron-dense structure marked by a *thin white arrow* inside the *white box* in (**B**) has a thickness of ∼3.9 nm, excluding an underlying flattened vesicular (i.e., lamellar body disc) morphology. *Solid white arrows* (**A–D**): transition desmosome cytoplasmic plaque; *solid black arrows* (**A–D**): cornified envelope; *thin black arrows* (**B,D**): very weak electron-dense lines associated with the transition desmosome cytoplasmic plaque (*thin white arrow* in inset box in **C**); *open white arrows* (**B,D**): electron-dense central double-layer pattern of the transition desmosome extracellular domain; *white asterisk* (**A,C**): widened areas; SG: uppermost stratum granulosum cell; SC1: lowermost stratum corneum cell; *open black arrows*: keratin intermediate filaments in keratinocyte (**A**) and corneocyte (**B**) cut approximately perpendicularly to their length axis; *oblique open white arrow* (**A**): microtubule; *open white double arrows* (**A–D**): section cutting direction. Section thickness (A–D) ∼50 nm. Scale bar (**A,C**) 100 nm and (**B,D**, inset box in **C**) 50 nm. *Source*: Adapted from Ref. 10.

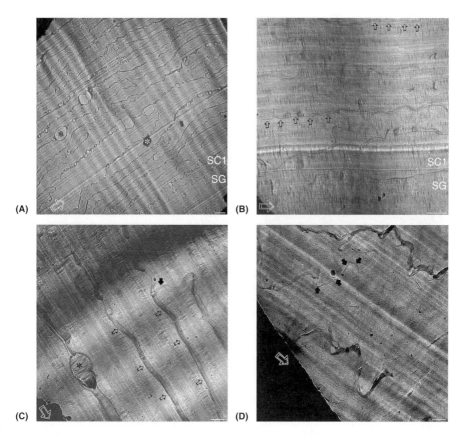

FIGURE 6 The stratum corneum extracellular space is dominated by ~44-nm-thick regions, interconnected by thinner linker regions. (**A–D**) Low magnification cryo-electron micrographs of stratum corneum of vitreous sections. (**A**) Overview of stratum corneum. (**B**) Lower stratum corneum. (**C, D**) Mid-portion of stratum corneum. The extracellular ~44-nm-thick regions (**B**, *open black arrows*) may extend over > 1 μm (**C**, *open black arrows*) and are interconnected by thinner linker regions (**C, D**, *solid black arrows*). At the cell edges (**D**), these linker regions may extend over distances of > 250 nm (cf. Fig. 13A). *Black asterisk* (**A,C**): apparent dilatations of the extracellular space; *white asterisk* (**A**): surface ice contamination; SG: uppermost stratum granulosum cell; SC1: lowermost stratum corneum cell; *open white double arrows* (**A–D**): section cutting direction. Section thickness (**A–D**) ~50 nm. Scale bars (**A,B**) 500 nm and (**C,D**) 200 nm. *Source*: Adapted from Ref. 10.

of the uppermost stratum granulosum cell. The transition desmosome single cornified envelope is characterized by an intracellular ~16- to 18-nm diffuse electron-dense band situated adjacent to two electron-dense lines representing the corneocyte lipid envelope (Fig. 5A–D, solid black arrows). The transition desmosome extracellular core domain contains a combination of (*i*) a multilamellar electron density pattern (inset box in Fig. 5C; Fig. 5D, region "3") of which a central electron-dense double-layer pattern is most prominent (inset box in Fig. 5C,D, open white arrow), (*ii*) a granular electron density pattern (Fig. 5D, region "2"), and (*iii*) a stack of four (in most cases) and up to six-paired electron-dense lines (Fig. 5A, open white arrow; cf. also Fig. 5D, region "1") (10).

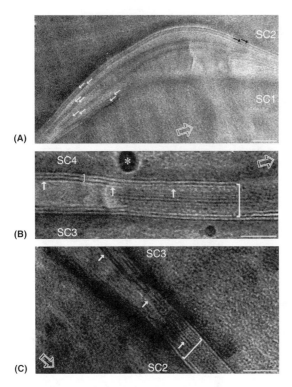

FIGURE 7 Loosely packed extended lipid bilayer-like structures are found in remaining widened areas of lower stratum corneum. High magnification cryo-transmission electron micrographs of lower stratum corneum of vitreous epidermis (**A–C**). The most peripheral double-layer patterns of remaining widened areas (**A**, pairs of *thin white arrows*) adhere closely to the corneocyte lipid envelope (**A**, pairs of *thin black arrows*). This is expressed as a characteristic trilamellar electron density pattern (**B**, *small white square bracket*) that seems to be continuous (**B**, *thin white arrows*) with the peripheral lines of adjacent eight-line ∼44-nm-thick regions (**B**, *large white square bracket*). More central double-layer patterns of remaining widened areas seem continuous (**C**, *thin white arrows*) with central lines of adjacent eight-line regions (**C**, *white square bracket*). SC1-4 (**A–C**): first to fourth stratum corneum cell; *open white double arrow* (**A–C**): section cutting direction. Section thickness (**A–C**) ∼50 nm. Scale bar (**A–C**) 50 nm. *Source*: Adapted from Ref. 10.

The detailed extracellular multilamellar electron density pattern of transition desmosomes (inset box in Fig. 5C) is characterized by a central electron-dense double-layer pattern paralleled on each side by three weaker electron-dense lines (thin black arrows). The outermost (as measured from the central electron-dense double layer) weak line runs adjacent to the outer electron-dense line of the two electron-dense lines forming either the corneocyte plasma membrane (or "lipid envelope") (upper side) or the stratum granulosum cell plasma membrane (lower side). The plasma membrane/lipid envelope line spacing (i.e., width) has been estimated to ∼4.4 nm and the line spacing of the two electron-dense lines forming the central electron-dense double-layer pattern to ∼4.9 nm. The first (peripheral-most) line of the transition desmosome extracellular space is situated at a distance of ∼4.7 nm from the outer electron-dense line of the double-layer pattern forming the corneocyte "lipid envelope" (upper side) or granular cell

TABLE 1 Dimensions of the Epidermal Extracellular Space

Description	Extracellular space thickness		Electron-dense central double-layer thickness		Number of electron-dense lines in the extracellular space
	Median (nm)	Range (nm)	Median (nm)	Range (nm)	
Viable desmosomes	32.6	27.9–38.7 ($n=12$)	—	—	—
Transition desmosomes	43.4	38.5–47.9 ($n=29$)	4.9	4.0–6.3 ($n=22$)	8
~9-nm-thick regions	9.0	8.2–11.6 ($n=5$)	—	—	1
~14-nm-thick regions	14.1	13.6–14.9 ($n=3$)	4.3	3.9–4.5 ($n=5$)	2
~25-nm-thick regions	25.3	23.7–28.9 ($n=3$)	4.3	4.0–4.5 ($n=3$)	4
~33-nm-thick regions	33.1	30.8–36.4 ($n=3$)	4.3	3.9–4.4 ($n=3$)	6
~39-nm-thick regions	39.0	38.7–40.0 ($n=5$)	4.3	3.9–4.7 ($n=5$)	8
~44-nm-thick regions	43.6	41.7–46.0 ($n=28$)	4.3	4.1–4.6 ($n=13$)	8
~48-nm-thick regions	48.3	47.9–49.3 ($n=3$)	4.4	4.0–4.7 ($n=3$)	10
~44-nm-thick region with cytoplasmic plaques	42.9	41.3–44.1 ($n=1$)	4.2	3.5–4.6 ($n=1$)	8
"Corneodesmosome"	34.3	33.3–35.1 ($n=1$)	—	—	—

plasma membrane (lower side). The second line of the transition desmosome extracellular space is situated at a distance of ~6.3 nm from the first line and ~4.3 nm from the third line. The third line is situated at a distance of ~4.3 nm from the adjacent line of the central electron-dense double-layer pattern (i.e., the fourth (strong) line of the transition desmosome extracellular space; inset box Fig. 5C). The extracellular space of transition desmosomes thus contains eight electron-dense lines with line spacings of approximately 4.5, 6.5, 4.5, 4.5, 5, 4.5, 4.5, 6.5, and 4.5 nm between the corneocyte "lipid envelope" (upper side) and the granular cell plasma membrane (lower side) (inset box Fig. 5C). The total thickness of the extracellular space varies between 39 and 48 nm (Table 1) (10).

Comparison between Conventional Data and Cemovis Data with Respect to the Structure of the Interface between Stratum Granulosum and Stratum Corneum

Desmosome Transformation

The fate of desmosomes is still an unresolved key issue in skin barrier research. The presence of desmosomes in the stratum corneum would imply the presence of direct protein links between the hydrated stratum corneum cells. If corneocytes were connected by a network of desmosomes, referred to as "corneodesmosomes," the stratum corneum cellular space would potentially offer a continuous pathway for the penetration of hydrophilic compounds, with important consequences for skin permeability. Also, stratum corneum desquamation, with its many implications for skin disease, is considered closely related to "corneodesmosome" degradation (21). Epidermal desmosomes undergo a pronounced reorganization at the interface between stratum granulosum and stratum corneum (Fig. 3) involving (*i*) a widening of the desmosome extracellular core domain from ~33 to ~43 nm (Table 1), (*ii*) the disappearance of the desmosome extracellular core domain transverse ~5 nm periodicity, (*iii*) the appearance of an eight-line electron density pattern of which a central double-layer pattern is the most electron dense (inset box in Fig. 5C) and in which the line spacings are the same as in the ~44-nm-thick regions of the extracellular space of cornified epidermis (cf. Fig. 8A), (*iv*) the disappearance of the cytoplasmic plaque (solid black arrow in Fig. 4A; solid white arrows in Fig. 5A–D), (*v*) the appearance of the cornified envelope (solid black arrows in Fig. 5A–D), and (*vi*) a decrease in plasma membrane electron density. Moreover, stacked lipid bilayer-like structures become closely associated laterally to the transition desmosome (Fig. 5D, region "1"), sometimes apparently penetrating into the transition desmosome extracellular core domain (Fig. 5A, open white arrow), as judged from the local presence of a remaining desmosome cytoplasmic plaque (Fig. 5A, solid white arrow). A close association between extra-desmosomal lipid bilayer structures and transition desmosome "plugs" has also been observed by conventional electron microscopy (22).

Conventional electron microscopy and immunocytochemistry studies have shown that non-peripheral desmosomes are gradually lost in the lower stratum corneum while "corneodesmosomes" on the corneocyte cell edges persist into the final desquamation (23–27). Our CEMOVIS data do not exclude this possibility. One high magnification micrograph obtained from the lower stratum corneum has shown a desmosome-like structure with a well-developed cytoplasmic plaque and electron-dense plasma membrane (Fig. 9A), which could correspond to a corneo-desmosome structure. The apparent lack of the characteristic desmosome cadherin

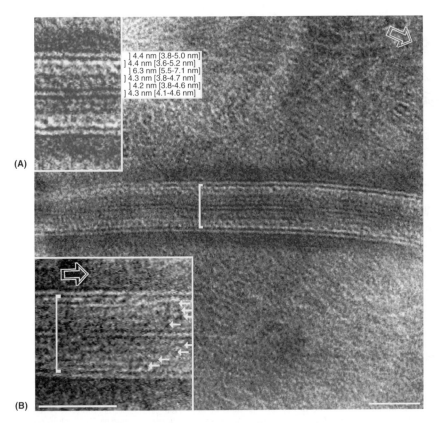

FIGURE 8 The ∼44-nm-thick regions **(A)** express a characteristic eight-line pattern between adjacent corneocyte lipid envelopes. High magnification cryo-transmission electron micrographs of vitreous mid-part stratum corneum. The dominating ∼44-nm-thick regions express eight parallel electron-dense lines with different, but characteristic, intensity, and spacing between adjacent corneocyte lipid envelopes (inset box **A**). Inset box **(A)** represents a magnification of the area marked by a *square bracket*. A relatively rare variant with a thickness of ∼48 nm (*white square bracket* in inset box **B**) expresses a 10-line pattern (inset box **B**, *thin white arrows*) instead of the more common eight-line pattern (inset box **A**). *Open white double arrows*: section cutting direction. Section thickness ∼50 nm. Scale bars 50 nm. *Source*: Adapted from Ref. 10.

∼5 nm periodicity (cf. Fig. 10) could, possibly, be due to a suboptimal orientation of the structure in the section. Nonetheless, at medium magnification, very few regions, even at the cell periphery, seem to express a characteristic cytoplasmic plaque electron density pattern (cf. Figs. 3 and 6B–D). However, a variant of the ∼44-nm-thick regions, retaining a cytoplasmic plaque structure, does exist in the lower stratum corneum (Fig. 9B, solid black arrows). Furthermore, the linker regions are both longer and more abundant at the corneocyte cell periphery (Fig. 6C,D, solid black arrows), which supports the notion of a morphological difference between flat and peripheral corneocyte areas. Freeze-substitution electron microscopy combined with immunocytochemistry [cf. (28)] could perhaps give quantitative insights into these matters.

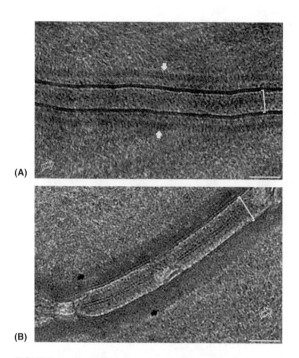

FIGURE 9 Corneodesmosomes? High magnification cryo-transmission electron micrographs of vitreous lower mid-part stratum corneum (**A,B**). (**A**) Desmosome-like structure (cf. Fig. 17) expressing a bilateral periodic cytoplasmic plaque pattern (*solid white arrows*). (**B**) Approximately 44-nm-thick region-like structure expressing a cytoplasmic plaque (*solid black arrows*) on the cytoplasmic sides of the cornified envelopes. Structures expressing cytoplasmic plaques (**A,B**) are rare in the stratum corneum (cf. Figs. 3 and 6B–D). *Open white double arrows* (**A,B**): section cutting direction. Section thickness (**A,B**) ∼50 nm. Scale bar (**A,B**) 50 nm. *Source*: Adapted from Ref. 10.

Formation of the Stratum Corneum Extracellular Lipid Matrix

Roughly half of the length of the extracellular space at the interface between stratum granulosum and stratum corneum of vitreous cryo-fixed epidermis is occupied by desmosomes at different stages of reorganization (Fig. 3, solid white arrows) and the remaining half by widened areas (Fig. 3, thin white arrows). The most frequently observed electron density patterns of the widened areas are stacked multilamellar, and diffuse granular, electron density patterns. Other characteristic structures are, however, also observed. Of these the most prevalent is an electron density check pattern marked by a white box in Figure 3A. The check pattern resembles, including its dimension, the cryo-electron density pattern of lipid/water in vitro phases with cubic symmetry (inset box in Fig. 4A) (10).

A second pattern is a bent multilamellar electron density (Fig. 4B) fully enclosing a granular electron density (white box). Figure 4B does not show a direct connection between the multilamellar complex and the extracellular space. However, it is probably connected outside of the section plane (solid white arrows in inset box). Its pattern shows global similarities (with the exception of the scale) to cubic-to-lamellar membrane transitions observed in myeloid bodies of retinal pigment epithelium (Fig. 11B) (29,32) and in the endoplasmatic reticulum of UT-1 cells (31) (Fig. 11A, white box; Fig. 11F). Further, similar electron density patterns

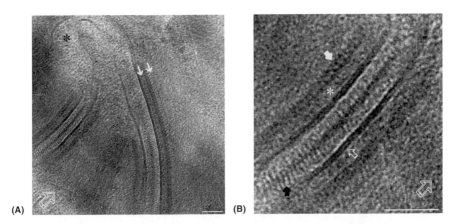

FIGURE 10 The desmosome extracellular core domain is characterized by an electron-dense transverse ~5 nm periodicity. High magnification cryo-electron micrograph of desmosomes at the midportion of the viable part of human epidermis. (**B**) Represents an enlargement of the middle left part of (**A**). The plasma membranes appear as ~4-nm-thick high-density double-layer patterns (**B**, *open white arrow*). The extracellular core domain is ~33-nm thick (cf. Table 1) and contains transverse electron-dense lines with a ~5 nm periodicity (**B**, *solid black arrow*), most probably corresponding to extracellular adhesion proteins (i.e., cadherins). On the cytoplasmic side, an ~11-nm-thick zone of medium electron density (**B**, *white asterisk*) separates the electron-dense plasma membrane from two parallel electron-dense layers, situated ~7 nm apart and interconnected by traversing electron-dense lines with a ~6 nm periodicity (**B**, *solid white arrow*). The inter-desmosomal space (*black asterisk*) showed no apparent internal fine structure. *Thin white arrows* (**A**) are very weak electron-dense lines associated with the desmosome cytoplasmic plaque. *Open white double arrows* (**A**, **B**): section cutting direction. Section thickness ~50 nm. Scale bar (**A**, **B**) 50 nm. *Source*: Adapted from Ref. 10.

have been reported in hamster cheek pouch stratum corneum (33) and in porcine palatal stratum corneum (34). Also, widened areas of the interface between stratum granulosum and stratum corneum of human epidermis have been reported to contain bent multilamellar lipid sheets associated with diffuse granular-like material (22).

The stacked, flattened multicircular electron density pattern of Figure 5B (white box) is remarkable by the complexity of the membrane-like structures and by the fact that, at several places, the line pattern seems to be closed on itself (thin white arrow). It is however evident that these apparently closed linear structures cannot represent flattened lipid vesicles [cf. "lamellar body discs" (19)] as their thickness (measured as the center-to-center distance between the two apposed electron-dense lines) is less than 4 nm, whereas a flattened lipid bilayer vesicle would be composed of two apposed ~4-nm lipid bilayers yielding a total thickness of at least ~8 nm. The complex electron density pattern observed may, however, be compatible with a single and coherent bicontinuous lipid structure (Fig. 12C,D). Other interpretations, e.g., that of a reversed oil-continuous micellar lipid morphology [Q227-like, cf. (36)] are also possible.

In the first to third extracellular space of stratum corneum, loosely packed extended lipid bilayer-like structures are observed in remaining widened areas (Fig. 7A). Similar loosely arranged extended lamellae have been observed previously in conventional electron microscopy preparations (22,37). The loosely packed lipid bilayer-like structures are sometimes observed to be in possible continuity both with

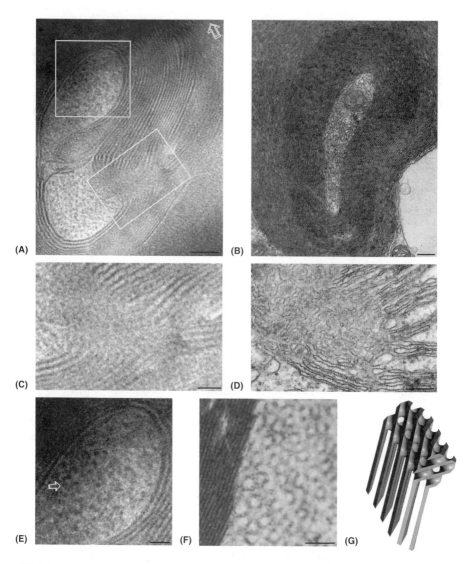

FIGURE 11 The electron density pattern of widened areas sometimes resembles cubic-to-lamellar membrane transitions. The overall shape of the cryo-electron density pattern of a widened area of the intercellular space between stratum granulosum and stratum corneum (**A**) is reminiscent of the overall shape of morphologically continuous cubic/lamellar membrane transitions of, e.g., myeloid bodies of retinal pigment epithelium of *Anguis fragilis*, as observed in conventional electron micrographs (**B**) [(29, p. 81), (32)] but with the difference that the scale differs about 10 times. In (**C**), which represents a magnification of the area marked by the *lower white box* in (**A**), the electron density pattern is reminiscent of the morphologically continuous cubic/lamellar membrane transitions in, e.g., the ER of spermatogenic cells of backswimmer (**D**) [(29, p. 79), (30)]. The lattice parameter of the central cubic membrane domain in (**D**) is ~100 to 200 nm, while the dimension of the central cubic-like membrane domain in (**C**) is roughly an order of magnitude smaller. Similarly, the electron density pattern in (**E**), which represents a magnification of the area marked by the *upper white box* in (**A**), is reminiscent (note, e.g., the sinusoidal electron density pattern marked by the *open white arrow* in **E**) of the cubic membrane domain (D^2-type) of the cubic/lamellar membrane transition in the ER of *(Continued)*

linker regions (Fig. 13A,C) and with ~44-nm-thick eight-line regions (Fig. 7B,C). No widened areas have been observed above the third stratum corneum extracellular space. Close packing of stacked lipid bilayers of widened areas may thus be at the origin of both linker (1-, 2-, 4-, and 6-line) and thick (8- and 10-line) regions of the mature (i.e., above the third) stratum corneum extracellular space (10).

Structure of the Stratum Corneum Extracellular Space as Observed by CEMOVIS

For a recent theoretical model on skin barrier structure and function, see (2,7).

Global Structure of the Stratum Corneum Extracellular Space

At low magnification, the extracellular space of fully differentiated stratum corneum (i.e., above the third cell layer) shows a seemingly identical morphology throughout the tissue (with the possible exception of the outermost desquamating cell layers; Fig. 6A). It is dominated by ~44-nm-thick regions (cf. Fig. 6B,C, open black arrows; Fig. 8; Table 1) interconnected by thinner linker regions (Fig. 6C,D, solid black arrows; Fig. 14A–H; Table 1). The ~44-nm-thick regions occupy the major portion of the extracellular space of both lower- (Fig. 6B, open black arrows) and mid-part (Fig. 6C, open black arrows) stratum corneum, often extending laterally over more than 1 μm (Fig. 6C, open black arrows). The measures of lateral extension may, however, be regarded with some reservation as close to perpendicular orientation of the extracellular space in the section is difficult to obtain over longer (μm) distances due to the undulated nature of the corneocyte surface. Linker regions are usually short (Fig. 6C,D, solid black arrows), but can extend laterally over more than 250 nm (Fig. 14A,C). Apparent dilatations of the extracellular space can be observed in many sections (Fig. 6A,C, black asterisk), both in lower and in mid-part stratum corneum. At high magnification, no internal structure has been observed in these dilatations (10).

Detailed Structure of the Stratum Corneum Extracellular Space

The ~44-nm-thick regions, dominating the stratum corneum extracellular space, contain eight electron-dense parallel lines with a characteristic pattern: a central electron-dense double-layer pattern paralleled on each side by three weaker electron-dense lines (inset box A in Fig. 8). The midline of the three weaker electron-dense lines is stronger than the two lines surrounding it. The outermost (as measured from the central electron-dense double-layer pattern) weak line runs adjacent to the outer electron-dense line of the two electron-dense lines forming the corneocyte plasma membrane (or "lipid envelope," which in turn separates the extracellular space from the diffuse electron-dense cornified envelope). All line spacings are shown in inset box A in

---

FIGURE 11   *(Continued)* conventionally resin-embedded UT-1 cells (**F**) (31). The cubic membrane of the UT-1 cells (**F**) has a lattice parameter of 245 nm [(29, p. 82)] while the dimension of the central cubic-like membrane domain in (**E**) is, again, about one order of magnitude smaller. (**G**) Schematic three-dimensional representation of 2×2×4 unit cells of a reversed (bilayer) bicontinuous membrane structure with balanced (central surface) diamond (D)-type cubic symmetry undergoing morphologically continuous lamellar "unfolding." *Open white double arrow* (**A**): section cutting direction. Section thickness ~50 nm (**A, C, E**). Scale bar (**A**) 50, (**B, D, F**) 200, and (**C, E**) 20 nm. *Abbreviation*: ER, endoplasmatic reticulum.

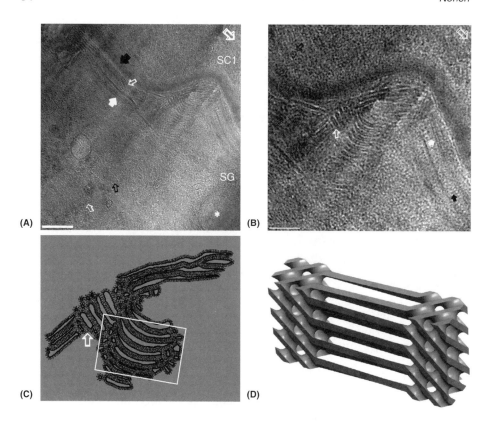

FIGURE 12   Disc-like pattern inconsistent with a stacked "lamellar body disk" morphology. (**A, B**) High magnification cryo-electron micrograph of the interface between stratum granulosum and stratum corneum of vitreous native epidermis (**B** represents an enlargement of the upper right part of **A**). (**C**) Two-dimensional interpretation of membrane-related optical density patterns of the stratum granulosum/stratum corneum intercellular space of (**B**). (**D**) Schematic three-dimensional interpretation of the area marked by a *white rectangle* in (**C**). In the vitreous cryo-fixed epidermis, the cellular, as well as intercellular, space appears densely packed with organic material (**A**). The intercellular space between stratum granulosum and stratum corneum contains lipid membrane material of highly variable appearance (**B**). Note that the "disc-like" electron-dense structure marked by an *open white arrow* in (**B**) has a thickness of ∼3.9 nm. This excludes an underlying flattened bilayer vesicle morphology [cf. "lamellar body disc" (19)]. The optical density pattern is, however, consistent with a *single and coherent* reversed lipid morphology (**C**) (cf. Figs. 5 and 17). Biological membranes with cubic-like symmetry represent reversed bicontinuous lipid morphologies (**D**). (**D**) Shows further schematically how a morphologically *continuous* cubic-to-lamellar membrane transition could proceed, via local expansion of the two subvolumes (or water-rich "tunnel systems") separated by a membrane surface with cubic (in this case D-type) symmetry, through lateral diffusion, or peripheral "alimentation", of highly dynamic liquid crystalline membrane lipids. Microtubule visible as dotted ring-like electron-dense structure in (**A**, lower left quadrant). *Solid white arrow* (**A**): "transition desmosome" cytoplasmic plaque; *solid white arrow* (**B**): emerging central electron-dense bilayer structure in "transition desmosome" "extracellular core domain"; *open white arrow* (**A**): multilamellar membrane structure stacked inside the "transition desmosome" extracellular "core domain"; *open white arrow* (**B, C**): "disc-like" electron density pattern; *solid black arrow* (**A**): newly formed protein "cell envelope"; *solid black arrow* (**B**): remnants of desmosome extracellular adhesion proteins in "transition desmosome" extracellular "core domain"; *open black arrow* (**A**): keratin intermediate filaments in viable keratinocyte cut approximately perpendicularly to their length axis; *open black arrow* (**B**): keratin intermediate filament in corneocyte with a central electron-dense dot, cut approximately   *(Continued)*

Figure 8. The line spacing of the two electron-dense lines forming the corneocyte "lipid envelope" is ~4.4 nm and the line spacing of the two electron-dense lines forming of the central double-layer pattern is ~4.3 nm. The first (weak) line of the extracellular space is situated at a distance of ~4.4 nm from the outer electron-dense line of the double-layer pattern forming the corneocyte lipid envelope. The second (medium electron dense) line of the stratum corneum extracellular space is situated at a median distance of ~6.3 nm from the first (weak) line and at a median distance of ~4.3 nm from the third (weak) line. The third (weak) line is situated at a median distance of ~4.2 nm from the adjacent line of the central electron-dense double-layer pattern (i.e., the fourth (strong) line of the extracellular space). The eight-line pattern of the ~44-nm-thick regions of the stratum corneum extracellular space thus closely resembles the eight-line pattern of the extracellular space of transition desmosomes (cf. inset box in Fig. 5C). In some stratum corneum eight-line regions, the total thickness of the extracellular space is smaller (38.7–40.0 nm, Table 1) than ~44 nm and the line spacings slightly different from the characteristic pattern (cf. Fig. 7C, white square bracket). Further, a minority of regions show a 10-line pattern with a thickness of the intercellular space of ~48.3 nm (inset box B in Fig. 8; Table 1) in which 4 (and not 3 as in the ~44-nm-thick regions) approximately equally spaced electron-dense lines are visible on each side of the central electron-dense double layer (thin white arrows) (10).

Four different types of linker regions have been observed, with a median thickness of the extracellular space of ~9.0, ~14.1, ~25.3, and ~33.1 nm, respectively (Table 1). The ~9-nm-thick linker regions contain one electron-dense line (Fig. 14E–G, thin white arrows), the ~14-nm-thick linker regions two lines (Fig. 14A,B, thin white arrows), the ~25-nm-thick linker regions four lines (Fig. 14C,D, thin white arrows), and the ~33-nm-thick linker regions six lines (Fig. 14H, thin black arrows; 7C, thin white arrows) with an approximately uniform line spacing of 4 to 5 nm. In addition to the smaller thickness of the extracellular space, the four- and six-line linker regions differ most typically from the dominating ~44-nm-thick eight-line regions in that all their lines are of approximately uniform electron density (10).

Comparison between Conventional Data and CEMOVIS Data with Respect to the Structure of Stratum Corneum Extracellular Space

Much model building for the structural organization of lipid matrix of the stratum corneum extracellular space has been based on a broad–narrow–broad electron lucent band pattern with a ~13 nm periodicity, as observed in conventional electron micrographs (38–40). Evidence for the presence of such a band pattern in native, hydrated stratum corneum is, however, lacking. No multilamellar ~13 nm

---

FIGURE 12 *(Continued)* perpendicularly to its axis; oblique *white arrow* (**A**): groups of diffuse electron-dense spots corresponding to the "polyribosome-like complex" observed in low and medium magnification cryo-transmission electron micrographs [cf. (8)]; *white asterisk* (**A**): optical density pattern corresponding to the new "organelle or branched tubular structure" reported in low and medium magnification cryo-transmission electron micrographs [cf. (8)], or alternatively, to the "lamellar body system," or "tubulo-reticular cisternal membrane system," reported in conventional resin-embedded samples [cf. (35)]; SG: stratum granulosum cell; SC1: first stratum corneum cell; *open white double arrow* (**A**, **B**): section cutting direction. Section thickness ~50 nm. Scale bar (**A**) 100 nm and (**B**) 50 nm.

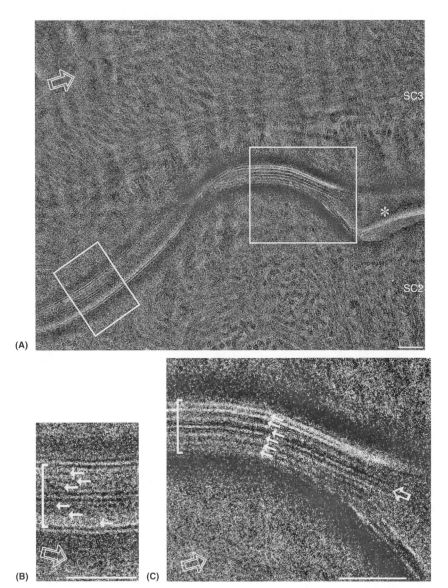

FIGURE 13 Loosely packed lipid bilayer-like structures are associated laterally to linker regions in addition to ~44-nm-thick regions. High magnification cryo-transmission electron micrograph of lower stratum corneum of vitreous epidermis (**A**). (**B**) Represents a magnification of the area marked by the *small left white box* in (**A**). (**C**) Represents a magnification of the area marked by the *large right white box* in (**A**). The loosely packed lipid bilayer-like patterns of a remaining widened area (**A**, *white asterisk*) seem to be in possible continuity (**C**, *open white arrow*) with parts of the six-line pattern (**C**, *thin white arrows*) of a ~33-nm-thick linker region (**C**, *white square bracket*). A ~44-nm-thick (**B**, *white square bracket*) eight-line (**B**, *thin white arrows*) region is seen adjacent to the six-line ~33-nm-thick linker region in (**A**). SC2-3 (**A**): second and third stratum corneum cell; *open white double arrows* (**A–C**): section cutting direction. Section thickness ~50 nm. Scale bar (**A–C**) 50 nm. *Source*: Adapted from Ref. 10.

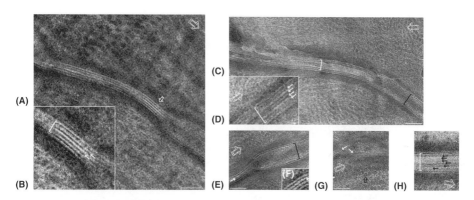

FIGURE 14 Linker regions express one, two, four, and six parallel electron-dense lines, respectively. High magnification cryo-transmission electron micrographs of vitreous mid-part stratum corneum (**A–H**). (**A, B**) Approximately 14-nm-thick (**B**, *white square bracket*) linker region containing two electron-dense lines (**B**, *thin white arrows*) between adjacent corneocyte lipid envelopes. (**B**) Represents a magnification of the area marked by an *open white arrow* in (**A**). (**C, D**) Approximately 25-nm-thick (*white brackets*) linker regions containing four lines (**D**, *thin white arrows*). In (**C**), the four-line linker region is associated with a ~44-nm-thick eight-line region (**C**, *black square bracket*). (**E–G**) Approximately 9-nm-thick linker regions containing one line (*thin white arrows*). Linker regions are particularly abundant in the cell periphery (**G**). In (**E**), the one-line linker region (*thin white arrow*) is associated with a ~44-nm-thick eight-line region (**E**, *black square bracket*). (**H**) Approximately 33-nm-thick (*white square bracket*) six-line (*thin black arrows*) linker region (cf. Fig. 13C). *Open black arrow* (**G**): individual keratin intermediate filaments cut perpendicularly. *Open white double arrows* (**A–H**): section cutting direction. Section thicknesses (**A–H**) ~50 nm. Scale bars (**A, C–E, G**) 50 nm. *Source*: Adapted from Ref. 10.

periodicity has been observed by CEMOVIS in cryo-preserved epidermis. This discrepancy may be due to morphological changes induced by fixation and/ or dehydration during conventional sample preparation for electron microscopy. However, as the optical density of conventional electron micrographs is directly related to the chemical ability to bind stain, whereas for cryo-electron micrographs of vitreous sections the optical density is directly related to the local density of biomaterial in the section, a direct comparison is not straightforward (10).

Small-angle X-ray diffraction on stratum corneum has shown 4.0 to 4.4, 5.8 to 6.6, and 12.9 to 13.6 nm reflections attributed to lipids (40–44). The direct linking of these results to the cryo-electron density patterns observed by CEMOVIS is difficult, as, except for the 4.0 to 4.4 nm periodicity, no periodic electron density pattern corresponding to the 5.8 to 6.6 and 12.9 to 13.6 nm reflections have been observed in the cryo-preserved stratum corneum. Again, stratum corneum dehydration during sample preparation for X-ray diffraction may partly explain these discrepancies (10).

Hypothetical Synthetic Model for the Formation of the Stratum Corneum Skin Barrier

Figure 15 presents a schematic view of the formation of the stratum corneum skin barrier as observed by CEMOVIS. The transformation starts in the upper part of viable epidermis where the extracellular space is constituted by desmosomes and their interspace. No fine structure has yet been resolved in the latter (10). A major change takes place in the extracellular space between viable and cornified

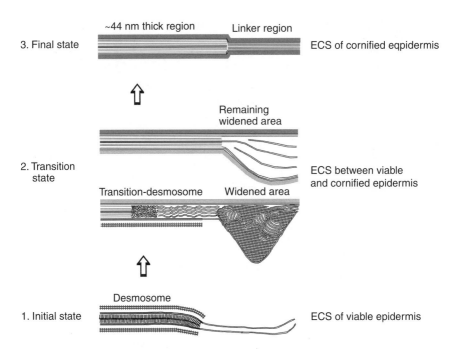

FIGURE 15 Schematic view of the transformation of the ECS during epidermal differentiation as observed by CEMOVIS. Initial state (1): The upper part of the viable epidermis is constituted by desmosomes and their interspace. Transition state (2): Desmosomes become transition desmosomes and the inter-desmosomal space becomes widened into a bag containing highly complex membrane-like material. In the first few layers of the cornified epidermis remaining widened areas contain loosely packed extended lipid bilayers, which subsequently are closepacked into multilamellar sheets. Final state (3): The mature corneocyte extracellular space is constituted by ~44-nm-thick eight-line regions interconnected by linker regions. The ~44-nm-thick regions may mainly be derived from transition desmosomes and possibly indirectly from widened areas. The linker regions may mainly be derived from widened areas. *Abbreviation*: ECS, extracellular space. *Source*: Adapted from Ref. 10.

epidermis. Here desmosomes become transition desmosomes, and the inter-desmosomal space becomes widened into a bag containing highly complex membrane-like material. Our CEMOVIS data do not support the view that this material represents stacks of flattened lipid bilayer vesicles [cf. (19)]. In contrast, all CEMOVIS observations made so far seem to fit with a membrane folding process involving cubic-like to lamellar lipid bilayer membrane transitions (Fig. 16) [cf. (18)].

The transformation continues in the first few layers of the cornified epidermis and ends with the formation of ~44-nm-thick eight-line regions, derived from transition desmosomes, interconnected by 1-, 2-, 4-, 6-line linker regions and 8-, 10-line regions, derived from lamellar close packing in remaining widened areas of 2, 3, 5, 7, 9, and 11 lipid bilayers, respectively (10). It is noteworthy that the desmosome transformation process seems morphologically continuous. Viable desmosomes do not simply become replaced by ~44-nm-thick regions. Instead, transition desmosomes keep many resemblances with their parent desmosomes.

Similarly, the final ~44-nm-thick regions are closely reminiscent of transition desmosomes. It is fair to say, however, that the close relationship between desmosomes and ~44-nm-thick regions is difficult to recognize without a detailed view of the complex nanostructure of transition desmosomes. Speculatively, the eight-line band pattern of the ~44-nm-thick regions may be related to the recently proposed arrangement of cadherin ectodomains of the desmosome extracellular core domain (45). The central double-layer pattern in Figure 10A and inset box in Figure 4C would then relate to the limit of desmosome EC1 ectodomains binding the cadherin molecules from both sides whereas the three bands on each side would relate to the limit between desmosome ectodomains EC2/3, EC3/4, and EC4/5, respectively. This observation could point to a new function of cadherin involving direct interactions between lipid and protein domains (10).

Structure of the Stratum Corneum Cellular Space

A recent theoretical model and detailed structural description of stratum corneum keratin organization and formation are available (14). The stratum corneum protein matrix, i.e., the corneocyte cellular space that is filled with a dense network of keratin intermediate filaments, represents a protective scaffold for the extracellular lipid matrix. The extraordinary rigidity of keratin thus allows for maintenance of the dimensions of the stratum corneum cellular, and thereby also the extracellular, space, unaffected by external (i.e., mechanical) as well as internal (i.e., osmotic) stress. This may in turn be vital, as the continuity of the "crystalline" (or gel) extracellular lipid matrix constituting the skin barrier (2,7,18,41,45) may not, under stress conditions, be preserved otherwise (14).

At high magnification (Fig. 17), corneocyte keratin intermediate filaments appear in vitreous epidermal sections as ~8 nm (measured as $2 \times$ peripheral to central subfilament center-to-center distance in a direction perpendicular to the section cutting direction) wide electron-dense structures with a median filament center-to-center distance of ~16 nm embedded in a comparatively electron lucent matrix (Fig. 17A,B). In perpendicular section planes, the electron density pattern corresponding to the subfilamentous intermediate filament architecture consists of one axial subfilament surrounded by an undetermined number of peripheral subfilaments, occasionally being reminiscent of a quasi-hexagonal arrangement of groups of ~6 electron dense ~1 nm spots surrounding a central electron dense ~1 nm spot (Fig. 17A,B, inset box in B). In fact, at closer inspection, the axial sub-filament structure could occasionally be distinguished in classical resin-embedded sections (Fig. 17C,D). Here the corneocyte keratin intermediate filaments appear as ~9-nm-wide electron lucent spots embedded in an electron-dense matrix (Fig. 17C). However, as no subfilamentous optical density pattern can unambi-guously be distinguished in resin-embedded sections and as the optical density of the recorded image here is not directly related to the local density of the biological material of the sample, as it is in vitreous sections, but to the local ability to bind stain, direct comparison of keratin intermediate filament diameter between chemically fixed and cryo-fixed samples is not straightforward. Nonetheless, in the dehydrated resin-embedded sample (Fig. 17C,D) the intermedi-ate filaments are clustered together with diminished interfilament distances when compared with the situation in the fully hydrated native sample (Fig. 17A,B) (14).

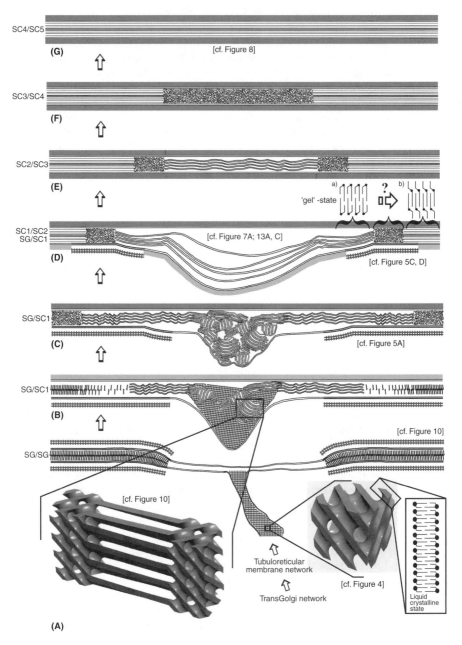

FIGURE 16 Tentative synthetic model for the formation of the skin barrier. It is proposed that the skin barrier formation process may be viewed as a lamellar "unfolding" of a small lattice parameter lipid "phase" with cubic-like symmetry (**A–C**) with subsequent "zipping" (i.e., "crystallization," or "condensation," including lamellar reorganization) of the intercellular lipid matrix (**D–F**). (**A**) Extrusion of a cubic lipid "phase" (i.e., membrane network with cubic-like symmetry with a lattice parameter of <30 nm) derived from the trans-Golgi network of the uppermost stratum granulosum cells (cf. Fig. 4). (**B, C**) Cubic-to-lamellar "phase" transition of the newly extruded cubic lipid "phase" in the *(Continued)*

EPIDERMAL TIGHT JUNCTIONS AND THE SKIN BARRIER

It was recently shown by freeze-fracture electron microscopy that stratum granulosum cells just beneath the stratum corneum seem connected laterally by a desmosome-interconnecting meshwork system of ridge structures, probably corresponding to tight junctions (46). In conventional transmission electron micrographs, tight junctions appear as plasma membrane contact sites referred to as "kissing points." Corresponding structures may also have been identified using CEMOVIS, but further studies are needed to confirm this. It has been claimed that claudin-based tight junctions are crucial for mammalian skin barrier function (47). How this tight junction-derived barrier function is mediated physically remains however unclear.

SKIN PERMEABILITY

It is generally believed that skin permeability is largely a function of the physical state and the structural organization of the stratum corneum intercellular lipid matrix [cf. (1,2)]. In this respect, two key issues are (*i*) whether water is present and (*ii*) whether liquid crystal forming lipids (normally medium chain, unsaturated lipids) are present, in the lipid matrix of the stratum corneum extracellular space (48).

In the mid-1970s Michaels et al. (49) launched the "brick and mortar model" characterizing the skin barrier as a two-compartment system with a discontinuous protein compartment embedded in a continuous lipid matrix. In an attempt to describe penetration through the skin, both compartments (protein and lipid) were, for simplicity reasons, treated as homogeneous and isotropic structures. Two possible penetration routes were sketched. One that required the alternate transit through protein and lipid domains, and one that regarded transit solely through the continuous lipid domain. In this second approach, the geometry of the protein and lipid elements would have large implications for the skin permeation rate of a specific substance, due to a considerable increase in permeation pathlength. It was concluded that compounds that are both water and oil soluble would generally display the highest diffusion rates (48).

A continuous multilamellar structure of alternating lipid and water regions most effectively hinders the diffusion of both polar and non-polar

---

FIGURE 16 *(Continued)* intercellular space between stratum granulosum and stratum corneum (cf. Fig. 12). Concomitant progressive reorganization of desmosome extracellular adhesion proteins and cytoplasmic desmosme plaques together with a widening of the desmosome extracellular core domain from ~30to ~43 nm (cf. Fig. 5) and the formation of the protein "cell envelope" beneath the cornocyte plasma membrane. (**D**) The newly "unfolded" (via the now completed cubic-to-lamellar "phase transition") loosely packed membrane bilayers of the intercellular space (cf. Figs. 7 and 13) have entered the "transition desmosome" extracellular "core domain" (cf. Fig. 5A, *open white arrow*), become close-packed and an internal lipid reorganization/"condensation"/"crystallization" has begun [cf. Fig. 5D ("1")-("3")]. Tentatively, this internal lipid reorganization may partly involve a flip-flop from hairpin-to-splayed chain conformation of a fraction of the stratum corneum ceramides (a, b). (**E**) Close-packing of newly "unfolded" loosely packed membrane bilayers of the intercellular space of lowermost stratum corneum (cf. Fig. 13A,C). (**F**) Final internal lamellar lipid reorganization/ "condensation"/"crystallization" of the intercellular lipid matrix (cf. **Da**, **Db**). (**G**) Mature "zipped" skin barrier lipid organization of the major part (i.e., ~43-nm wide regions) of the intercellular space of stratum corneum (cf. Fig. 8).

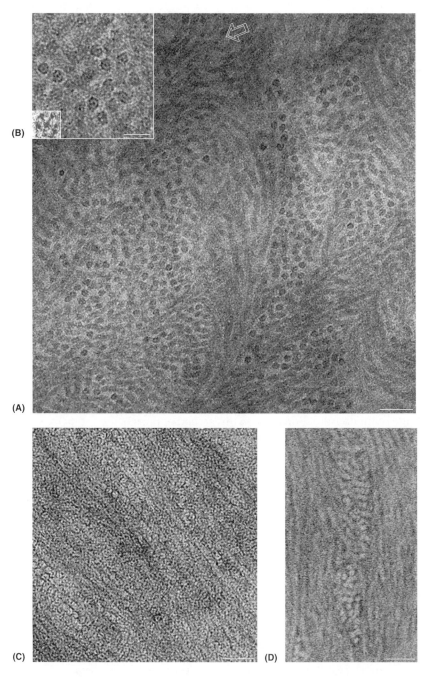

FIGURE 17 Cryo-electron microscopy reveals the native keratin intermediate filament organization at the nanometer level. High magnification electron micrographs of keratin intermediate filaments filling out the cell cytoplasm at the midportion of the cornified part of human epidermis. (**A,B**) Cryo-electron micrograph of vitreous section. (**C,D**) Conventional electron micrograph of resin-embedded section. The subfilamentous molecular architecture can only be guessed in (**C,D**), while in (**A,B**) it *(Continued)*

substances [4]. Thus, slow permeation rate through the stratum corneum extra-cellular lipid matrix for different compounds may primarily be a consequence of the partition of the substance between the aqueous and lipid compartment of the multilamellar regions, and to a much lesser degree to their molecular mobility within each compartment (50,51). The equation for the normal component ($D_\perp$) of the diffusion coefficient in a multilamellar lipid/water system is (4):

$$D_\perp = D_{aq}(d_{aq} + d_{lip})^2/(d_{aq} + Kd_{lip})(d_{aq} + d_{lip}(D_{aq}/KD_{lip})) \tag{1}$$

where D_{aq} and D_{lip} are the diffusion coefficients of a molecule in the aqueous and lipid regions, respectively, and d_{aq} and d_{lip} are the thicknesses of the aqueous and lipid regions. K is the bilayer/aqueous partition coefficient. If, for simplicity reasons, it is assumed that $D_{aq} \approx D_{lip} = D$, then:

$$D_\perp = D(d_{aq} + d_{lip})^2/(d_{aq} + Kd_{lip})(d_{aq} + K^{-1}d_{lip}) \tag{2}$$

where $D_\perp$ has its maximum for $K=1$. It is evident that $D_\perp$ is very low for $K \ll 1$ or $K \gg 1$. In fact, molecules such as dimethyl sulfoxide (DMSO) that is both water and oil soluble show very high penetration rates through the skin (4). These results underline the need for further studies to solve the longstanding question whether water is present or not in the stratum corneum extracellular space (48).

The permeability of a substance across a membrane depends not only on its partition coefficient, but also on the physical state of the bilayer. In addition, the gel-phase bilayer/aqueous partition coefficient for penetrating molecules is expected to be considerably lower than the corresponding liquid crystalline bilayer/aqueous partition coefficient (52). Since there is a large gradient in water chemical potential over the skin it is reasonable to assume that transdermal solute and water flux not only is a function of the solute/membrane interaction and the physical state of the bilayer, but also of structural changes along the transmembrane water gradient (51). Consequently, the diffusional transport across the stratum corneum is expected to be nonlinear. In addition, other gradients (e.g., of small solutes or amphiphilic molecules) could exert an influence on the phase behavior of the intercellular multilamellar lipid matrix of the skin barrier (48).

In the early 1990s, evidence was accumulating that the intercellular lipid matrix may exhibit phase separation at physiological skin temperature (53,54). At the same time, Forslind formulated the "domain mosaic model" for the skin barrier, where the intercellular lipid matrix was treated as a multilamellar two-phase system with a discontinuous lamellar crystalline structure embedded in a continuous liquid crystalline structure (1). To support this model, the heterogeneity of the lipid population constituting the intercellular lipid matrix, the predominantly crystalline character of the intercellular lipid matrix of stratum corneum in vitro, and the

---

FIGURE 17 *(Continued)* appears as groups of peripheral electron-dense spots surrounding a central dense dot (**A,B**, inset box in **B**). In (**A,B**) keratin intermediate filaments appear as ~7.8-nm wide (2×center-to-center distance between peripheral and central electron-dense dots in a direction perpendicular to the section cutting direction) structures with a center-to-center distance of ~16 nm, embedded in a comparatively electron lucent matrix. In the dehydrated embedded samples (**C,D**) the intermediate filaments are clustered together, with consequent diminished interfilament distances. *Open white double arrow* (**A**): section cutting direction. Section thicknesses ~50 nm (**A,B**). Scale bars 50 nm (**A,C,D**), 20 nm (**B**), 10 nm (side-length inset box in **B**). Figure (**D**) adapted from Brody (1960). *Source:* Adapted from Ref. 14.

proposed stacked bilayer nature of the "lamellar bodies" involved in skin barrier formation were invoked. If (*i*) the crystalline areas are regarded as effectively impermeable and the liquid crystalline areas as permeable to diffusing substances and (*ii*) the water primarily is located to the liquid crystalline zones [lipid liquid crystals swell more readily than lipid crystals (13)], then the diffusion of both hydrophilic and hydrophobic compounds would be allocated to the liquid crystalline structure. Consequently, penetrating molecules would perform a one-dimensional "random walk" in the "channels" of liquid crystalline structure separating two crystalline domains. The only way of going up one step to the next layer would then be when two "channels" cross. The diffusing molecules would thus have to follow a highly tortuous pathway on their journey along the concentration gradient through the skin (55).

The presence of liquid crystalline structures could allow formation of structures other than flat bilayers (L_α), such as oil-continuous or bicontinuous morphologies (e.g., H_{II}, L_2, or V_2) [cf. (13)] locally or more generally over the liquid crystalline "grain borders." If bicontinuous structures are present in the intercellular space of stratum corneum, a direct penetration pathway for both hydrophilic and lipophilic substances is present normal to the skin surface. For substances with a bilayer/aqueous partition coefficient (K) equal to one (i.e., the permeating substance prefers neither the bilayer nor the water domain), the presence of a bicontinuous structure would not affect the penetration rate through the skin. However, for $K \ll 1$ or $K \gg 1$, the skin permeability of a substance may be enhanced more than two orders of magnitude even when relatively low fractions (<10%) of the intercellular lipid bilayers have undergone transition into a bicontinuous structure (50). Thus, more studies focusing on the question of whether or not liquid crystal forming lipids are present in the stratum corneum extracellular space are welcomed (48).

SKIN BARRIER LIPID COMPOSITION

The outcome of biophysical computer simulation experiments and in vitro experiments using mixtures of synthetic or extracted skin lipids as skin barrier models ultimately depend on the chosen lipid composition. For such experiments, it is a prerequisite to have access to accurate and precise (within a few molar percent) compositional skin lipid data.

Contaminants in Skin Lipid Analysis Experiments

Many published accounts of the composition of lipids from human stratum corneum have been complicated by the presence of sebaceous lipids as well as exogenous contaminants (56–58). When stratum corneum samples are obtained from excised skin, there is almost always massive contamination with triglycerides from subcutaneous fat. In addition, fatty acids are derived from the subcutaneous triglycerides through the action of lipases on the skin surface. The human skin surface is also generally coated with sebaceous lipids (59). This is a major source of squalene, wax esters, and triglycerides, and again the triglycerides undergo hydrolysis to yield fatty acids. The sebaceous fatty acids are mostly 16 and 18 carbons in length and contain high proportions of monounsaturated species and variable proportions of branched chains. This is in contrast to the stratum corneum fatty acids, which are mostly longer than 20 carbons, saturated and straight chained. The omnipresence of medium chain free fatty acid contamination is exemplified by the measured extreme experimental and interindividual variation in the human forearm stratum corneum medium chain free fatty acid fraction (<20 C) as compared to the long chain free fatty acid fraction (≥20 C) (60). The medium chain free fatty acid fraction was shown to be dominated by C16:0, C16:1, C18:0, C18:1 and was invariably present in the blank of each of the 22 subjects analyzed (while no long chain free fatty acids were present in any of the 22 blanks). The extremely large interindividual variation and the almost complete absence (<1 mol%) in 3 out of the 22 subjects of unsaturated medium chain free fatty acids strongly speaks in favor of the notion that the medium chain free fatty acid fraction is mainly of extra-endogenous origin (60). Reports claiming the presence in the lower stratum corneum of significant amounts of unsaturated medium chain free fatty acids may therefore be viewed with some reservation (56).

The "True" Lipid Composition of the Stratum Corneum Extracellular Space

In a paper by Wertz et al. (57), the lipid composition of epidermal cysts, containing by comparison enormous amounts of stratum corneum lipids, thereby limiting to a minimum the effect of contamination, was analyzed. A result very close to that of Wertz et al. (57) was obtained using quantitative high-performance liquid chromatography/light scattering detector on lipids extracted from the forearm of 22 healthy subjects after 15 tape strippings to remove two-third of the stratum corneum thickness (61). Largely based on these results it was recently proposed that the population mean total (non-polar + polar fraction) lipid composition (in wt%) (covalently bound lipids of human stratum corneum not included; wt% of total ceramide fraction given between square brackets for the individual ceramide subfractions) can be found within the following "confidence intervals" (56).

Non-Polar Fraction

Alkanes	[0–0]
Squalene	[0–0]
Wax esters	[0–0]
Cholesteryl esters	[0–20]
Triacylglycerols	[0–0]
Unsaturated FFA	[0–?]
Saturated FFA	[7–13]
Cholesterol	[20–33]
Total ceramides	[40–50]
N-(triacontanoyl-ω-*O*-linoleyl)-sphingosine (EOS, Ceramide 1)	[6–12]
N-(stearoyl)-sphingosine (NS, Ceramide 2)	[12–25]
N-(stearoyl)-4-hydroxysphinganine (NP, Ceramide 3)	[11–34]
N-(triacontanoyl-ω-*O*-linoleyl)-6-hydroxysphingosine (EO, Ceramide 4)	[4–9]
N-(2-hydroxystearoyl)-sphingosine (AS, Ceramide 5) + *N*-(stearoyl)-6-hydroxysphingosine (NH)	[17–27]
N-(2-hydroxystearoyl)-4-hydroxysphinganine (AP, Ceramide 6)	[4–11]
N-(2-hydroxystearoyl)-6-hydroxysphingosine (AH, Ceramide 7)	[10–27]

Polar Fraction

Total cerebrosides	[0–1]
Total phospholipids	[0–0]
Cholesterol sulfate	[0–7]

Skin Barrier Ceramide Composition

Until recently, skin ceramide analysis relied on gas chromatography/mass spectrometry, necessitating ceramide hydrolysis, derivatization, and subsequent separate analysis of the resulting sphingoid bases and fatty acids, with consequent increased risks for lipid contamination. The introduction of electrospray ionization mass spectrometry (ESI-MS) in the late 1980s allowed for direct detection of stratum corneum ceramide species, thereby avoiding most contamination sources. ESI-MS analysis has shown that ω-esterified human skin ceramides (EOS, EOP, and EOH) contain amide bound fatty acids with chain lengths between 28 and 36 carbons peaking at 32 and 34 carbons, and that remaining ceramides (NS, NdS, NP, NH, AS, AP, and AH) have chain lengths between 20 and 36 carbons peaking at 26 and 28 carbons (62,63). The only ceramide species with reported medium chain lengths (C15–C18) is ceramide AS (63). However, this conflicts with the results of Vietzke et al. (62) who reported chain lengths between C22 and C36 for ceramide AS. Further studies are needed to resolve this discrepancy, which could have important consequences for the structural organization of the stratum corneum extracellular lipid matrix and thus for skin barrier function.

REFERENCES

1. Forslind B. A domain mosaic model of the skin barrier. Acta Derm Venereol (Stockh) 1994; 74:1–6.
2. Norlén L. Skin barrier structure and function: the single gel-phase model. J Invest Dermatol 2001; 117:830–6.
3. Guldbrand L, Jönsson B, Wennerström H. Hydration forces and phase equilibria in the dipalmitoyl phosphatidylcholine–water system. J Colloid Interface Sci 1982; 89:532–41.
4. Evans FD, Wennerström H. The Colloidal Domain: Where Physics, Chemistry, Biology and Technology Meet. New York: VCH Publishers, 1994.
5. Sparr E, Wennerström H. Diffusion through a lamellar liquid crystal: a model of molecular transport across stratum corneum. Colloids Surf B Biointerfaces 2000; 19: 103–16.
6. Peacocke AR. An Introduction to the Physical Chemistry of Biological Organization. New York: Oxford University Press, 1983:1–72.
7. Norlén L. Does the single gel-phase exist in stratum corneum? Reply J Invest Dermatol 2002; 118:899–901.
8. Norlén L, Al-Amoudi A, Dubochet J. A cryo-transmission electron microscopy study of skin barrier formation. J Invest Dermatol 2003; 120:555–60.
9. Masich S, Ostberg T, Norlen L, et al. A procedure to deposit fiducial markers on vitreous cryo-sections for cellular tomography. J Struct Biol 2006; 156:461–8.
10. Al-Amoudi A, Dubochet J, Norlén L. Nanostructure of the epidermal extracellular space as observed by cryo-electron microscopy of vitreous sections of human skin. J Invest Dermatol 2005; 124:764–77.
11. Small DM. The Physical Chemistry of Lipids. Handbook of Lipid Research. New York: Plenum Press, 1986.
12. Israelachvili JN. Intermolecular and Surface Forces. 2nd ed. San Diego: Academic Press, 1992.
13. Larsson K. Lipids: Molecular Organisation, Physical Functions and Technical Applications. Dundee, Scotland: The Oily Press, 1994.
14. Norlén L, Al-Amoudi A. Stratum corneum keratin structure, function, and formation: the cubic rod-packing and membrane templating model. J Invest Dermatol 2004; 123:715–32.
15. Dubochet J, Adrian M, Chang J-J, et al. Cryo-electron microscopy of vitrified specimens. Q Rev Biophys 1988; 21:129–228.
16. Al-Amoudi A, Chang J-J, Leforestier A, et al. Cryo-electron microscopy of vitreous sections. EMBO J 2004; 1523(18):3583–8.

17. Brody I. Ultrastructure of the stratum corneum. Int J Dermatol 1977; 16:245–56.
18. Norlén L. Skin barrier formation: the membrane folding model. J Invest Dermatol 2001; 117:823–9.
19. Landmann L. Epidermal permeability barrier: transformation of lamellar granule-disks into intercellular sheets by a membrane-fusion process, a freeze-fracture study. J Invest Dermatol 1986; 87:202–9.
20. Spicer PT, Hayden KL, Lynch ML, et al. Novel process for producing cubic liquid crystalline nanoparticles (cubosomes). Langmuir 2001; 17:5748–56.
21. Rawlings A. Stratum corneum moisturization at the molecular level: an update in relation to the dry skin cycle. J Invest Dermatol 2005; 124:1099–110.
22. Fartasch M, Bassukas ID, Diepgen T. Structural relationship between epidermal lipid lamellae, lamellar bodies and desmosomes in human epidermis: an ultrastructural study. Br J Dermatol 1993; 128:1–9.
23. Lundström A, Egelrud T. Cell shedding from human plantar skin in vitro: evidence on its dependence on endogenous proteolysis. J Invest Dermatol 1988; 91:340–3.
24. Skerrow CJ, Clelland DG, Skerrow D. Change to desmosomal antigens and lecithin-binding sites during differentiation in normal human epidermis: a quantitative study. J Cell Sci 1989; 92:667–77.
25. Chapman SJ, Walsh A. Desmosomes, corneosomes and desquamation. An ultrastructural study of adult pig epidermis. Arch Dermatol Res 1990; 282:304–10.
26. Mils V, Vincent C, Croute F, et al. The expression of desmosomal and corneodesmosomal antigens shows specific variations during terminal differentiation of epidermis and hair follicle epithelia. J Histochem Cytochem 1992; 40:1329–37.
27. Haftek M, Teillon M-H, Schmitt D. Stratum corneum, corneodesmosomes and ex-vivo percutaneous penetration. Microsc Res Tech 1998; 43:242–9.
28. Pfeiffer S, Vielhaber G, Vietzke J-P, et al. High-pressure freezing provides new information on human epidermis: simultaneous protein antigen and lamellar lipid structure preservation. Study on human epidermis by cryoimmobilization. J Invest Dermatol 2000; 114:1030–8.
29. Landh T. Cubic cell membrane architectures—taking another look at membrane bound cell spaces. Thesis, Department of Food Technology, Lund University, Sweden, 1996.
30. Tandler B, Moribier LG. Ultrastructure of pseudochromosomes and calottes in spermatogenic cells of the backswimmer. Notonecta undulata (Say). Tissue Cell 1974; 6:557–72.
31. Pathak RK, Luskey KL, Anderson RGW. Biogenesis of the crystalloid endoplasmic reticulum in UT-1 cells: evidence that the newly formed endoplasmatic reticulum emerges from the nuclear envelope. J Cell Biol 1986; 102:2158–68.
32. Ahn JNH. Les corps myéloïdes de l'épithelium pigmentaire rétinien. I Répartition, morphologie et rapports avec les organites cellulaires. Z Zellforsch 1971; 115:508–23.
33. Hayward AF. Ultrastructural changes in contents of membrane-coating granules after extrusion from epithelial cells of hamster cheek pouch. Cell Tissue Res 1978; 187:323–31.
34. Swartzendruber DC, Manganaro A, Madison KC, et al. Organization of the intercellular spaces of porcine epidermal and palatal stratum corneum: a quantitative study employing ruthenium tetroxide. Cell Tissue Res 1995; 279:271–6.
35. Elias PM, Cullander C, Mauro T, et al. The secretory granular cell: the outermost granular cell as a specialized secretory cell. J Invest Dermatol Symp Proc 1998; 3(2): 87–100.
36. Luzzati V. Biological significance of lipid polymorphism: the cubic phases. Curr Opin Struct Biol 1997; 7:661–8.
37. Menon GK, Feingold KR, Elias P. Lamellar body secretory response to barrier disruption. J Invest Dermatol 1992; 98:279–89.
38. Madison KC, Swartzendruber DC, Wertz PW, et al. Presence of intact intercellular lamellae in the upper layers of the stratum corneum. J Invest Dermatol 1987; 88:714–8.
39. Swartzendruber DC, Wertz PW, Kitko DJ, et al. Molecular models of the intercellular lipid lamellae in mammalian stratum corneum. J Invest Dermatol 1989; 92:251–7.
40. Hou SYE, Mitra AK, White SH, et al. Membrane structures in normal and essential fatty acid-deficient stratum corneum: characterization by ruthenium tetroxide staining and X-ray diffraction. J Invest Dermatol 1991; 96:215–23.

41. Garson J-C, Doucet J, Lévêque J-L, et al. Oriented structure in human stratum corneum revealed by x-ray diffraction. J Invest Dermatol 1991; 96:43–9.
42. Bouwstra JA, Gooris GS, Van der Spek JA, et al. Structural investigations of human stratum corneum by small-angle x-ray scattering. J Invest Dermatol 1991; 97:1005–12.
43. Schreiner V, Gooris GS, Pfeiffer S, et al. Barrier characteristics of different human skin types investigated with X-ray diffraction, lipid analysis, and electron microscopy imaging. J Invest Dermatol 2000; 114:654–60.
44. Ohta N, Ban S, Tanaka H, et al. Swelling of the intercellular lipid lamellar structure with short repeat in hairless mouse stratum corneum as studied by X-ray diffraction. Chem Phys Lipids 2003; 123:1–8.
45. Garrod DR, Merritt AJ, Nie Z. Desmosomal cadherins. Curr Opin Cell Biol 2002; 14:537–45.
46. Schlüter H, Wepf R, Moll I, et al. Sealing the live part of the skin: the integrated meshwork of desmosomes, tight junctions and curvilinear ridge structures in the cells of the uppermost granular layer of the human epidermis. Eur J Cell Biol 2004; 83:655–65.
47. Furuse M, Hata M, Furuse K, et al. Claudin-based tight-junctions are crucial for the mammalian epidermal barrier: a lesson from claudin-1-deficient mice. J Cell Biol 2002; 156:1099–111.
48. Norlén L. Molecular skin barrier models and some central problems for the understanding of skin barrier structure and function. Skin Pharm Appl Physiol 2003; 16:203–11.
49. Michaels AS, Chandrasekaran SK, Shaw JE. Drug permeation through human skin: theory and in vitro experimental measurements. AICHE J 1975; 21:985–96.
50. Engström S, Forslind B, Engblom J. Lipid polymorphism—a key to the understanding of skin penetration. In: Brain KR, James VJ, Walters KA, eds. Prediction of Percutaneous Penetration. Vol. 4b. Cardiff: STS Publishing, 1995:163–6.
51. Sparr. Responding model membranes—lipid phase behaviour, domain formation and permeability. Thesis, Department of Physical Chemistry I, Lund University, Sweden 2001.
52. Mesquita R, Melo E, Thompson TE, et al. Partitioning of amphiphiles between coexisting ordered and disordered phases in two-phase lipid bilayer membranes. Biophys J 2000; 78:3019–25.
53. Kitson N, Thewalt J, Lafleur M, et al. A model membrane approach to the epidermal permeability barrier. Biochemistry 1994; 33:6707–15.
54. Ongpipattanakul B, Francoeur ML, Potts RO. Polymorphism in stratum corneum lipids. Biochim Biophys Acta 1994; 1990:115–22.
55. Forslind B, Engström S, Engblom J, et al. A novel approach to the understanding of human skin barrier function. J Dermatol Sci 1997; 14:115–25.
56. Wertz P, Norlén L. "Confidence intervals" for the "true" lipid composition of the human skin barrier. In: Forslind B, Lindberg M, eds. Skin, Hair and Nails—Structure and Function. New York: Marcel Dekker, 2003:85–106.
57. Wertz PW, Swartzendruber DC, Madison KC, et al. Composition and morphology of epidermal cyst lipids. J Invest Dermatol 1987; 89:419–24.
58. Bortz JT, Wertz PW, Downing DT. On the origin of alkanes found in human skin surface lipids. J Invest Dermatol 1989; 93:723–7.
59. Wertz PW, Michniak BB. Sebum. In: Elsner P, Maibach HI, eds. Cosmeceuticals. New York: Marcel Dekker, 2000:45–56.
60. Norlén L, Nicander I, Lundsjö A, et al. A new HPLC-based method for the quantitative analysis of inner stratum corneum lipids with special reference to the free fatty acid fraction. Arch Dermatol Res 1998; 290:508–16.
61. Norlén L, Nicander I, Lundh-Rozell B, et al. Inter and intra individual differences in human stratum corneum lipid content related to physical parameters of skin barrier function in-vivo. J Invest Dermatol 1999; 112:72–7.
62. Vietzke J-P, Brandt O, Abeck D, et al. Comparative investigation of human stratum corneum ceramides. Lipids 2001; 36:299–304.
63. Farwanah H, Wohlrab J, Neubert RHH, et al. Profiling of human stratum corneum ceramides by means of normal phase LC/APCI-MS. Anal Bioanal Chem 2005; 383:632–7.

4 Morphology of Epidermal Lipids

Jennifer R. Hill and Philip W. Wertz

Dows Institute, University of Iowa, Iowa City, Iowa, U.S.A.

HISTORICAL BACKGROUND OF SKIN MORPHOLOGY

Light Microscopy

Histologic examination of skin reveals relatively cuboidal cells at the base of the epidermis (1). This is the replicative compartment and occasionally basal cells are seen in the process of cell division. However, most of the cells in the basal layer are quiescent and serve to anchor the epidermis onto the basal lamina, which is a specialized interface between the epidermis and the dermis. Several layers of cells immediately above the basal layer have a prickly or spiny appearance and are collectively called the spinous layer. This appearance reflects the shrinkage of cell bodies away from the many desmosomal plaques in these suprabasal layers. Above the spinous cells are several layers of cells that contain dark granular material. The grainy material is composed of several protein components, which make up the keratohyalin granules. In the uppermost cells within this compartment there are no nuclei.

The outermost portion of the epidermis is the stratum corneum. This consists of extremely flat keratin-filled cells embedded in a lipid matrix. In frozen sections, the stratum corneum is very compact, and individual cells cannot be discerned. However, after alkali expansion, individual cells can be seen and are often arranged in very orderly stacks (2). In more routine paraffin-embedded sections, the cells of the stratum corneum separate into a basket weave pattern that is considered normal by dermatopathologists (1). A compact stratum corneum in a paraffin-embedded section would be considered pathologic. When viewed *en face* after silver staining, the corneocytes have a very geometric shape (3). Most are hexagonal with only a narrow overlap at the edges of adjacent corneocytes.

Transmission Electron Microscopy

With the advent of transmission electron microscopy (TEM), much more detail about the structures of the membranous organelles of the epidermis became available. The viable cells of the epidermis contain all of the usual organelles including mitochondria, endoplasmic reticulum, and Golgi apparatus. One organelle, unique to keratinizing epithelia, was originally mistaken for a shrunken and degenerating mitochondrion (4). However, George Odland subsequently recognized that this was a unique organelle (5). This organelle has been given many names in the literature including membrane coating granule, Odland body, lamellar body, cementsome, and lamellar granule. Lamellar granules are generally round to ovoid in shape and contain one, or sometimes several, internal stacks of lamellae. They are approximately 200 nm in diameter (6). An array of lamellar granules is shown in Figure 1.

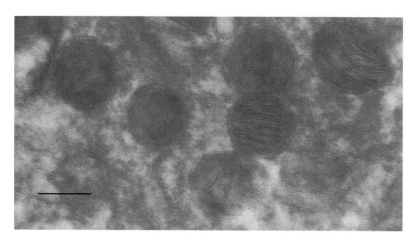

FIGURE 1 Lamellar granules in the upper portion of the epidermal granular layer. The bar equals 200 nm.

Based on TEM images, it was proposed that the lamellar granules arose from the Golgi (7). Several groups have subsequently isolated lamellar granules by exploiting either their low buoyant density or their fairly unique size (8–13). Consistent with their being derived from the Golgi, the isolated lamellar granules were shown to be rich in glucosylceramides, ceramide galactosyltransferase, and ceramide glucosyltransferase, which are considered to be biochemical markers for the Golgi (13).

The most abundant of the glucosylceramides associated with the epidermal lamellar granules is a structurally unusual acylglucosylceramide consisting of 30- through 34-carbon chain ω-hydroxyacids amide-linked to sphingosine with linoleate ester-linked to the ω-hydroxyl group and glucose β-glycosidically linked to the primary hydroxyl group of the long-chain base (Fig. 2) (14–16). It has been argued that the acylglucosylceramide is essential for the formation of the lamellar granules (17). It has been estimated that about two-thirds of the lamellar granule-associated acylglucosylceramide is in the bounding membrane, and this pool of acylglucosylceramide is the precursor for the covalently bound ω-hydroxyceramide at the surface of the cornified envelope (18–20). The remaining one-third is associated with the internal lamellae, and this is the precursor of the acylceramide found in the stratum corneum. The significance of the covalently bound hydroxyceramide is still under investigation, although there is evidence that it is important for normal barrier function as well as for cell cohesion and desquamation (21,22). It is more generally accepted that the linoleate-containing acylceramide is essential for physical organization of the lipids in the intercellular spaces of the stratum corneum, and thereby the barrier function of the skin (20,23–25). In essential fatty acid deficiency, oleate replaces linoleate in the acylglucosylceramide (26,27). This still supports the formation of lamellar granules and delivery of lipid to the intercellular space; however, the oleate-containing acylceramide does not provide for proper barrier function. Likewise, in the keratinizing oral epithelium from the hard palate, saturated fatty acids replace linoleate in

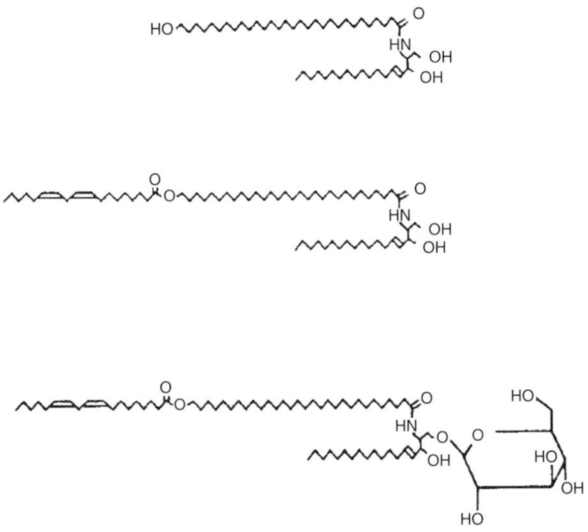

FIGURE 2 Representative structures of ω-hydroxyacid-containing epidermal sphingolipids. These include linoleate-rich acylglucosylceramides (*bottom*), analogous acylceramides (*middle*), and ω-hydroxyceramides (*top*).

the ω-hydroxysphingolipids (28). Lamellar granules form and deliver lipid to the intercellular space of the oral mucosa, but the barrier function is relatively poor (29).

In the uppermost granular cells, the lamellar granules migrate to the apical end of the cell, and the bounding membrane of the lamellar granule fuses with the cell plasma membrane (30–32). At this point, the linoleate is removed from the acylglucosylceramide that was in the bounding membrane and is recycled in the viable epidermis (33). Evidence indicates that the acylglucosylceramide in the bounding membrane of lamellar granules is oriented with the glucose moiety on the inside (34). The fusion event and removal of the linoleate would result in ω-hydroxyglucosylceramide with the ω-hydroxyl group adjacent to the nascent cornified envelope. The transglutaminase 1 that is involved in polymerizing proteins into the envelope has also been implicated in attaching the hydroxyceramide to the outer surface of the cornified envelope through formation of ester linkages to acidic side chains (35). Finally, the glucose is removed, and the cornified envelope has a covalently linked coat of ω-hydroxyceramide.

It is noteworthy that in the human, there are three acylglucosylceramides that differ in the long-chain base component. This can be sphingosine, phytosphingosine or 6-hydroxysphingosine. Accordingly, this gives rise to three different hydroxyceramides (19,36) and three acylceramides (37). The acylglucosylceramides that were associated with the internal lamellae of the lamellar granules are deglycosylated on passing into the stratum corneum to yield acylceramides.

The fact that intact lamellar granules could be isolated from frozen tissue (13) indicates that they have a low water content, and ice crystals cannot form. In fact, when viewed by TEM, lamellar granules are the only intact membranous organelle that can be identified in frozen epidermis. The low internal free water content may, in part, be related to the glucose moieties of the acylglucosylceramides on the inside of the bounding membrane, which could hydrogen bond with water molecules to prevent ice formation.

In addition to delivering a lipid mixture rich in phospholipids, glycolipids, and cholesterol to the interface between the stratum granulosum and the stratum corneum, the lamellar granules deliver a battery of hydrolytic enzymes to the intercellular space (9,11,13). Once in the intercellular space these hydrolases rapidly convert sphingomyelin and glucosylceramides to the corresponding ceramides. The phosphoglycerides are catabolized to release fatty acids, and oleate is transferred to cholesterol to make cholesterol esters (38). This lipid processing results in the ceramide–cholesterol–fatty acid mixture of the intercellular space of the stratum corneum. That lipid processing does not take place within the lamellar granules is at least partly due to the lack of free water. Spatial segregation may also be a significant factor. In this regard, caveolins capable of binding various hydrolases to a fixed membrane domain have been noted in isolated lamellar granules (13).

The intercellular spaces of the stratum corneum appear empty as judged by TEM using conventional osmium tetroxide fixation (30–32). Initially, this was thought to reflect lipid extraction during processing of specimens. However, with the introduction of the more reactive ruthenium tetroxide (39), the lamellae of the intercellular spaces could be visualized throughout the stratum corneum (Fig. 3). The lamellae appeared to consist of multiple trilaminar units with an overall thickness of 13 nm. This same periodicity is found by X-ray diffraction of stratum corneum or reconstituted stratum corneum lipids (24,40–42). In addition, the lucent band components of the trilaminar units appeared to alternate in thickness with a broad–narrow–broad pattern. At the ends of adjacent cells in the same layer of stratum corneum, a single trilamellar unit was most frequently observed (20,25).

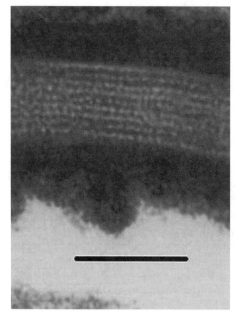

FIGURE 3 Intercellular lipid lamellae in epidermal stratum corneum. The bar equals 60 nm.

However, between the flat surfaces of adjacent cell layers, the number of trilamellar units was most frequently two or three and occasionally more (20,25).

Freeze fracture

The freeze fracture technique was first applied to skin in 1973 (43). This method revealed for the first time that the intercellular spaces of the stratum corneum do contain multiple lipid lamellae (30,31,43). In a series of studies employing largely the freeze fracture method, Lucas Landmann (6) deduced that the lamellae within the lamellar granules are approximated as stacks of flattened lipid vesicles. After extrusion into the intercellular space, the flattened vesicles align and fuse in an edge-to-edge manner to produce the multilamellar structures of the intercellular spaces of the stratum corneum.

cryo-TEM

Most recently, Lars Norlen and co workers have applied the cryo-TEM method to studies of epidermal structure (44,45). This method, like the freeze fracture technique, is less subject to artifacts than any chemical fixation method. The results are consistent with formation of 13 nm trilamellar structures; however, the component membranes would not alternate broad–narrow–broad in thickness, but would all be roughly 4.3 nm thick. There may be a greater number of lamellae across the intercellular space than seen with the ruthenium tetroxide method. Other aspects of epidermal structure revealed by cryo-TEM have been discussed (46).

BARRIER FUNCTION OF NORMAL HUMAN SKIN
Composition and Structure of the Barrier

The evolution of life on dry land required a water tight skin to prevent desiccation, and this requirement is met by the stratum corneum and the lipids contained therein (47). All mammalian species examined contain primarily ceramides, cholesterol, and fatty acids as the principal lipids of the stratum corneum. Although there is some variation in the structural types of ceramides, all species evaluated contained acylceramides, suggesting fundamental significance of this lipid in determining barrier function. This lipid is also found in the epidermis of birds.

There are currently two molecular models for the 13 nm trilaminar units that are formed by free stratum corneum lipids. In each of these models, the ω-hydroxyacyl chains of acylceramides are located in the outer two lamellae of the trilamellar units with the linoleates inserting into the central lamella. In the "sandwich model" of Bouwstra et al. (42), the linoleate tails of the acylceramides are inserted into the central lamella, and the lipids in this central lamella are interdigitated, so that the lamellar thicknesses are broad–narrow–broad. This arrangement is consistent in all of the X-ray diffraction data and is also supported by the impression of the trilaminar units from TEM using ruthenium tetroxide.

The second model is similar except that the lipids in the central lamella are not interdigitated, and all three lamellae are approximately 4.3 nm thick. This model was based on densitometric measurements of TEMs, and information of the reactivity of different lipids. Basically, it is thought that the linoleates in the central lamella will reduce more ruthenium than the mostly saturated chains in the outer lamellae. This additional reduced ruthenium accumulates beneath the planes of the polar head group regions associated with the central lamella. This results in thickening of the electron-dense boundaries of the central lamella and artifactual narrowing of the electron lucent part of this membrane. As noted above, cryo-TEM results support the presence of uniformly 4.3 nm thick lamellae. In addition, with keratinized epithelium from the hard palate, the acylceramide contains saturated fatty acids instead of linoleate, so it cannot reduce ruthenium. In this case only uniformly spaced lamellae are seen.

BARRIER FUNCTION IN DISEASE
Atopic Dermatitis
Atopic dermatitis is an inflammatory skin disease that usually has an onset early in life. It appears to be driven by a Th2 response to a combination of airborne antigens in combination with an endogenous epidermal component. This disease often resolves by early adulthood but, in some cases, it is a lifetime condition. Atopic dermatitis is often accompanied by food allergies and/or asthma. At any given time, the skin of an atopic individual may have uninvolved regions that are essentially normal in terms of stratum corneum lipids and barrier function. Involved regions appear rough and dry and display transepidermal water loss (TEWL) levels approximately twice that of normal skin (ca. 1.0 vs. 0.5 mg/cm^2 per hour). There are significant reductions in the ceramide content of involved versus uninvolved or normal stratum corneum. Most notably, there is a reduction in the amount of acylceramide in the involved stratum corneum. Inappropriate enzymatic deacylation of sphingomyelin and glucosylceramides is at least partly responsible for the decrease in ceramides. Lesional regions are erythematous, papulovesicular, and crusted. TEWL is very much elevated in these eczematous lesions because the barrier is physically breached. These lesions often become infected with *Staphylococcus aureus*.

The intercellular lamellae of the stratum corneum appear normal in specimens fixed with ruthenium tetroxide; however, it appears that the extrusion of lipid from the lamellar granules is aberrant, resulting in some retention of lamellar granule lipids within corneocytes (48,49).

Psoriasis
Psoriasis is a hyperproliferative epidermal scaling disease that affects approximately 1% of the population in the United States. It is thought to be mediated by a Th1 immune reaction directed against autoantigens. Motta et al. (50) have found that acylceramide and several other specific ceramide species are present in reduced amounts in psoriatic scale, and there was a roughly 50% reduction in free fatty acids.

Ultrastructurally, psoriatic scale contains numerous parakeratotic corneocytes that, in addition to nuclei or nuclear fragments, also contain lipid droplets (49). The extruded lamellar granule contents are not converted into the broad multiple lamellae until several layers into the stratum corneum, and the intercellular lamellae seem sparse and disordered (49,51).

Ichthyoses
The ichthyoses are a group of relatively rare disorders of keratinization which result in various degrees of skin scaliness. In ichthyosis vulgaris and recessive X-linked ichthyosis, TEWL is slightly but significantly elevated compared to normal, and in autosomal recessive ichthyosis TEWL is elevated 50% above normal (52). Altered

barrier function as indicated by elevated TEWL suggests some alteration of either lipid composition, distribution, or organization.

In the specific case of recessive X-linked ichthyosis, the enzyme sterol sulfatase is defective, and cholesterol sulfate accumulates to high levels in the stratum corneum and elsewhere (53). This is directly related to skin scaliness in that cholesterol sulfate inhibits serine proteases and thereby prevents normal desquamation. At an ultrastructural level, the retention of desmosomes into the superficial layers of the stratum corneum is a notable feature. The lamellar bodies, secretion of lamellar body contents, and formation and structure of intercellular lamellae all appear normal (49,54).

In Harlequin ichthyosis, there are essentially no lamellar granules or intercellular lamellae (55). A similar but less extreme defect in barrier formation has been described for congenital ichthyosiform erythroderma (56). In ichthyosis vulgaris, profillagrin is not synthesized and, accordingly, there are no normal keratohyalin granules (57).

Gaucher's disease

Gaucher's disease is an inherited disorder in which glucocerebrosidase is either absent or defective such that glucosylceramides cannot be deglycosylated. The most serious symptoms are neurologic; however, it has recently been recognized that the skin barrier is also defective. In this sphingolipidosis, the lamellar granule contents appear to be extruded normally, but the inability to convert the initially extruded glucosylceramide-rich lipid mixture into ceramides largely prevents maturation of the lipid system into the broad multilamellar sheets. The short stacks of lipid lamellae are found in the intercellular spaces, even in the outer layers of the stratum corneum (58).

REFERENCES

1. Holbrook KA, Wolff K. The structure and development of skin. In: Fitzpatrick TB, Eisen AZ, Wolff K et al, eds. Dermatology in General Medicine. 4th ed. New York: McGraw-Hill Inc., 1993:97–144.
2. Christophers E. Cellular architecture of the stratum corneum of mammalian skin. J Invest Dermatol 1971; 56:165–9.
3. Mackenzie IC. An examination of cellular organization within the stratum corneum by a silver staining method. J Invest Dermatol 1973; 61:245–50.
4. Selby CC. An electron microscope study of thin sections of human skin. J Invest Dermatol 1957; 29:131–49.
5. Odland GF. A submicroscopic granular component in human epidermis. J Invest Dermatol 1960; 34:11–5.
6. Landmann L. The epidermal permeability barrier. Anat Embryol 1988; 178:1–13.
7. Matoltsy AG, Parakkal PF. Membrane-coating granules of keratinizing epithelia. J Cell Biol 1965; 24:297–307.
8. Freinkel RK, Traczyk TN. A method for partial purification of lamellar granules from fetal rat epidermis. J Invest Dermatol 1981; 77:478–82.
9. Freinkel RK, Traczyk TN. Lipid composition and acid hydrolase content of lamellar granules of fetal rat epidermis. J Invest Dermatol 1985; 85:295–8.
10. Grayson S, Johnson-Winegar AD, Elias PM. Isolation of lamellar bodies from neonatal mouse epidermis by selective sequential filtration. Science 1983; 221:962–4.
11. Grayson S, Johnson-Winegar AG, Wintraub BU, et al. Lamellar body-enriched fractions from neonatal mice: preparative techniques and partial characterization. J Invest Dermatol 1985; 85:289–94.

12. Wertz PW, Downing DT, Freinkel RK, et al. Sphingolipids of the stratum corneum and lamellar granules of fetal rat epidermis. J Invest Dermatol 1984; 83:193–5.
13. Madison KC, Sando GN, Howard EJ, et al. Lamellar granule biogenesis: a role for ceramide glucosyltransferase, lysosomal enzyme transport, and the Golgi. J Investig Dermatol Symp Proc 1998; 3:80–6.
14. Gray GM, White RJ, Majer JR. 1(3'-Oacyl)-β-glucosyl-N-dihydroxypenta-triacontadie-noyl-sphingosine, a major component of the glucosylceramides of pig and human epidermis. Biochim Biophys Acta 1978; 528:127–37.
15. Wertz PW, Downing DT. Acylglucosylceramides of pig epidermis: structure determination. J Lipid Res 1983; 24:753–8.
16. Abraham W, Wertz PW, Downing DT. Linoleate-rich acylglucosylceramides from pig epidermis: structure determination by proton magnetic resonance. J Lipid Res 1985; 26:761–6.
17. Wertz PW, Downing DT. Glycolipids in mammalian epidermis: structure and function in the water barrier. Science 1982; 217:1261–2.
18. Swartzendruber DC, Wertz PW, Madison KC, et al. Evidence that the corneocyte has a chemically bound lipid envelope. J Invest Dermatol 1987; 88:709–13.
19. Wertz PW, Madison KC, Downing DT. Covalently bound lipids of human stratum corneum. J Invest Dermatol 1989; 91:109–11.
20. Wertz PW. Lipids and barrier function of the skin. Acta Derm Venereol 2000; 208:7–11.
21. Wertz PW, Swartzendruber DC, Kitko DJ, et al. The role of the corneocyte lipid envelopes in cohesion of the stratum corneum. J Invest Dermatol 1989; 93:169–72.
22. Elias PM, Fartasch M, Crumrine D, et al. Origin of the corneocyte lipid envelope (CLE): observations in harlequin ichthyosis and cultured human keratinocytes. J Invest Dermatol 2000; 115:765–9.
23. Wertz PW. Integral lipids of hair and stratum corneum. In: Jolles P, Zahn H, Hocker H, eds. Formation and Structure of Human Hair. Berlin: Birkhauser, 1997:227–38.
24. Bouwstra JA, Gooris GS, Dubbelaar FE, et al. Role of ceramide 1 in the molecular organization of the stratum corneum lipids. J Lipid Res 1998; 39:186–96.
25. Hill JR, Wertz PW. Molecular models of the intercellular lipid lamellae from epidermal stratum corneum. Biochim Biophys Acta 2003; 1616:121–6.
26. Wertz PW, Cho ES, Downing DT. Effects of essential fatty acid deficiency on the epidermal sphingolipids of the rat. Biochim Biophys Acta 1983; 753:350–5.
27. Melton JL, Wertz PW, Swartzendruber DC, et al. Effects of essential fatty acid deficiency on O-acylsphingolipids and transepidermal water loss in young pigs. Biochim Biophys Acta 1987; 921:191–7.
28. Hill JR, Wertz PW. Chemical structures of ceramides from palatal stratum corneum. J Dent Res 2005; 84A:1255.
29. Lesch CA, Squier CA, Cruchley A, et al. The permeability of human oral mucosa and skin to water. J Dent Res 1989; 68:1345.
30. Elias PM, Friend DS. The permeability barrier in mammalian epidermis. J Cell Biol 1975; 65:180–91.
31. Elias PM, McNutt NS, Friend DS. Membrane alterations during cornification of mammalian squamous epithelia: a freeze-fracture, tracer and thin-section study. Anat Rec 1977; 189:577–94.
32. Elias PM, Goerke J, Friend DS. Mammalian epidermal barrier layer lipids: composition and influence on structure. J Invest Dermatol 1977; 69:535–46.
33. Madison KC, Swartzendruber DC, Wertz PW, et al. Murine keratinocyte cultures grown at the air/medium interface synthesize stratum corneum lipids and "recycle" linoleate during differentiation. J Invest Dermatol 1989; 93:10–7.
34. Slater J, Hill JR, Wertz PW. Evidence indicating that the acylglucosylceramide in the bounding membrane of the lamellar granule is oriented with the glucosyl moiety on the inside. J Dent Res 2003; 82A:760.
35. Nemes Z, Steinert PM. Bricks and mortar of the epidermal barrier. Exp Mol Med 1999; 31:5–19.
36. Hill JR, Paslin D, Wertz PW. A new covalently bound ceramide from human stratum corneum—ω-hydroxyacylphytosphingosine. Int J Cosmet Sci 2006; 28:225–30.

37. Ponec M, Weerheim A, Lankhorst P, et al. New acylceramide in native and reconstructed epidermis. J Invest Dermatol 2003; 120:581–8.
38. Wertz PW, Swartzendruber DC, Madison KC, et al. The composition and morphology of epidermal cyst lipids. J Invest Dermatol 1987; 89:419–25.
39. Madison KC, Swartzendruber DC, Wertz PW, et al. Presence of intact intercellular lamellae in the upper layers of the stratum corneum. J Invest Dermatol 1987; 88:714–8.
40. Bouwstra JA, Gooris GS, van der Spek JA, et al. The lipid and protein structure of mouse stratum corneum: a wide and small angle diffraction study. Biochim Biophys Acta 1994; 1212:183–92.
41. Bouwstra JA, Gooris GS, Dubbelaar FE, et al. pH, cholesterol sulfate, and fatty acids affect the stratum corneum lipid organization. J Invest Dermatol Symp Proc 1998; 3:69–74.
42. Bouwstra JA, Gooris GS, Dubbelaar FE, et al. Phase behavior of lipid mixtures based on human ceramides: coexistence of crystalline and liquid phases. J Lipid Res 2001; 42:1759–70.
43. Breathnach AS, Goodman T, Stolinski C, et al. Freeze fracture replication of cells of stratum corneum of human epidermis. J Anat 1973; 114:65–81.
44. Norlen L. Skin barrier formation: the membrane folding model. J Invest Dermatol 2001; 117:823–9.
45. Norlen L. Skin barrier structure and function. J Invest Dermatol 2001; 117:830–6.
46. Norlen L, Al-Amoudi A. Stratum corneum keratin structure, function, and formation: the cubic rod-packing and membrane templating model. J Invest Dermatol 2004; 123:715–32.
47. Attenborough D. Life on Earth. Boston: Little, Brown and Company, 1980.
48. Fartasch M, Diepgen TL. The barrier function in atopic dry skin. Disturbance of membrane-coating granule exocytosis and formation of epidermal lipids? Acta Derm Venereol Suppl 1992; 176:26–31.
49. Fartasch M. Epidermal barrier in disorders of the skin. Microsc Res Tech 1997; 38:361–72.
50. Motta S, Monti M, Sesana S, et al. Ceramide composition of the psoriatic scale. Biochim Biophys Acta 1993; 1182:147–51.
51. Menon GK, Elias PM. Ultrastructural localization of calcium in psoriatic and normal human epidermis. Arch Dermatol 1991; 127:57–63.
52. Lavrijsen APM, Oestmann E, Hermans J, et al. Barrier function parameters in various keratinization disorders: transepidermal water loss and vascular response to hexyl nicotinate. Br J Dermatol 1993; 129:547–54.
53. Williams ML. Epidermal lipids and scaling diseases of the skin. Semin Dermatol 1992; 11:169–75.
54. Menon G, Ghadially R. Morphology of lipid alterations in the epidermis: a review. Microsc Res Tech 1997; 37:180–92.
55. Milner ME, O'Guin WM, Holbrook KA, et al. Abnormal lamellar granules in harlequin ichthyosis. J Invest Dermatol 1992; 99:824–9.
56. Ghadially R, Williams ML, Hou SY, et al. Membrane structural abnormalities in the stratum corneum of the autosomal recessive ichthyoses. J Invest Dermatol 1992; 99:755–63.
57. Fartasch M, Haneke E, Anton-Lamprecht I. Ultrastructural study of the occurrence of autosomal dominant ichthyosis vulgaris in atopic dermatitis. Arch Dermatol Res 1987; 279:270–2.
58. Holleran WM, Ginns EI, Menon GK, et al. Consequences of β-glucocerebrosidase deficiency in epidermis. J Clin Invest 1994; 93:1756–64.

Stratum Corneum as a Biosensor

Peter M. Elias and Kenneth R. Feingold
*Dermatology and Medical (Metabolism) Services, Veterans Affairs Medical Center,
and Departments of Dermatology and Medicine, University of California,
San Francisco, California, U.S.A.*

Mitsuhiro Denda
Shiseido Research Center, Yokohama, Japan

Genes expressed in the vertebrate brain and spinal cord show up on the
surface...*Could this mean that brains started out on the body surface?*

Thurston Lacalli

INTRODUCTION

The principal role of the nucleated layers of the epidermis in terrestrial mammals is
to form a protective layer, the stratum corneum (SC), which interfaces with a
potentially hostile, desiccating external environment. This outermost layer
subserves a large set of distinct, defensive, or protective functions, serving not
only as regulator of permeability barrier homeostasis but also a large set of other
defensive functions (Table 1). Implicit in this set of functions is an emerging
awareness that the SC, though anucleate, possesses a wide array of metabolic
activities (concept of the "living stratum corneum"), and it is also now becoming
apparent that the outer epidermis is the initial sensor of changes in osmotic
pressure, pH, and thermal stimuli, serving as a critical environmental "biosensor"
(Table 2).

SIGNALS OF BARRIER HOMEOSTASIS

The biosensor concept implies signaling mechanisms between the SC and the
underlying epidermis and deeper skin layers. Although our knowledge of these
signals is still incomplete, they include the following.

Cytokines

The SC contains a substantial pool of preformed, primary cytokines, IL-1α and
IL-1β, which are released from the corneocyte cytosol, when the SC is injured (1).
Recent studies have shown that these primary cytokines initiate metabolic
responses in the underlying epidermis, including increased lipid and DNA
synthesis that lead to barrier repair (Fig. 1). Yet, if external injury to the SC is
sufficiently great, or if it is repetitive, the cytokine cascade can be sustained,
eventually leading to inflammation. Detailed studies of this signal cascade lead to
the "outside–inside" concept of the pathogenesis of inflammatory dermatoses.

TABLE 1   Localization of Functions of Outer Epidermis and SC

Function	Localization
Permeability barrier	Extracellular + corneocyte
Hydration	Extracellular, corneocyte, and outer epidermis: osmoreceptors/AQP3, 9
SC integrity/cohesion → desquamation	Extracellular
Antimicrobial barrier (innate immunity)	Extracellular
Toxic chemical/antigen exclusion, selective absorption	Extracellular
Mechanical (impact and shear resistance)	Corneocyte
UV barrier	Corneocyte
Initiation of inflammation (cytokine activation)	Corneocyte
Neurosensory interface	Outer epidermis: plasma membrane TRPVs

Abbreviations: SC, stratum corneum; TRPV, transient receptor potential vanilloid receptor; UV, ultraviolet.

Ionic Gradients

Barrier insults also change intraepidermal ionic gradients (Ca^{++}, K^+), and these alterations, in turn, stimulate a different set of downstream metabolic responses (Table 3). Best understood is signaling via changes in the epidermal calcium gradient. Since the integrity of the Ca^{++} gradient is dependent upon barrier status, acute barrier disruption allows Ca^{++} (and presumably K^+ ions as well) to escape outward through the SC. This reduction in extracellular Ca^{++} and K^+, in turn, stimulates the immediate secretion of a preformed pool of lamellar bodies (LB) from the outermost stratum granulosum layer. The rapid LB secretory response is the initial event in a prolonged cascade that is followed sequentially by an increase in epidermal lipid synthesis, extracellular processing of secreted lipids, and increased DNA synthesis. Together, these orchestrated, sequential responses rapidly normalize permeability barrier homeostasis (Fig. 2). Although the Ca^{++} gradient is largely restored by six hours, its further restoration parallels the return of barrier function toward normal, a sequence that requires about three days in humans (Fig. 3).

pH-Serine Proteases

The SC processes a highly acidic pH, which regulates several key functions by divergent mechanisms (Fig. 4). Acute and chronic barrier insults disrupt not only

TABLE 2   Evolving Concepts of Stratum Corneum

Outdated
   Disorganized, no functional significance ("basket weave")
   Homogenous film ("Saran Wrap")
Current
   Two-compartment organization ("bricks and mortar")
   Microheterogeneity within extracellular spaces ("There is more to the mortar than lipid")
   Persistent metabolic activity (dynamic changes in cytosol, cornified envelope, and interstices from inner to outer SC)
   Homeostatic links to the nucleated cell layers (changes in permeability barrier function signal epidermal DNA and lipid synthesis, antimicrobial peptide expression, and angiogenesis)
   Pathophysiologic links to deeper skin layers (sustained barrier abrogation stimulates cytokine cascade, initiating epidermal hyperplasia and inflammation)
   Stratum corneum as a biosensor (changes in external humidity regulate proteolysis of filaggrin, epidermal DNA/lipid synthesis)

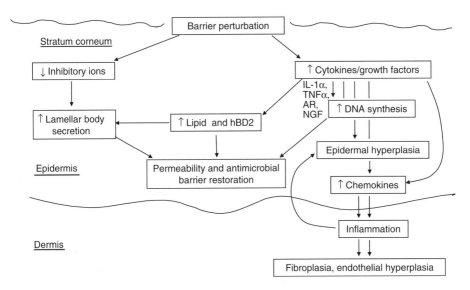

FIGURE 1 The cytokine cascade restores barrier function, but it can also lead to inflammation. *Abbreviations*: AR, amphiregulin; hBD2, human beta defensin-2; IL, interleukin; NGF, nerve growth factor; TNF, tumor necrosis factor.

ionic gradients, but also the normally acidic pH of the SC, shown further by the elevated pH in inflammatory dermatoses. The pH elevation that accompanies experimental barrier perturbations and inflammation, in turn, has negative consequences for barrier function, SC cohesion (i.e., it results in increased desquamation), antimicrobial function, and perhaps inflammation (Fig. 4). Yet, how elevations in the pH of SC signal downstream events is not yet well understood. Elevations in pH alone suffice to activate serine proteases (SP), including two largely epidermis-specific kallikreins, SC tryptic and SC chymotryptic enzymes (klk5 and klk7, respectively). Increased SP activity then impacts permeability

TABLE 3 Stratum Corneum as Biosensor: Signaling Mechanisms and Responses

Perturbation	Signal	Sensors/receptors	Consequences
Acute barrier disruption	Cytokine and growth factor generation	Multiple autocrine and paracrine	Lipid and DNA synthesis, cytokine cascade
	↓ Extracellular Ca^{++}/K^+	VDR CaR	↑ Secretion of preformed lamellar bodies
	↑pH → ↑ serine protease activity PAR2	TRPV1 (pH sensor)	Terminal differentiation and ↓ lamellar body secretion
	↓O_2 → ↑ VEGF	VEGFr	Vasodilation and angiogenesis
↑ or ↓ Humidity	Water gradient	TRPV4 (osmotic sensor)	↓ or ↑ lipid synthesis, respectively

Abbreviations: PAR2, plasminogen activator receptor type 2; TRPV, transient receptor potential vanilloid receptor; VDR, vitamin D receptor; VEGFr, vascular endothelial growth factor receptor.

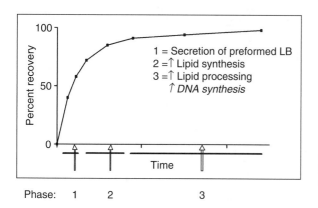

FIGURE 2 Rapid restoration of normal function after acute insults to the permeability barrier. *Source*: From Ref. 1.

barrier function by two different mechanisms: (*i*) sustained activation of SP directly degrades at least two LB-derived, lipid-processing enzymes, β-glucocerebrosidase, and acidic sphingomyelinase, contributing to permeability barrier dysfunction and (*ii*) SP activate the plasminogen activator receptor type 2 (PAR2) leading to blockade of lamellar body secretion and cornification. But sustained activation of SP-PAR2 activation can provoke premature apoptosis, causing epidermal thinning and entombment of LB in nascent corneocytes, as shown in an animal model of atopic dermatitis.

The pH-induced increase in SP activity impacts another key epidermal function, i.e., SC integrity by different mechanisms: SP activity normally initiates

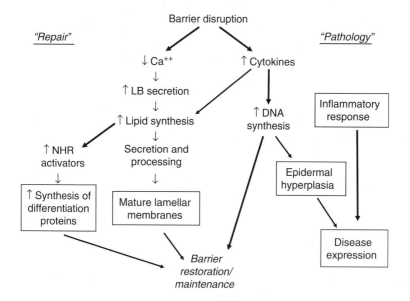

FIGURE 3 Coordinate signaling of permeability barrier homeostasis by calcium and cytokines. *Abbreviations*: LB, lamellar bodies; NHR, nuclear hormone receptor.

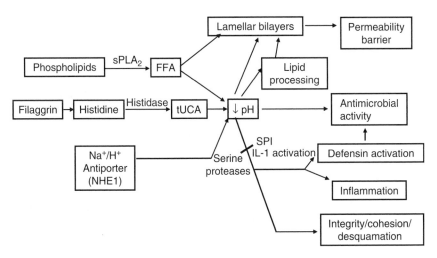

FIGURE 4 Endogenous pathways of stratum corneum acidification: regulated functions. *Abbreviations*: FFA, free fatty acids; NHE1, Na^+/H^+ antiporter; SPI, serine protease inhibitors; *t*-UCA, *trans*-urocanic acid. *Source*: From Ref. 1.

degradation of corneodesmosomes, allowing SC to be shed more easily (Fig. 4). Yet, again, if SC activation is sustained, as in the case in certain inherited skin conditions (e.g., Netherton syndrome), accelerated degradation of corneodesmosomes can compromise SC integrity and cohesion, accompanied by macroscopic evidence of excess scale.

HUMIDITY-INDUCED CHANGES IN PERMEABILITY BARRIER FUNCTION

Perhaps the most dramatic example of the biosensor concept is the cutaneous metabolic response of normal skin to variations in environmental humidity alone. As the external humidity falls below 80%, a proteolytic cascade is initiated within the corneocyte cytosol that initially generates constituent amino acids from filaggrin. These amino acids are further deiminated by both enzymatic and nonenzymatic mechanisms, generating osmotically active molecules, such as pyrrolidone carboxylic acid and *trans*-urocanic acid (UCA) (Fig. 5). These products together comprise the osmotically active "natural moisturizing factor" (NMF) that binds water within corneocytes. But certain of these deiminated molecules have functions that extend beyond moisturization, e.g., UCA is one potential endogenous source of SC acidification (Fig. 5), and it absorbs UV-B, in the process generating its immunosuppressant metabolite, *cis*-UCA. Thus, the filaggrin proteolytic cascade provides another eloquent example of the living stratum corneum (Table 2).

How does this proteolytic cascade operate in vivo? Recent studies suggest that the initial, responsible protease that attacks filaggrin is an aspartate protease, cathepsin D; hence, the severe xerosis suffered by HIV+ patients who receive prolonged therapy with the aspartate protease inhibitor group of antiretroviral drugs. At typical ambient humidities, filaggrin proteolysis begins in the mid-SC, thereby insuring adequate hydration of corneocytes in the outer SC (i.e., no

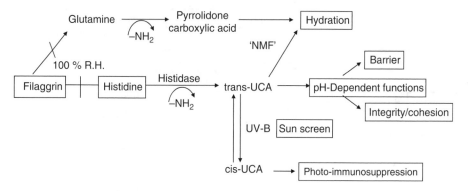

FIGURE 5 Functional consequences of the filaggrin proteolytic cascade. *Abbreviations*: NMF, natural moisturizing factor; UCA, urocanic acid.

visible xerosis). Conversely, at high ambient humidities, and presumably also with the use of occlusive moisturizers, filaggrin proteolysis should be down-regulated, because NMF is not needed. In contrast, at very low ambient humidities, proteolysis should accelerate, guaranteeing the generation of additional amounts of NMF.

Fluctuations in external humidity alter not only rates of filaggrin proteolysis but also metabolic processes that regulate permeability barrier homeostasis. Studies in hairless mice have shown that shifts from a normal (e.g., 40–70% RH) to a dry environment (RH <10%) provoke a progressive improvement in permeability barrier homeostasis, attributable to acceleration of lipid synthesis and lamellar body production (Fig. 6). Yet, exposure to a dry environment simultaneously stimulates epidermal hyperplasia, and if sustained, can initiate early signs of inflammation, such as mast cell degradation. Conversely, shifts to a humid (>80% RH) environment downregulate permeability barrier function, because with lesser barrier requirements, metabolic processes that maintain barrier function can be conserved. Surprisingly, extreme shifts in environmental humidity, i.e., from a humid to a dry environment, provoke a paradoxical, but transient barrier abnormality (Fig. 6). Apparently, humid-adapted cells can no longer upregulate their metabolic machinery in response to the demands of a dry environment. Whether these studies, performed in hairless mice, have clinical relevance still remains to be determined. Finally, though the water gradient across the SC changes in response to altered external humidities, how changes in the water gradient, in turn, signal downstream metabolic changes in the underlying epidermis remains unknown (Table 3).

THE EPIDERMIS AS A NEUROSENSOR

Our capacity to perceive external stimuli, such as changes in temperature, humidity, chemical stimuli and light touch, have long been attributed to peripheral arborization of cutaneous sensory neurons (Fig. 7). The most peripheral extensions of these nerve fibers have been shown to reach into the epidermis. Yet since, these nerve termini are widely separated, they cannot

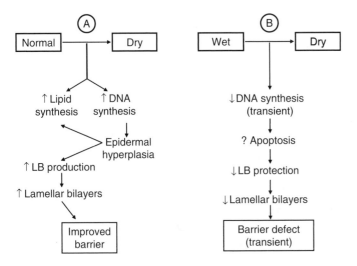

FIGURE 6 Downstream response to changes in environmental humidity. *Abbreviation*: LB, lamellar bodies.

account for fine discrimination. Moreover, this traditional view ignores the embryologic co-origins of neurons and keratinocytes, downplaying another important, potential, protective function of the epidermis, i.e., in sensory perception. Recent studies, primarily from the laboratory of one of the coauthors (M. Denda), have shown that keratinocytes form the initial interface of cutaneous perception. Keratinocytes, largely in the outer epidermis, express three receptors of the transient receptor potential vanilloid receptor (TRPV) family, TRPV1, 3, and 4, which all have been shown to transducer responses to a variety of sensations, including temperature, osmotic pressure, mechanical stress, and certain chemical stimuli (Table 4). The existence of these outwardly poised receptors provides an important link between modulations in barrier function and metabolic responses in the underlying epidermis. For example, TRPV1 is activated by reductions in pH, which could accompany Na^+/H^+ antiporter–

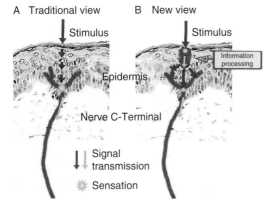

FIGURE 7 Old versus current view of epidermis as a distal outpost of the somatosensory system. *Source*: From Ref. 2.

TABLE 4 Barrier Repair Signaling: Homeostatic and Pathophysiologic Consequences

Signal	Homeostatic response	Potential pathogenic signal?
Ions		
Ca^{++}, K$^+$	Lamellar body secretion	No
Primary cytokines		
IIα/β, IL1ra, GM-CSF, TNFα, IL-6	DNA, lipid synthesis	Yes, if sustained
Serine proteases—PAR2	Terminal differentiation	Yes[a]
Growth factors	DNA synthesis	Yes[b]
NGF, TGFβ1, Amphiregulin, VEGF	Vasodilatation, angiogenesis	Yes[c]

[a] SP-PAR2 signaling → atopic dermatitis.
[b] Amphiregulin overexpression → inflammation.
[c] VEGF overexpression → psoriasiform dermatitis.
Abbreviations: NGF, nerve growth factor; SP-PAR2, serine protease-plasminogen activator receptor type 2.

mediated proton production, necessary to maintain SC acidity. It therefore could serve as a negative feedback regulator, downregulating epidermal metabolic responses once SC acidity is reestablished. Conversely, TRPV3 is activated not only by heat and chemical stimuli, but also apparently by mechanical stress, an inevitable accompaniment of barrier perturbations. Finally, TRPV4 is activated by changes in osmotic pressure, suggesting that it could be humidity sensor that response both to changes in permeability barrier stratus, but also external

TABLE 5 Neuroreceptors and Transmitters in Epidermis

Receptor type	Barrier recovery	Reference
Cholinergic		
Muscarinic (acetylcholine)	?	Grando et al. (1997)
Nicotinic (acetylcholine) activator	Delay	Grando et al. (1997) and Denda et al. (2003a)
Ionotropic		
NMDA		
Activators	Delay	Fuziwara et al. (2003)
Antagonists	Accelerate	Fuziwara et al. (2003)
Purinergic (P2X)		
Activators	Delay	Denda et al. (2002a)
Antagonists	Accelerate	Denda et al. (2002a)
GABA (A)		
Activators	Accelerate	Denda et al. (2002b)
Glycine		
Activators	Accelerate	Denda et al. (2003a)
G-protein–coupled metabotropic receptor		
β-Adrenergic (β-2)		
Activators	Delay	Denda et al. (2003b)
Antagonists	Accelerate (↑ cAMP)	Denda et al. (2003b)
Gi/O protein–coupled neurotransmitter		
Dopaminic (D2)		
Activators	Accelerate(↓ cAMP)	Fuziwara et al. (2005)
Antagonists	Delay (↑ cAMP)	Fuziwara et al. (2005)

Abbreviations: cAMP, cyclic adenosine monophosphate; GABA, gamma-aminobutyric acid; NMDA, N-methyl-D-aspartate; ?, unknown.

humidity. At the present time, these possibilities remain highly speculative. Moreover, the metabolic responses that are signaled by TRPV1, 3, and 4 activation remain unknown.

Further evidence for the epidermis as a distal outpost of the nervous system comes from the identification of ATP and neurotransmitter receptors in keratino-cytes, again largely from the Denda lab (Table 5). The ATP receptors could regulate downstream metabolic response following TPRV activation, or they could respond directly to alterations in barrier function, such as the ATP receptors, P2X, a ligand-gated ion channel, and P2Y, a G-protein–coupled receptor. Moreover, keratinocytes also contain several neurotransmitter receptors, including ionotropic and G-protein–coupled receptors that regulate ion channels and cyclic adenosine monophosphate levels, respectively (Table 5). In fact, using highly specific inhibitors of these receptors, the Denda group has shown that most of these receptors are both regulated by and important for, permeability barrier homeostasis (2), and there is also evidence that these receptors further signal the peripheral nervous system. Finally, expression of neurohormone and neuropeptide receptors in epidermis suggests a mechanism whereby the epidermis could interface with the endocrine system.

REFERENCES

1. Wood LC, Elias PM, Calhoun C, et al. Barrier disruption stimulates interleukin-1 alpha expression and release from a pre-formed pool in murine epidermis. J Invest Dermatol 1996; 106(3):397–403.
2. Denda M, Sokabe T, Fukumi-Tominaga T, et al. Effects of skin surface temperature on epidermal permeability barrier homeostasis. J Invest Dermatol 2007; 127(3):654–9.

6 Cutaneous Metabolism

Simon C. Wilkinson
Medical Toxicology Research Centre, Newcastle University, Newcastle upon Tyne, U.K.

Faith M. Williams
Medical Toxicology Research Centre and Institute for Research on Environment and Sustainability, Newcastle University, Newcastle upon Tyne, U.K.

INTRODUCTION

The skin is now recognized as more than an inert barrier capable of limiting chemical entry and exit. Numerous enzyme activities have been identified in cutaneous tissues, which are capable of a wide range of chemical transformations of both endo- and xenobiotic compounds. These activities may modulate toxicity and in certain cases percutaneous absorption, and are hence potentially of great importance in the response of the skin (and the whole body) to environmental, occupational, and therapeutic exposure to chemicals via the dermal route. Xenobiotic metabolism is regarded as a multistage process. In Phase I metabolism, xenobiotics are subject to "functionalization," in which functional groups (especially oxygen-containing groups) are introduced as a result of oxidation, reduction, or hydrolysis. In Phase II metabolism, these functionalized compounds are conjugated to water soluble compounds such as glucuronic acid, sulfate, glycine, and glutathione (GSH) or further metabolized by epoxyhydrases and other oxidoreductases, in order to increase their molecular weight and water solubility (to facilitate the removal from the cell). While Phase I metabolism can result in an increase in toxicity by generating reactive intermediates capable of binding to macromolecules, Phase II generally results in detoxification, though an intermediate may be formed that may undergo further Phase I metabolism. This chapter will summarize reports of expression and activity of enzymes in cutaneous tissues and will cover the consequences of enzyme activity for percutaneous penetration, absorption, and toxicity of topical xenobiotics; how expression and/or catalytic activity in tissue homogenates relate to whole cells and "intact" skin; and the ability to predict cutaneous metabolism in vivo using model systems, such as cell cultures, reconstructed skin models, and ex vivo models.

PHASE I ENZYMES
Cytochromes P-450
The cytochromes P-450 (CYP), considered as the most important Phase I enzymes for the activation of toxic chemicals, comprise a ubiquitous group of hem-containing, mixed-function oxidases, present in organisms in both prokaryotic and eukaryotic domains. In eukaryotes, they are membrane-bound to endoplasmic reticulum. CYP may utilize a broad range of endogenous chemicals as substrates, including prostaglandins, leukotrienes, vitamin D, corticosteroids, testosterone, fatty acids and cholesterol, as well as a wide range of xenobiotics. The general

equation for a chemical reaction catalyzed by CYP [equation (1)] involves the insertion of a single oxygen atom (from molecular oxygen) in the substrate.

$$RH + O_2 + NAD(P)H + H^+ \rightarrow ROH + H_2O + NAD(P)^+ \tag{1}$$

CYP have low substrate specificity and can thus utilize a wide range of substrates, and hence catalyze a broad range of reactions, including hydroxylation (both aliphatic and aromatic), N-hydroxylation and N-oxidation, oxidative and reductive dehalogenation, and O-, N- and S-dealkylation (1). The CYP are part of a gene superfamily coding for various isoforms. Our knowledge of the presence of specific CYP isoforms in skin has increased following the application of immuno-histochemical and molecular [polymerase chain reaction (PCR)-based] techniques, though while these methods may indicate the presence of mRNA or protein for specific isoforms, they do not necessarily indicate the presence of catalytic activity.

Measurements of Total and Specific CYP Isoform Activity in Cutaneous Tissues
Various experimental approaches have been used to identify and quantify expression and activity of cutaneous CYP, ranging from spectroscopic studies through selective probe substrates and immunohistochemical studies to molecular techniques, such as RT-PCR (semi quantitative and real time) and RNAse inhibition. Systems studied have included skin microsomes (derived from whole skin, epidermis, or dermis), keratinocytes, transformed keratinocyte cell lines, and cultured human hair follicles, in the presence and absence of classical CYP inducers such as 3-methyl-cholanthrene and phenobarbitone. The amount of CYP in skin microsomes was estimated to be about 6% of that in liver by spectroscopic studies (2). Both CYP1A1/2 and CYP2B were detected by immunochemical methods in rat skin, and both isoforms showed aryl hydrocarbon hydroxylation (AHH) and 7-ethoxycoumarin-O-deethylase (ECOD), both markers for CYP2B. CYP2B was described as "constitutive" in rat skin, while CYP1A1/2 was "very low or absent in uninduced skin" but "preferentially expressed following induction with 3-methyl-cholanthrene (3-MC)" (3–5). A considerable body of evidence has accumulated for the expression of numerous CYP isoforms from the application immunological techniques such as Western blotting (Table 1). More recently, single, immuno-reactive bands corresponding to CYP2B12, CYP2C13, CYP2D1, CYP2D4, CYP2E1, CYP3A1, and CYP3A2 were detected in rat (Fischer F344) and whole skin microsomes using a panel of monospecific antibodies directed toward small defined regions of respective CYP enzymes, whose specificity was demonstrated by immunoassay (14). CYP1A1, CYP1A2, and CYP2C12 were absent from whole skin microsomes but clearly identified in liver. Skin isoform protein expression levels ranged from 0.1% (CYP2D1) to 4.7% (CYP3A1) of those in liver (based on relative staining intensity), though 2D4 was not expressed in liver. Expression levels of proteins were lower in freshly isolated keratinocytes but increased in culture to levels comparable with whole skin.

Selective Probe Substrates
Several investigations on cutaneous CYP activity have utilized classical probe substrates, known to be metabolized, specifically or selectively, by different hepatic CYPs. The enzyme activities which utilize these probe substrates include 7-ethoxyresorufin-O-deethylase (EROD), a marker for CYP1A1/2, 7-ECOD, 7-pentoxyresorufin-O-deethylase (PROD), both markers for CYP2B, coumarin-7-hydroxylase (CYP2A6), *p*-nitrophenol hydroxylase (CYP2E1) and

TABLE 1 Reports of CYP Expression and Activity in Cutaneous Tissues

Main isoform(s)	Species/tissue	Detection	Remarks	Reference
1A1	SENCAR mouse microsomes	Monoclonal antibody	Constitutive expression (no 2B1 or 3A detected)	6
1A1/2	Mouse skin microsomes	Protein (immunoblotting)	Constitutive expression, lower levels of 2B1/2 and 3A	7
1A1, 1B1, 3A1, 3A2	Sprague–Dawley rat microsomes	Specific antipeptide antibodies		8
3A	Mouse epidermal microsomes, human keratinocytes	Western blotting (polyclonal antibodies raised versus liver isoform)	Constitutive expression	7
3A, 2E1	BALB1c mouse whole skin microsomes	Specific antipeptide antibodies	Constitutive expression	9
2E1	Human whole skin microsomes	Specific antipeptide antibodies		10
3A	Human skin	Specific antibody against human isoform		11
3A	Human keratinocytes, SVK14 cell line	Specific antibody against human isoform	Not detected in cultured hair follicles	12
Aromatase	Human sebaceous glands and hair follicles	Immunohisto-chemistry		13
2B12, 2C13, 2D1, 2D4, 2E1, 3A1, 3A2	Fischer 344 rat whole skin microsomes	Specific antipeptide antibodies	1A1, 1A2, 2C12 absent from skin	14
Epoxide hydrase 2C9	Human epidermis microarrays	Immunohisto-chemistry	2C8, 2J2 not detected	15

erythromycin-*N*-demethylase (CYP3A4). These substrates have been used to demonstrate the presence of a range of CYP activities in human and rodent skins, especially CYP1A1/2 (7,16–19), one of the highest CYP activities measurable in cutaneous tissues. CYP2B activity has also been measured using PROD and ECOD as markers, and appears to be constitutively expressed in skin (7), though cultured human keratinocytes appeared to lack PROD and 7-benzoxyresorufin activities (20). CYP2A6 was not detected by enzyme activity in human cutaneous tissues or rodent skins (21). CYP2E1 and CYP3A (7,21) have also been detected. Comparison of CYP probe substrate activity between skin and liver have shown considerable variation. EROD and benzo[*a*]pyrene epoxidase activities in skin range from 0.1% to 15% and 0.1% to 12% of hepatic activity respectively, while ECOD activity ranges from 0.5%

to 7% and PROD activity ranges from 20% to 27% of hepatic activity respectively (22). The 7-EROD activity in primary murine keratinocytes was approximately 2000-fold lower compared with hepatocytes on a per cell basis (23). However, basal EROD activity in HepG2 cells was only about 2.5-fold higher than in HaCaT cells (24).

Measurement of Cutaneous CYP Expression Using Molecular Biological Techniques

The application of molecular biological techniques, such as RT-PCR and especially quantitative (real-time) RT-PCR, for the measurement of cutaneous CYP expression has further increased the number of CYP isoforms detected in cutaneous tissues compared with immunological techniques and measurement of catalytic activity (Table 2). Of particular interest is CYP2S1, which appears to be relatively highly expressed in skin compared to the liver. It must be stressed, however, that measurement of CYP mRNA and protein expression levels do not necessarily correlate with catalytic activity.

Localization of CYP in Cutaneous Tissues

A number of immunohistochemical studies have indicated that cutaneous CYPs are localized in the epidermis, especially in basal keratinocytes, hair follicles, and vascular endothelium (35,36). Other studies based on measurement of catalytic activity (AHH and EROD) have confirmed this (37). The localization of CYP2E1 protein in normal human epidermis (assessed using immunochemical staining) was reported to be mainly in the upper layers, with weaker staining in the basal layer. In the dermis, vascular endothelium and eccrine sweat glands were well stained. Involved psoriatic skin showed a similar pattern (38). Lee et al. (39) showed that the main portion of cutaneous CYP protein expression was in the lower epidermis, while the appendages were more highly stained that the other dermal tissues. Janmohamed et al. (34) used in situ hybridization (ISH) using antisense mRNA probes to localize expression of CYP2A6, CYP2B6, and CYP3A4 in adult human breast skin. All three mRNAs were expressed uniformly in the epidermis of fixed sections of skin, as well as in sebaceous- and sweat-producing glands. Enayetallah et al. (15) demonstrated the expression of soluble epoxide hydrolase and CYP2C9 in tissue microarrays of epidermal skin using immunohistochemistry, though neither CYP2C8 nor CYP2J2 were detected. One of the more recently discovered cutaneous CYPs, CYP2S1, has low expression levels in liver but high and constitutive expression in many other tissues including skin, and is also dioxin-inducible under the control of aryl hydrocarbon receptor (AhR) and aryl hydrocarbon receptor nuclear translocator (ARNT) (29). Saarikoski et al. (40) performed ISH, using a 160-base pair RNA probe spanning a specific region on the $3'$ end of CYP2S1 cDNA, and immunohistochemistry (using a peptide-directed antibody) on cDNA tissue microarrays, in order to localize expression of this isoform. Staining intensity in human skin microarrays was comparable with that in nasal cavity and bronchus/bronchiolar tissue, and greater than that in liver. Two skin samples were analyzed, and both mRNA and protein expression were strong throughout the epidermis (apart from in the stratum corneum). Epithelial cells in sweat glands and hair follicles exhibited strong staining, and ISH especially indicated higher grain densities in basal cells than in upper layers of the epidermis.

TABLE 2 Selected Reports of CYP Expression in Cutaneous Tissues Based on mRNA Detection

Main isoform(s) reported (Ref.)	Species/ tissue	Detection	Findings	Remarks
3A subfamily members (25)	Human skin biopsies	RT-PCR (3A specific primers)	3A mRNA detected in all adults tested. Expression did not increase in response to clobetasol treatment	Only 3A5 protein detected using antibodies to conserved epitopes (in all individuals tested), suggesting 3A3 and 3A4 not significantly expressed in skin
1A1, 1B1, 2B6, 2E1, 3A4, 3A5 (26)	Human proliferating epidermal keratinocytes (obtained from fresh skin)	RT-PCR	Constitutive expression of all but 3A4. 3A4 inducible by dexamethasone. 1A1 expression increased in presence of benzanthracene	Findings confirmed by immuno-reactive protein and catalytic activity
1A1, 1B1, 2A6, 2E1, 2C, 2D6, 3A5, 3A7, 4B1 (27)	Freshly obtained cultured human Langerhans cells, keratinocytes, fibroblasts and melanocytes from six individuals	RT-PCR	1A1, 1B1, 2E1 expressed in all cell types and individuals 2A6, 2C, 2D6, 3A5, 3A7, 4B1 expressed in some cell types or individuals 1A2, 2A7, 2B6, 3A4 not detected	
1B1, 2B6, 2D6, 2C18, 3A4, 2C19, 3A5 (28)	Human skin biopsies (healthy volunteers)	Real-time RT PCR	Main isoforms expressed were 1B1, 2B6, 2D6, 3A4 Lower level expression of 2C18, 2C19, 3A5	Considerable interindividual variation in expression (some individuals apparently lacked 2B6)
1B1, 1A1, 2E1, 2S1, 3A4, 3A5 (29,30)	Human skin biopsies (healthy volunteers and psoriasis patients)	Real-time RT PCR	1B1 most expressed isoform in healthy volunteers, 1A1, 2S1 consistently expressed. 2E1 expressed in some individuals at levels comparable with 1B1. 3A4 levels much lower. 2S1 expression inducible by UV radiation and coal tar	Marked individuality of expression for 1B1, 2E1 and 2S1. Lower overall expression levels in non-lesional skin in randomly selected psoriasis patients. 2E1 and 2S1 expression significantly increased in lesional versus non-lesional skin, 1B1 and 3A5 decreased

(Continued)

TABLE 2 Selected Reports of CYP Expression in Cutaneous Tissues Based on mRNA Detection (*Continued*)

Main isoform(s) reported (Ref.)	Species/ tissue	Detection	Findings	Remarks
1A1, 1B1, 2E1, 2C, 3A5 (31)	Commercial organotypic skin models (with and without classical inducers)	Real-time RT PCR and cDNA microarrays	1A1 and 1B1 highly inducible by liquor carbons detergens	Expression localized using immunofluorescent staining
2B19 (32)	Primary and differentiating mouse epidermal keratinocytes	Real-time RT PCR	Expression increased 39-fold in differentiating keratinocytes	Confirmed by protein immunoreactivity and 11,12-EET activity
CYP1 and 2 subfamily members, 3A4 and 4B1 (33)	Human epidermal keratinocytes (proliferating and differentiating)	Real-time RT PCR	4B1, 2S1, 2J2 most abundant in pooled phenotypes. 2B6 undetectable. Significant increases in 4B1 (356-fold), 2W1 (27-fold) and 2C18 (113-fold) in differentiating cells	Overall range of expression covered five orders of magnitude. Expression of nearly half isoforms studied varied twofold or less between proliferating and differentiating states, majority less than 10-fold different
2A6, 2B6, 3A4 (34)	Adult human breast skin	RNAse protection assay	All skin samples expressed 2B6, some expressed 2A6 and 3A4	
	Primary keratinocytes		Expression of 2B6 and 3A4 was 75–100% lower in cultured primary keratinocytes. 3A4 absent	
	HaCaT cells		Expression of 2B6 in HaCaT more comparable to human skin than primary keratinocytes, but 2A6 and 3A4 absent	

Activation of Xenobiotics by CYP Activities
Polyaromatic Hydrocarbons
The ability of cutaneous CYP to activate xenobiotics to more reactive (and potentially more toxic) compounds is now well established. In 1775, Sir Percival Pott reported an increased incidence of scrotal cancer in chimney sweeps. Subsequent research showed that certain polyaromatic hydrocarbons, such as benzo[*a*]pyrene and dimethyl-benzanthracene, may form genotoxic metabolites in the skin following activation by CYP1A1/2 (and others) to epoxides and subsequent conversion to diol epoxides catalyzed by epoxide hydrolase (41,42). The CYP involved in polycyclic aromatic hydrocarbon (PAH) metabolism, CYP1A1 and CYP1B1, are substrate inducible, as well as being under the control of the AhR. This cytosolic receptor binds readily to planar PAHs such as benzo[*a*]pyrene, and after dimerization with the ARNT, enters the nucleus, where the complex binds to regions of DNA known as xenobiotic response elements. This results in the upregulation or induction of genes involved in response to xenobiotic insult, such as CYPs (43). Numerous studies have since been undertaken to establish the nature and toxicity of DNA adducts formed from the products of CYP activity and the contributions of the different CYP isoforms to this process in a variety of tissues (44). Studies with knockout mice, lacking particular genes for CYP isoforms and the AhR (see below), have been of special importance in this process. Kleiner et al. (45) investigated the role of different CYP isoforms in the formation of epidermal PAH–DNA adducts using CYP2A1 ($-/-$), CYP2B1 ($-/-$) and AhR ($-/-$) knockout mice, following topical treatment with one of several PAHs. In mice treated with dibenz[*a,h*]pyrene, DNA adduct levels were significantly lower in CYP1A2 ($-/-$), and CYP1B1 ($-/-$) mice compared to wild-type mice (57% and 46% lower respectively). There was no significant difference in DNA adduction with AhR ($-/-$) mice. In contrast, DNA adduct levels in CYP1A2 ($-/-$) mice treated with dimethylbenzanthracene (DMBA) were not significantly different to wild-type mice, but DNA adduct levels were significantly lower in both CYP1B1 ($-/-$) and AhR ($-/-$) mice (64% and 52% lower respectively). In benzo[*a*]pyrene-treated mice, DNA adduct levels were significantly lower (73%) in AhR ($-/-$) compared to wild-type mice, but no significant difference was found between either CYP1A2 ($-/-$) or CYP1B1 ($-/-$) and wild-type mice. The results suggested that different CYP isoforms had roles in bioactivation of different PAHs, and that CYP1B1 preferentially forms syn-DMBA-diol epoxides, while 1A1 preferentially formed anti-DMBA-diol epoxides. Ide et al. (46) demonstrated the same cutaneous tumor incidence and latency in both AhR ($-/-$) and AhR ($+/+$) 8-week-old female mice following treatment with 7,12-dimethylbenz[*a*]anthracene (DMBA, 50 µg weekly for 20 weeks applied to shaved dorsal skin). CYP1A1 expression was absent in the epidermis of AhR ($-/-$) mice, but was slightly induced in AhR ($+/+$) mice exposed to DMBA. In both mice strains, CYP1B1 expression was constitutive at approximately equivalent levels, as was microsomal epoxide hydrolase (mEH), regardless of DMBA treatment, though CYP1A2 expression was not detectable. The authors concluded that CYP1B1 and mEH maintained the response of cutaneous tissues to DMBA in AhR ($-/-$) mice.

N-Hydroxylation of Amines
Reports of N-hydroxylation of amines in skin or skin models are rare. The majority of reports have identified N-acetylation as the major pathway in skin for amines (see below). Reilly et al. (47) reported that neonatal and adult human keratinocytes

were able to generate hydroxylamine derivatives of sulfamethoxazole and dapsone as well as *N*-acetyl derivatives. The derivatives of dapsone were cytotoxic, while sulfamethoxazole derivatives were less cytotoxic but resulted in considerable depletion of GSH. More recently, Vyas et al. (48) showed that the contribution of CYP to the enzyme-mediated haptenation of dapsone and sulfamethoxazole in human keratinocytes was apparently limited, as addition of demonstrable CYP inhibitors failed to attenuate protein adduction with either substrate.

Species Differences in CYP Expression and Activity

There have been relatively few comparisons of CYP expression in animal models and humans. Recent studies based on the detection of mRNA have concentrated on skin biopsies, primary keratinocytes, or cell lines (Table 2). Investigations using probe substrates demonstrated that CYP1A1 activity in rodent models ranged from 1.5 to 20.6 pmol/min/mg (7,19), compared with, for example, 62 fmol/min/mg for human skin biopsies (16). Similarly, CYP1A/2B activity measured using 7-ECOD was not detectable in human skin (49) and was 0.11 pmol/min/mg in reconstructed human epidermis (50) compared with 24.3 pmol/min/mg in mouse skin (51). Some reports of enzyme activity appear to contradict findings based on protein expression. For example, CYP1A1 protein was apparently not detected in the skin of Fischer 344 rats (14), though measurable activity was reported by Pham et al. (19). Pig skin has received very little attention regarding CYP expression and activity. The pig is accepted as a good model for dermal penetration studies although information is lacking for many enzyme systems in pig skin, despite characterization of hepatic CYP in mini-pigs (52–54). Measurement of cutaneous CYP activity requires skin to be freshly isolated, as the enzymes degrade rapidly after removal of skin from the animal or volunteer. Since human skin is in short supply, and additional logistical problems arise from the need to collect fresh skin, a suitable animal model should be found.

Model Systems: Keratinocytes, Cell Lines, and Organotypic Cell Cultures

Although a great many studies have measured CYP expression levels (via mRNA and protein) in cell cultures, cell lines and organotypic cell cultures (Table 2), measures of activity have been scarcer. Gelardi et al. (55) reported that ECOD (10 pmol/min/mg), EROD (2 pmol/min/mg), and PROD (0.6 pmol/min/mg) activities were easily detectable in NCTC 2544 human keratinocytes under basal conditions. These levels were rather higher than those previously reported by Cotovio et al. (56) for this cell line.

CYP Activity During Percutaneous Absorption

Although there have been numerous reports of CYP activity in skin microsomal preparations (either from whole skin, keratinocytes or cell lines), measurement of CYP-catalyzed biotransformations during percutaneous penetration has been more rarely reported in peer reviewed literature. Testosterone was metabolized during in vitro percutaneous absorption though human, rat, and mouse skin to a range of hydroxylated metabolites (21), suggesting the presence of CYP3A activity.

Regulation of CYP Expression and Activity

Agarwal et al. (6) demonstrated induction of CYP1A1, CYP2B1, and CYP3A activities (measured using classical probe substrates) following a single topical administration of pyridine (30 or 50 mg/kg) to Sencar mice. This was also reflected in reactivity to specific antibodies to these proteins. Northern blotting indicated a significant increase in CYP1A1 mRNA following pyridine treatment. As mentioned above, CYP1A1 and CYP1B1 are known to be regulated by the AhR and ARNT system. Jones and Reiners (57) showed that 2,3,7,8-tetrachlorodibenzo-p-dioxin (TCDD) preferentially induced EROD activities in differentiating murine keratinocytes, despite demonstrating that both proliferating and differentiating cells exhibited constitutive mRNA expression of CYP1A1 and CYP1B1 (as well as Ahd4 and Nmo1 genes). Both AhR and ARNT were found in both cell types and were located in the nucleus in both cases, regardless of TCDD treatment. The authors concluded that AhR activation was regulated as a function of keratinocyte differentiation in murine skin. Cotovio et al. (56) compared CYP activity using probe substrates in normal human keratinocytes (NHK) with spontaneously immortalized cell lines (NCTC 2544 and HaCaT), and keratinocytes immortalized with simian virus 40 (SV40) transfection simian virus keratinocyte 14 (SVK14). After subculture, NHK retained EROD and ECOD activities, and these activities were inducible by 3-MC as in primary culture. Similar basal activity for EROD and ECOD was found in the immortalized cell lines (PROD activity was not found in any cell line), but these activities were not inducible by 3-methylchoanthrene to the same extent as in NHK. Gelardi et al. (55) noted that addition of classical inducers of CYP such as β-naphthoflavone (BNF), phenobarbital (PB), and 3-MC resulted in significant and considerable increases in EROD, PROD, and ECOD activities in NCTC 2544 human keratinocytes. MC-induced ECOD and EROD activities were inhibited by α-naphthoflavone in a dose-dependent manner, while PB-induced PROD activity could be inhibited by the CYP2B inhibitor metapyrone. Harris et al. (58) showed that CYP1A1 activity (measured by EROD activity) was induced by BNF and 3-MC in cultured keratinocytes; the level of induction increased with increasing confluence. Induced EROD activity was inhibited by clomitrazole in a dose-dependent manner. Basal EROD activity was not detected in hair follicles or epidermis but could be induced with 3-MC; the ability to induce EROD activity in reconstituted epidermal models varied from batch to batch, and induced EROD activity was inhibited by clomitrazole. Rastogi et al. (59) reported that twice weekly topical application of Alfatoxin B1 (16 nmol in acetone vehicle) to Swiss albino mice for 24 weeks in vivo caused significant induction of cutaneous CYP1A monooxygenase activity, measured by AHH (increased 162%) and EROD activity (increased 108%), without significantly affecting hepatic CYP1A activity. In contrast, glutathione-S-transferase (GST) activity was significantly induced in liver and skin, and NAD(P)H quinone reductase (NQR) activities were unaffected in both tissues. Lipid peroxidation increased in both tissues in response to Alfatoxin B1 treatment, and this was accompanied by a concomitant decrease in both hepatic and cutaneous GSH levels. The flavonolignans silybin and dehydrosilybin, prospective UV-protective agents, both significantly inhibited basal CYP1A1 activity (measured by 7-EROD) in HaCaT cells at 100 μM (the highest concentration tested) after 48 hours, though the decreases were numerically small. However, TCDD-induced CYP1A1 activity was significantly reduced by silybin at 10 and 100 μM after both 24- and 48-hours exposure, and by dehydrosilybin at all concentrations and both time-points, the decrease in activity being especially marked with dehydrosilybin (this latter compound was cytotoxic to HaCaT cells). Studies on recombinant CYP1A1 showed that the potency of inhibition of dehydrosilybin was two orders of magnitude greater than silybin (60).

There have been several studies of the effects of UV-radiation on the induction of CYP expression and activity. Gonzalez et al. (61) reported that mRNA for CYP2E1, CYP1A1, and CYP3A5 was detected in UVA-, UVB-, and non-irradiated keratinocytes obtained from primary culture; 19Aro, 2C19, and 2C26 were not expressed constitutively but some induction of 19Aro was measured after irradiation with UVB and UVA. CYP3A4 and CYP3A7 were not detected; although mRNA for CYP4A11 was measured in non-irradiated keratinocytes, two protein bands were immunoreactive with anti-CYP4A11 antibodies. Smith et al. (30) showed modest induction of CYP1B1 expression (mean 1.48-fold) following exposure to UVA [1–4 times minimal erythma dose (MED)] in human volunteers, but no significant induction for other genes measured (see above). In psoriasis patients treated with psoralen-UVA, significant induction of CYP1B1, CYP2E1, and CYP2S1 was measured. Katiyar et al. (62) showed that UVB exposure (1–4 times MED) resulted in enhanced staining for CYP1A1 and CYP1B1 in keratome biopsies, which was both dose- and time-dependent (maximal at 48 hours after exposure), compared with unexposed skin. RT-PCR confirmed that CYP1A1 (threefold) and CYP1B1 (2.5-fold) were both induced following UVB exposure. Expression of CYP protein was confirmed with Western blotting of microsomal protein; catalytic activity of CYP1A1 was also higher following UVB exposure.

Smith et al. (63) showed that topical application of coal tar preparation to human skin in vivo resulted in significant inductions of CYP1A1 (mean 212-fold), CYP1A2 (32.8-fold), and CYP1B1 (27.0-fold) and to a lesser but still significant extent, CYP2C18 (2.03-fold). The NAD(P)H quinone oxidoreductase 1 was also significantly induced (5.76-fold). The authors cautioned, however that constitutive expression of CYP1A1 was extremely low and that the fold induction observed with coal tar may have been an overestimation. There was marked interindividual variation in response. All trans retinoic acid resulted in a significant suppression of CYP1A1 (0.09-fold) and CYP1B1 expressions (0.03-fold), while significantly inducing CYP26 expression (33.8-fold).

Esterases

Esterases are ubiquitously expressed in mammalian tissues including, liver, blood, kidney, intestines, testes, brain, central nervous system, skin, and lung (64). Both cytosolic- and membrane-bound forms have been characterized, and the most significant group with respect to xenobiotic metabolism are the carboxyl esterases (formerly categorized among a group known as B esterases), which catalyze the hydrolysis of carboxylic acid esters to the organic acid and alcohol. The nature of microsomal esterases in liver and gut have been most extensively studied (65) and differing proportions of the three human isoforms, hCE1, and hCE2 (corresponding to CES1 and CES2, respectively) and hCE3 have been detected. Cloning of hCE1, hCE2, and hCE3 has allowed ranking of the specificity. Skin has long been known to possess a considerable nonspecific esterase activity, which has been exploited for the delivery of ester pro-drugs (66–70). However, characterization of isoforms of esterase in cutaneous tissues remains comparatively rudimentary at present.

Protein Expression of Esterases in Cutaneous Tissues

Reports detailing quantitation of esterase protein in skin have been relatively scarce. Protein cross reacting with carboxylesterase pI 6.0 (hCE1) was detected in rat skin cytosol and microsomes (71). Esterase staining with naphthylacetate has identified two staining bands in human skin and one major band with different properties in mini-pig skin (72). Zhu et al. (73) found a higher expression of hCE2 than hCE1 in human skin.

Reports of Esterase Activity with Probe Substrates and Inhibitors—Localization of Activity

The majority reports of cutaneous enzyme activity are based on hydrolysis of specific substrates and the effects of modulators such as inducers and inhibitors. Histochemical studies of mini-pig, human, and rat skin showed carboxylesterase activity (using naphthyl acetate as a substrate) was located in the basal keratinocytes of epidermis and hair follicles and sebaceous glands with little activity in the dermis (71,74). Beisson et al. (75) also found esterase activity in the stratum corneum, identified using methylumbelliferyl esters as substrates and demonstrating lipase activity. McCracken and coworkers (76) confirmed esterase activity in cytosol and microsomal fractions from rat skin and that they were inducible. Ahmed and coworkers (68) found higher levels of skin cytosolic esterase activity compared to microsomal activity in hairless mouse skin. It was also shown that the nature of skin esterases was different to liver based on the inhibition profile, and that distribution varied according to location (epidermis, dermis, or subcutaneous tissue) (77). Esterase activity measured in skin microsomes and cytosol with *p*-nitrophenol acetate, phenyl valerate, phenylacetate, and procaine was lower than liver for human, mini-pig, and rat. (78,79). Overall, ester hydrolysis by human skin was closer to mini-pig and lower than rat whereas for methyl umbelliferyl acetate, mini-pig skin had the highest activity. For all species, there was higher activity in skin cytosol compared to microsomes when expressed per gram of tissue. There was a variation in esterase activities between different sites on mini-pig and sexes but this was less than between species as observed here (80). Inhibition by loperamide suggested that hCE2 was present in human skin microsomes and cytosol. Cytosolic esterases may have particular importance in skin during percutaneous penetration as the diffusing ester must be taken up into the cell, where it will come into contact with cytosolic enzymes before uptake into the lumen of the endoplasmic reticulum, where microsomal esterases are located, occurs.

Esterase Activity During Percutaneous Absorption

Esterases are known to be robust enzymes, and esterase activity has been detected in previously frozen skin. Consequently, reports of hydrolysis of esters during percutaneous absorption studies are common. Clark et al. (81) and Hewitt et al. (82) showed that hydrolysis of ester herbicides occurred during dermal absorption through skin in vitro in a diffusion cell. Parabens (*p*-hydroxybenzoic acid esters) are found in many skin products, range in molecular size and lipophilicity (methyl paraben to benzyl paraben) and are substrates for skin carboxylesterases (83,84). They are hydrolyzed to *p*-hydroxybenzoic acid during absorption. Application of range of parabens to the surface of human or pig skin in short-term culture resulted in hydrolysis during absorption. Metabolism was greater for the methyl and ethyl esters than for butyl and benzyl esters. Inhibition studies with loperamide (specific for hCE2) differential response for hydrolysis of methyl and ethyl esters (which we not affected by loperamide) to butyl and benzyl esters, for which hydrolysis was inhibited, indicating involvement of hCE2 (72). Skin esterases have also been shown to be stereoselective in the affinity for substrates (68). Ethyl nicotinate applied topically was converted by esterases to nicotinic acid in a range of species (85).

Species Differences

There have been numerous reports of species differences in esterase activity, for example toward corticosteroid esters (86), fluazifop butyl (71,81), and soman (87). A survey of several species showed that esterase activity toward ethyl nicotinate during percutaneous absorption was higher in rodent species and rabbits than in monkey, human, and snake skin (85). In contrast, a number of other studies have found extensive esterase activity to certain substrates in several diverse species, for example toward the phthalic acid esters (88). Overall enzyme activity is believed to be higher in rat skin than human skin (see, for example, Ref. 89).

Esterase Activity in Keratinocytes and Cell Lines

There have been a number of reports of esterase activity in keratinocytes. Barker and Clothier (90) demonstrated esterase activity using methyl umbelliferyl heptanoate as a model substrate in NCTC 2544 and SVK-14 cell lines, as well as in freshly isolated breast keratinocytes, with activity in the latter decreasing during differentiation. Lobemeier et al. (83) showed evidence of esterase activity toward parabens in extracts of transformed keratinocytes, while Kubota et al. (91) demonstrated the capacity to hydrolyze betamethasone-21-valerate in homogenates of a living skin equivalent. Esterase activity in cultured keratinocytes developed markedly during growth of both humans and rats (89). However, the isoforms of carboxylesterases in keratinocyte cell lines and organotypic skin models remain to be characterized fully.

Role of Esterase Activity in Toxicity

The general consensus among researchers is that hydrolysis resulting from esterase activity will reduce the systemic absorption of the parent compound, so this will result in detoxification if the parent compound is systemically or locally toxic (see, for example, Ref. 92). It must be mentioned, however, that the products of hydrolytic cleavage of an ester are a carboxylic acid and an alcohol, either of which may be subsequently metabolized by Phase I enzymes alcohol dehydrogenase (ADH) and/or aldehyde dehydrogenase (ALDH) to more reactive metabolites (see below). Hydrolysis of benzyl acetate to benzyl alcohol was followed by oxidation of the alcohol to benzoic acid in human and rat skin during percutaneous absorption (93).

Alcohol and Aldehyde Dehydrogenases

The alcohol dehydrogenases (ADH) and aldehyde dehydrogenases (ALDH) have received particular attention recently, due to the possible role of alcohol oxidation to aldehydes in the mechanism of skin sensitization. ADH activity may result in the formation of aldehydes from alcohols, which may subsequently react with, and bind covalently to, proteins in the epidermis resulting in haptenization. Benzyl alcohol was oxidized to benzoic acid in human and rat skin (93), while cinnamaldehyde was oxidized to cinnamic acid as well being reduced to cinnamic alcohol in human skin (94). Tonge (95) reported that hydroxycitronellal was both reduced to hydrocitronellol and oxidized to hydroxycitronellic acid in human skin.

Phenoxyethanol was metabolized to phenoxyacetic acid in skin postmitochondrial fractions (96). These findings provided evidence of both ADH and ALDH activities in skin.

Protein Expression of ADH and ALDH in Cutaneous Tissues

Cheung et al. (97) demonstrated constitutive expression of ADH1, ADH2, and ADH3, as well as ALDH1 and ALDH3, in human foreskin, breast, and abdomen skin using Western-blot analysis. Densitometric analysis showed that staining intensity was significantly lower in foreskin for ADH1 and ADH2 and significantly greater in foreskin for ALDH1 and ALDH3, than breast or abdomen skin. Immunohistochemistry showed that ADH1 and ALDH3 were localized mainly in the epidermis with some expression in the dermal appendages, while staining for ADH2 in skin sections was much less intense. ALDH1 and ALDH3 were also localized mainly in the epidermis, with some highly localized expression in the dermal appendages.

ADH and ALDH Activity Measurements in Skin Homogenates and Subcellular Fractions

The cutaneous metabolism of cinnamic alcohol and cinnamaldehyde has been studied in skin cytosol (98). Measurements of ADH activity showed the apparent V_{max} of this enzyme to be higher in liver (6.02–16.67 nmol/mg protein/min) than in skin (0.32–1.21 nmol/mg protein/min), and higher in mouse skin (1.07–1.21 nmol/mg protein/min) than in human skin (0.34–0.41 nmol/mg protein/min). ADH activity in skin appeared to be less sensitive to inhibition by 1 mM 4-methyl pyrazole than ADH in liver (activity was reduced to 30–40% and 2–10% of control values in skin and liver respectively). Cheung et al. (99) demonstrated that cutaneous transformation of cinnamic alcohol into cinnamaldehyde, and of cinnamic acid, and cinnamaldehyde into cinnamic alcohol and cinnamic acid occurred principally in human skin cytosolic fractions, with less metabolic activity being measured in mitochondrial and microsomal fractions. When cinnamic alcohol (1 mM) was used as the parent compound, 26% to 31% was converted to cinnamic acid in both whole skin and cytosolic preparations after 30 and 90 minutes; in mitochondrial and microsomal fractions, only 1% to 9% was converted. No cinnamaldehyde was measured. When cinnamaldehyde (1 mM) was the parent compound, complete conversion into cinnamic alcohol (at earlier timepoints) and/or cinnamic acid was measured with whole skin and cytosolic fractions. With 5 mM cinnamaldehyde, the proportion of remaining parent compound was 19% in whole skin and 32% in cytosolic fraction after 90 minutes. In contrast, metabolism of cinnamaldehyde in mitochondrial and microsomal fractions was limited (up to 19% conversion). Conversion of cinnamic alcohol to cinnamic acid was significantly reduced by 4-methylpyrazole in whole skin and cytosolic fractions, while conversion of cinnamaldehyde to cinnamic alcohol was about eightfold higher in the presence of the inhibitor. In cytosolic fractions, conversion of cinnamaldehyde to cinnamic acid was significantly reduced following pretreatment with 4-methyl pyrazole, though there was no effect in microsomal or mitochondrial fractions. The ALDH inhibitor disulfiram significantly reduced conversion of cinnamic alcohol to cinnamic acid in cytosolic fractions, but again, there was no influence on microsomal or mitochondrial fractions. In contrast, disulfiram affected metabolism of cinnamldehyde in all fractions, and completely inhibited conversion in mitochondrial fractions.

ADH and ALDH Activity During Percutaneous Penetration

When neat cinnamaldehyde (243.8 $\mu mol/cm^2$) was applied to freshly excised human skin in flow through cells, penetration of cinnamic alcohol (321.4 $\pm$ 250.3 $nmol/cm^2/h$) and cinnamic acid (238.0 $\pm$ 164.0 $nmol/cm^2/h$) exceeded that of the parent compound (132.9 $\pm$ 24.6 $nmol/cm^2/h$) in the first two hours of study (100). Penetration of the two metabolites was maximal after four to eight hours then decreased, while penetration of the parent compound was maximal after 18 hours. Preincubation of skin with pyrazole increased the penetration rate of the parent compound, though preincubation with water vehicle also caused this effect. However, pyrazole pretreatment significantly reduced penetration of the alcohol and acid metabolites compared to vehicle controls. When cinnamic alcohol was applied as the parent compound, the penetration rate of the acid metabolite (52.3 $\pm$ 18.5 $nmol/cm^2/h$) was approximately half that of the parent compound (128.6 $\pm$ 47.9 $nmol/cm^2/h$) and no cinnamaldehyde was detected. Pretreatment with pyrazole did not significantly affect penetration of the parent compound compared to vehicle control, but 320 μmol pyrazole significantly reduced penetration of the acid metabolite. Again, none aldehyde metabolite was detected. The authors proposed that they had observed conversion of cinnamaldehyde to cinnamic alcohol by ADH, and by ADH (acting as an aldehyde dismutase) and ALDH to cinnamic acid, as pyrazole reduced penetration of cinnamldehyde metabolites, but not the parent compound. The greater extent of metabolism to acid from the aldehyde compared to the alcohol suggested that the latter process was slower. The fact that no aldehyde metabolites were detected was not unexpected, as rapid further metabolism, conjugation, or protein adduction would have occurred. Gelardi et al. (55) reported that ALDH activity (detected spectrophotometrically using benzaldehyde and propionaldehyde as substrates) was easily detectable in cell homogenates of NCTC 2544 keratinocytes (up to 28.7 $\pm$ 0.7 $nmol/min/mg$ protein, depending on the substrate and cofactor used).

Species Differences

Species differences in expression of cutaneous ADH and ALDH classes have been demonstrated. ADH1 and ADH3, as well as ALDH1 and ALDH2, were expressed constitutively in the skin and liver of rat, mouse, and guinea pig (demonstrated by Western-blot analysis), while ADH2 was not expressed in any rodent skin but was present in the liver of all rodent species (98). ALDH3 was constitutively expressed in rat and mouse skin (though not in guinea pig), and was not expressed in the liver of any rodent species tested. Immunohistochemistry showed that expression of ADH and ALDH was localized mainly in the epidermis, sebaceous glands, and hair follicles, with similar patterns of expression measured in all rodent species tested and in humans. Lockley et al. (101) compared rates of ADH oxidation of a range of alcohols in rat skin cytosol with those measured in rat liver cytosol: in the latter tissue, the highest oxidation rate was measured with ethanol, followed by 2-ethoxyethanol, ethylene glycol, 2-phenoxyethanol, and 2-butoxyethanol, while this order was reversed for skin cytosol. Activity in dermatomed skin was twice that in full thickness skin when expressed in terms of protein content. ADH oxidation of all alcohols tested was completely inhibited by 1 mM pyrazole in rat liver cytosol, while pyrazole only inhibited ADH activity by 40% in skin cytosol at the same concentration, and did not inhibit oxidation of the other alcohols in skin cytosol (a similar difference in inhibition between cutaneous and hepatic ADH activities was demonstrated by Cheung et al. (98) for 4-methyl pyrazole). Furthermore,

Lockley et al. (101) showed that disulfiram completely inhibited metabolism of all alcohols in skin cytosol at 500 μM. These data suggested that different isoforms of ADH were present in skin and liver. Although skin has the capacity to metabolize 2-butoxyethanol to 2-butoxyacetic acid, the rapid percutaneous penetration of 2-butoxyethanol in vivo and in vitro prevented local metabolism (102). Similar findings were reported for 2-ethoxyethanol (103).

Regulation of ADH/ALDH Activity

Compared to other oxidation enzymes (especially CYPs), there have been few investigations of the regulation of cutaneous ADH and ALDH activity. Gelardi et al. (55) reported that ALDH activity was inducible (resulting in a significant 3.8- to 4.2-fold increase) by 3-MC (2.5 μM) but not significantly influenced by PB (2 mM). Lockley et al. (101) showed that multiple topical application of ethanol or 2-butoxyethanol (2-BE) to rat skin in vivo resulted in a preferential increase in oxidation activity of these respective substrates in skin cytosol, suggesting that the two substrates may induce different isoforms of ADH with affinities for alcohols of differing chain lengths. Topical treatment with a classical inducer (dexamethasone) resulted in enhanced activity with both ethanol and 2-BE as substrates, indicating the induction of several isoforms simultaneously. The ALDH activity is well known to be involved in the synthesis of retinoic acid (see below). Ulrich et al. (104) showed the treatment of keratinocytes in a skin equivalent model with all-trans retinoic acid (10^{-6} M) resulted in a significant (up to 30-fold) and rapid induction of ALDH1A3 (measured by real-time PCR and confirmed by Northern blotting and ISH). However, other Class 1 family members and the Class 2 and 3 family members tested of this enzyme were not induced, and no upregulation was measured with fibroblasts. ALDH1A3 was also significantly induced by TCDD, suggesting a general detoxification role for this enzyme as well as involvement in retinoid metabolism.

Flavin-Containing Monooxygenases

Flavin-containing monooxygenases (FMOs) are another group of multi-substrate enzymes of critical importance in detoxification of xenobiotics in both hepatic and extrahepatic systems (105), though little is known about their expression and activity in cutaneous systems (106,107). Janmohamed et al. (34) measured expression of genes encoding FMOs (using RNAse protection techniques) in adult human skin and primary keratinocytes, as well as in HaCaT cells. In whole human skin, FMO expression was considerably lower than that in kidney and liver. FMO1 expression was the only FMO detected in all nine individuals tested, and mRNA levels ranged from 9 to 163 mol/ng total RNA in skin, compared to 80 to 850 mol/ng total RNA in the kidney. FMO5 expression was detected in seven out of eight individuals tested, with mRNA levels ranging from 23 to 128 mol/ng total RNA (compared with 500–5700 mol/ng total RNA in liver). FMO3 and FMO4 were expressed in only half the individuals tested, at a maximum of 111 and 9 mol/ng total RNA respectively, again considerably lower than expression levels in liver. In cultured keratinocytes, expression of FMO3, FMO4, and FMO5 was 75% to 100% lower than in primary skin, and FMO1 was not detected. Expression of FMO4 mRNA was at least threefold higher in HaCaT cells than in primary skin, while expression levels of FMO3 and FMO5 were similar to primary skin. FMO1 expression was, again, not detected in HaCaT cells. The ISH with anitsense RNA probes showed that cutaneous expression of all four genes was localized in the epidermis (uniformly distributed, not restricted to a particular layer), the sweat producing cells of sebaceous glands and hair follicles. More recently, Vyas et al. (108) showed that protein adduction of dapsone and sulfamethoxazole in human keratinocytes could be inhibited by the addition of a prototypical substrate for FMOs. While recombinant FMO1 and FMO3 were capable of activating both substrates, FMO1 was absent from keratinocytes when assessed by mRNA expression. The authors suggested that FMO3, along with as yet unidentified peroxidises, was responsible for haptenization of dapsone and sulfamethoxazole, and that these enzymes may have a role in the predisposition to cutaneous drug reactions.

NAD(P)H Quinone Reductase

The NQR activity has been detected in rodent epidermal cytosol at higher levels than those measured hepatically (109), and similar findings have been reported for human skin (110,111). This enzyme may well play a role in stable reduction of quinones to hydroquinones, this detoxifying quinones and preventing oxidative stress due to quinone redox cycling (112). Subsequent studies have suggested that NQR is involved in reduction of the semiquinone anthralin to danthrone (111), and the enzyme was found to be dose dependently induced by danthrone itself (110). Gelardi et al. (55) reported the basal-specific activity of NQR as 134 ± 0.05 nmol/min/mg in NCTC 2544 human keratinocytes. This activity was increased by 146% in the presence of 2.5 µM of 3-MC, but phenobarbitone had no effect. Despite the relative activity of this enzyme compared to the liver, it remains surprisingly unresearched in cutaneous tissues.

PHASE II ENZYMES

Cutaneous tissues are known to have a high capacity to detoxify dermally applied chemicals, and this capacity is believed to exceed the skin's basal capacity to generate activated toxins as a result of Phase I metabolism. This evidenced in higher skin: liver activity ratios for Phase II enzymes compared to CYPs, for example (113). This detoxification capacity may well originate in the need to detoxify reactive oxygen species, which result from UV exposure. Indeed, the skin maintains a battery of detoxification mechanisms designed to remove harmful reactive oxygen species, such as the superoxide anion, hydroxyl radical, and singlet oxygen [reviewed by Afaq and Mukhtar (114)]. The transferases [GSH, glucuronide, acetyl, and sulfotransferases (SULT)] comprise the major group of Phase II enzymes.

Glutathione Transferases

Reduced glutathione (GSH) is a cysteine-containing tripeptide present in all eukaryotic cells. GSH plays a central role in detoxification of reactive oxygen species, both directly and as a dimer, GSSG (GSH disulfide or oxidized GSH), and the skin has considerable capacity to recycle GSSG to GSH (115). The glutathione-S-transferases (GSTs) are mainly cytosolic enzymes that catalyze the conjugation of reduced GSH with electrophilic chemicals. Five human isoforms of GST have been characterized: α(GST A), μ(GST M), π(GST P), θ(GST T), and ζ(GST Z) (116,117). Immunochemical studies have shown that human and rodent skins contain predominately π isoforms, with some α present only in humans, and μ

present only in skin from rodent species. Immunohistochemical studies showed the presence of π and μ forms in sebaceous glands and the outer root sheath of hair follicles in murine skin (118) and π and α in the hair follicles of human skin (119). GST activities are greater compared with liver that some Phase I enzymes e.g., specific activity of conjugation of *cis*-stilbene oxide in rat skin was 49% of hepatic rates (2). Human and rodent skins have been shown to metabolize a range of substrates (2,4-dinitro chlorobenzene (DNCB), benzo[*a*]pyrene-4,5-oxide, styrene-7,8-oxide, and others) (118,120). GSH depletion has been reported in skin during percutaneous absorption and metabolism of DNCB (120). Smith et al. (30) showed GST P1 to be induced by UV radiation and to be significantly more expressed in lesional psoriatic skin. Recent studies of GST in skin have been scarce however. GST is a polymorphic enzyme, and there has been some discussion of the role of GST polymorphisms in susceptibility to certain skin cancers (121–123).

GST Expression and Activity in Keratinocytes and Cell Lines
Class p GST was found to be the major isoform in cultured rat keratinocytes. Irradiation of keratinocytes with UV light resulted in a decrease in class p GST mRNA (124). GST activity was detected in cultured keratinocytes, reconstructed epidermis, and hair follicles at levels greater than or equal to levels in human epidermis (58). Zhu et al. (14) reported significant basal GST activity in human epidermal keratinocytes (up to 261.3 nmol/min/mg in crude cell lysates), while activity in HaCaT cells was only 62% of that in NHK, and activity in melanocytes was much lower.

Glucuronyl Transferases
The uridine diphosphate glucuronyl transferases (UGT) are a family of microsomal enzymes that catalyze the glucuronidation of a range of substrates, using the cosubstrate uridine diphosphate glucuronic acid (UDPGA). Such transformations have been reported in cutaneous tissues, and cutaneous activity measurements are relatively high compared to other cutaneous enzymes systems, with activities ranging from 0.6% to 50% of hepatic-specific activity (2,113,125). Naphthol, propofol, morphine, and androstanediol have also been used as probes and have been shown to be specific for UGT1A6, UGT1A9, UGT2B7, and UGT2B15 isoforms (126). More recently specific substrates for UGT1A1, UGT1A4, UGT1A6, UGT1A9, UGT2B7, and UGT2B15 have been described (127). Glucuronyltransferases have been shown to be expressed in the skin but despite their role in conjugating hydroxylated metabolites and free acids, their role in the skin has been poorly evaluated. UGT2B7, UGT2B15, and UGT2B17 that carry out conjugation of androgens as well as other drugs and xenobiotics have been shown to be expressed in the skin (128).

Sulfotransferases
The sulfotransferases (SULTs) catalyze the transfer of sulfate [activated to 5′-phosphoadenosine phosphosulfate (PAPS) by ATP] to phenol and amines. The SULTs are mainly cytosolic enzymes. The SULTs have been shown to comprise at least five classes. Human SULTs have been classified on their ability to catalyze sulfate transfer to particular substrates, namely class P-ST (phenol sulfotransferase, isoforms ST1A1, ST1A2, and ST1A3), class M-ST (monoamine sulfotransferase, isoform ST1A5), and class HST [hydroxysteroid sulfotransferase,

isoforms HST and EST (estrogen sulfotransferase, also referred to as ST1E4)] (129,130). A number of marker substrates have been used for SULTs; 4-nitrophenol, dopamine, dihydroxyepiandrosterone, lithocholic acid, and β-estradiol have been used as marker substrates for P-PST (p-nitrophenol sulfotransferase), M-PST (monoamine-preferring sulfotransferase), HST, and EST classes, respectively, in human and rat skin. Cutaneous activities were approximately 10- to 20-fold lower than in liver (131,132). SULTs in the experimental animals studied have shown less variability than humans and similarity to human ST1A3 rather than ST1A5. Activity was measured by consumption of S^{35} PAPS. The SULT2B gene encodes two isoforms, SULT2B1a and SULT2B1b. Only SUL2B1b is expressed in the skin (133). Higashi et al. (134) also showed that SULT2B1b which sulfate cholesterol is expressed in NHK and expression is increased with differentiation.

N-Acetyltransferases

The N-acetyltransferases (NATs) catalyze the N-acetylation of nitrogen-containing xenobiotics using acetyl coenzyme A as a cosubstrate. There are two classes, NAT-1 and NAT-2, both of which exhibit polymorphisms. NAT activity has been previously demonstrated in cutaneous tissues using a range of substrates, including azo dyes, 2-acetylaminofluorene, benzocaine, p-aminobenzoic acid, and others (see Ref. 135). More recently, Kawakubo et al. (136) investigated the capacity for human skin to acetylate p-phenylenediamine (PPD). Both mono- and diacetylated metabolites of PPD were detected in cytosolic fractions of human skin and cultured NHK. The rate of formation of the mono- and diacetyl metabolites was 0.41 to 3.68 nmol/mg/min and 0.65 to 3.25 nmol/mg/min respectively for whole human skin, and rates were similar for keratinocytes. Formation of both products was competitively inhibited by p-aminobenzoic aicd (a substrate for NAT1) but not by sulfamethazine. However, RT-PCR showed the presence of both NAT1 and NAT2 mRNA. Reilly et al. (47) showed that both neonatal and adult human keratinocytes were able to metabolize sulfamethoxazole and dapsone to 4-hydroxylamine and N-acetyl derivatives in a time-dependent manner. Both cell types expressed mRNA for NAT1 but apparently not NAT2. Nohynek et al. (137) reported that there was no significant difference in the metabolic profile between NAT2 slow and intermediate acetylators among human volunteers exposed to oxidative hair dyes containing radiolabeled PPD in vivo. The major urinary metabolites identified in all samples were N-monoacetylated and N,N'-diacetylated PPD, which collectively accounted for 80% to 95% of urinary radioactivity. Overall, the results indicated that acetylation of PPD in humans following topical application was independent of NAT2 status, probably due to epidermal metabolism by NAT1. Nohynek et al. (138) compared biotransformation of p-aminophenol (PAP) and PPD in EPISKIN reconstructed human epidermis (compounds applied to the epidermal surface) with that in human hepatocytes (compounds added directly to culture medium). The reconstructed human epidermis quantitatively converted PAP to N-acetyl-aminophenol, while hepatocytes converted PAP to sulfate and glucuronyl deriva-tives of N-acetyl-aminophenol and PAP, as well as the free N-acetylated metabolite. Both epidermis and hepatocytes converted PPD to N-monoacetylated and N,N'-diacetylated derivatives of PPD, with formation of diacetylated metabolites favored at lower concentrations of PPD (up to 250 µM). Conversion of PPD applied at 10 µM in epidermis was approximately 80%. The capacity for conversion to monoacety-lated metabolites was threefold lower in the reconstructed epidermis than in hepatocytes, and the capacity to form the diacetylated metabolites was eightfold lower. No N-hydroxylated derivatives were detected in either tissue from either PPD or PAP. Studies of dermal metabolism of PAP and PPD in rats in vivo showed that neither parent compound was detectable in plasma following dermal application of 12.5 mg/kg of PAP or 50 mg/kg of PPD. Three metabolites were detected in plasma following dermal application of PAP; these were tentatively identified as paracetamol (acetylated PAP) and were tentatively identified as paracetamol (acetylated PAP) and O-glucuronide and O-sulfate conjugates of paracetamol. Paracetamol was not detected at two hours after application, while the glucuronide and sulfate conjugates represented 30% and 70% of total plasma radioactivity after two hours. Between four and eight hours after application, paracetamol in plasma increased to 11.7% to 17.7% of total radioactivity, while the conjugates amounted to 27.6% to 45.0% (glucuronide) and 46.9% to 59.0% (sulfate). Dermal application of PPD resulted in a single metabolite in plasma, corresponding to N,N'-diacetylated PPD. No free or monoacetylated PPD was detected. The authors concluded that the metabolites originated from dermal transformation, as parent compound would have been detected in plasma if the metabolites had originated from hepatic enzyme activity. Again, no N-hydroxylated metabolites were detected (139).

Glycine Conjugation

There have been very few reports of glycine conjugation in cutaneous tissues. Some glycine conjugation of benzoic acid (1 μmol/L) to hippuric acid was detected in rat and human keratinocytes after eight hours (about 10% and 2% conversion respectively), but none was detected in primary keratinocytes (140).

CUTANEOUS METABOLISM OF ENDOGENOUS COMPOUNDS

The skin is being increasingly recognized as an organ with a distinct endobiotic biochemistry (141). There has been considerable progress in research into metabolism of endogenous compounds in cutaneous tissues. Some examples of these include:

■ *Vitamin D3*: This originates from the precursor steroid 7-dehydrocholesterol (located mainly in the plasma membrane of basal keratinocytes). The product of the *CYP11A1* gene is responsible for hydroxylation of cholesterol, followed by cleavage of the cholesterol side chain, and CYP17 and CYP21A2 have also been identified in a variety of cutaneous tissues (142,143). Thiboutot and coworkers (144) demonstrated the expression of the CYP side chain cleavage enzyme and the CYP 17-hydroxylase, as well as other steroidogenic enzymes and cofactors, in epidermis, hair follicles, sebaceous glands, and sebaceous ducts in sections of human facial skin.

■ *Arachidonic acids:* Keeney et al. (145) showed that CYP2B12 mRNA was expressed solely in sebocytes in rat anogenital skin, with CYP2B15 expressed at similar levels. The product of CYP2B12 was almost exclusively 11,12-epoxyeicosatrienoic acid (EET), though other EETs were detected in sebocytes, suggesting that other CYP enzymes might be involved.

■ *Retinoic acid and retinoids:* Vitamin A (retinol) is converted to retinoic acid (the biologically active form in epidermis) via a two-step oxidative pathway. The first step involves enzymatic conversion of retinol to retinaldheyde by retinol dehydrogenase/reductase. Markova et al. (146) reported the characterization of a retinol dehydrogenase activity, hRoDH-E2, which was abundantly expressed in epidermis, epidermal appendages, and cultured human keratinocytes. The enzyme was able to utilize both free and protein-bound retinol as a substrate, and protein was principally detected in the basal and viable differentiated epidermis.

■ *Serotonin and melatonin:* Slominski et al. (147) demonstrated expression of tryptophan hydroxylase (TPH), which catalyzes one of the first steps in serotonin synthesis from tryptophan, in a variety of cutaneous tissues, though not in HaCaT cells. The mRNA for amino acid N-acetyltransferase (AANAT) and 5-hydroxyindole-O-methyl transferase (HIOMT), which are involved in subsequent metabolism of serotonin to melatonin, was also detected in a variety of cutaneous tissues, including HaCaT cells. Expression of TPH was subsequently demonstrated in C57BL/6 mouse skin in anagen and catagen phases (though not in telogen skin) and in immortalized melanocytes. Furthermore, mRNA for amino acid AANAT was also expressed in mouse skin and immortalized melanocytes, though subsequent investigation showed the majority of transcripts to be of aberrant isoforms, devoid of catalytic activity (148). Serotonin was acetylated in rat skin homogenates in the presence of acetyl coenzyme A. This activity was suppressed by Cole bisubstrate inhibitor. The metabolite of serotonin, 5-hydroxyindole acetic acid, was also detected; accumulation of this metabolite was almost completely eliminated by a monoamine oxidase inhibitor (149). Slominski et al. (150) reviewed the synthesis and possible biological actions of serotonin and melatonin in skin.

CONCLUSIONS

Considerable progress has been made in our understanding of the skin as a metabolic organ as a result of the application of modern molecular biological techniques to cutaneous tissues, especially with regard to the expression of CYP isoforms in human skin and other cutaneous tissues. We are gaining a better understanding of the differences in enzyme expression and activity in different model systems (experimental animals, cell cultures, transformed cell lines, and reconstructed epidermal models). Our knowledge of endobiotic biochemistry in the skin is increasing greatly. However, there is still much work to be done in certain areas, including (among others):

■ The functional significance of CYP activity in human skin for xenobiotic metabolism and activation for a range of chemicals
■ The relationship between skin metabolism and skin sensitization is gradually being explored, but more work is needed
■ A suitable model organism for studying CYP expression, activity, and activation of xenobiotics
■ The application of microdialysis to study skin metabolism in vivo
■ Characterization of the different classes of carboxylesterases in human and animal skin, as well as cell cultures and cell lines
■ The effects of environmental stresses on metabolism of xenobiotics
■ Metabolic activity in damaged and irritated skin
■ The influence of xenobiotic metabolism on cutaneous detoxification pathways for reactive oxygen species, as well as on endobiotic metabolism, especially steroidogenesis, and the functional consequences of these effects.

REFERENCES

1. Correia MA. Drug biotransformation. In: Katzung BG, ed. Basic and Clinical Pharmacology. 8th ed. New York: McGraw Hill, 2001:51–63.
2. Pham MA, Magdalou J, Totis M, et al. Characterization of distinct forms of cytochromes P-450, epoxide metabolising enzymes and UDP-glucuronyltransferases in rat skin. Biochem Pharmacol 1989; 38:2187–94.
3. Bickers DR, Mukhtar H. Skin as a portal for entry for systemic effect: xenobiotic metabolism. In: Galli CL, Hensby CN, Marinovich M, eds. Skin Pharmacology and Toxicology, Recent Advances. New York: Plenum Press, 1990:85–97.
4. Khan WA, Park SS, Gelboin HV, et al. Epidermal cytochrome P-450: immunochemical characterization of isoform induced by topical application of 3-methylcholanthrene to neonatal rat. J Pharmacol Exp Thera 1989; 249:921–7.
5. Khan WA, Park SS, Gelboin HV, et al. Monoclonal antibodies directed characterization of epidermal and hepatic cytochrome P-450 isoforms induced by skin application of therapeutic crude coal tar. J Invest Dermatol 1989; 93:40–5.
6. Agarwal R, Jugert FK, Khan SG, et al. Evidence for multiple inducible cytochrome P450 ioszymes in Sencar mouse skin by pyridine. Biochem Biophys Res Commun 1994; 199:1400–6.
7. Jugert FK, Agarwal R, Khun A, et al. Multiple cytochrome P450 isozymes in murine skin: induction of P450 1A, 2B, 2E and 3A by dexamethasone. J Invest Dermatol 1994; 102:970–5.
8. James HL, Hotchkiss SAM, Edwards RJ. Developmental changes in cytochrome P450 expression in Sprague–Dawley rat skin and liver. Human Exp Toxicol 1997; 16:404.
9. Hotchkiss SAM, Hewitt PG, Edwards R. Immunochemical detection of specific cytochrome P450 enzymes in uninduced BALB/c mouse skin. Proc ISSX 1996; 10 (Abstract 172).
10. Ashcroft JA, Flint MS, Hotchkiss SAM. Constitutive expression and localization of CYP2E1 mRNA in BALB/c mouse skin determined by in situ hybridization. Proc ISSX 1997; 11 (Abstract 56).
11. Murray GI, Barnes TS, Sewell HF, et al. The immunocytochemical localisation and distribution of cytchrome P-450 in normal human hepatic and extrahepatic tissues with a monoclonal antibody to human cytochrome P-450. Br J Clin Pharmacol 1988; 25:465–75.
12. van Pelt FNAM, Olde Meierink YJM, Blaauboer BJ, et al. Immunohistochemical detection of cytochrome P450 iosenzymes in cultured human epidermal cells. J Histochem Cytochem 1990; 38:1847–51.
13. Sawaya ME, Penneys NS. Immunohistochemical distribution of aromatase and 3B-hydroxysteroid dehydrogenase in human hair follicle and sebaceous gland. J Cutan Pathol 1992; 19:309–14.
14. Zhu ZY, Hotchkiss SA, Boobis AR, et al. Expression of P450 enzymes in rat whole skin and cultured epidermal keratinocytes. Biochem Biophys Res Commun 2002; 297:65–70.
15. Enayetallah AE, French RA, Thibodeau MS, et al. Distribution of soluble epoxide hydrolase and of cytochrome P4502C8, 2C9, and 2J2 in human tissues. J Histochem Cytochem 2004; 52:447–54.
16. Bickers DR, Mukhtar H, Dutta-Choudhury T, et al. Aryl hydrocarbon hydroxylase, epoxide hydrolase and benzo[a]pyrene metabolism in human epidermis: comparative studies in normal subjects and patients with psoriasis. J Invest Dermatol 1984; 83:51–6.
17. Rettie AE, Williams FM, Rawlins MD, et al. Major differences between lung, skin and liver in the microsomal metabolism of homologous series of resorufin and coumarin ethers. Biochem Pharmacol 1986; 35:3495–500.
18. Finnen MJ. Skin metabolism by oxidation and conjugation. In: Shroot B, Schaefer H, eds. Pharmacology and the Skin. Skin Pharmacokinetics. Vol. 1. Basel: Karger, 1987:163–9.
19. Pham MA, Magdalou J, Siest G, et al. Reconstituted epidermis: a novel model for the study of drug metabolism in human epidermis. J Invest Dermatol 1990; 94:749–52.
20. Raffali F, Rougier A, Rouget R. Measurement and modulation of cytochrome P450 dependent enzyme activity in cultured human keratinocytes. Skin Pharmacol 1994; 7:345–54.

21. Beckley-Kartey SAJ, Hotchkiss SAM, Capel M. Comparative in vitro skin absorption and metabolism of coumarin (1,2-benzopyrone) in human, rat and mouse. Toxicol Appl Pharmacol 1997; 145:34–42.

22. Mukhtar H, Khan WA. Cutaneous cytochrome P-450. Drug Metab Rev 1989; 20:657–73.

23. Reiners JJ, Amador RC, Pavone A. Modulation of constitutive cytochrome P450 expression in vivo and in vitro in murine keratinocytes as a function of differentiation and extracellular Ca^{2+} concentration. Proc Natl Acad Sci 1990; 87:1825–9.

24. Ledirac L, Delescluse C, de Sousa G, et al. Carbaryl induces CYP1A1 gene expression in HepG2 and HaCaT cells but is not a ligand of the human hepatic Ah receptor. Toxicol Appl Pharmacol 1997; 144:178–82.

25. Li X-Y, Duell EA, Qin L, et al. Cytochrome P450 3A5 is the major 3A subfamily member expressed in normal human skin in vivo. J Invest Dermatol 1994; 102:624.

26. Baron JM, Holler D, Schiffer R, et al. Expression of multiple cytochrome P450 enzymes and multidrug resistance-associated transport proteins in human skin keratinocytes. J Invest Dermatol 2001; 116:541–8.

27. Saeki M, Saito Y, Nagano M, et al. mRNA expression of multiple cytochrome P450 isozymes in four types of cultured skin cells. Int Arch Allergy Immunol 2002; 127:333–6.

28. Yengi LG, Xiang Q, Pan JM, et al. Quantitation of cytochrome P450 mRNA levels in human skin. Anal Biochem 2003; 316:103–10.

29. Smith G, Deeni YY, Dawe RS, et al. Cytochrome P450 CYP2S1 expression in human skin: individuality in regulation by therapeutic agents for psoriasis and other skin diseases. Br J Dermatol 2003; 148:853.

30. Smith G, Dawe RS, Clark C, et al. Cytochrome P450 quantitative real-time reverse transcription-polymerase chain reaction analysis of drug metabolizing and cytoprotective genes in psoriasis and regulation by ultraviolet radiation. J Invest Dermatol 2003; 121:390–8.

31. Neis MM, Marquard Y, Joussen S, et al. Cytochrome P450 characterisation of cytochrome P450 expression in organotypic skin models. J Invest Dermatol 2005; 125:A83.

32. Du LP, Yermalitsky V, Ladd PA, et al. Evidence that cytochrome P450 CYP2B19 is the major source of epoxyeicosatrienoic acids in mouse skin. Arch Biochem Biophys 2005; 435:125–33.

33. Du LP, Neis MM, Ladd PA, et al. Effects of the differentiated keratinocyte phenotype on expression levels of CYP1-4 family genes in human skin cells. Toxicol Appl Pharmacol 2006; 213:135–44.

34. Janmohamed A, Dolphin CT, Phillips IR, et al. Quantification and cellular localization of expression in human skin of genes encoding flavin-containing monooxygenases and cytochromes P450. Biochem Pharmacol 2001; 62:777–86.

35. Jugert FK, Frankenberg S, Junginger H, et al. Multiple cytochrome P450 isozymes are present in human keratinocytes. In: 13th European Drug Metabolism Workshop. Bergamo, Italy, 1992.

36. Frankenberg S, Jugert FK, Merk HF. Multiple cytochrome P450 isozymes present in human hair follicle derived keratinocytes. J Invest Dermatol 1993; 100:518.

37. Merk HF, Mukhtar H, Schutte B, et al. Human hair follicle benzo[a]pyrene and enzo[a]pyrene-7,8-diol metabolism: effect of exposure to a coal tar-containing shampoo. J Invest Dermatol 1987; 88:71–6.

38. Kawakubo Y, Tamiya S, Umezawa Y, et al. Distribution of cytochrome p450 (CYP) 2e1 in the skin: a novel marker for keratinocyte differentiation? J Invest Dermatol 2001; 117:792.

39. Lee A, Choi W, Ko D, et al. Constitutive expression and distribution of cytochrome P450 isozymes in normal human skin. J Invest Dermatol 2001; 117:528.

40. Saarikoski ST, Wikman HAL, Smith G, et al. Localization of cytochrome P450CYP2S1 expression in human tissues by in situ hybridization and immunohistochemistry. J Histochem Cytochem 2005; 53:549–56.

41. Rogan EG, Devanesan PD, Ramakrishna NVS, et al. Identification and quantitation of benzo[a]pyrene dna adducts formed in mouse skin. Chem Res Toxicol 1993; 6:356–63.

42. Bronaugh RL, Collier SW, Macpherson SE, et al. Influence of metabolism in skin on dosimetry after topical exposure. Environ Health Persp 1994; 102:71–4 (Suppl.).
43. Whitlock JP. Induction of cytochrome P4501A1. Ann Rev Pharmacol Toxicol 1999; 39:103–25.
44. Baird WM, Hooven LA, Mahadevan B. Carcinogenic polycyclic aromatic hydrocarbon-DNA adducts and mechanism of action. Environ Mol Mutagen 2005; 45:106–14.
45. Kleiner HE, Vulimiri SV, Hatten WB, et al. Role of cytochrome P4501 family members in the metabolic activation of polycyclic aromatic hydrocarbons in mouse epidermis. Chem Res Toxicol 2004; 17:1667–74.
46. Ide F, Suka N, Kitada M, et al. Skin and salivary gland carcinogenicity of 7,12-dimethylbenz[a]anthracene is equivalent in the presence or absence of aryl hydrocarbon receptor. Cancer Lett 2004; 214:35–41.
47. Reilly TP, Lash LH, Doll MA, et al. A role for bioactivation and covalent binding within epidermal keratinocytes in sulfonamide-induced cutaneous drug reactions. J Invest Dermatol 2000; 114:1164–73.
48. Vyas PM, Roychowdhury S, Khan FD, et al. Enzyme-mediated protein haptenation of dapsone and sulfamethoxazole in human keratinocytes: I. Expression and role of cytochromes P450. J Pharm Exp Thera 2006; 319:488–96.
49. Storm JE, Collier SW, Stewart RF, et al. Metabolism of xenobiotics during percutaneous absorption: role of absorption rate and cutaneous enzyme activity. Fund Appl Toxicol 1990; 15:132–41.
50. Cotovio J, Roguet R, Pion FX, et al. Effect of imidazole derivatives on cytochrome P-450 enzyme activities in a reconstructed human epidermis. Skin Pharmacol 1996; 9:242–9.
51. Moloney SJ, Fromson JM, Bridges JW. Cytochrome P-450 dependent deethylase activity in rat and hairless mouse skin microsomes. Biochem Pharmacol 1982; 31:4011–8.
52. Fujimori KA, Takahashi H, Numata BS, et al. Drug metabolizing systems of Gottingen miniature pigs. Swine in Biomedical Research 1986; Vol. 1:533–48.
53. Skaanild MT, Friis C. Characterization of the P450 system in Gottingen minipigs. Pharmacol Toxicol 1997; 80(Suppl.):28–33.
54. Skaanild MT, Friis C. Cytochrome P450 sex differences in minipigs and conventional pigs. Pharmacol Toxicol 1999; 85:174–80.
55. Gelardi A, Morini F, Dusatti F, et al. Induction by xenobiotics of phase I and phase II enzyme activities in the human keratinocyte cell line NCTC 2544. Toxicol In Vitro 2001; 15:701–11.
56. Cotovio J, Leclaire J, Roguet R. Cytochrome P450-dependent enzyme activities in normal adult human keratinocytes and transformed human keratinocytes. In Vitro Toxicol 1997; 10:207–16.
57. Jones CL, Reiners JJ. Differentiation status of cultured murine keratinocytes modulates induction of genes responsive to 2,3,7,8-tetrachlorodibenzo-p-dioxin. Arch Biochem Biophys 1997; 347:163–73.
58. Harris IR, Siefken W, Beck-Oldach K, et al. NAD(P)H: quinone reductase activity in human epidermal keratinocytes and reconstructed epidermal models. Skin Pharmacol Appl Skin Physiol 2002; 15(S1):58–73.
59. Rastogi S, Dogra RKS, Khanna SK, et al. Skin tumorigenic potential of aflatoxin B1 in mice. Food Chem Toxicol 2006; 44:670–7.
60. Dvorak Z, Vrzal R, Ulrichova J. Silybin and dehydrosilybin inhibit cytochrome P450 1A1 catalytic activity: a study in human keratinocytes and human hepatoma cells. Cell Biol Toxicol 2006; 22:81–90.
61. Gonzalez MC, Marteau C, Franchi J, et al. Cytochrome P450 4A11 expression in human keratinocytes: effects of ultraviolet irradiation. Br J Dermatol 2001; 145:749–57.
62. Katiyar SK, Matsui MS, Mukhtar H. Ultraviolet-B exposure of human skin induces cytochromes P450 1A1 and 1B1. J Invest Dermatol 2000; 114:328–33.
63. Smith G, Ibbotson SH, Comrie MM, et al. Regulation of cutaneous drug-metabolizing enzymes and cytoprotective gene expression by topical drugs in human skin in vivo. Br J Dermatol 2006; 155:275–81.
64. Satoh T, Hosokawa M. The mammalian carboxylesterases: from molecules to function. Annu Rev Pharmacol Toxicol 1998; 38:257–88.

65. Huang TL, Shiotsuki T, Uematsu T, et al. Structure-activity relationships for substrates and inhibitors of mammalian liver microsomal carboxylesterases. Pharm Res 1996; 13:1495–500.
66. Williams FM. Clinical significance of esterases in man. Clin Pharmacokinet 1985; 10:392–403.
67. Higuchi WI, Yu C-D. Prodrugs in transdermal delivery. In: Kydonius AF, Berner B, eds. Transdermal Delivery of Drugs. Vol. 3. Boca Raton, FL: CRC Press, 1987:43–83.
68. Ahmed ST, Imai T, Yoshigae Y, et al. Stereospecific activity and nature of metabolizing esterases for propanolol prodrug in hairless mouse skin, liver and plasma. Life Sci 1997; 61:1879–87.
69. Bando HS, Mohri S, Yamashita S, Takakura Y, Hashida M. Effects of skin metabolism on percutaneous penetration of lipophilic drugs. J Pharm Sci 1997; 86:759–61.
70. Liederer BM, Borchardt RT. Enzymes involved in the bioconversion of ester-based prodrugs. J Pharm Sci 2006; 95:1117–95.
71. Clark NWE. Cutaneous xenobiotic metabolism and its role in percutaneous absorption. PhD thesis, University of Newcastle, U.K., 1992.
72. Jewell C, Prusakiewicz JJ, Ackermann CA, et al. Hydrolysis of a series of parabens by skin microsomes and cytosol from human and minipigs and in whole skin in short-term culture. Toxicol Appl Pharmacol 2007 (in press).
73. Zhu QG, Hu JH, Zeng HW. Stereoselectivity of skin carboxylesterase metabolism. Yao Xiue Xue Bao 2005; 40:322–6.
74. Mayer W, Neurand K. The distribution of enzymes in the skin of the domestic pig. Lab Anim 1976; 10:237–47.
75. Beisson F, Aoubala M, Marull S, et al. Use of tape stripping technique for directly quantifying esterase activity in human stratum corneum. Anal Biochem 2001; 290:179–85.
76. McCracken NW, Blain PG, Williams FM. Nature and role of xenobiotic metabolising esterases in rat liver, lung, skin and blood. Biochem Pharmacol 1993; 45:31–6.
77. Heymann E, Hoppe W, Krusselmann A, et al. Organophosphate sensitive and insensitive carboxylesterases in human skin. Chem Biol Interact 1993; 87:217–26.
78. Prusakiewicz JJ, Ackermann C, Voorman R. Comparison of skin esterase from different species. Pharm Res 2006; 23:1517–24.
79. Jewell C, Ackermann C, Payne NA, et al. Specificity of procaine and ester hydrolysis by human, minipig and rat skin and liver. Drug Metab Dispos 2007; 35(11) (in press).
80. Jewell C, Prusakiewicz JJ, Ackermann C, et al. The distribution of esterases in the skin of the minipig. Toxicol Lett 2007; 173:118–23.
81. Clark NWE, Scott RC, Blain PG, et al. Fate of fluazifop butyl in rat and human skin in vitro. Arch Toxicol 1993; 67:44–8.
82. Hewitt PG, Perkins J, Hotchkiss SAM. Metabolism of fluroxypyr, fluroxypyr methyl ester, and the herbicide fluroxypyr methylheptyl ester. I: during percutaneous absorption through fresh rat and human skin in vitro. Drug Metab Dispos 2000; 28:748–54.
83. Lobemeier C, Tschoetschel C, Westie S, et al. Hydrolysis of parabenes by extracts from differing layers of human skin. Biol Chem 1996; 377:647–51.
84. Harville HM, Voorman R, Prusakiewicz JJ. Comparison of paraben stability in human and rat skin. Drug Metab Lett 2007; 1:17–21.
85. Ngawhirunpat T, Opanasopit P, Prakongpan S. Comparison of skin transport and metabolism of ethyl nicotinate in various species. Eur J Pharm Biopharm 2004; 58:645–51.
86. Tauber U, Rost KL. Esterase activity of the skin including species variation. In: Shroot B, Schaefer H, eds. Pharmacology and the Skin. Skin Pharmacokinetics. Vol. 1. Basel: Karger, 1987:170–83.
87. van Hooidonk C, Ceulen BI, Kienhuis H, et al. Rate of skin penetration of organophosphates measured in diffusion cells. In: Holmstedt B, Lauwerys R, Mercier M et al., eds Mechanisms of Toxicity and Hazard Evaluation. Amsterdam: Elsevier, 1980:643–6.
88. Mint A. Investigation into the topical disposition of the phthalic acid esters, dimethyl phthalate, diethyl phthalate and dibutyl phthalate in rat and human skin. PhD thesis, University of London, U.K., 1995.

89. Ngawhirunpat T, Kawakami J, Hatanaka T, et al. Age dependency of esterase activity in rat and human keratinocytes. Biol Pharm Bull 2003; 26:1311–4.

90. Barker CL, Clothier RH. Human keratinocyte cultures as models of cutaneous esterase activity. Toxicol In Vitro 1997; 11:637–40.

91. Kubota K, Ademola J, Maibach HI. Metabolism and degradation of betamethasone 17-valerate in homogenized living skin equivalent. Dermatology 1994; 188:13–7.

92. Boogaard PJ, van Elburg PA, de Kloe KP, et al. Metabolic inactivation of 2-oxiranyl-methyl 2-ethyl-2,5-dimethylhexanoate (C10GE) in skin, lung and liver of human, rat and mouse. Xenobiotica 1999; 29:987–1006.

93. Garnett A. Investigation of the in vitro percutaneous absorption and skin metabolism of benzyl acetate and related compounds. PhD thesis, University of London, U.K., 1992.

94. Weibel H, Hansen J. Interaction of cinnamaldehyde (a sensitiser in fragrance) with protein. Contact Dermatitis 1989; 20:161–6.

95. Tonge RP. The cutaneous disposition of the sensitizing chemicals hydroxycitronellal and dinitrochlorobenzene. PhD thesis, University of London, U.K., 1995.

96. Roper CS, Howes D, Blain PG, et al. Percutaneous penetration of 2-phenoxyethanol through rat and human skin. Food Chem Toxicol 1997; 35:1009–16.

97. Cheung C, Smith CK, Hoog JO, et al. Expression and localization of human alcohol and aldehyde dehydrogenase enzymes in skin. Biochem Biophys Res Commun 1999; 261:100–7.

98. Cheung C, Davies NG, Hoog JO, et al. Species variations in cutaneous alcohol dehydrogenases and aldehyde dehydrogenases may impact on toxicological assessments of alcohols and aldehydes. Toxicology 2003; 184:97–112.

99. Cheung C, Hotchkiss SAM, Pease CKS. Cinnamic compound metabolism in human skin and the role metabolism may play in determining relative sensitisation potency. J Dermatol Sci 2003; 31:9–19.

100. Smith CK, Moore CA, Elahi EN, et al. Human skin absorption and metabolism of the contact allergens, cinnamic aldehyde, and cinnamic alcohol. Toxicol Appl Pharmacol 2000; 168:189–99.

101. Lockley DJ, Howes D, Williams FM. Cutaneous metabolism of glycol ethers. Arch Toxicol 2005; 79:160–8.

102. Lockley DJ, Howes D, Williams FM. Percutaneous penetration and metabolism of 2-butoxyethanol. Arch Toxicol 2004; 78:617–28.

103. Lockley DJ, Howes D, Williams FM. Percutaneous penetration and metabolism of 2-ethoxyethanol. Toxicol Appl Pharmacol 2002; 180:74–82.

104. Ulrich K, Amatschek S, Uthman A, et al. Treatment of human skin with retinoic acid strongly induces aldehyde dehydrogenase 1A3. J Invest Dermatol 2004; 122:A87.

105. Ziegler DM. Flavin-containing monooxygenases—enzymes adapted for multisubstrate specificity. Trends Pharm Sci 1990; 11:321–4.

106. Hodgson E, Levi PE. The role of the flavin-containing monooxygenase (ec 1.14.13.8) in the metabolism and mode of action of agricultural chemicals. Xenobiotica 1992; 22:1175–83.

107. Hotchkiss SAM. Cutaneous toxicity: kinetic and metabolic determinants. Toxicol Ecotoxicol News 1995; 2:10–8.

108. Vyas PM, Roychowdhury S, Koukouritaki SB, et al. Enzyme-mediated protein haptenation of dapsone and sulfamethoxazole in human keratinocytes: II. Expression and role of flavin-containing monooxygenases and peroxidises. J Pharmacol Exp Thera 2006; 319:497–505.

109. Khan WA, Das M, Stick S, et al. Induction of epidermal NAD(P)H: quinone reductase by chemical carcinogens: a possible mechanism for detoxification. Biochem Biohpys Res Commun 1987; 146:126–33.

110. Merk HF, Jugert FK, Bonnekoh B, et al. Induction and inhibition of NAD(P)H: quinone reductase in murine and human skin. Skin Pharmacol 1991; 4:183–90.

111. Merk HF, Jugert FK. Cutaneous NAD(P)H: quinone reductase: a xenobiotic metabolizing enzyme with potential cancer and oxidative stress protecting properties. Skin Pharmacol 1991; 4:95–100.

112. Smith M. Quinones as mutagens, carcinogens, and anticancer agents: introduction and overview. J Toxicol Environ Health 1985; 16:665–72.
113. Lilienblum W, Irmscher G, Fusenig NE, et al. Induction of UDP-glucuronyltransferase and arylhydrocarbon hydroxylase activity in mouse skin and in normal and transformed skin cells in culture. Biochem Pharmacol 1986; 35:1517.
114. Afaq F, Mukhtar H. Effects of solar radiation on cutaneous detoxification pathways. J Photochem Photobiol B 2001; 63:61–9.
115. Connor MJ, Wheeler LA. Depletion of cutaneous glutathione by ultraviolet radiation. Photochem Photobiol 1987; 46:239–45.
116. Mannervik B, Awasthi YC, Board PG, et al. Nomenclature for human glutathione transferases. Biochem J 1992; 282:305–6.
117. Board PG, Baker RT, Chelvanayagam G, et al. Zeta, a novel class of glutathione transferases in a range of species from plants to humans. Biochem J 1997; 328:929–35.
118. Raza H, Awasthi YC, Zaim MT, et al. Glutathione S-trasnferases in human and rodent skin: multiple forms and species specific expression. J Invest Dermatol 1991; 96:463–7.
119. Campbell JA, Corrigall AV, Guy A, et al. Immunohistologic localization of alpha, mu and pi class glutathione S-transferases in human tissues. Cancer 1991; 67:1608–13.
120. Jewell C, Williams F. Absorption and metabolism of dinitrochlorobenzene through mouse skin in vitro. In: Brain KR, James VJ, Walters KA, eds. Prediction of Percutaneous Penetration. Vol. 4b. Cardiff: STS Publishing, 1996:218–21.
121. Strange RC, Spiteri MA, Ramachandran S, et al. Glutathione-S-transferase family of enzymes. Mutat Res Fundam Mol Mech Mutagen 2001; 482(special issue):21–6.
122. Ramachandran S, Fryer AA, Strange RC. Genetic factors determining cutaneous basal cell carcinoma phenotype. Med Ped Oncol 2001; 36:559–63.
123. Lear JT, Smith AG, Strange RC, et al. Detoxifying enzyme genotypes and susceptibility to cutaneous malignancy. Br J Dermatol 2000; 142:8–15.
124. Nakano H, Kimura J, Kumano T, et al. Decrease in class pi glutathione transferase mRNA levels by ultraviolet irradiation of cultured rat keratinocytes. Jpn J Cancer Res 1997; 88:1063–9.
125. Bock KW, Clausbruch UCV, Kaufmann R, et al. Functional heterogeneity of glucuronyltransferase in rat tissues. Biochem Pharmacol 1980; 29:495–500.
126. Soars MG, Ring BJ, Wrighton SA. The effect of incubation conditions on the enzyme kinetics of UDP-glucuronosyltransferases. Drug Metab Dispos 2003; 31:762–7.
127. Court MH. Isoform-selective probe substrates for in vitro studies of human UDP-glucuronosyltransferases. Methods Enzymol 2005; 400:104–16.
128. Belanger A, Pelletier G, Labrie F, et al. Inactivation of androgens by UDP-glucuronosyltransferase enzymes in humans. Trends Endocrinol Metab 2003; 14:473–9.
129. Honma W, Kamiyama Y, Yoshinari K, et al. Enzymatic characterisoation and interspecies difference of phenol sulfotransferases, ST1A forms. Drug Metab Dispos 2001; 29:274–81.
130. Honma W, Shimada M, Sasano H, et al. Phenol sulphotransferase ST1A3, as the main enzyme catalyzing the sulfation of troglitazone in human liver. Drug Metab Dispos 2002; 30:944–9.
131. Moss T, Howes D, Williams FM. Characteristics of sulphotransferases in human skin. In: Brain KR, James VR, Walters KA, eds. Predictions of Percutaneous Penetration. Vol. 4b. Cardiff: STS Publishing, 1996:307–11.
132. Moss T. Phase II metabolism during percutaneous penetration. PhD thesis, University of Newcastle, U.K., 1997.
133. Kohjitani A, Fuda H, Hanyu O, et al. Cloning, characterization and tissue expression of rat SULT2B1a and SULT2B1b steroid/sterol sulfotransferase isoforms: divergence of the rat SULT2B1 gene structure from orthologous human and mouse genes. Gene 2006; 367:66–73.
134. Higashi Y, Fuda H, Yania H, et al. Expression of cholesterol sulfotransferase (SULT2B1b) in human skin and primary cultures of human epidermal keratinocytes. J Invest Dermatol 2004; 122:1207–13.
135. Hotchkiss SAM. Dermal metabolism. In: Roberts MS, Walters KA, eds. Dermal Absorption and Toxicity Assessment. New York: Marcel Dekker, 1996:43–101.

136. Kawakubo Y, Merk HF, Al Masaoudi T, et al. N-acetylation of paraphenylene-diamine in human skin and keratinocytes. J Pharmacol Exp Thera 2000; 292:150–5.
137. Nohynek GJ, Skare JA, Meuling WJA, et al. Urinary acetylated metabolites and N-acetyltransferase-2 genotype in human subjects treated with a *para*-phenylenediamine-containing oxidative hair dye. Food Chem Toxicol 2004; 42:1885–91.
138. Nohynek GJ, Duche D, Garrigues A, et al. Under the skin: biotransformation of *para*-aminophenol and *para*-phenylenediamine in reconstructed human epidermis and human hepatocytes. Toxicol Lett 2005; 158:196–212.
139. Dressler WE, Appelqvist T. Plasma/blood pharmacokinetics and metabolism after dermal exposure to *para*-aminophenol or *para*-phenylenediamine. Food Chem Toxicol 2006; 44:371–9.
140. Nasseri-Sina P, Hotchkiss SAM, Caldwell J. Cutaneous xenobiotic metabolism: glycine conjugation in human and rat keratinocytes. Food Chem Toxicol 1997; 35:409–16.
141. Tobin DJ. Biochemistry of human skin—our brain on the outside. Chem Soc Rev 2006; 35:52–67.
142. Slominski A, Ermak G, Mihm M. ACTH receptor, CYP11A1, CYP17 and CYP21A2 genes are expressed in skin. J Clin Endocrinol Metab 1996; 81:2746–9.
143. Slominski A, Zjawiony J, Wortsman J, et al. A novel pathway for sequential transformation of 7-dehydrocholesterol and expression of the P450scc system in mammalian skin. Eur J Biochem 2004; 271:4178–88.
144. Thiboutot S, Jabara S, McAllister JM, et al. Human skin is a steroidogenic tissue: steroidogenic enzymes and cofactors are expressed in epidermis, normal sebocytes, and an immortalized sebocyte cell line (SEB-1). J Invest Dermatol 2003; 120:905–14.
145. Keeney DS, Skinner C, Weii S, et al. A keratinocyte-specific epoxygenase, CYP2B12, metabolizes arachidonic acid with unusual selectivity, producing a single major epoxyeicosatrienoic acid. J Biol Chem 1998; 273:9279–84.
146. Markova NG, Pinkas-Sarafova A, Karaman-Jurukovska N, et al. Expression pattern and biochemical characteristics of a major epidermal retinol dehydrogenase. Mol Gen Metab 2003; 78:119–35.
147. Slominski A, Pisarchik A, Semak I, et al. Serotoninergic and melatoninergic systems are fully expressed in human skin. FASEB J 2002; 16:896–8.
148. Slominski A, Pisarchik A, Semak I, et al. Characterization of the serotoninergic system in the C57BL/6 mouse skin. Eur J Biochem 2003; 270:3335–44.
149. Semak I, Korik E, Naumova M, et al. Serotonin metabolism in rat skin: characterization by liquid chromatography-mass spectrometry. Arch Biochem Biophys 2004; 421:61–6.
150. Slominski AJ, Wortsman J, Tobin DJ. The cutaneous serotoninergic/melatoninergic system: securing a place under the sun. FASEB J 2005; 19:176–94.

7 Formulation Issues

U. F. Schaefer
Biopharmaceutics and Pharmaceutical Technology, Saarland University, Saarbruecken, Germany

B. C. Lippold
Institute of Pharmaceutics and Biopharmaceutics, Heinrich Heine University, Duesseldorf, Germany

C. S. Leopold
Department of Pharmaceutical Technology, Institute of Pharmacy, University of Hamburg, Hamburg, Germany

SEMISOLID FORMULATIONS
Effects of Vehicles and Penetration Enhancers

After cutaneous administration of formulations such as ointments or creams, drug, vehicle, and the skin may affect the penetration process and thus drug action in different ways. Tronnier's triangle (Fig. 1) (1) serves as model to illustrate these relationships. Drug and vehicle are the components of cutaneous formulations, which may be divided into those intended for transdermal absorption and systemic action of the drug, those for regional effects in deeper tissue layers (e.g., joints) and those for action on or in the skin (local action) (2). Formulations intended for systemic drug action require therapeutic plasma levels of the drug. The use of transdermal patches, which remain on the skin for an extended period of time, allows in most cases a zero-order drug input kinetic and thus constant plasma levels over the whole application time period (3). While formulations with regional action require drug penetration into deeper skin tissues with minimal systemic action, for formulations with local action systemic action is undesired. In the latter case, drug penetration into the skin may be slow but accompanied by a high substantivity.

The efficacy of topically applied drugs is often limited by poor skin penetration (2,4,5). To improve the cutaneous absorption of drugs, various methods have been developed such as optimization of the thermodynamic activity of the drug, chemical penetration enhancers, novel vehicle systems, and physical enhancement techniques including iontophoresis, sonophoresis, and electroporation (2,5,6).

Thermodynamic Vehicle Effects

The thermodynamic activity of a drug in a vehicle represents the affinity of the drug to the vehicle and its tendency to penetrate into the stratum corneum. As a measure of the thermodynamic drug activity, the ratio of the drug concentration in the vehicle (c_V) and its solubility in this vehicle (c_{sV}) may be used. The thermodynamic drug activity therefore depends on the solubility of the drug in its vehicle (2,7). The highest thermodynamic activity of a drug is reached at the saturation level of

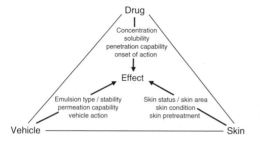

FIGURE 1 Triangular relationship between drug, vehicle, and skin status on the effect of a cutaneously applied drug formulation according to Tronnier. *Source*: From Ref. 1.

the drug c_{sV} in the vehicle. At the saturation level, the maximum drug flux J_{max} may be observed [equation (1)] (8):

$$J = \frac{D_B c_{sB}}{d_B} \frac{c_V}{c_{sV}} \rightarrow J_{max} = \frac{D_B c_{sB}}{d_B} \tag{1}$$

where D_B, diffusion coefficient of the drug in the barrier stratum corneum; d_B, thickness of the stratum corneum; c_{sB}, drug saturation concentration in the stratum corneum; c_{sV}, drug saturation concentration in the vehicle; c_V, drug concentration in the vehicle.

If a test formulation (T) is compared to a standard formulation (S), the relative effective activity coefficient $\gamma_{T/S}$ may be calculated as the ratio of the drug solubilities in the standard and test vehicle, respectively, provided that the solubilities are low because at low solubilities partition coefficients may be calculated as concentration ratios instead of activity ratios [equation (2)]. In the case of high drug solubilities, $\gamma_{T/S}$ may be calculated as the ratio of the drug partition coefficients between the vehicles and an aqueous phase ($PC_{S/T}$) (9):

$$\gamma_{T/S} = \frac{c_{sS}}{c_{sT}} = \frac{PC_{S/W}}{PC_{T/W}} \tag{2}$$

where $\gamma_{T/S}$, relative effective activity coefficient; c_{sS}, drug solubility in the standard vehicle; c_{sT}, drug solubility in the test vehicle; $PC_{S/W}$, partition coefficient standard vehicle/aqueous phase; $PC_{T/W}$, partition coefficient test vehicle/aqueous phase.

Saturated or supersaturated formulations with a high thermodynamic drug activity lead to higher penetration rates than unsaturated systems. A supersaturated state can be created by various methods just before or during application. Generally, the following three methods are available to obtain a supersaturated system: water uptake from the skin, evaporation of a volatile formulation component during application, and by using mixed cosolvent systems wherein vehicle changes are produced immediately prior to administration of the formulation (6). As a limiting factor for drug permeation from a supersaturated system, optimization of the degree of saturation in the basal formulation is important. The degree of saturation can increase by increasing the drug concentration or by decreasing the overall solubility of drugs in the cosolvent mixture (6). Both approaches can enhance the thermodynamic activity of drugs in the supersaturated systems and thus force drugs out of the vehicle and into the membrane. However, such solutions are thermodynamically unstable and can result in recrystallization of drugs even in the short term (6,10–12) leading to a decrease of the thermodynamic drug activity (5,13). Therefore, the use of penetration enhancers to improve drug penetration is often preferred over supersaturated systems.

Penetration-Enhancing Effects

Drug penetration can be improved by physical or chemical methods to break up the rigid structure of the stratum corneum, for example, by fluidization of the intercellular lipids (Fig. 2) (14–16). Because of the effect of penetration enhancers on the stratum corneum the lag time of drug diffusion through the stratum corneum is altered. This lag time is affected by the drug partition coefficient stratum corneum/vehicle, the length of the penetration pathway, and drug permeability [equation (3)] (17,18).

$$PCh = 6PL \tag{3}$$

where PC, drug partition coefficient stratum corneum/vehicle; h, length of the penetration pathway; P, drug permeability; L, lag time of drug diffusion through the stratum corneum.

The ratio of the activity coefficients with and without enhancer corresponds to the relative activity parameter K_r.

Penetration enhancers are compounds that alter the barrier properties of the stratum corneum by reversibly affecting the lipid bilayers (Fig. 2) or the protein structures in the corneocytes (14,19–21). The fluidization process leads to so-called kink isomers by movement of the CH-chains and the resulting change in conformation causing structural defects with mobile free space (15). In this mobile free space, small molecules may be deposited, which can permeate the barrier together with the kinks (15). Thereby, the lag time of drug diffusion into the skin is reduced and drug penetration is enhanced. The penetration-enhancing effect results from the increase of the diffusion coefficient in the barrier and the improved partitioning of the drugs into the stratum corneum (5,21,22).

Using differential scanning calorimetry (DSC), the phase transitions of untreated stratum corneum lipids are located at 70°C and 85°C. A fluidization of the lipids leads

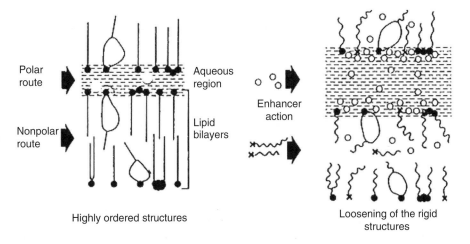

FIGURE 2 Polar and apolar routes of penetration through stratum corneum lipid bilayers according to Barry. *Source*: From Ref. 14.

to a shift of these phase transitions to lower temperatures as a result of a breakdown in lipid structure, which ultimately leads to an increase of the drug flux through the barrier (23). From a chemical point of view, polar penetration enhancers are bound to the polar head groups of the stratum corneum lipids through hydrogen bonds as well as ionic interactions (8) and/or the volume of bulk water within the bilayers is increased (24). In contrast, lipophilic enhancers induce the fluidization of the lipophilic chains in the lipid bilayers. The combination of hydrophilic and lipophilic penetration enhancers (e.g., ethanol and Azone®; Aderis Pharmaceuticals, Richmond, Virginia, U.S.A.) often leads to a synergistic enhancing effect (8,25).

Chemical penetration enhancers are therefore divided into compounds that interact with the lipids, for instance alcohols (propylene glycol), lipids (oleic acid), or surfactants (sodium lauryl sulfate) and substances that alter the protein structures in the corneocytes such as dimethyl sulfoxide (DMSO), urea, and water.

The following properties are required from penetration-enhancing compounds (26,27):

1. Physiologically inert,
2. No irritating or toxic action,
3. No allergic potential,
4. Reversibility of the effect,
5. Specificity with regard to the drug, and
6. Chemical and physical stability and compatibility.

Penetration-enhancing compounds can induce skin irritation and may significantly alter the stratum corneum lipids, in some cases irreversibly. Therefore, enhancers are used at the lowest possible concentrations or in combination. The calculation of enhancement ratios (ER), enhancement factors (EF), or enhancement indices (EI) allows a comparison of the effect of different penetration enhancers (28) [equation (4a–c)]. All three are described in the literature (7,8,29,30):

$$\mathrm{ER} = \frac{P_{\mathrm{B(E)}}}{P_{\mathrm{B(0)}}} \tag{4a}$$

where ER, enhancement ratio; $P_{\mathrm{B(E)}}$, permeability of the stratum corneum after enhancer treatment; $P_{\mathrm{B(0)}}$, permeability of the stratum corneum before enhancer treatment

$$\mathrm{EF} = \frac{J_{\mathrm{aT}}}{J_{\mathrm{aS}}} = \frac{f}{\gamma_{\mathrm{T/S}}} \tag{4b}$$

where EF, enhancement factor; f, bioavailability factor; $\gamma_{\mathrm{T/S}}$, relative effective activity coefficient; $J_{\mathrm{aT}}/J_{\mathrm{aS}}$, flux ratio of test and standard formulation at equal thermodynamic drug activities

$$\mathrm{EI}_{\mathrm{ER_{max}}}^{\log \mathrm{PC_{Oct/W}\ (drug)}}[\%] = \frac{\mathrm{ER_E} - 1}{\mathrm{ER_{max}} - 1} 100 \tag{4c}$$

where $\mathrm{ER_{max}}$, maximum ER; $\mathrm{ER_E}$, ER after enhancer treatment; $\log \mathrm{PC_{Oct/W}}$, logarithm of the partition coefficient octanol/water of the drug.

The EI is of interest mainly during tape-stripping studies, where it gives information on the percentage of the maximal possible penetration enhancement after pretreatment with an enhancer. The maximum ER ($\mathrm{ER_{max}}$) is the quotient of the permeability of the stripped skin, i.e., stratum corneum-free epidermis, and the permeability of the epidermis with stratum corneum (8).

Many compounds or compound classes, such as DMSO, diethylene-glycol-monoethylether (DGME, Transcutol P®; Gattfossé, Luzern, Switzerland), fatty acid esters, terpenes, and surfactants are penetration enhancers.

The simplest penetration enhancer is water. It is well-known that occlusive vehicles increase the hydration state of the stratum corneum and ultimately cause changes in the stratum corneum structure (Fig. 2) (31). DMSO is a widely used penetration enhancer (32) that improves the permeation of many drugs, particularly those with a molecular weight less than 3000 Da (5). The concentration required for enhancement usually exceeds 50% (5,29). After cutaneous penetration, DMSO is taken up in a concentration-dependent manner by the corneocytes and alters the conformation of the keratin from the α-helix to the β-pleated sheet structure (14,32,33). Moreover, due to the formation of larger shells of water molecules around the polar head groups a general change of the lipid bilayer structure takes place (14,29,32,33). After treatment of the skin with DMSO, Smith et al. (29) observed the formation of a depot of DMSO in the stratum corneum. Neat DMSO may cause skin irritation within minutes after application and a metabolite, dimethylsulfide, causes an unpleasant, garlic-like breath (29).

Another type of enhancing mechanism has been observed with DGME (34). Its hygroscopic properties improve water transport through the skin. Solubilization effects lead to enhanced drug penetration (5,21,34,35). DGME increases drug solubility in the stratum corneum and does not affect the lipid-phase transitions (35,36). After application of DGME a depot is formed within the epidermis, which may cause swelling of the stratum corneum (34). The increase in permeation is concentration dependent but the stratum corneum uptake capacity for DGME may be a limiting factor (37). The combination of DGME and oleic acid may improve the penetration process synergistically and increase the ER (38).

Fatty alcohols, fatty acids, and fatty acid esters are known penetration enhancers for hydrophilic and lipophilic drugs because of their amphiphilic nature (39,40). The penetration-enhancing effects lead to the following changes in the stratum corneum: (i) perturbation of the barrier properties, (ii) interactions with cellular proteins, (iii) improvement of drug partitioning into the stratum corneum, and (iv) formation of fatty acid–drug complexes with a higher octanol/water partition coefficient than the drug itself (41). The optimum chain lengths are between C10 and C12, because of their ability to significantly decrease the ceramide–cholesterol or cholesterol–cholesterol interactions (42). Unsaturated fatty acids and alcohols are more effective than the corresponding saturated species (43). With lauric acid, the alkyl chain length of 12 carbon atoms is crucial, as the compound shows an optimum balance between hydrophilic and lipophilic properties with this chain length leading to an improved partitioning into the skin and skin affinity (44). In contrast, oleic acid is a component of skin lipids (6%) and may easily be deposited in the stratum corneum. Interactions with the intercellular lipids and the formation of domains (micropores) lead to a decrease in viscosity and a fluidization of the lipid bilayers (39,45–49). The conformation of these lipids remains almost unchanged (48,49). If oleic acid causes a shift of the lipid-phase transitions after application to the skin remains unclear. Whereas Potts et al. observed a shift of the phase transitions to lower temperatures (50), Green et al. could not confirm this shift (46). If the conformation of the lipids remains unchanged, mainly the transport of charged molecules through the forming micropores is improved (51).

Among the polar solvents ethanol causes lipid fluidization at low concentrations by displacing water (15). In addition, lipids are extracted from the intercellular space, which further compromises the barrier (5). As a consequence, the transport of lipophilic substances is enhanced (52) but an increase of the ethanol concentration to over 50% causes the formation of micropores as a result of a conformation change of the keratin structures (53).

Laurocapram (1-dodecylazacycloheptane-2-one, Azone) belongs to the class of N-alkylated, cyclic amides (54). Its chemical structure, consisting of a polar head group connected to a long alkyl chain (5), and the spoon conformation are responsible for its effect as a penetration enhancer (15). It is deposited in the lipid bilayers and increases their fluidity (14). In addition, hydration of the stratum corneum takes place resulting from water retention and an increase of the diffusion coefficient in the barrier (35,54). In contrast to the enhancers discussed previously, a shift of the first three lipid-phase transitions to lower temperatures is observed. The reduction of the barrier function of the stratum corneum leads to an improved penetration of lipophilic and hydrophilic compounds (55–58). A major disadvantage of Azone is its skin irritating potential (59). Phosphatidylcholine also alters the structure of the lipid bilayers and enhances cutaneous drug penetration but without the disadvantage of skin irritation (59,60).

Propylene glycol is a well-known penetration enhancer for lipophilic drugs (61). It causes a conformation change of keratin from the α-helix to the β-pleated sheet structure (15,59). This conformation change facilitates the transcellular route of penetration (62). However, compared to DMSO, propylene glycol is an inferior penetration enhancer, as its influence on the structure of the intercellular lipids is less pronounced (43,63). Therefore, it is often used in combination with other enhancers and acts synergistically (14). At propylene glycol concentrations above 40% skin irritation may occur (64).

Surfactants, e.g., sodium lauryl sulfate, also have penetration-enhancing properties with a mode of action similar to that of laurocapram. Cationic surfactants have a high skin irritation potential and they would not be used as enhancers. In contrast, electron microscopic investigations by Gloor et al. revealed no significant damage to the stratum corneum after treatment with the anionic surfactant sodium lauryl sulfate (65). The observed dehydration of the stratum corneum was explained by the decrease of the water-binding amino acids. Nonionic surfactants such as sucrose esters have not caused skin irritation (66) but are capable of fluidizing stratum corneum lipids.

Ingredients of essential oils, e.g., terpenes, can enhance the permeation of hydrophilic and lipophilic drugs (67). They are characterized by a low systemic toxicity and negligible skin irritation. Monoterpenes and sesquiterpenes are used, but whether alcohols or ketones are more efficient enhancers is still under discussion (47,68). The most frequently used terpenes are D-limonene, (−) carvone, (−)menthone, R(+)pulegone, nerolidole, and 1,8-cineole (17,69). According to DSC data they shift the lipid-phase transitions to lower temperatures and swell the lipid structures. They do not affect the keratin structure. With D-limonene a melting point depression of the lipid bilayers was observed (69). If terpene uptake by the lipid bilayers were only dependent on their solubility, terpenes with low melting points would be more efficient as penetration enhancers because of their higher solubility (70). Finally, some drugs themselves may act as penetration enhancers. For instance, with local anesthetic bases effects on the stratum corneum structure were shown (71).

Depletion Effects

With solution-type drug formulations applied to the skin depletion effects in the vehicles may be observed under finite-dose conditions. Drug depletion may result from a high thermodynamic activity of the drug in the vehicle and/or from pronounced penetration enhancement caused by vehicle components or by the vehicle itself. The extent of this effect depends on the thickness of the applied ointment layer. Because ointments are usually applied to the skin as thin films, decreased drug penetration rates have to be taken into consideration (72). Drug depletion may lead to a reduction of the drug-induced response and thus has a major impact on the quantification of vehicle effects using pharmacodynamic response data. Mathematical models have been developed to describe drug depletion (73–78).

Using Fick's First Law of diffusion, bioavailability factors f may be obtained by calculating the ratios of the first-order penetration rate constants of a test vehicle k_T and a standard vehicle k_S [equation (5)].

$$f = k_T/k_S \tag{5a}$$

where the penetration rate constant k is defined as follows:

$$k = D_B A PC_{B/V}/(d_B V) \tag{5b}$$

where D_B, diffusion coefficient of the drug in the barrier stratum corneum; A, application area; $PC_{B/V}$, stratum corneum/vehicle partition coefficient of the drug; d_B, thickness of the stratum corneum; V, volume of the applied formulation.

The ratio V/A is an expression of the thickness h of the ointment layer.

From the horizontal distance between the parallel portions of dose–response curves of a standard (S) and a test formulation (T) at a certain response level Resp% the bioavailability factor f is determined as follows [equation (6)] (8,79,80):

$$\log f = \log \text{dose}_{\text{Resp\%S}} - \log \text{dose}_{\text{Resp\%T}} \tag{6a}$$
$$f = \text{dose}_{\text{Resp\%S}}/\text{dose}_{\text{Resp\%T}} \tag{6b}$$

In practice, the shape of the dose–response curves is often sigmoidal. A plateau is reached as soon as the permeant solubility limit in the vehicle is exceeded. This plateau may be elevated under the influence of penetration enhancers (8).

The bioavailability factor f also depends on the volume of the applied vehicles. The use of concentration–response curves mathematically eliminates the influence of the preparation volume on f and, assuming equal areas of application for test and standard formulations, also the thickness of the formulation. After elimination of the ointment film thickness, the resulting bioavailability factors are called f_h:

$$\log f_h = \log c_{\text{Resp\%S}} - \log c_{\text{Resp\%T}} \tag{7a}$$
$$f_h = c_{\text{Resp\%S}}/c_{\text{Resp\%T}} \tag{7b}$$
$$f_h = k_T h_T/(k_S h_S) = P_{B(T)}/P_{B(S)} \tag{7c}$$

Any increase of k leads to a more or less pronounced drug depletion. This phenomenon is not described by the above equations. With the data of penetration studies performed under both infinite- and finite-dose conditions, drug depletion which usually occurs under finite-dose conditions and which manifests itself in a significant decrease of the drug penetration rate and thus in an insufficient parallelism of dose–response or concentration–response curves, can be quantified. In order to do so, a so-called depletion factor (DF) has been introduced and can be calculated from the infinite-dose (inf) and finite-dose (fin) EF as follows (81):

$$DF = EF_{inf}/EF_{fin} \qquad (8)$$

Depending on which vehicle is chosen as standard, these DFs can reach values greater or smaller than unity. A standard vehicle, which shows pronounced penetration-enhancing properties, leads to values ≤ 1 whereas an inert standard vehicle leads to values ≥ 1. It has to be mentioned that not only the diffusion coefficient and the solubility in the barrier as described by the EF but also every single factor included in k contributes to the extent of drug depletion (81).

Changes in the Vehicle on Application to the Skin

Normally semisolid cutaneous formulations will be applied to the skin in a thin layer. However, during application the formulation undergoes many changes in composition due to mechanical agitation, e.g., rubbing, and evaporation of ingredients. As a result the properties of the formulation may change and the active moiety will be influenced in different ways. In addition, these processes of change will continue as long as the formulation remains on the skin. This phenomenon is described by Surber et al. (82) as metamorphosis of the vehicle. For example, evaporation of water will result in a more lipophilic matrix, which will influence the partition between the stratum corneum and the formulation. Moreover, depending on the physicochemical properties of the active ingredient changes in phase distribution within the formulation may occur leading to modifications in the thermodynamic activity of the drug within the formulation. If supersaturation takes place the drug is delivered to the skin in higher amounts.

SPECIAL DELIVERY SYSTEMS

Transdermal Patches

Transdermal drug delivery systems have been developed since the 1970s. The first commercial available product was a scopolamine patch that was approved by the FDA in 1979. The patch delivered scopolamine at a constant rate for three days to treat motion sickness. Today transdermal patches exist for many drugs such as clonidine, estradiol, fentanyl, lidocaine, nicotine, nitroglycerine, oxybutynin, testosterone, and norelgestrone in combination with ethinylestradiol (83). However, not every drug is suitable for formulation as a transdermal patch. In addition to liopophilicity and molecular size of the drug, parameters influencing skin permeation, high pharmacological potency (efficacy) of the drug is needed so that only small amounts of drugs need be delivered. If the necessary drug amount exceeds a certain magnitude the required patch size would be too large. Often skin penetration enhancers are needed, and those most often used are ethanol, oleic acid, and propylene glycol or a combination. Two different types of transdermal patch are presently marketed; the reservoir type and the matrix type. Characteristic of the reservoir type is a rate-controlling membrane, which encloses the reservoir containing the drug usually in suspension, often dispersed in a gel. Thus, zero-order release is maintained for a longer time period. In contrast, matrix-type patches consist of the drug embedded in the adhesive resulting in a $\sqrt{t}$-delivery. However, in many cases, skin permeation is determined by skin permeability and not by drug delivery. From safety aspects, matrix-type patches are preferable to reservoir types as there is no problem with dose dumping. A major drawback of both types of patches is the potential for local irritation (84,85) but this can be minimized by changing the site after each application. Relatively large patches with drugs for regional action such as erythema inducing substances have been in use for a long time. Modern antirheumatic patches contain nonsteroidal anthitheumatic drugs, e.g., diclofenac.

Thin Polymeric Films for Cutaneous Use

Polymeric solutions with film-forming properties may serve as an alternative to transdermal patches. In contrast to patches, film-forming solutions provide many advantages, e.g., highly flexible dosing and improved cosmetic appearance. More-over, film-forming solutions are superior to semisolid preparation with regard to adhesion to the skin and therefore prolonged residence on the skin surface. Polymeric film-forming solutions have been used in skin care for a long time, however, they are normally applied for nonsurgical care of minor skin injury (86,87) or for skin protection around wounds (88). Misra et al. (89) report on the use of a testosterone formulation containing polyvinylpyrrolidone and polyvinyl alcohol in isopropanol, which results in biphasic drug delivery. More information on poly-meric drug loaded film-forming solutions for application to the skin is given by Zurdo Schroeder et al. (90) who evaluate different groups of polymers, such as acrylates, polyurethane acrylates, cellulose derivatives, polyvinylpyrrolidones, and silicones, for suitability. It was found that no correlation existed between transepi-dermal water loss in vivo and water permeability in vitro. The same authors showed (Fig. 3) that the permeation of the drug ethinylestradiol is enhanced from the film-forming polymeric solution with DynamX® (National Starch and Chemical Co., Bridgewater, New Jersey, U.S.A.; polyurethane-14 and AMP-acrylates copolymer) and Klucel® LF (Hercules, Inc., Wilmington, Delaware, U.S.A.; hydroxypropyl cellulose) when compared with a 5% solution of ethinylestradiol in ethanol using in vitro human heat separated epidermis (91). Furthermore, it was shown that Eudragit® RLPO (Roehm Pharma Polymers, Darmstadt, Germany; ammonio methacrylate copolymer type A) reduced the amount of drug permeated whereas with SMG36® (Dow Corning SA, Seneffe, Belgium; silicon gum) more or less the same values were obtained as for the reference vehicle.

A new film-forming formulation composed of terbinafine (Lamisil Once®, Novartis, Germany) is available as an antimycotic skin treatment. The manufacturer claims that using this application a depot will build up in the stratum corneum for over a week with drug concentration levels higher than the minimal active concentration.

Vesicular Carriers

Liposomes

Normally liposomes consist of phospholipids and in some cases cholesterol is added. They are widely used as colloidal carriers with a double-layer structure especially for drug targeting. First reports on the use of liposomes in cutaneous

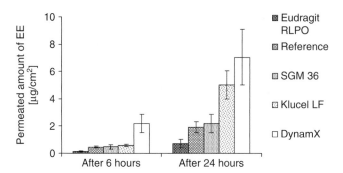

FIGURE 3   Influence of polymer type on the permeated amount of ethinylestradiol (EE) through heat separated human epidermis (Franz diffusion cell experiments).

application were those of Mezei et al. (92). Using triamcinolone acetonide and other steroids (93) they found that liposomes reduced drug absorption but there was significant enrichment in the epidermis and dermis, the site of drug's action. The modulation of drug delivery by liposomal preparations was also shown for many other drugs including betamethasone diproprionate (94), tretinoin (95), dyphilline (96), caffeine (97), tetracaine (98), cyclosporin (99), and interferon-γ (100). The mode of interaction of liposomes with the skin is unclear but it is generally accepted that liposomes do not permeate the stratum corneum intact. Liposomes may fuse with stratum corneum lipids and deliver their drug content to the skin. Furthermore, liposome permeation of the hair follicles has been discussed (101–103).

Niosomes
In contrast to classical liposomes, niosomes are composed of nonionic surfactants such as polyoxyethylene alkyl ethers. Their potential as a cutaneous delivery system was investigated by Bouwstra et al. (104) using estradiol. Two mechanisms were postulated for the improvement of drug delivery: a penetration enhancement effect of the individual surfactant molecules and an interaction of the vesicular structure with the stratum corneum lipids at the interface. Skin interactions of liposomes and niosomes are reviewed (105).

Transfersomes
The term transfersome was introduced by Cevc et al. (106) to describe vesicles consisting of a mixture of phosphatidylcholine, sodium cholate, and ethanol. They postulated that their flexible structure allowed transfersomes to penetrate the skin as intact vesicles as a result of the hydration gradient within the stratum corneum. Transfersomes, composed of polysorbate surfactants and containing a variety of steroids, had more prolonged activity and were 10-fold more potent in their anti-inflammatory response to arachidonic acid-induced murine ear edema compared with classical cream application (107,108).

Ethosomes
Ethosomes are phospholipid vesicular systems containing high amounts of ethanol and are suggested to enhance skin penetration of lipophilic and hydrophilic drugs. Ethosomes dramatically enhanced the skin permeation of minoxidil when

compared to ethanolic, hydroethanolic, or phospholipid ethanolic micellar solutions, and testosterone when compared to commercial testosterone patches (109). Horwitz et al. (110) investigated the clinical efficacy of ethosomal acyclovir and reported improved efficacy compared to a standard cream. The potential of this carrier system was also shown for trihexyphenidyl HCl (111), azelaic acid (112), finasteride (113), erythromycin (114), and ammonium glycyrrhizinate (115).

Nanoparticles
Solid Lipid Nanoparticles
In the early 1990s, solid lipid nanoparticles (SLN) were introduced as drug carriers in pharmaceutical formulations. In general, SLN are composed of physiological solid lipids and an emulsifier and are manufactured by a high-pressure homogenization process. Prednicarbate loaded SLNs in an aqueous dispersion were compared to prednicarbate cream (Dermatop® cream; Sanofi-Aventis, Frankfurt, Germany) using human skin in vitro (flow through diffusion cells) (116). It was shown that the SLN dispersions were superior to the cream with a 30% increase in prednicarbate penetration. Cytotoxicity of the SLNs, evaluated by MTT (3-[4,5-dimethylthiazol-2-yl]-2,5-diphenyltetrazolium bromide) assay with keratinocyte monolayers, showed a clear dependency on SLNs composition.

Jenning et al. (117) demonstrated the time dependence of drug distribution in porcine skin in vitro from SLNs loaded with vitamin A. After 6-hour exposure to the SLN, there was an increased targeting to the upper skin layers compared to that obtained with a nano-emulsion preparation. In contrast to these findings, the concentration was reduced after an incubation period of 24 hours. The authors stated that this is related to polymorphic transformation of the SLN. Furthermore, incorporation of the SLN dispersion in a xanthan gum hydrogel or an o/w cream had an influence. With the hydrogel preparation, similar effects to the dispersion were detected. However, incorporation of the SLN into an o/w cream delayed the polymorphic transformation leading to similar drug distributions at 6 and 24 hours. There were no SLN occlusive effects. This is in contrast to Wissing et al. (118) who reported an occlusive effect for sunscreen systems based on SLN incorporated with tocopherol acetate. These different results may be attributed to different experimental conditions. While Jenning et al. (117) used skin-based models, Wissing et al. (118) measured evaporation from a water reservoir covered with a membrane either treated or not treated with the SLN preparation. In a further study, Wissing et al. (119) investigated the effect of SLN on the penetration of oxybenzone, a sunscreen, in humans using a tape-stripping technique. They demonstrated that oxybenzone incorporated into SLN gave a sustained release, resulting in a longer duration of sunscreen on the skin surface. A similar effect was reported by Yener et al. (120) for the sunscreen octyl methoxycinnamate (OMC).

Chen et al. (121) incorporated podophyllotoxin into SLN to reduce systemic side effects after cutaneous application. In comparison to podophyllotoxin in an ethanolic solution no drug transport through porcine skin was observed with the SLN preparations over 8 hours but, depending on the SLN composition, enrichment of podophyllotoxin in the skin was detected.

Nanostructured Lipid Carriers
A recent development of the SLNs are nanostructured lipid carriers (NLC) which have an additional lipophilic liquid nanophase embedded in the lipophilic solid.

Advantages of these carriers are their higher drug load and higher physical stability (122). Ricci et al. (123) reported a delayed and sustained activity for indomethacin loaded NLC after cutaneous application in vitro and in vivo.

Polymeric Nanoparticles

Self-assembling nanoparticles containing minoxidil were prepared from poly(ε-capro-lactone-)block-poly(ethylenglycol) copolymer by a solvent evaporation technique and applied in vitro and in vivo to the skin of hairy and hairless guinea pigs and hairless mice (124). For hairy guinea pigs, it was clearly demonstrated that minoxidil permeation was enhanced using nanoparticles compared to an ethanolic solution and a liposomal preparation. This effect was not seen in the hairless species. The authors suggested that permeation enhancement was due to facilitated nanoparticle penetration to hair follicles. These findings are in accordance with several other reports (125–128) but are in contrast to other publications. Shim et al. (124) demonstrated by means of ^{1}H-NMR spectroscopy that minoxidil loaded nanoparticles were found in the receptor phase and therefore must have permeated the skin. Small nanoparticles (40 nm) penetrated faster than larger nanoparticles (130 nm).

Nanoencapsulation of highly lipophilic OMC, a sunscreen, into the biodegradable polymer poly(ε-caprolactone) resulted in a 3.4-fold increased OMC level within porcine stratum corneum compared with an OMC emulsion whereas penetration into deeper porcine skin layers was not affected (128). The same authors showed, using confocal laser microscopy, that nile red encapsulated in poly(ε-caprolactone) resulted in deeper penetration of the dye into porcine skin compared to a solution in propylene glycol. This effect was attributed to a higher thermodynamic activity of the drug in the nanoparticulate preparation. Using human skin, Luengo et al. (129) showed that permeation of flufenamic acid encapsulated in PLGA [poly(DL-lactide-co-glycolide)] was enhanced and that higher amounts were found in deeper skin layers over 12 hours compared to an aqueous solution, possibly mediated by pH alterations due to polymer degradation. Stracke et al. (130), using fluorescent-labeled PLGA nanoparticles and multiphoton microscopy, showed that nanoparticles accumulated in skin furrows with prolonged residence on the stratum corneum surface.

The potential use of nanoparticles for the delivery of vaccines and DNA to the skin has been discussed (131,132). Briefly, negatively charged particles with a size less than 50 nm appear feasible for vaccine and DNA delivery. However, for each application, the system has to be optimized (133).

Microparticles: Inorganic Microfine Particles

Microfine metallic oxides such as titanium dioxide and zinc oxide are powerful protecting agents against UV radiation. Although widely used, there are few reports on their behavior after application to the skin. Using spectroscopic and microscopic techniques, Lademann et al. (134) demonstrated that, although titanium dioxide particles did not penetrate into the viable skin tissue in vivo, enrichment in the follicular regions was observed. Similar data were obtained by Pfluecker et al. (135) using light and electron microscopy. Gamer et al. (136) confirmed these results in vitro using titanium dioxide and zinc oxide.

REFERENCES

1. Tronnier H. Arzneitherapie an der Haut. Pharm Ztg 1977; 45:2021–7.
2. Lippold BC. How to optimize drug penetration through the skin. Pharm Acta Helv 1992; 67:294–300.
3. Schiller M, Schmidt PC. Transdermale therapeutische Systeme—Arzneistoffe zum Aufkleben. Pharm Ztg 2002; 22:18–24.
4. Moser K, Kriwet K, Fröhlich C, et al. Supersaturation: enhancement of skin penetration and permeation of a lipophilic drug. Pharm Res 2001; 18:1006–11.
5. Moser K, Kriwet K, Naik A, et al. Passive skin penetration enhancement and its quantification in vitro. Eur J Pharm Biopharm 2001; 52:103–12.
6. Moser K, Kriwet K, Fröhlich C, et al. Permeation enhancement of a highly lipophilic drug using supersaturated systems. J Pharm Sci 2001; 90:605–14.
7. Leopold CS. Enhancer-Effekte von lipophilen Salbengrundstoffen auf die Steady-State-Penetration von Methylnicotinat durch die Haut. PhD Thesis, University of Düsseldorf, 1992.
8. Bach M, Lippold BC. Percutaneous penetration enhancement and its quantification. Eur J Pharm Biopharm 1998; 46:1–13.
9. Lippold BC, Reimann H. Wirkungsbeeinflussung bei Lösungssalben durch Vehikel am Beispiel von Methylnicotinat. Teil I: relative thermodynamische aktivität des Arzneistoffs in verschiedenen Vehikeln und Freisetzungsverhalten. Acta Pharm Technol 1989; 35:136–9.
10. Iervolino M, Raghavan SL, Hadgraft J. Membrane penetration enhancement of ibuprofen using supersaturation. Int J Pharm 2000; 198:229–38.
11. Moser K, Kriwet K, Kalia YN, et al. Stabilization of supersaturated solutions of a lipophilic drug for dermal delivery. Int J Pharm 2001; 224:169–76.
12. Raghavan SL, Kiepfer B, Davis AF, et al. Membrane transport of hydrocortisone acetate from supersaturated solutions; the role of polymers. Int J Pharm 2001; 221:95–105.
13. Iervolino M, Cappello B, Raghavan SL, et al. Penetration enhancement of ibuprofen from supersaturated solutions through human skin. Int J Pharm 2001; 212:131–41.
14. Barry BW. Mode of action of penetration enhancers in human skin. J Control Release 1987; 6:85–97.
15. Suhonen TM, Bouwstra JC, Urtti A. Chemical enhancement of percutaneous absorption in relation to stratum corneum structural alterations. J Control Release 1999; 59:149–61.
16. Wotton PK, Mollgaard B, Hadgraft JW, et al. Vehicle effect on topical drug delivery. III: effect of azone on the cutaneous permeation of metronidazole and propylene glycol. Int J Pharm 1985; 24:19–26.
17. Vaddi HK, Ho PC, Chan SY. Terpenes in propylene glycol as skin-penetration enhancers: permeation and partition of haloperidol, fourier transform infrared spectroscopy, and differential scanning calorimetry. J Pharm Sci 2002; 91:1639–51.
18. Potts RO, Francoeur ML. The influence of stratum corneum morphology on water permeability. J Invest Dermatol 1991; 96:495–9.
19. Hadgraft J. Modulation of the barrier function of the skin. Skin Pharmacol Appl Skin Physiol 2001; 14:72–81.
20. Loth H. Vehicular influence on transdermal drug penetration. Int J Pharm 1991; 68:1–10.
21. Hadgraft J. Skin deep. Eur J Pharm Biopharm 2004; 58:291–9.
22. Yamane MA, Williams AC, Barry BW. Effects of terpenes and oleic acid as skin penetration enhancers towards 5-fluorouracil as assessed with time; permeation, partitioning and differential scanning calorimetry. Int J Pharm 1995; 116:237–51.
23. Pilgram GSK, van der Meulen J, Gorris GS, et al. The influence of two azones and sebaceous lipids on the lateral organization of lipids isolated from human stratum corneum. Biochim Biophys Acta 2001; 1511:244–54.
24. Barry BW. Lipid-protein-partitioning theory of skin penetration enhancement. J Control Release 1991; 15:237–48.
25. Bouwstra JA, Pilgram G, Gooris GS, et al. New aspects of the skin barrier organization. Skin Pharmacol Appl Skin Physiol 2001; 14:52–62.

26. Akimoto T, Aoyagi T, Minoshima J, et al. Polymeric percutaneous drug penetration enhancer: synthesis and enhancing property of PEG/PDMS block copolymer with a cationic end group. J Control Release 1997; 49:229–41.
27. Godwin DA, Michniak BB. Influence of drug lipophilicity on terpenes as transdermal penetration enhancers. Drug Dev Ind Pharm 1999; 25:905–15.
28. Cornwell PA, Barry BW. Effects of penetration enhancer treatment on the statistical distribution of human skin permeabilities. Int J Pharm 1995; 117:101–12.
29. Smith EW, Maibach HI. Percutaneous Penetration Enhancers. Boca Raton, FL: CRC Press, 1995.
30. Wilhelm KP, Surber C, Maibach HI. Effect of sodium lauryl sulfate-induced skin irritation on in vivo percutaneous absorption of four drugs. J Invest Dermatol 1991; 96:927–32.
31. Frömder A, Lippold BC. Water vapour transmission and occlusivity in vivo of lipophilic excipients used in ointments. Int J Cosmet Sci 1993; 15:113–24.
32. Anigbogu ANC, Williams AC, Barry BW, et al. Fourier transform raman spectroscopy of interactions between the penetration enhancer dimethyl sulfoxide and human stratum corneum. Int J Pharm 1995; 125:265–82.
33. Puttnam NA. Attenuated total reflectance studies of the skin. J Soc Cosmet Chem 1972; 23:209–26.
34. Godwin DA, Kim N-H, Felton LA. Influence of Transcutol® CG on the skin accumulation and transdermal permeation of ultraviolet absorbers. Eur J Pharm Biopharm 2002; 53:23–7.
35. Harrison JE, Watkinson AC, Green DM, et al. The relative effect of Azone® and Transcutol® on permeant diffusivity and solubility in human stratum corneum. Pharm Res 1996; 13:542–6.
36. Gwak HS, Oh IS, Chun IK. Transdermal delivery of ondansetron hydrochloride: effects of vehicles and penetration enhancers. Drug Dev Ind Pharm 2004; 30:187–94.
37. Panchagnula R, Ritschel WA. Development and evaluation of an intracutaneous depot formulation of corticosteroids using transcutol as a cosolvent: in-vitro, ex-vitro and in-vivo rat studies. J Pharm Pharmacol 1991; 43:609–14.
38. Touitou E, Levi-Schaffer F, Dayan N, et al. Modulation of caffeine skin delivery by carrier design: liposomes versus penetration enhancers. Int J Pharm 1994; 103:131–6.
39. Yamashita F, Koyama Y, Kitano M, et al. Analysis of in vivo skin penetration enhancement by oleic acid based on two-layer diffusion model with polar and nonpolar routes in the stratum corneum. Int J Pharm 1995; 117:173–9.
40. Cornwell PA, Tubek J, van Gompel HAHP, et al. Glycerol monocaprylate/caprate as a moderate skin penetration enhancer. Int J Pharm 1998; 171:243–55.
41. Wang Y, Fan Q, Song Y, et al. Effects of fatty acids and iontophoresis on the delivery of midodrine hydrochloride and the structure of human skin. Pharm Res 2003; 20:1612–8.
42. Kanikkannan N, Singh M. Skin permeation enhancement effect and skin irritation of saturated fatty alcohols. Int J Pharm 2002; 248:219–28.
43. Tanojo H, Boelsma E, Junginger HE, et al. In vivo human skin permeability enhancement by oleic acid: a laser Doppler velocimetry study. J Control Release 1999; 58:97–104.
44. Stott PW, Williams AC, Barry BW. Mechanistic study into the enhanced transdermal permeation of a model β-blocker, propranolol, by fatty acids: a melting point depression effect. Int J Pharm 2001; 219:161–76.
45. Menon GK. New insights into skin structure: scratching the surface. Adv Drug Deliv Rev 2002; 54:3–17.
46. Green PG, Guy RH, Hadgraft J. In vitro and in vivo enhancement of skin permeation with oleic and lauric acids. Int J Pharm 1988; 48:103–11.
47. Meidan VM, Al-Khalili M, Michniak BB. Enhanced iontophoretic delivery of buspirone hydrochloride across human skin using chemical enhancers. Int J Pharm 2003; 264:73–83.
48. Tanojo H, Junginger HE, Bodde HE. In vivo skin permeability enhancement by oleic acid: transepidermal water loss and Fourier-transform infrared spectroscopy studies. J Control Release 1997; 47:31–9.

49. Naik A, Pechthold LARM, Potts RO, et al. Mechanism of oleic acid-induced skin penetration enhancement in vivo in humans. J Control Release 1995; 37:299–306.
50. Potts RO, Golden GM, Francoeur ML, et al. Mechanism and enhancement of solute transport across the stratum corneum. J Control Release 1991; 15:249–60.
51. Ongpipattanakul B, Burnette RR, Potts RO, et al. Evidence that oleic acid exists in a separate phase within stratum corneum lipids. Pharm Res 1991; 8:350–4.
52. Kurihara-Bergstrom T, Knutson K, DeNoble LJ, et al. Percutaneous absorption enhancement of an ionic molecule by ethanol–water systems in human skin. Pharm Res 1990; 7:762–6.
53. Megrab NA, Williams AC, Barry BW. Oestradiol permeation across human skin, silastic and snake skin membranes: the effects of ethanol/water co-solvent systems. Int J Pharm 1995; 116:101–12.
54. Szolar-Platzer C, Patil S, Maibach HI. Effect of topical laurocapram (Azone®) on the in vitro percutaneous permeation of sodium lauryl sulfate using human skin. Acta Derm Venereol 1996; 76:182–5.
55. Dias M, Raghavan SL, Hadgraft J. ATR–FTIR spectroscopic investigation on the effect of solvents on the permeation of benzoic acid and salicylic acid through silicone membranes. Int J Pharm 2001; 216:51–9.
56. Bouwstra JA, Peschier LJC, Brussee J, et al. Effect of N-alkyl-azocycloheptan-2-ones including Azone® on the thermal behaviour of human stratum corneum. Int J Pharm 1989; 52:47–54.
57. Harrison JE, Groundwater PW, Brain KR, et al. Azone®, induced fluidity in human stratum corneum. A fourier transform infrared spectroscopy investigation using the perdeuterated analogue. J Control Release 1996; 41:283–90.
58. Degim IT, Uslu A, Hadgraft J, et al. The effects of azone and capsaicin on the permeation of naproxen through human skin. Int J Pharm 1999; 179:21–5.
59. Fang J-Y, Hwang T-L, Fang CL, et al. In vitro and in vivo evaluations of the efficacy and safety of skin permeation enhancers using flurbiprofen as a model drug. Int J Pharm 2003; 255:153–66.
60. Bonina FP, Montenegro L, Scrofani N, et al. Effects of phospholipid based formulations on in vitro and in vivo percutaneous absorption of methyl nicotinate. J Control Release 1995; 34:53–63.
61. Touitou E, Levi-Schaffer F, Shaco-Ezra N, et al. Enhanced permeation of theophylline through the skin and its effect on fibroblast proliferation. Int J Pharm 1991; 70:159–66.
62. Bendas B, Schmalfuß U, Neubert R. Influence of polypropylene glycol as cosolvent on mechanisms of drug transport from hydrogels. Int J Pharm 1995; 116:19–30.
63. Morimoto Y, Sugibayashi K, Hosoya K, et al. Penetration enhancing effect of azone on the transport of 5-fluorouracil across the hairless rat skin. Int J Pharm 1986; 32:31–8.
64. Funk JO, Maibach HI. Propylene glycol dermatitis: re-evaluation of an old problem. Contact Dermatitis 1994; 31:236–41.
65. Gloor M, Hauth A, Gehring W. O/W emulsions compromise the stratum corneum barrier and improve drug penetration. Pharmazie 2003; 58:709–15.
66. Ayala-Bravo HA, Quintanar-Guerrero D, Naik A, et al. Effects of sucrose oleate and sucrose laureate on in vivo human stratum corneum permeability. Pharm Res 2003; 20:1267–73.
67. El-Kattan AF, Asbill CS, Kim N, et al. The effects of terpene enhancers on the percutaneous permeation of drugs with different lipophilicities. Int J Pharm 2001; 215:229–40.
68. Arellano A, Santoyo S, Martin C, et al. Enhancing effect of terpenes on the in vitro percutaneous absorption of diclofenac sodium. Int J Pharm 1996; 130:141–5.
69. Cornwell PA, Barry BW, Bouwstra JA, et al. Modes of action of terpene penetration enhancers in human skin; differential scanning calorimetry, small-angle X-ray diffraction and enhancer uptake studies. Int J Pharm 1996; 127:9–26.
70. Mackay KMB, Williams AC, Barry BW. Effect of melting point of chiral terpenes on human stratum corneum uptake. Int J Pharm 2001; 228:89–97.

71. Roemmen C, Leopold CS, Lippold BC. Do local anesthetics have an influence on the percutaneous penetration of a model corticosteroid? An in vivo study using the vasoconstrictor assay Eur J Pharm Sci 1999; 9:227–34.

72. Zatz JL. Percutaneous absorption: computer simulation using multicompartmented membrane models. In: Bronaugh RL, Maibach HI, eds. Percutaneous Absorption. New York: Marcel Dekker, 1985:165–81.

73. Guy RH, Hadgraft J. A theoretical description relating skin penetration to the thickness of the applied medicament. Int J Pharm 1980; 6:321–32.

74. Cooper ER, Berner B. Finite dose pharmacokinetics of skin penetration. J Pharm Sci 1985; 74:1100–2.

75. Zatz JL. Influence of depletion on percutaneous absorption characteristics. J Soc Cosmet Chem 1985; 36:237–49.

76. Addicks WJ, Flynn G, Weiner N, et al. A mathematical model to describe drug release from thin topical applications. Int J Pharm 1989; 56:243–8.

77. Addicks W, Weiner N, Flynn G, et al. Topical drug delivery from thin applications: theoretical predictions and experimental results. Pharm Res 1990; 7:1048–54.

78. Walker M, Chambers LA, Hollingsbee DA, et al. Significance of vehicle thickness to skin penetration of halcinonide. Int J Pharm 1991; 70:167–72.

79. Lippold BC, Teubner A. Biopharmazeutische Qualität von Arzneiformen, insbesondere für lokale Anwendung, abgeleitet aus Wirkungsmessungen. Pharm Ind 1981; 43:71–3.

80. Lippold BC. Selection of the vehicle for topical administration of drugs. Pharm Acta Helv 1984; 59:166–71.

81. Leopold CS. Quantification of depletion in solution-type topical preparations in vivo. J Cosmet Sci 1998; 49:165–74.

82. Surber C, Smith EW. The mystical effects of dermatological vehicles. Dermatology 2005; 210:157–68.

83. Schulmeister L. Transdermal drug patches: medicine with muscle. Nursing 2005; 35:48–52.

84. Stricker T, Sennhauser FH. Allergic contact dermatitis due to transdermal contraception patch. J Pediatr 2006; 148:845.

85. Hadgraft J, Lane ME. Passive transdermal drug delivery systems: recent considerations and advances. Am J Drug Deliv 2006; 4:153–60.

86. Foroutan SM, Ettehadi HA, Torabi HR. Formulation and in vitro evaluation of silver sulfadiazine spray. Iran J Pharm Res 2002; 1:47–9.

87. Eaglstein WH, Sullivan TP, Giordano PA, Miskin BM. A liquid adhesive bandage for the treatment of minor cuts and abrasions. Dermatol Surg 2002; 28:263–7.

88. Campbell K, Woodbury MG, Whittle H, Labate T, Hoskin A. A clinical evaluation of 3M no sting barrier film. Ostomy Wound Manage 2000; 46(1):24–30.

89. Misra A, Pal R, Majumdar SS, Talwar GP, Singh O. Biphasic testosterone delivery profile observed with two different transdermal formulations. Pharm Res 1997; 14(9):1264–8.

90. Zurdo Schroeder I, Franke P, Schaefer UF, Lehr CM. Development and characterization of film forming polymeric solutions for skin drug delivery. Eur J Pharm Biopharm 2007; 65(1):111–21.

91. Zurdo Schroeder I, Franke P, Schaefer UF, Lehr CM. Poster presentation. CRS, Annual Meeting, Vienna, 2006.

92. Mezei M, Gulasekharam V. Liposomes—a selective drug delivery system for the topical route of administration. I. Lotion dosage form. Life Sci 1980; 26:1473–7.

93. Mezei M, Gulasekharam V. Liposomes. A selective drug delivery system for the topical route of administration: gel dosage form. J Pharm Pharmacol 1982; 34:473–4.

94. Korting HC, Zienicke H, Schäfer-Korting M, Braun-Falco O. Liposome encapsulation improves efficacy of betamethasone dipropionate in atopic eczema but not in psoriasis vulgaris. Eur J Clin Pharmacol 1990; 39(4):349–51.

95. Schaefer-Korting M, Korting HC, Ponce-Poschl E. Liposomal tretinoin for uncomplicated acne vulgaris. Clin Invest 1994; 72:1086–91.

96. Touitou E, Shaco-Ezra N, Dayan N, Jushynski M, Rafaeloff R, Azoury R. Dyphylline liposomes for delivery to the skin. J Pharm Sci 1992; 81:131–4.

97. Touitou E, Levi-Schaffer F, Dayan N, et al. Modulation of caffeine skin delivery by carrier design: liposomes versus permeation enhancers. Int J Pharm 1994; 103:131–6.

98. Foldvari M. In vitro cutaneous and percutaneous delivery and in vivo efficacy of tetracaine from liposomal and conventional vehicles. Pharm Res 1994; 11:1593–8.

99. Egbaria K, Ramachandran C, Weiner N. Topical delivery of ciclosporin: evaluation of various formulations using in vitro diffusion studies in hairless mouse skin. Skin Pharmacol 1990; 3(1):21–8.

100. Short SM, Rubas W, Paasch BD, Mrsny RJ. Transport of biologically active interferon-gamma across human skin in vitro. Pharm Res 1995; 12(8):1140–5.

101. Lieb LM, Flynn G, Weiner N. Follicular (pilosebaceous unit) deposition and pharmacological behavior of cimetidine as a function of formulation. Pharm Res 1994; 11(10):1419–23.

102. Lieb LM, Ramachandran C, Egbaria K, Weiner N. Topical delivery enhancement with multilamellar liposomes into pilosebaceous units: I. In vitro evaluation using fluorescent techniques with the hamster ear model. J Invest Dermatol 1992; 99(1):108–13.

103. Weiner N, Lieb L, Niemiec S, Ramachandran C, Hu Z, Egbaria K. Liposomes: a novel topical delivery system for pharmaceutical and cosmetic applications. J Drug Target 1994; 2:405–10.

104. Hofland HE, van der Geest R, Bodde HE, Junginger HE, Bouwstra JA. Estradiol permeation from nonionic surfactant vesicles through human stratum corneum in vitro. Pharm Res 1994; 11(5):659–64.

105. Schreier H, Bouwstra J. Liposomes and niosomes as topical drug carriers: dermal and transdermal drug delivery. J Control Release 1994; 30:1–15.

106. Cevc G, Blume G. Lipid vesicles penetrate into intact skin owing to the transdermal osmotic gradients and hydration force. Biochim Biophys Acta Biomembr 1992; 1104:226–32.

107. Cevc G, Blume G. Biological activity and characteristics of triamcinolone-acetonide formulated with the self-regulating drug carriers, Transfersomes®. Biochim Biophys Acta Biomembr 2003; 1614:156–64.

108. Cevc G, Blume G. Hydrocortisone and dexamethasone in very deformable drug carriers have increased biological potency, prolonged effect, and reduced therapeutic dosage. Biochim Biophys Acta Biomembr 2004; 1663:61–73.

109. Touitou E, Dayan N, Bergelson L, Godin B, Eliaz M. Ethosomes—Novel vesicular carriers for enhanced delivery: characterization and skin penetration properties. J Control Release 2000; 65:403–18.

110. Horwitz E, Pisanty S, Czerninski R, Helser M, Eliav E, Touitou E. A clinical evaluation of a novel liposomal carrier for acyclovir in the topical treatment of recurrent herpes labialis. Oral Surg Oral Med Oral Pathol Oral Radiol Endod 1999; 87(6):700–5.

111. Dayan N, Touitou E. Carriers for skin delivery of trihexyphenidyl HCl: ethosomes vs. liposomes. Biomaterials 2000; 21(18):1879–85.

112. Esposito E, Menegatti E, Cortesi R. Ethosomes and liposomes as topical vehicles for azelaic acid: a preformulation study. J Cosmet Sci 2004; 55(3):253–64.

113. Rao YF, Li F, Liang WQ. Study on transdermal permeation and skin accumulation of finasteride ethosomes. Chin Pharm J 2004; 39(12):923–5.

114. Godin B, Touitou E, Rubinstein E, Athamna A, Athamna M. A new approach for treatment of deep skin infections by an ethosomal antibiotic preparation: an in vivo study. J Antimicrob Chemother 2005; 55(6):989–94.

115. Paolino D, Lucania G, Mardente D, Alhaique F, Fresta M. Ethosomes for skin delivery of ammonium glycyrrhizinate: in vitro percutaneous permeation through human skin and in vivo anti-inflammatory activity on human volunteers. J Control Release 2005; 106:99–110.

116. Maia CS, Mehnert W, Schaefer-Korting M. Solid lipid nanoparticles as drug carriers for topical glucocorticoids. Int J Pharm 2000; 196:165–7.

117. Jenning V, Gysler A, Schäfer-Korting M, Gohla SH. Vitamin a loaded solid lipid nanoparticles for topical use: occlusive properties and drug targeting to the upper skin. Eur J Pharm Biopharm 2000; 49(3):211–8.

118. Wissing SA, Mueller RH. A novel sunscreen system based on tocopherol acetate incorporated into solid lipid nanoparticles. Int J Cosmet Sci 2001; 23(4):233–43.
119. Wissing SA, Mueller RH. Solid lipid nanoparticles as carrier for sunscreens: in vitro release and in vivo skin penetration. J Control Release 2002; 81(3):225–33.
120. Yener G, Inceguel T, Yener N. Importance of using solid lipid microspheres as carriers for UV filters on the example octyl methoxy cinnamate. Int J Pharm 2003; 258:203–7.
121. Chen H, Chang X, Du D, et al. Podophyllotoxin-loaded solid lipid nanoparticles for epidermal targeting. J Control Release 2006; 110(2):296–306.
122. Mueller RH, Radtke M, Wissing SA. Solid lipid nanoparticles (SLN) and nanostructured lipid carriers (NLC) in cosmetic and dermatological preparations. Adv Drug Deliv Rev 2002; 54(Suppl.):S131–55.
123. Ricci M, Puglia C, Bonina F, Di Giovanni C, Giovagnoli S, Rossi C. Evaluation of indomethacin percutaneous absorption from nanostructured lipid carriers (NLC): in vitro and in vivo studies. J Pharm Sci 2005; 94:1149–59.
124. Shim J, Seok Kang H, Park WS, Han SH, Kim J, Chang IS. Transdermal delivery of mixnoxidil with block copolymer nanoparticles. J Control Release 2004; 97(3):477–84.
125. Lademann J, Richter H, Schaefer UF, et al. Hair follicles—a long-term reservoir for drug delivery. Skin Pharmacol Physiol 2006; 19(4):232–6.
126. Alvarez-Román R, Naik A, Kalia YN, Fessi H, Guy RH. Visualization of skin penetration using confocal laser scanning microscopy. Eur J Pharm Biopharm 2004; 58:301–16.
127. Alvarez-Román R, Naik A, Kalia YN, Guy RH, Fessi H. Enhancement of topical delivery from biodegradable nanoparticles. Pharm Res 2004; 21:1818–25.
128. Alvarez-Román R, Naik A, Kalia YN, Guy RN, Fessi H. Skin penetration and distribution of polymeric nanoparticles. J Control Release 2004; 99(1):53–62.
129. Luengo J, Weiss B, Schneider M, et al. Influence of nanoencapsulation on human skin transport of flufenamic acid. Skin Pharmacol Physiol 2006; 19:190–7.
130. Stracke F, Weiss B, Lehr CM, König K, Schaefer UF, Schneider M. Multiphoton microscopy for the investigation of dermal penetration of nanoparticle-borne drugs. J Invest Dermatol 2006; 126:2224–33.
131. Hammond SA, Tsonis C, Sellins K, et al. Transcutaneous immunization of domestic animals: opportunities and challenges. Adv Drug Deliv Rev 2000; 43(1):45–55.
132. Hammond SA, Walwender D, Alving CR, Glenn GM. Transcutaneous immunization: T cell responses and boosting of existing immunity. Vaccine 2001; 19:2701–7.
133. Kohli AK, Alpar HO. Potential use of nanoparticles for transcutaneous vaccine delivery: effect of particle size and charge. Int J Pharm 2004; 275:13–7.
134. Lademann J, Weigmann H, Rickmeyer C, et al. Penetration of titanium dioxide microparticles in a sunscreen formulation into the horny layer and the follicular orifice. Skin Pharmacol Appl Skin Physiol 1999; 12:247–56.
135. Pflücker F, Wendel V, Hohenberg H, et al. The human stratum corneum layer: an effective barrier against dermal uptake of different forms of topically applied micronised titanium dioxide. Skin Pharmacol Appl Skin Physiol 2001; 14(Suppl. 1):92–7.
136. Gamer AO, Leibold E, Van Ravenzwaay B. The in vitro absorption of microfine zinc oxide and titanium dioxide through porcine skin. Toxicol In Vitro 2006; 20(3):301–7.

Interpretation of In Vitro Skin Absorption Studies of Lipophilic Chemicals

Robert L. Bronaugh
Office of Cosmetics and Colors, Food and Drug Administration, College Park, Maryland, U.S.A.

INTRODUCTION

The major issue of concern in the accuracy of in vitro skin absorption studies is the way in which absorption of a lipophilic (hydrophobic) compound is determined. Lipophilic chemicals that penetrate into the skin may not freely partition into the receptor fluid beneath the skin. Therefore, skin absorption values for lipophilic chemicals determined from receptor fluid samples may underestimate skin absorption. The problem was alluded to over 30 years ago by Franz who, in selecting compounds for study, omitted highly lipophilic compounds to avoid results that were "artificially limited due to insolubility in the dermal bathing solution" (1). In the early in vivo and in vitro absorption comparisons made by Tsuruta, lower than expected in vitro absorption values were noted for organic solvents with the lowest water solubility (2,3). Brown and Ulsamer found that the skin permeation of the lipophilic compound hexachlorophene increased twofold when normal saline was replaced with 3% bovine serum albumin (BSA, in a physiological buffer) in the diffusion cell receptor (4).

APPROACHES TO DETERMINE THE ABSORPTION OF LIPOPHILIC CHEMICALS

An initial approach in our laboratory was to systematically examine various lipophilic receptor fluids to determine if receptor fluid levels at the end of an in vitro absorption study agreed with systemic absorption measured in vivo (5,6). Use of a 6% solution in water of the nonionic surfactant Volpo 20 (PEG 20 oleyl ether) resulted in substantial increases in penetration of model ^{14}C-labeled lipophilic ingredients (Table 1). Damage to the skin with the surfactant solutions was assessed using ^{3}H-cortisone absorption as a control in dual-label studies. With dermatomed rat skin (350 μm), cinnamyl anthranilate absorption into the receptor fluid was enhanced fivefold and acetyl ethyl tetramethyl tetralin (AETT) absorption was enhanced 30-fold without damage to the skin compared to the use of normal saline in the receptor fluid (Table 1). However, absorption was still 1.6- or 3-fold less than observed during in vivo absorption studies with cinnamyl anthranilate and AETT, respectively. The use of 6% PEG 20 oleyl ether with rat skin dermatomed to 200 μm resulted in damage to the barrier properties of skin presumably due to the reduced protection of the epidermis from the thinner dermal tissue layer present (6). Use of either 40:60 ethanol–water or 50:50 methanol–water receptor fluids resulted in damage to the skin barrier as evidenced by increased penetration of the cortisone control (5). A 3% solution of BSA more than doubled the absorption of cinnamyl anthanilate compared to saline; however,

TABLE 1 Effect of Diffusion Cell Conditions of the Absorption of Cinnamyl Anthranilate and AETT (Cortisone Control)

Receptor fluid	Percent applied dose absorbed in five days	Cortisone permeability constant $\times 10^5$
Cinnamyl anthranilate		
Normal saline (4)[a]	5.0 ± 0.3	3.8 ± 0.7
1.5% PEG 20 oleyl ether (4)[a]	5.4 ± 0.9	N.D.
Normal saline (4)	5.8 ± 0.4	7.1 ± 0.5
1.5% PEG 20 oleyl ether (10)	15.5 ± 1.2^b	6.1 ± 0.5
6% PEG 20 oleyl ether (8)	27.9 ± 1.8^b	7.0 ± 0.9
20% PEG 20 oleyl ether (8)	18.3 ± 1.8^b	9.3 ± 0.9
Rabbit serum (4)	8.8 ± 0.6^b	6.8 ± 0.8
3% Bovine serum albumin (4)	12.1 ± 1.2^b	5.4 ± 0.2
50:50 Methanol–water (4)	27.1 ± 2.0^b	17.2 ± 0.2^b
1.5% Octoxynol 9 (4)	17.9 ± 1.1^b	10.8 ± 0.5^b
6% Octoxynol 9 (4)	38.4 ± 2.9^b	14.5 ± 1.3^b
6% Poloxymer 188	7.3 ± 1.8	9.8 ± 0.6^b
AETT		
Normal saline (6)[a]	0.08 ± 0.01	3.8 ± 0.7^c
1.5% PEG 20 oleyl ether (6)[a]	0.23 ± 0.07	N.D.
Normal saline (4)	0.20 ± 0.06	6.3 ± 0.3
1.5% PEG 20 oleyl ether (4)	2.3 ± 0.4^b	4.9 ± 0.2
6% PEG 20 oleyl ether (4)	6.0 ± 0.9^b	7.0 ± 0.9^c
50:50 Glycerol–water (3)	0.14 ± 0.03	4.7 ± 0.9
40:60 Ethanol–water (4)	$6.1 \pm 1.2^{b,d}$	21.7 ± 3.3^b

Values are the mean $\pm$ SEM of the number of determinations in parentheses. For most experiments, a 350-μm section from the surface of rat skin was prepared with a dermatome. Compounds were applied to skin in a petrolatum vehicle. In vivo absorption of cinnamyl anthranilate and AETT was 45.6% and 18.9%, respectively.
[a] Full thickness skin.
[b] Significant increase when compared with results from the appropriate saline control (dermatomed skin) by one-tailed Student's *t*-test, $p < 0.05$.
[c] Value determined in experiments with cinnamyl anthranilate.
[d] Value determined at four days.
Abbreviation: AETT, acetyl ethyl tetramethyl tetralin.

absorption of the compound was less than that observed with 6% PEG 20 oleyl ether as the receptor fluid (5).

The use of solvents and surfactants in the receptor fluid should raise concerns about the potential for skin barrier damage. It also presents a problem in studies where skin metabolism is an issue since a physiological buffer is required to maintain viability of skin (7). Another approach to determining absorption of a lipophilic compound is, therefore, to use a physiological buffer such as a tissue culture media or a balanced salt solution and add BSA to this receptor fluid to improve lipid solubility. However, skin may still contain amounts of lipophilic compounds that have been artificially retained because of lack of free partitioning of these compounds from the skin.

An attempt was made to address this problem by extending the absorption study for an additional period of time to see if the material remaining in the skin at the end of the initial study would subsequently diffuse into the receptor fluid. An extended study was first conducted with musk xylol. Skin levels at the end of a 24-hour study significantly declined when, in separate diffusion cells, the amount of unabsorbed material was washed off the skin and the study was continued for an additional period of time (Fig. 1) (8). At the end of 72 hours, the amount of musk

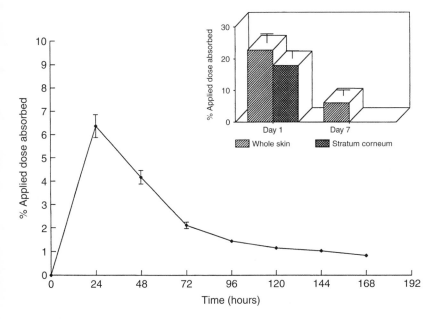

FIGURE 1 Time course of percutaneous absorption of musk xylol into the receptor fluid. *Inset*: Skin levels of musk xylol. Values are the mean $\pm$ SEM of determinations in excised skin from two human subjects.

xylol absorbed from human skin into the receptor fluid approximately doubled from about 6% (at 24 hours) to 12%. This suggested that skin levels of musk xylol should be included as being potentially able to be systemically absorbed.

Disperse Blue 1 (DB1) is a coal tar hair dye that is poorly soluble in oil and water and is used in temporary and semi-permanent (non-oxidative) hair dyes, colors, and rinses (9). The compound was incorporated into a hair dye formulation and applied to excised human skin. Only about 0.2% of the applied dose was found in the receptor fluid at the end of 24 hours and more that 10 times that amount remained in skin at that time (9). A 72-hour extended absorption study found that the DB1 did not appreciably diffuse into the receptor fluid beyond what was absorbed in the 24 hours studies. Therefore, it was concluded that skin levels of DB1 should probably not be included as test material that could eventually be systemically absorbed.

Another approach at determining the accuracy of in vitro measurements of chemicals that form a skin reservoir is to compare the in vitro results with absorption data from in vivo experiments. The skin absorption of retinol was measured through fuzzy rat skin from a gel and an emulsion formulation. Preliminary 24-hour absorption data showed that receptor fluid levels from in vitro studies agreed closely with in vivo systemic absorption (10).

SKIN RESERVOIR FORMATION WITH HYDROPHILIC COMPOUNDS

However, some compounds like diethanolamine (DEA) are water soluble and also found extensively in skin at the end of a 24-hour study (Table 2) (11). A 72-hour

TABLE 2   DEA Penetration in Human Skin from a Lotion

	% of applied dose penetrated		
	24 hr[a]	48 hr[a]	72 hr[a]
Receptor fluid	0.7±0.1	1.2±0.1	1.7±0.5
Stratum corneum	4.2±0.2	3.3±0.1	3.7±0.3
Epidermis and dermis	7.7±0.9	7.4±1.3	7.4±0.9
Total in skin	11.9±0.7	10.7±0.3	11.1±0.6
Total penetration	12.5±0.5	11.9±1.3	12.8±1.1
Recovery	95.2±3.0	93.3±3.4	96.6±3.0

Values are the mean ± SEM of three replicates in skin from each of three subjects. DEA dose applied at 24 hours was 1.0 μg/cm². Corresponding values at the different study times are not significantly different (ANOVA, $p < 0.05$).
[a] Duration of study.
Abbreviation: DEA, diethanolamine.

extended study conducted on DEA found that there was no significant increase in receptor fluid levels over the additional 48 hours. One explanation for the reservoir of DEA in skin would be that the compound was bound to skin and not retained in skin because of its solubility properties. When DEA was applied to skin for 24 hours on three successive days, the daily amount of DEA found in the receptor fluid did not significantly increase (Table 3). However, the total amount of DEA in skin at the end of the three-day experiment increased 2.3-fold over the value found in a 24-hour single application study (Table 2). Daily application of DEA cannot be continued longer than three days in an in vitro study because of concerns about skin barrier integrity. The skin penetration of DEA following long-term daily applications is unknown.

Lawsone is another chemical that appears to be more soluble in water than in oil and yet formed a significant reservoir in skin during a percutaneous absorption study (12). There was a small but significant increase in receptor fluid levels of lawsone at the end of the extended studies when four different lawsone-containing cosmetic products were examined. This suggests that the receptor fluid levels of lawsone alone might be a reasonable estimate of systemic absorption.

GUIDELINES AND REGULATORY OPINIONS

The recently adopted Organization for Economic Cooperation and Development (OECD) guideline for in vitro skin absorption studies addresses the issue of

TABLE 3   DEA Penetration in Human Skin from Multiple Lotion Doses

	% of applied dose penetrated		
	Day 1	Day 2	Day 3
DEA dose applied (μg/cm²)	1.0	1.0	1.0
Receptor fluid	0.5±0.1	0.8±0.1	0.9±0.2
Stratum corneum	—	—	8.0±0.2
Epidermis and dermis	—	—	21.2±2.4
Total in skin	—	—	29.2±2.2
Total penetration	—	—	30.1±2.4

Values are the mean ± SEM of three replicates in skin from each of two subjects.
Abbreviation: DEA, diethanolamine.

accountability of test chemicals remaining in the skin at the end of a study (13). The amount remaining in the skin may need to be included in the total amount absorbed unless additional studies are conducted to demonstrate the systemic fate of this material. No specific information is provided as to the types of additional studies that could be done in the referenced OECD Guidance Document for the Conduct of Skin Absorption Studies (14).

The Scientific Committee on Cosmetics and Non-Food Products (SCCNFP) gave an opinion on basic criteria for the in vitro assessment of percutaneous absorption in 1999 (15). Test material remaining in the skin at the end of an experiment was considered systemically absorbed if it was found in viable tissue (the viable epidermis or dermis). Test material found in the stratum corneum layer of skin was not considered to contribute to the systemic dose. The SCCNFP's updated opinion in 2003 stated that irreversible binding of an ingredient to the epidermis (which includes the stratum corneum) would need to be demonstrated in a separate experiment. An ingredient bound irreversibly to the epidermis in vivo would eventually be removed due to desquamation of the skin and would not be available for systemic absorption (16). No change in opinion on the contribution of the skin reservoir to systemic absorption is found in the most recent criteria by the Scientific Committee on Consumer Products (SCCP, formerly the SCCNFP) (17).

CONCLUSIONS

There are differences in the international guidelines cited above in how ingredients remaining in the skin at the end of a study should be treated with regard to the potential availability for systemic absorption. Additional studies focused on comparison of in vivo and in vitro absorption of lipophilic chemicals should help answer the remaining uncertainties. One purpose for conducting a 24-hour absorption study is to determine the daily amount of chemical absorbed through skin. Results obtained for systemic absorption from a 24-hour in vivo study would be the "gold standard." Then in vitro diffusion cell data can be examined to see if test chemical in one or more of the skin layers needs to be included with receptor fluid as systemically absorbed. For some chemicals that form a skin reservoir in vitro, the skin reservoir observed in vivo will likely be similar and therefore no inclusion of skin levels in the in vitro determination of systemic absorption will be necessary.

REFERENCES

1. Franz TJ. Percutaneous absorption. On the relevance of in vitro data. J Invest Dermatol 1975; 52:190–5.
2. Tsuruta H. Percutaneous absorption of organic solvents: comparative study of the in vivo percutaneous absorption of chlorinated solvents in mice. Ind Health 1975; 13:227–36.
3. Tsuruta H. Percutaneous absorption of organic solvents: a method for measuring the penetration rate of chlorinated solvents through excised rat skin. Ind Health 1977; 15:131.
4. Brown DWC, Ulsamer AG. Percutaneous absorption of hexachlorophene as related to receptor solutions. Food Cosmet Toxicol 1975; 13:81–6.
5. Bronaugh RL, Stewart RF. Methods for in vitro percutaneous absorption studies. III. Hydrophobic compounds. J Pharm Sci 1984; 73:1255–8.
6. Bronaugh RL, Stewart RF. Methods for in vitro percutaneous absorption studies VI. Preparation of the barrier layer. J Pharm Sci 1986; 75:487–91.

7. Collier SW, Sheikh NM, Sakr A, et al.. Maintenance of skin viability during in vitro percutaneous absorption/metabolism studies. Toxicol Appl Pharmacol 1989; 99:522–33.
8. Hood HL, Wickett RR, Bronaugh RL. The in vitro percutaneous absorption of the fragrance ingredient musk xylol. Food Chem Toxicol 1996; 34:483–8.
9. Yourick JJ, Koenig ML, Yourick DL, et al.. Fate of chemicals in skin after dermal application: does the in vitro skin reservoir affect the estimate of systemic absorption? Toxicol Appl Pharmacol 2004; 195:309–20.
10. Yourick JJ, Jung CT, Bronaugh RL. Percutaneous absorption of retinol in fuzzy rat (in vivo and in vitro) and human skin (in vitro) from cosmetic vehicles. Toxicologist 2006; 90(S1):164 (Abstract Number 810).
11. Kraeling MEK, Yourick JJ, Bronaugh RL. Percutaneous absorption of diethanolamine in human skin in vitro. Food Chem Toxicol 2004; 42:1553–61.
12. Kraeling MEK, Jung CT, Bronaugh RL. Absorption of lawsone through human skin. Cutaneous Ocular Toxicol 2007; 26(1):45–56.
13. Anon. OECD Guideline for the Testing of Chemicals: skin Absorption (in vitro method), Test Guideline 428, Organization for Economic and Cooperation and Development, Paris, 2004.
14. Anon. Guidance Document for the Conduct of Skin Absorption Studies, OECD Series on Testing and Assessment Number 28, Organization for Economic and Cooperation and Development, Paris, 2004.
15. Anon. SCCNFP Opinion Concerning Basic Criteria for the In Vitro Assessment of Percutaneous Absorption of Cosmetic Ingredients, Scientific Committee on Cosmetic Products and Non-Food Products, European Commission, 1999.
16. Anon. SCCNFP Opinion Concerning Basic Criteria for the In Vitro Assessment of Dermal Absorption of Cosmetic Ingredients, Scientific Committee on Cosmetic Products and Non-Food Products, European Commission, 2003.
17. Anon. SCCP Opinion on Basic Criteria for the In Vitro Assessment of Dermal Absorption of Cosmetic Ingredients, Scientific Consumer Products, European Commission, 2006.

9 | Use of Skin Equivalents for Dermal Absorption and Toxicity

Monika Schäfer-Korting and Sylvia Schreiber
Institut für Pharmazie (Pharmakologie und Toxikologie) der Freien Universität Berlin, Berlin, Germany

INTRODUCTION

Building up a three-dimensional (3D) human skin tissue was initially stimulated by the idea of an improved healing of severe wounds and, in fact, skin equivalents for transplantation purposes are now commercially available. Importantly, human skin equivalents are also used in the risk assessment of chemicals and safety tests of cosmetics. The Organisation of Economic Cooperation and Development (OECD) has adopted a test guideline (TG) for the assessment of skin corrosion [TG 431; (1)], which is based on reconstructed human epidermis (RHE). TG 431 also defines quality parameters for RHE which are important for alternative uses such as risk assessment linked to the absorption of chemicals and drugs through the skin and in the development of dermatological and topical antirheumatic drugs. The OECD technical guidance document 28 [TGD 28, (2)] that accompanies TG 428 (3) states that skin equivalents can be used for in vitro assays of percutaneous absorption, given that the obtained results are equivalent to those obtained with the accepted matrices of human and animal skin. Thus, in principle, relevant aspects of skin toxicity can be studied using the same matrix. The various aspects of in vitro tests based on skin equivalents are described below.

HUMAN SKIN MODELS

A rather simplistic model is the monolayer culture, e.g., of keratinocytes or fibroblasts. Moreover, keratinocytes can also host other cell types, e.g., melanocytes or dendritic cells. Skin equivalents in the stricter sense encompass 3D matrices, RHE, and full-thickness (FT) models, in which a reconstructed epidermis overlays a dermis equivalent. These, too, may host other cell types.

For the safety assessment of chemicals and cosmetics, as well as for drug penetration and permeation, excised human or animal skin can also be used. With respect to the latter, pig and rat (furry and nude) skin are most often selected (4–6). The skin is either used as FT or split skin (< 1000 µm). Moreover, the epidermis can be removed from human skin or the skin of the pig ear by applying heat. More rarely trypsinization can be used to isolate the horny layer.

Monolayer Cultures

Monolayer cultures of human cells as well as human derived cell lines have been used for many years. Most often, fibroblasts and keratinocytes are isolated from juvenile or adult foreskin and are cultivated submerged (Fig. 1B,C) to form a monolayer (7–10). Besides primary keratinocytes, the HaCaT cell line,

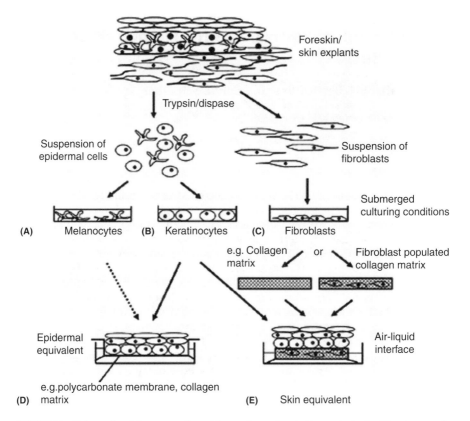

FIGURE 1 Schematic of the generation of three-dimensional skin equivalents. Monolayer cultures are established from fresh skin specimens. After trypsinization, epidermal keratinocytes (**B**) and/or melanocytes (**A**) are seeded onto an acellular (e.g., polycarbonate membrane or structures of collagen) or a cellular (e.g., fibroblast-populated collagen matrix) compartment. Depending on the presence of fibroblasts (**C**), epidermal (**D**) or skin equivalents (**E**) can be generated.

a spontaneously transformed human keratinocyte (11), SZ94 cells, which are transformed human sebocytes (12), and dendritic cells [e.g., XS52; (13–15)] are used to study skin physiology and pharmacological effects. Melanocytes are cultivated to study pigment cell biology (16). Cocultured with keratinocytes (17) the regulation of melanogenesis under different culture conditions may be investigated (18).

Cultivation of Skin Equivalents and Culture Conditions

The cultivation of RHE (Fig. 1D) is carried out by seeding dissociated primary keratinocytes, derived from, e.g., foreskin or abdominal skin, onto an appropriate substrate. Such substrates include polycarbonate membranes, as in the EpiDerm™ (MatTek Corporation, Ashland, Massachusetts, U.S.A.; Fig. 2) and SkinEthic® model (Laboratoire SkinEthic, Nice, France), or structures of collagen types I and III coated with collagen type IV, as in the EPISKIN® model (L'Oreal, Paris, France). A rat keratinocyte cell line can also be used to form a structured tissue (19).

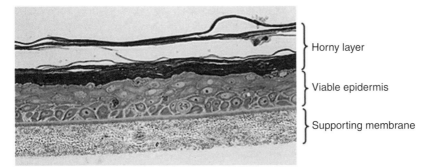

FIGURE 2 Histological appearance of a reconstructed human epidermis model (EpiDerm). After fixation in Karnovsky solution, several washing steps, and a gradual dehydration procedure, the sample was embedded in epoxy resin, cut into 1 to 2 μm semi-thin sections, stained with 1% toluidine/1% pyronine G, and visualized by light optical microscopy (original magnification 400×).

The culture is incubated for several days, submerged in culture medium to stimulate proliferation (Fig. 1). After formation of a thin multilayered tissue, the cultures are exposed to an air–liquid interface to induce differentiation. Thus, under approximately physiological conditions, the cells are supplied with nutrients by the subjacent substrate. Air exposure of the epidermal cells is crucial for the development of a multilayered tissue with a coherent stratum corneum (20–23).

For cultivation of FT models, other substrates, such as a fibroblast-populated collagen matrix, are used (Fig. 1E). Also, an incorporation of dermal fibroblasts into the skin models, e.g., by culturing the cells on the bottom of the plate, by cultivation on the basolateral side of de-epidermized dermis with maintained basal membrane components (22,24,25), or by cultivation on inert filters before the keratinocytes are inserted, are the common techniques. Fibroblasts synthesize collagen fibrils and incorporate them into the dermal compartment (26,27). The function of fibroblasts in the dermal compartment is mainly to regulate keratinocyte proliferation. As direct contact of keratinocytes and fibroblasts does not seem to be of vital importance, diffusible dermal products, like growth factors and/or cytokines, are regarded as eminent signals of intercellular communication (28,29).

Besides epithelial–mesenchymal cocultures, keratinocytes and melanocytes (30–32) can be cultivated together in the epidermal compartment (Fig. 1). This allows, for example, the investigation of controlled UV-induced melanogenesis or the testing of bleaching substances and their effect on melanin production. Treatment of stable vitiligo by cultured epidermal autografts bearing melanocytes seems to be possible (33–35).

The extracellular milieu, consisting of ambient temperature and atmosphere, composition of the growth medium, matrix, and substrate are crucial in skin model cultivation. With commercial models (e.g., SkinEthic), the addition of serum, which was thought to be essential due to its growth promoting properties, was discontinued because of its biological variability and poor standardization. To compensate for the lack of serum, supplements, such as hormones, growth factors, vitamins, transport and lipid-binding proteins, trace elements, antioxidants, stabilizing factors, and other low molecular weight (MW) nutrients, are included (36–38). A gradual modification of the culture conditions resulted in the creation of skin models with high resemblance to native epidermis (36,37). The most important changes, apart from the omission of serum, were the reduction of growth factor concentration and supplementation of vitamins. In particular, vitamin C is crucial for the formation of a competent skin barrier (36).

Commercially Available 3D Skin Models

If keratinocyte cultures are allowed to build up to form a multilayered tissue which is then lifted to the air–liquid interface, cornification is induced (Figs. 1 and 2). The general and functional conditions of several commercially available 3D skin equivalents have been well defined. This is true for the EpiDerm, EPISKIN, and SkinEthic models. These models have been extensively and repeatedly characterized with respect to morphology, lipids, and barrier function. A most recent comparison extended the spectrum of applicable models for the hazard analysis of chemicals (39). In fact, an improvement of the barrier function has become possible using ascorbic acid supplementation of the medium (36).

Recently other models have been introduced to the market, including EST-1000 (Cell Systems, St. Katharinen, Germany) and Euroskin (Euroderm, Leipzig, Germany). Commercially available for transplantation purposes is the autologous EpiDex™ skin model [Euroderm (40,41)]. The EST-1000 model is derived from proliferating and differentiating keratinocytes (42). Interestingly, the Euroskin and the EpiDex models are built up from epidermal stem cells, isolated from hair plugs, which allows the generation of skin equivalents from the cells of a single donor for many years (43,44).

For full-tissue models, AST-2000 (Cell Systems), EpiDerm-FT (MatTek), SkinEthic-FT (Laboratoire SkinEthic), and Phenion®-FT Skin Model (Phenion, Düsseldorf, Germany) are available. Fundamental parameters describing commercially available human skin equivalents are summarized in Table 1.

In-House 3D Models

Several in-house 3D models have also been developed and are based on primary skin cells or cell lines from different species. Suhonen et al. built up an organotypic epidermal model derived from rat epidermal keratinocytes. A rat epidermal keratinocyte cell line was grown for three weeks on collagen gel in the absence of feeder cells in culture inserts at an air–liquid interface. A good correlation of the permeability characteristics of the model compared with human cadaver epidermis was shown by testing 18 compounds covering a large range of physicochemical parameters (46).

A skin model closely resembling native human skin and based on autologous dermal fibroblasts, collagen, keratinocytes derived from freshly plucked hair follicles, and medium enriched with serum of the respective donor, was developed by Hoeller et al. (47). The autologous material may enable skin grafting and thereby reduces the risk of rejection of the graft.

Augustin et al. developed a dermal and a skin equivalent model that included a collagen–glycosaminoglycans–chitosan porous matrix populated by normal human fibroblasts (dermal equivalent). The skin model was made by seeding normal human keratinocytes onto the dermal equivalent after 14 days of incubation, leading to a fully differentiated epidermis after 7 days of cultivation and 14 days at the air–liquid interface. The models were tested for screening the phototoxic

TABLE 1 Basic Characteristics of Human Skin Equivalents

Skin equivalent	Typical histology	Size (cm^2)	Purposes, e.g., testing for:	Origin of cells (donors)	Membrane
Epidermis models (39):					
EpiDerm EPI-200; 606	9–12 layers (45)	0.63; 4	Skin corrosion, irritation (validated), phototoxicity, skin absorption	Foreskin/abdomen (single)	Collagen coated
EPISKIN	8–10 layers (45)	1.07	Skin corrosion (validated), histology	Abdomen, adults (several)	Collagen I sheet
EST-1000	Not yet published	0.63	Skin corrosion (42)	Foreskin/abdomen (neonatal/adult)	Polycarbonate
SkinEthic	5–7 layers (45)	0.5; 4	Skin corrosion, irritation, absorption	Foreskin/abdomen (neonatal/adult single)	Polycarbonate
EpiDex	3–8 layers	0.8	(Grafting)	Epidermal stem cells (single)	None
Full-tissue models:					
AST-2000	4–6 layers	0.63	Pharmacotoxicology	Foreskin (several)	Polycarbonate, collagen coated
EpiDerm-FT	8–12 layers	0.5; 1.0; 3.8	Pharmacotoxicology	Foreskin/breast skin (neonatal/adult) (keratinocytes), neonatal/adult skin (fibroblasts) (single)	Collagen matrix
Euroskin	3–8 layers	0.5; 0.8; 3.1	Pharmacotoxicology	Epidermal stem cells (single)	Polycarbonate
Phenion	8–10 layers	1.1	Pharmacotoxicology	Foreskin (single)	Collagen matrix
SkinEthic-FT	Not published	0.5	Pharmacotoxicology	Foreskin (keratinocytes), adult breast skin (fibroblasts, single)	(Wire gauze)

Abbreviations: AST, advanced skin test; EST, Epidermal-skin-test; FT, full-thickness.
Source: From Ref. 39.

potential of new compounds (48) and the protective efficacy of new sunscreen molecules and formulations (49).

A skin model suitable for storage under nitrogen freezing, consisting of dermal and epidermal layers that were derived from human dermal fibroblasts and spontaneously transformed human epidermal cells from the HaCaT cell line, was evaluated for permeability. In comparison with excised human stratum corneum, it showed higher drug permeability (50).

CHARACTERIZATION OF SKIN EQUIVALENTS
Morphology and Immunohistochemistry
The histological evaluation of the commercially available skin models EPISKIN, EpiDerm, and SkinEthic showed a fully stratified epithelium consisting of an organized stratum basale, stratum spinosum, stratum granulosum, and stratum corneum in all epidermal models (45). The manufacturers of the epidermal and "FT" skin models describe the existence of a fully developed basal membrane and the expression of important basal membrane markers, such as collagen IV and VII, laminin I and V, integrin α6 and β4, as well as antigen BP. Characteristic epidermal ultrastructures were detected (36,37,51) as well as the expression of epidermal differentiation markers (52–54). However, a more detailed inspection of expression and localization of a multitude of differentiation specific protein markers revealed some features of abnormal differentiation. For instance, an aberrant expression of keratin-6, which is missing in healthy human epidermis and is often associated with hyperproliferation and wound healing, was shown. Also, skin-derived antileuko-proteinase, which physiologically does not occur in human skin, was expressed in the skin models. Moreover, an abnormal expression of small proline-rich proteins and involucrin appeared together with an early expression of transglutaminase (45). This results in an imbalance of proliferation and differentiation that contributes to an impaired barrier function of the skin models.

Lipid Composition
From the early days of RHE research, lipid analysis proved the existence of all important epidermal lipid classes. Nevertheless, the ceramide profile was, and still is, incomplete in all skin models inspected (EPISKIN, EpiDerm, and SkinEthic). With the early models, the contents of the polar ceramides 5 and 6 were lower than in human skin and ceramide 7 was missing completely. The content of free fatty acids also appeared to be very low (55), yet the addition of ascorbic acid promoted synthesis of ceramides 6 and 7 (36). A recent comparison of three commercially available skin equivalents showed well-developed lipid profiles. The SkinEthic cultures had the highest amount of ceramides (29% of total lipid content), ceramides amounted to 23.3% of the lipids recovered from the EPISKIN model and 18.5% of the EpiDerm culture. In fact, the SkinEthic model contained ceramide 6 as one of the dominating ceramides amounting to 9.5% to 13% of the total lipid content. In contrast, the EpiDerm model had the highest content of the ceramide precursors, the glucosylceramides, which amounted to 30% of the total lipid content. With EPISKIN, glucosylceramides were about 12% and with SkinEthic about 7% of the total lipid content, which corresponds with the higher age of these cultures when shipped. Free fatty acids made up 7.3% (EpiDerm), 9.7% (EPISKIN), and 12.1% (SkinEthic) (39), which is close to the free fatty acid content of native human epidermis (55,56). The crystalline nature of the epidermal lipid layers influences the

barrier function. Dense packing by orthorhombic structure in healthy human skin is deemed essential for the normal permeability barrier of the stratum corneum. In fact, there is a predominating hexagonal packing in lesional skin from atopic dermatitis and lamellar ichthyosis (57), and similar aberrations may contribute to the impaired barrier function of the skin models.

Gene Expression
Recently it has been demonstrated that gene expression in the SkinEthic model is close to that in native human skin while the transcriptome of monolayer cultures is clearly different (58). This makes the skin equivalent an interesting matrix in which to study pharmacodynamic and toxic effects but also skin metabolism in vitro, given that the gene expression profile is reproducible.

QUALITY PARAMETERS OF SKIN EQUIVALENTS

To allow the future use of skin equivalents in the assessment of potential risks due to skin contact, TG 431 defines general and functional conditions that skin equivalents have to fulfill before they are eligible to be subjected to formal validation of assay procedures for testing in regulatory toxicology. These conditions include a multilayered, functional stratum corneum with an adequate lipid profile, no microbial contamination, stable, and sufficiently high viability [derived from its metabolic conversion capacity, e.g., 3-(4,5-dimethylthiazol-2-yl)-2,5-diphenyltetra-zolium bromide (MTT) reduction], and sufficient resistance to slowly penetrating cytotoxic marker chemicals (1% Triton X). Generated data have to be reproducible over time and between laboratories. With respect to corrosivity, skin equivalents have to be able to correctly classify the 12 marker chemicals specified in TG 431 (1).

These quality criteria are met by the EpiDerm, EPISKIN, and SkinEthic models (45,55,59–63). Moreover, EST-1000 has been subjected to corrosivity testing and correctly predicted the test compounds of TG 43 except for those reducing MTT (42).

PERCUTANEOUS ABSORPTION IN SKIN EQUIVALENTS

Human and animal skin are accepted as an in vitro approach for determining percutaneous absorption. A test procedure was first established by the The European Cosmetic, Toiletry and Perfumery Association (4) and subsequently TG 428 was adopted by the OECD (3) accompanied by the TGD 28 (2). Conforming to these documents, a ring trial was performed using the OECD reference compounds caffeine, benzoic acid, and testosterone. However, the test matrix, human skin, varied widely in thickness (300–1800 μm), and was obtained both following surgical intervention and from cadaver skin. Additionally, Franz cell surface areas varied by 10-fold and receptor volumes even more. Thus, although this study fully agreed with TG 428 and TGD 28, a high variability of the generated permeation data (64) showed the need for higher degree of standardization of test conditions as proposed by the OECD to allow a comparison of data obtained in different laboratories.

Rat skin is a frequently used option for absorption testing in vitro because this species is also used for the corresponding in vivo experiment (65) and to quantify acute dermal toxicity (66). Rat skin, however, overestimates absorption in human skin by a factor not related to MW, lipophilicity, and/or aqueous solubility (67). If this is due to penetration of a significant fraction of the test material via hair follicles, which are abundant in rat skin, RHE may be a valid alternative despite the clear overestimation of skin permeation compared with native human skin. Despite an overestimation of caffeine absorption (∼20-fold), the first comprehensive studies using in-house RHE (68) and commercially available RHE (69–71) stimulated a comparison of absorption between heat-separated human epidermis and RHE. Interestingly, using reconstructed rat epidermis, a close correlation with the permeation of human cadaver epidermis was shown. Permeation data were obtained for 18 compounds, many of them rather close in structure (β-blockers) and generated in a single laboratory (19). Moreover, a formal validation of skin absorption by RHE has been started (72–76).

Fundamentals of Validation of Nonanimal Experiments

In 2004, the European Centre for the Validation of Alternative Methods (ECVAM) outlined a stepwise approach for validation studies of nonanimal experiments to ensure that the alternative approach can replace the in vivo study (77). First, the test matrix has to reflect all the important features. Next, a protocol has to be established and transferred to participating laboratories. The agreed protocol is then tested using a limited number of test agents (prevalidation). For the formal validation process, the number of test agents has to be increased and the experiments should be run under blinded conditions. Finally, a prediction model has to be established.

Validation of RHE-Based Test Procedures for Percutaneous Absorption

The validation study of skin absorption conforms to these aspects. This was facilitated by the statement of TGD 28 that skin equivalents can be applicable for absorption testing, given that the results of percutaneous absorption are comparable to those obtained with approved in vitro procedures. Moreover, quality criteria are met by several commercially available RHE models.

Following the principles of TG 428 and TGD 28, a protocol was established, testing with human skin, pig skin, and bovine udder skin in the Franz cell, and making use of OECD reference compounds that were applied as aqueous solutions. Aspects of the experimental variables were carefully studied by the project partners. These included a comparison of static and dynamic diffusion cells, the origin of pig skin, the choice of the donor and receptor medium, and the influence of heat separation of human epidermis on permeability (75). Importantly, the use of transepidermal water loss (TEWL) as a skin integrity test was evaluated. TEWL proved insufficient to detect minor damage (73); transepidermal electrical resistance measurement and the application of a radiolabeled tracer were also rejected, so the study management group decided to rely on visual inspection of the skin (74) to assure integrity.

Following the successful transfer of the test procedure into the partner laboratories (75) and some protocol refinements, a prevalidation study was run. The RHE included in the study were those commercially available in 2002 (EpiDerm, EPISKIN, and SkinEthic models). The OECD reference compounds (2) caffeine and testosterone were applied using an infinite dose approach to unravel matrix effects. For both substances, permeability of the RHE, in particular of the SkinEthic model, exceeded the permeability of heat-separated human epidermis

TABLE 2 Summary of Permeation Data: P_{app} Values and Drug Permeated into the Receptor Medium after 6 Hours for Caffeine 0.1% and Testosterone 0.004% Solution Applied to HES, Reconstructed Epidermis, and Pig and Bovine Udder Skin

Skin type	Permeation 6 hr ($\mu g/cm^2$) $\bar{x} \pm s$	P_{app} (10^{-6} cm/sec) $\bar{x} \pm s$
Caffeine		
HES	1.1 ± 1.2	0.1 ± 0.0
Pig skin	0.5 ± 0.4	0.1 ± 0.1
Udder skin	8.2 ± 3.9	0.6 ± 0.2
EpiDerm	4.9 ± 2.7	0.2 ± 0.1
SkinEthic	73.7 ± 36.6	3.6 ± 1.9
EPISKIN	51.3 ± 9.8	2.8 ± 0.8
Testosterone		
HES	0.3 ± 0.3	0.4 ± 0.4
Pig skin	0.1 ± 0.2	0.1 ± 0.0
Udder skin	0.1 ± 0.2	0.3 ± 0.3
EpiDerm	2.4 ± 0.9	2.9 ± 1.1
SkinEthic	4.5 ± 0.6	6.00 ± 1.17
EPISKIN	1.5 ± 0.5	2.11 ± 0.63

Abbreviation: HES, human epidermal sheets.
Source: From Ref. 74.

and animal (pig, bovine udder, 1000 μm) skin (Table 2). Of note is the short lag time of RHE permeation (74).

After a final protocol refinement, a formal validation study was performed. In contrast to the ECVAM principles, blinded conditions were excluded for analytical purposes. The test compounds were extended to include very hydrophilic (mannitol, log P −4.67) to highly lipophilic agents (clotrimazole, log P 5.76) as well as those of a MW exceeding 500 Da. For the larger molecules, ivermectin (MW 875.1 Da) permeation was not detected with any matrix, and digoxin (MW 780.9 Da) permeated RHE (any type), human epidermis, and pig skin only in very low amounts. Therefore, the cutoff limit of RHE appeared to reflect the limit of normal human stratum corneum (78). Nevertheless, RHE is more permeable than human and pig skin. The improved skin equivalents commercially available today remain overpredictive in terms of normal skin permeability (79).

Vehicle Effects

Independently of the validation study described above, the influence of vehicles on the penetration and permeation of EpiDerm and EPISKIN models were compared to uptake by cryopreserved human abdominal skin. Finite doses of caffeine (MW 194; log P −0.1) and α-tocopherol (MW 431 Da; log P 12.2) were applied in oil-in-water (o/w) emulsion, water-in-oil (w/o) emulsions, an ethanol containing hydrogel and an aqueous solution (caffeine only), and α-tocopherol loaded in liposomes. Caffeine penetrated both skin and RHE to a much greater extent over 24 hours than α-tocopherol (71). This is in agreement with the detection of the hydrophilic dye, patent blue V, in the deeper stratum corneum, and the retention of the lipophilic dye, curcumin, in the most superficial layers when applied to human volunteers (80). Caffeine and α-tocopherol penetrated and permeated RHE more rapidly than human split skin (300–500 μm). Solute permeability rank order was correctly predicted while vehicle effects appeared less clearly predictable. In particular, uptake from the hydrogel differed for skin and RHE (71). This was also the case for estradiol (81). Ethanol appears to damage reconstructed tissue, possibly due to the less well-developed barrier.

Miscellaneous Topics

When evaluating the permeation of agents that may be subject to cutaneous metabolism, viability of the skin equivalents is very important. The continuous decline of the applied substance may be essential for further penetration. Therefore, a careful selection of the receptor medium is of high relevance. For example, addition of 5% albumin to the receptor medium, as suggested for the testing of lipophilic agents (2,82), induced necrosis of the RHE (SkinEthic), reducing hydrolysis, and thus penetration of a topical glucocorticoid ester (72).

Skin models may also be used in cutaneous microdialysis investigations (83). At first this technique was only applied in vivo, but it now allows a direct comparison of drug penetration or metabolism in vivo and in vitro using the same test and the same endpoint. Using an in-house epidermal model generated from adult human keratinocytes and excised human breast skin, methyl nicotinate permeation was compared using microdialysis probes inserted superficially into the human skin, de-epidermized dermis or just below the RHE. Drug levels sampled from the RHE exceeded those in superficial skin by only twofold, while drug levels increased by 20-fold when methyl nicotinate was applied to isolated dermis (83).

TOXICITY TESTING IN SKIN EQUIVALENTS

According to the OECD TG 404, which describes in vivo tests for skin corrosion and irritation (84), skin corrosion characterizes irreversible severe skin damage (ulcers, bleeding) following contact with a substance. For health protection in occupational settings and the use of consumer products, compounds are EU classified R34 or R35, which means they cause burns or severe burns, respectively. While skin corrosion relates to severe damage of the skin and scar formation during healing, skin irritation (R38 classification) is less severe and reversible.

All chemicals introduced into the market have to be subjected to skin corrosivity testing according to international regulatory requirements. Thus, while skin equivalents (RHE) have only recently been subjected to a validation study for cutaneous absorption testing, toxicity assays have been developed and validated over a longer period of time. In fact, TG 431 describing skin corrosion tests using skin equivalents has already been adopted by the OECD (2004) (1) and the outcome of validation or prevalidation studies for phototoxicity and skin irritation has been published. Thus, in Europe testing of chemicals for skin corrosion in laboratory animals is no longer permitted.

Corrosivity Testing (Skin Corrosion)

Since in vivo tests for skin corrosion can cause severe pain to the animal, alternative methods have been developed. According to the outcome of a validation study, coordinated by ECVAM in 1996 to 1998, two assays [quantification of the transcutaneous electrical resistance (TER) of excised rat skin TER assay; decline in MTT dye reduction by the EPISKIN skin equivalent, EPISKIN assay] appeared to have the potential for full replacement of the animal experiment (85). Following the ECVAM principles of the modulatory approach of test validation (77), a catch-up validation was established and successfully completed using the EpiDerm model

(86). Thus, all three procedures have been accepted as full replacement for animal testing in the assessment of skin corrosion [TER assay: TG 430, (87); RHE assays: TG 431, (1)].

Irritancy Testing

Other than skin corrosivity, minor effects have to be detected by an in vitro procedure based on skin equivalents when studying irritant potential. While the outcome of a first ECVAM funded prevalidation study based on the EpiDerm and EPISKIN model revealed insufficient predictivity [sensitivity, specificity, accuracy (88,89)], an improved protocol (15-minute exposure, 18- or 42-hour post-incubation period) allowed classification of nonirritant and irritant compounds by correct MTT dye reduction in a validation study (90,91). When studying the SkinEthic model, IL-1α release into the culture medium served as an additional parameter of irritancy (39).

Phototoxicity Testing

Cosmetic ingredients and their mixtures should be tested for acute phototoxic and photogenotoxic potential while photosensitization testing is not specifically required (92). For phototoxicity, in vitro testing performed using a validated stepwise approach is sufficient. First, 3T3 fibroblast monolayers exposed to the test compounds are irradiated with UV light. Viability is checked by membrane integrity; damaged cells are less able for neutral red uptake (phototoxicity assay, 3T3 NRUPT assay) (93–95). This test is also accepted by the European Medicines Evaluation Agency (Annex V to Directive 67/548/EEC). Because of the lack of a penetration barrier, however, the test is clearly overpredictive. A second step for positive substances, an adjunct test, is possible using skin equivalents (EpiDerm). This procedure also permits testing of final products. After UVA irradiating the tissues exposed to the test compounds, RHE are incubated for another 21 hours, and then viability is determined by MTT dye reduction. Nonirradiated cultures, treated with the substance of interest, serve as control (92). In principle, the test procedure is also applicable to the SkinEthic model (96).

Sensitization

Chemicals from the environment, from professional exposure, or from the application of cosmetics or topical drugs for skin disease, may induce contact sensitization. This potential hazard has to be investigated with the relevant agents. However, the complex mechanism, including skin penetration, skin metabolism, chemical reactivity, and immune recognition, requires a multistep approach. An accepted in vitro predictive procedure is not yet available.

ADDITIONAL FIELDS OF APPLICATION

While the use of skin equivalents is well established for skin toxicity testing and is of increasing importance in skin absorption measurements of chemicals, cosmetic ingredients, and drugs, their use for studies of skin metabolism is emerging only recently.

Investigation of Metabolism in Skin Equivalents

To date, the metabolic capacity of skin models has only been investigated to a small extent. Harris and coworkers compared the three models, EPISKIN, EpiDerm, and SkinEthic, with monolayer cultures and human excised epidermis for Phase I (CYP1A1) and Phase II (glutathione S-transferase) activity and showed a high variability of enzyme activities depending on the donor/batch and the skin model (97). They further determined the NAD(P)H:quinone reductase activity in primary keratinocyte cultures, human epidermis and the three cultured skin models, and found similar activity in reconstructed epidermis and human epidermis that was lower than in the monolayer cultures (98).

An in-house epidermal model contained active membrane-bound mixed-function oxidases [cytochrome P-450 (CYP-450) dependent], NADPH cytochrome c (P450) reductases, testosterone-5α-reductase, glucuronosyl-transferases, glutathione S-transferase, steroid- and arylsulfatases, and two distinct forms of epoxide hydrolases (99).

An in-house full-tissue model showed a metabolite profile of testosterone that was very similar to that of neonatal foreskin (100). Regarding testosterone metabolism, foreskin fibroblasts were more active than foreskin keratinocytes (101). The SkinEthic model formed estron and estradiol conjugates when estradiol gel was applied (81). Further studies will show whether this also holds true with respect to RHE from other sources.

Investigations of the beta-methasone 17-valerate biotransformation in an artificial skin equivalent showed higher esterasic activity of the model compared with the control culture medium and an accelerated conversion of beta-methasone-21-valerate to beta-methasone by the skin homogenate (102). Pharmacokinetic investigations of skin metabolism using RHE (SkinEthic) confirmed the high esterasic activity when topical glucocorticoid diesters in addition to beta-methasone valerate were included (103,104). In addition, primary human keratinocytes showed a distinctively higher esterasic enzyme activity than dermal fibroblasts in metabolic studies with prednicarbate (9). When studying a nonsteroidal antiandrogen ester prodrug, relevant cleavage was also seen in the sebocyte cell line SZ95 (105). In contrast, cyproterone acetate resisted hydrolysis of the 17α ester group (106).

Biotransformation studies with caffeine and theophylline in primary keratinocyte and fibroblast cultures revealed low conversion to the respective xanthine metabolites (Table 3). Both qualitatively and quantitatively, the two skin models

TABLE 3 Metabolism of Caffeine and Theophylline (% of the Applied Amount) by Primary Human Keratinocytes, Fibroblasts, Epidermal Model (EpiDerm™), and Full-Tissue Model (EpiDerm™-FT) after an Incubation Time of 48 Hours

	Keratinocytes	Fibroblasts	ED	ED-FT
Metabolism of caffeine to:				
Theophylline	0.07 ± 0.01	0.15 ± 0.06	0.13	0.26 ± 0.13
13U	—	0.17 ± 0.06	—	0.04 ± 0.05
Metabolism of theophylline to:				
13U	—	0.2 ± 0.09	—	0.06 ± 0.01

The data represent the mean values ± SD from three (monolayer cultures) or two (skin models) independent experiments.
Abbreviations: ED, EpiDerm™; ED-FT, EpiDerm™ full-tissue model; 13U, 1,3-dimethylurate.

investigated, the epidermal model EpiDerm and the full-tissue model EpiDerm-FT, showed a metabolite pattern comparable to that of the primary cultures. Theophylline, a substance extensively metabolized by CYP1A2 in the liver (107,108), showed a minor biotransformation in skin. In keratinocytes and in the epidermal model exclusively based on primary keratinocytes at different stages of differentiation, an oxidative (CYP-450 dependent) transformation of theophylline to its metabolite 1,3-dimethylurate did not occur in contrast to fibroblasts and the full-tissue model confirming earlier findings of a higher oxidative capacity of fibroblasts compared with keratinocytes (101). These studies exclude a nameable metabolism of the xanthine caffeine which is recommended as a reference substance for testing percutaneous absorption by the OECD (2) and a consequent impact on its permeation behavior in human skin material. Thus, there is a metabolite activity of the skin which is, however, clearly less than foreign substance biotransformation in the liver (109,110).

Genotoxicity

An additional field of application for human skin models is the determination of genotoxicity and of the mechanism of action of mutagens/carcinogens in skin material of human origin that was established by Zhao et al. using the EpiDerm model. The application of different carcinogenic agents such as benzo[a]pyrenes, UVB and UVA radiation and psoralen-UVA-radiation for instance increased the expression of c-fos and p53-proteins in the skin equivalent as already shown in human and murine skin (111).

Miscellaneous Use in Skin Research

In-house FT models and coculture models, built up by seeding human keratinocytes and melanocytes or Langerhans cells onto de-epidermized dermis, were used to study UV-induced damage and sunscreen efficacy. In fact, using an FT model, UVA- and UVB-induced biological markers were detected at the keratinocyte and fibroblast level, while the keratinocyte/melanocyte cocultures allowed detection of UV-induced pigmentation and immunosuppression (112). Moreover, the SkinEthic model has been used to monitor glutathione redox status following UVB irradiation.

CONCLUSION

At present several skin equivalents of well-defined morphology and lipid composition are commercially available. Some of these have been subjected to formal validation studies to allow the replacement of animal experimentation in the skin hazard analysis of chemical compounds. More commercially available models fulfilling these criteria should follow. In addition, skin equivalents have the potential to enhance the optimization of vehicles for dermatological products and thus reduce the need for clinical studies. The increasing use, however, requires additional testing in comparison to established procedures in vivo and/or in relation to approved tests using human or animal skin ex vivo.

ACKNOWLEDGMENT

Financial support of the German Ministry of Education and Research (BEO 0313343-0313338) is gratefully acknowledged.

REFERENCES

1. OECD. Test Guideline 431: In Vitro Skin Corrosion: Human Skin Model Test. Adopted on 13th April 2004.
2. OECD. Guidance Document No 28 for the Conduct of Skin Absorption Studies. Adopted at 35th Joint Meeting August 2003.
3. OECD. Test Guideline 428: Skin Absorption: In Vitro Method. Adopted on 13th April 2004.
4. Diembeck W, Beck H, Benech-Kieffer F, et al. Test guidelines for in vitro assessment of dermal absorption and percutaneous penetration of cosmetic ingredients. European Cosmetic, Toiletry and Perfumery Association. Food Chem Toxicol 1999; 37(2–3): 191–205.
5. Wagner H, Kostka KH, Lehr CM, et al. Drug distribution in human skin using two different in vitro test systems: comparison with in vivo data. Pharm Res 2000; 17(12):1475–81.
6. Jacobi U, Gautier J, Sterry W, et al. Gender-related differences in the physiology of the stratum corneum. Dermatology 2005; 211(4):312–7.
7. Dubertret L, Coulomb B. Reconstruction of human skin in culture. C R Seances Soc Biol Fil 1994; 188(3):235–44.
8. Rheinwald JG, Green H. Serial cultivation of strains of human epidermal keratinocytes: the formation of keratinizing colonies from single cells. Cell 1975; 6(3):331–43.
9. Gysler A, Lange K, Korting HC, et al. Prednicarbate biotransformation in human foreskin keratinocytes and fibroblasts. Pharm Res 1997; 14(6):793–7.
10. Lange K, Gysler A, Bader M, et al. Prednicarbate versus conventional topical glucocorticoids: pharmacodynamic characterization in vitro. Pharm Res 1997; 14(12):1744–9.
11. Fusenig NE, Boukamp P. Multiple stages and genetic alterations in immortalization, malignant transformation, and tumor progression of human skin keratinocytes. Mol Carcinog 1998; 23(3):144–58.
12. Zouboulis CC, Seltmann H, Neitzel H, et al. Establishment and characterization of an immortalized human sebaceous gland cell line (SZ95). J Invest Dermatol 1999; 113(6):1011–20.
13. Kitajima T, Ariizumi K, Bergstresser PR, et al. T cell-dependent loss of proliferative responsiveness to colony-stimulating factor-1 by a murine epidermal-derived dendritic cell line, XS52. J Immunol 1995; 155(11):5190–7.
14. Kitajima T, Ariizumi K, Mohamadazadeh M, et al. T cell-dependent secretion of IL-1 beta by a dendritic cell line (XS52) derived from murine epidermis. J Immunol 1995; 155(8):3794–800.
15. Radeke HH, von Wenckstern H, Stoidtner K, et al. Overlapping signaling pathways of sphingosine 1-phosphate and TGF-beta in the murine Langerhans cell line XS52. J Immunol 2005; 174(5):2778–86.
16. Gilchrest BA, Vrabel MA, Flynn E, et al. Selective cultivation of human melanocytes from newborn and adult epidermis. J Invest Dermatol 1984; 83(5):370–6.
17. Staiano-Coico L, Hefton JM, Amadeo C, et al. Growth of melanocytes in human epidermal cell cultures. J Trauma 1990; 30(8):1037–42 (discussion 1043).
18. Kippenberger S, Bernd A, Bereiter-Hahn J, et al. Transcription of melanogenesis enzymes in melanocytes: dependence upon culture conditions and co-cultivation with keratinocytes. Pigment Cell Res 1996; 9(4):179–84.
19. Marjukka Suhonen T, Pasonen-Seppanen S, Kirjavainen M, et al. Epidermal cell culture model derived from rat keratinocytes with permeability characteristics comparable to human cadaver skin. Eur J Pharm Sci 2003; 20(1):107–13.

20. Asselineau D, Bernhard B, Bailly C, et al. Epidermal morphogenesis and induction of the 67 kD keratin polypeptide by culture of human keratinocytes at the liquid–air interface. Exp Cell Res 1985; 159(2):536–9.
21. Bodde HE, Holman B, Spies F, et al. Freeze-fracture electron microscopy of in vitro reconstructed human epidermis. J Invest Dermatol 1990; 95(1):108–16.
22. Ponec M, Weerheim A, Kempenaar J, et al. Lipid composition of cultured human keratinocytes in relation to their differentiation. J Lipid Res 1988; 29(7):949–61.
23. Regnier M, Schweizer J, Michel S, et al. Expression of high molecular weight (67 K) keratin in human keratinocytes cultured on dead de-epidermized dermis. Exp Cell Res 1986; 165(1):63–72.
24. Freeman AE, Igel HJ, Herrman BJ, et al. Growth and characterization of human skin epithelial cell cultures. In Vitro 1976; 12(5):352–62.
25. Regnier M, Asselineau D, Lenoir MC. Human epidermis reconstructed on dermal substrates in vitro: an alternative to animals in skin pharmacology. Skin Pharmacol 1990; 3(2):70–85.
26. Bell E, Ivarsson B, Merrill C. Production of a tissue-like structure by contraction of collagen lattices by human fibroblasts of different proliferative potential in vitro. Proc Natl Acad Sci USA 1979; 76(3):1274–8.
27. Naughton G, Jacob L, Naughton B. A Physiological Skin Model for In Vitro Toxicity Studies. New York: Mary Ann Liebert, 1989.
28. Coulomb B, Lebreton C, Dubertret L. Influence of human dermal fibroblasts on epidermalization. J Invest Dermatol 1989; 92(1):122–5.
29. Mackenzie IC, Fusenig NE. Regeneration of organized epithelial structure. J Invest Dermatol 1983; 81(Suppl. 1):189s–94.
30. Bertaux B, Morliere P, Moreno G, et al. Growth of melanocytes in a skin equivalent model in vitro. Br J Dermatol 1988; 119(4):503–12.
31. Nakazawa K, Nakazawa H, Collombel C, et al. Keratinocyte extracellular matrix-mediated regulation of normal human melanocyte functions. Pigment Cell Res 1995; 8(1):10–8.
32. Todd C, Hewitt SD, Kempenaar J, et al. Co-culture of human melanocytes and keratinocytes in a skin equivalent model: effect of ultraviolet radiation. Arch Dermatol Res 1993; 285(8):455–9.
33. Pellegrini G, Bondanza S, Guerra L, et al. Cultivation of human keratinocyte stem cells: current and future clinical applications. Med Biol Eng Comput 1998; 36(6):778–90.
34. Pianigiani E, Risulo M, Andreassi A, et al. Autologous epidermal cultures and narrow-band ultraviolet B in the surgical treatment of vitiligo. Dermatol Surg 2005; 31(2):155–9.
35. Andreassi L, Pianigiani E, Andreassi A, et al. A new model of epidermal culture for the surgical treatment of vitiligo. Int J Dermatol 1998; 37(8):595–8.
36. Ponec M, Weerheim A, Kempenaar J, et al. The formation of competent barrier lipids in reconstructed human epidermis requires the presence of vitamin C. J Invest Dermatol 1997; 109(3):348–55.
37. Gibbs S, Vicanova J, Bouwstra J, et al. Culture of reconstructed epidermis in a defined medium at 33°C shows a delayed epidermal maturation, prolonged lifespan and improved stratum corneum. Arch Dermatol Res 1997; 289(10):585–95.
38. Ponec M, Gibbs S, Weerheim A, et al. Epidermal growth factor and temperature regulate keratinocyte differentiation. Arch Dermatol Res 1997; 289(6):317–26.
39. Kandarova H. Evaluation and Validation of Reconstructed Human Skin Models as Alternatives to Animal Tests in Regulatory Toxicology. Berlin: Free University of Berlin, 2006.
40. Hafner J, Kuhne A, Trueb RM. Successful grafting with EpiDex in pyoderma gangrenosum. Dermatology 2006; 212(3):258–9.
41. Tausche AK, Skaria M, Bohlen L, et al. An autologous epidermal equivalent tissue-engineered from follicular outer root sheath keratinocytes is as effective as split-thickness skin autograft in recalcitrant vascular leg ulcers. Wound Repair Regen 2003; 11(4):248–52.

42. Hoffmann J, Heisler E, Karpinski S, et al. Epidermal-skin-test 1000 (EST-1000)—a new reconstructed epidermis for in vitro skin corrosivity testing. Toxicol In Vitro 2005; 19(7):925–9.
43. Limat A, Noser FK. Serial cultivation of single keratinocytes from the outer root sheath of human scalp hair follicles. J Invest Dermatol 1986; 87(4):485–8.
44. Limat A, Breitkreutz D, Hunziker T, et al. Restoration of the epidermal phenotype by follicular outer root sheath cells in recombinant culture with dermal fibroblasts. Exp Cell Res 1991; 194(2):218–27.
45. Boelsma E, Gibbs S, Faller C, et al. Characterization and comparison of reconstructed skin models: morphological and immunohistochemical evaluation. Acta Derm Venereol 2000; 80(2):82–8.
46. Marjukka Suhonen T, Pasonen-Seppanen S, Kirjavainen M, et al. Epidermal cell culture model derived from rat keratinocytes with permeability characteristics comparable to human cadaver skin. Eur J Pharm Sci 2003; 20(1):107–13.
47. Hoeller D, Huppertz B, Roos TC, et al. An improved and rapid method to construct skin equivalents from human hair follicles and fibroblasts. Exp Dermatol 2001; 10(4):264–71.
48. Augustin C, Collombel C, Damour O. Use of dermal equivalent and skin equivalent models for identifying phototoxic compounds in vitro. Photodermatol Photoimmunol Photomed 1997; 13(1–2):27–36.
49. Augustin C, Collombel C, Damour O. Measurements of the protective effect of topically applied sunscreens using in vitro three-dimensional dermal and skin equivalents. Photochem Photobiol 1997; 66(6):853–9.
50. Hoffmann C, Müller-Goymann CC. Use of artificial skin constructs in permeation studies of clindamycin phosphate. Pharmazie 2005; 60(5):350–3.
51. Rosdy M, Clauss LC. Terminal epidermal differentiation of human keratinocytes grown in chemically defined medium on inert filter substrates at the air–liquid interface. J Invest Dermatol 1990; 95(4):409–14.
52. Gibbs S, Boelsma E, Kempenaar J, et al. Temperature-sensitive regulation of epidermal morphogenesis and the expression of cornified envelope precursors by EGF and TGF alpha. Cell Tissue Res 1998; 292(1):107–14.
53. Ponec M. Reconstruction of human epidermis on de-epidermized dermis: expression of differentiation-specific protein markers and lipid composition. Toxicol In Vitro 1991; 5:597–606.
54. Tinois E, Tiollier J, Gaucherand M, et al. In vitro and post-transplantation differentiation of human keratinocytes grown on the human type IV collagen film of a bilayered dermal substitute. Exp Cell Res 1991; 193(2):310–9.
55. Ponec M, Boelsma E, Weerheim A, et al. Lipid and ultrastructural characterization of reconstructed skin models. Int J Pharm 2000; 203(1–2):211–25.
56. Bouwstra JA, Honeywell-Nguyen PL, Gooris GS, et al. Structure of the skin barrier and its modulation by vesicular formulations. Prog Lipid Res 2003; 42(1):1–36.
57. Pilgram GS, Vissers DC, van der Meulen H, et al. Aberrant lipid organization in stratum corneum of patients with atopic dermatitis and lamellar ichthyosis. J Invest Dermatol 2001; 117(3):710–7.
58. Gazel A, Ramphal P, Rosdy M, et al. Transcriptional profiling of epidermal keratino-cytes: comparison of genes expressed in skin, cultured keratinocytes, and reconstituted epidermis, using large DNA microarrays. J Invest Dermatol 2003; 121(6):1459–68.
59. Faller C, Bracher M. Reconstructed skin kits: reproducibility of cutaneous irritancy testing. Skin Pharmacol Appl Skin Physiol 2002; 15(Suppl. 1):74–91.
60. Faller C, Bracher M, Dami N, et al. Predictive ability of reconstructed human epidermis equivalents for the assessment of skin irritation of cosmetics. Toxicol In Vitro 2002; 16(5):557–72.
61. Ponec M, Boelsma E, Weerheim A. Covalently bound lipids in reconstructed human epithelia. Acta Derm Venereol 2000; 80(2):89–93.
62. Ponec M, Boelsma E, Gibbs S, et al. Characterization of reconstructed skin models. Skin Pharmacol Appl Skin Physiol 2002; 15(Suppl. 1):4–17.

63. Kandarova H, Liebsch M, Spielmann H, et al. Assessment of the human epidermis model SkinEthic RHE for in vitro skin corrosion testing of chemicals according to new OECD TG 431. Toxicol In Vitro 2006; 20(5):547–59.
64. van de Sandt JJ, van Burgsteden JA, Cage S, et al. In vitro predictions of skin absorption of caffeine, testosterone, and benzoic acid: a multi-centre comparison study. Regul Toxicol Pharmacol 2004; 39(3):271–81.
65. OECD. Test Guideline 427: Skin Absorption: In Vivo Method. Adopted on 13th April 2004.
66. OECD. Test Guideline 402: Acute Dermal Toxicity. Updated Guideline, adopted on 24th February 1987.
67. van Ravenzwaay B, Leibold E. The significance of in vitro rat skin absorption studies to human risk assessment. Toxicol In Vitro 2004; 18(2):219–25.
68. Regnier M, Caron D, Reichert U, et al. Barrier function of human skin and human reconstructed epidermis. J Pharm Sci 1993; 82(4):404–7.
69. Schmook FP, Meingassner JG, Billich A. Comparison of human skin or epidermis models with human and animal skin in in-vitro percutaneous absorption. Int J Pharm 2001; 215(1–2):51–6.
70. Lotte C, Patouillet C, Zanini M, et al. Permeation and skin absorption: reproducibility of various industrial reconstructed human skin models. Skin Pharmacol Appl Skin Physiol 2002; 15(Suppl. 1):18–30.
71. Dreher F, Fouchard F, Patouillet C, et al. Comparison of cutaneous bioavailability of cosmetic preparations containing caffeine or alpha-tocopherol applied on human skin models or human skin ex vivo at finite doses. Skin Pharmacol Appl Skin Physiol 2002; 15(Suppl. 1):40–58.
72. Haberland A, Schreiber S, Maia CS, et al. The impact of skin viability on drug metabolism and permeation—BSA toxicity on primary keratinocytes. Toxicol In Vitro 2006; 20(3):347–54.
73. Netzlaff F, Kostka KH, Lehr CM, et al. TEWL measurements as a routine method for evaluating the integrity of epidermis sheets in static Franz type diffusion cells in vitro. Limitations shown by transport data testing. Eur J Pharm Biopharm 2005; 63:44–50.
74. Schafer-Korting M, Bock U, Gamer A, et al. Reconstructed human epidermis for skin absorption testing: results of the German prevalidation study. Altern Lab Anim 2006; 34(3):283–94.
75. Schreiber S, Mahmoud A, Vuia A, et al. Reconstructed epidermis versus human and animal skin in skin absorption studies. Toxicol In Vitro 2005; 19(6):813–22.
76. Netzlaff F, Schaefer UF, Lehr CM, et al. Comparison of bovine udder skin with human and porcine skin in percutaneous permeation experiments. ATLA 2006; 34:499–513.
77. Hartung T, Bremer S, Casati S, et al. A modular approach to the ECVAM principles on test validity. Altern Lab Anim 2004; 32(5):467–72.
78. Bos JD, Meinardi MM. The 500 Dalton rule for the skin penetration of chemical compounds and drugs. Exp Dermatol 2000; 9(3):165–9.
79. Haltner-Ukomadu E, Vuia A, Bock U, et al. Reconstructed human epidermis versus native skin for skin absorption testing—results of the German validation study. In: CRS-Meeting, 22nd–26th July. Vienna, 2006.
80. Jacobi U, Tassopoulos T, Surber C, et al. Cutaneous distribution and localization of dyes affected by vehicles all with different lipophilicity. Arch Dermatol Res 2006; 297(7):303–10.
81. Mahmoud A, Haberland A, Dürrfeld M, et al. Cutaneous estradiol permeation, penetration and metabolism in pig and man. Skin Pharmacol Physiol 2005; 18(1):27–35.
82. Cross SE, Anissimov YG, Magnusson BM, et al. Bovine-serum-albumin-containing receptor phase better predicts transdermal absorption parameters for lipophilic compounds. J Invest Dermatol 2003; 120(4):589–91.
83. Boelsma E, Anderson C, Karlsson AM, et al. Microdialysis technique as a method to study the percutaneous penetration of methyl nicotinate through excised human skin, reconstructed epidermis, and human skin in vivo. Pharm Res 2000; 17(2):141–7.
84. OECD. Test Guideline 404: Acute Dermal Irritation/Corrosion. Updated Guideline, adopted on 24th April 2002.

85. Fentem JH. Validation of in vitro tests for skin corrosivity. Altex 1999; 16(3):150–3.
86. Liebsch M, Traue D, Barrabas C, et al. The ECVAM prevalidation study on the use of EpiDerm for skin corrosivity testing. Altern Lab Anim 2000; 28:371–401.
87. OECD. Test Guideline 430: In Vitro Skin Corrosion: Transcutaneous Electrical Resistance Test (TER). Adopted on 13th April 2004.
88. Fentem JH, Botham PA. ECVAM's activities in validating alternative tests for skin corrosion and irritation. Altern Lab Anim 2002; 30(Suppl. 2):61–7.
89. Zuang V. ECVAM's research and validation activities in the fields of topical toxicity and human studies. Altern Lab Anim 2002; 30(Suppl. 2):119–23.
90. Kandarova H, Liebsch M, Genschow E, et al. Optimisation of the EpiDerm test protocol for the upcoming ECVAM validation study on in vitro skin irritation tests. Altex 2004; 21(3):107–14.
91. Kandarova H, Liebsch M, Gerner I, et al. The EpiDerm test protocol for the upcoming ECVAM validation study on in vitro skin irritation tests—an assessment of the performance of the optimised test. Altern Lab Anim 2005; 33(4):351–67.
92. Liebsch M, Spielmann H, Pape W, et al. UV-induced effects. Altern Lab Anim 2005; 33(Suppl. 1):131–46.
93. OECD. Test Guideline 432: In Vitro 3T3 NRU Phototoxicity Test. Adopted on 13th April 2004.
94. Spielmann H, Balls M, Dupuis J, et al. The international EU/COLIPA in vitro phototoxicity validation study: results of phase II (blind trial), part 1: the 3T3 NRU phototoxicity test. Toxicol In Vitro 1998; 12:305–27.
95. Spielmann H, Balls M, Dupuis J, et al. A study on UV filter chemicals from Annex VII of EU Directive 76/768/EEC in the 3T3 NRU phototoxicity test. ATLA 1998; 26:679–708.
96. Bernard FX, Barrault C, Deguercy A, et al. Development of a highly sensitive in vitro phototoxicity assay using the SkinEthic reconstructed human epidermis. Cell Biol Toxicol 2000; 16(6):391–400.
97. Harris IR, Siefken W, Beck-Oldach K, et al. Comparison of activities dependent on glutathione *S*-transferase and cytochrome P-450 IA1 in cultured keratinocytes and reconstructed epidermal models. Skin Pharmacol Appl Skin Physiol 2002; 15(Suppl. 1):59–67.
98. Harris IR, Siefken W, Beck-Oldach K, et al. NAD(P)H:quinone reductase activity in human epidermal keratinocytes and reconstructed epidermal models. Skin Pharmacol Appl Skin Physiol 2002; 15(Suppl. 1):68–73.
99. Pham MA, Magdalou J, Siest G, et al. Reconstituted epidermis: a novel model for the study of drug metabolism in human epidermis. J Invest Dermatol 1990; 94(6):749–52.
100. Slivka SR, Landeen LK, Zeigler F, et al. Characterization, barrier function, and drug metabolism of an in vitro skin model. J Invest Dermatol 1993; 100(1):40–6.
101. Münster U, Hammer S, Blume-Peytavi U, et al. Testosterone metabolism in human skin cells in vitro and its interaction with estradiol and dutasteride. Skin Pharmacol Appl Skin Physiol 2003; 16(6):356–66.
102. Kubota K, Ademola J, Maibach HI. Metabolism and degradation of betamethasone 17-valerate in homogenized living skin equivalent. Dermatology 1994; 188(1):13–7.
103. Gysler A, Kleuser B, Sippl W, et al. Skin penetration and metabolism of topical glucocorticoids in reconstructed epidermis and in excised human skin. Pharm Res 1999; 16(9):1386–91.
104. Santos Maia C, Mehnert W, Schaller M, et al. Drug targeting by solid lipid nanoparticles for dermal use. J Drug Target 2002; 10(6):489–95.
105. Munster U, Nakamura C, Haberland A, et al. RU 58841-myristate–prodrug development for topical treatment of acne and androgenetic alopecia. Pharmazie 2005; 60(1):8–12.
106. Stecova J, Mehnert W, Blaschke T, et al. Cyproterone acetate loading to lipid nanoparticles for topical acne treatment: particle characterisation and skin uptake. Pharm Res 2007; 24:991–1000.
107. Kizu J, Watanabe S, Yasuno N, et al. Development and clinical application of high performance liquid chromatography for the simultaneous determination of plasma levels of theophylline and its metabolites without interference from caffeine. Biomed Chromatogr 1999; 13(1):15–23.

108. Ha HR, Chen J, Freiburghaus AU, et al. Metabolism of theophylline by cDNA-expressed human cytochromes P-450. Br J Clin Pharmacol 1995; 39(3):321–6.
109. Ademola JI, Wester RC, Maibach HI. Cutaneous metabolism of theophylline by the human skin. J Invest Dermatol 1992; 98(3):310–4.
110. Bronaugh RL, Stewart RF, Storm JE. Extent of cutaneous metabolism during percutaneous absorption of xenobiotics. Toxicol Appl Pharmacol 1989; 99(3):534–43.
111. Zhao JF, Zhang YJ, Kubilus J, et al. Reconstituted 3-dimensional human skin as a novel in vitro model for studies of carcinogenesis. Biochem Biophys Res Commun 1999; 254(1):49–53.
112. Duval C, Schmidt R, Regnier M, et al. The use of reconstructed human skin to evaluate UV-induced modifications and sunscreen efficacy. Exp Dermatol 2003; 12(Suppl. 2):64–70.

10 Skin Absorption as Studied by Spectroscopic Methods

Ulrike Günther
Institute of Pharmaceutics and Biopharmaceutics, Martin Luther University of Halle-Wittenberg, Halle, Germany

Siegfried Wartewig
Institute for Applied Dermatopharmacy, Halle, Germany

Hendrik Metz and Reinhard H. H. Neubert
Institute of Pharmaceutics and Biopharmaceutics, Martin Luther University of Halle-Wittenberg, Halle, Germany

INTRODUCTION

Vibrational spectroscopy has been extensively used in both qualitative and quantitative pharmaceutical analyses. In dermatopharmaceutics, these spectroscopic methods can be applied in the following way:

1. For studying the structure of the stratum corneum (SC) lipids on a molecular level and
2. For investigating the substance penetration into and through the skin.

Depending on the experimental conditions, spectroscopic studies can be performed dynamically (with the possibility of online detection) or statically (like tape-stripping procedure in conjunction with different analytical methods).

Standard methods employed to study the structure of SC are Fourier transform infrared (FTIR) and Raman spectroscopy. In particular, FTIR spectroscopy can be used to investigate the structure of polar submolecular groups of SC lipids, e.g., the head groups. On the other hand, Fourier transform (FT)-Raman spectroscopy was intensively used to study hydrocarbon chains of the SC lipids. Vibrational microspectroscopy may be useful in this field.

In recent years, research interest has been intensively focused on the development of spectroscopic techniques for online monitoring of substance penetration into and through the skin and SC. For this purpose, FTIR attenuated total reflection (ATR) spectroscopy and the FTIR photoacoustic spectroscopy (PAS) were utilized. The challenge in this field is to create spectroscopic methods that allow measurement of drug penetration noninvasively in vivo. There are also literature reports on the application of fiber optic evanescent wave FTIR spectroscopy (FEWS) and confocal Raman spectroscopy for such measurement. Variations of photothermal spectroscopy might be a powerful alternative to measure drug penetration online in vivo.

This chapter covers both standard and modern spectroscopic methods used in dermatopharmaceutics. Spectroscopic methods, which are used to study the structure of the SC lipids, are presented as well as those used to measure substance penetration into and through the skin. UV/VIS and fluorescence methods are not included. After a short introduction to the basic principles of vibrational spectroscopic methods, we address the following issues:

1. Evaluation of the penetration of substances into skin
2. Characterization of the influence of penetration modifier on the properties of the SC
3. Determination of water content and natural moisturizing factor (NMF) of skin.

BASIC PRINCIPLES OF VIBRATIONAL SPECTROSCOPY

Infrared (IR) and Raman spectroscopy deal with the vibrations of the atoms of a molecule. IR spectroscopy is based on the absorption of electromagnetic radiation, whereas Raman spectroscopy relies upon inelastic scattering of light by matter. In vibrational spectroscopy, it is common to use the wave number unit $\tilde{\nu}$, which is expressed in cm^{-1}, instead of the frequency.

Mid-infrared (MIR) spectra provide images of fundamental vibrations of molecules in the region between 400 and 4000 cm^{-1}, while near-infrared (NIR) spectra give those of overtone and combinatory modes of these fundamental vibrations in the range 4000 to 12,500 cm^{-1}. A standard Raman spectrum comprises the spectral range 100 to 3500 cm^{-1}.

The position and intensity of a vibrational band are characteristic of the underlying molecular motion and consequently of the atoms participating in the chemical bond, their conformation and immediate environment. Thus, a certain submolecular group produces bands in a characteristic spectral region. These characteristic bands form the empirical basis for the interpretation of vibrational spectra.

Whereas MIR and Raman spectra are directly related to molecular properties, the molecular information derived from a NIR spectrum is restricted due to the lack of specificity and scattering effects.

The reader interested in details of the basic principles of vibrational spectroscopy and the interpretation of vibrational spectra is referred to relevant books (1–7).

ATR Spectroscopy

FTIR ATR spectroscopy has emerged as one of the standard tools utilized to study the structure of SC on the molecular level, to evaluate the influence of penetration enhancers on the SC barrier function, and to analyze the penetration of substances through skin or SC. It is a nondestructive sampling technique for obtaining the IR spectra of a material's surface and can provide online data in penetration experiments.

In ATR, the sample is placed in optical contact against an internal reflection element (IRE), usually a crystal consisting of ZnSe. The use of ATR in spectroscopy is based upon the fact that although complete internal reflection occurs at the sample–crystal interface, radiation does in fact penetrate a short distance into the sample. The sample interacts with this evanescent wave resulting in the absorption of radiation by the sample, which closely resembles its transmission spectrum. Because the typical range of sampling depth is 1 to 2 μm, information obtained from an ATR spectrum only pertains to the immediate layer in contact with the crystal.

Therefore, an intimate constant optical contact between the sample and the ATR crystal during the entire experiment is crucial but often difficult to guarantee.

In a common ATR penetration setup for online monitoring, the SC as an acceptor is sandwiched between the crystal and a reservoir of penetrant, the donor. Drug diffuses through the SC, initially devoid of the diffusant, until it reaches the impermeable ATR crystal and thus, there will be a build up of penetrant concentration at the interface between SC and crystal. Unfortunately, due to the roughness of the SC, a constant optical contact is not guaranteed during the penetration experiments. In the case of diffusion from a solution, there will be an additional decrease of the optical contact due to formation of a thin solute layer between the crystal and the SC. Obviously, the common ATR penetration setup is not ideal for diffusion experiments on the SC.

An improved FTIR-ATR diffusion cell, which combines the advantages of the ATR technique with the Franz-type diffusion cell, has been developed by Hartmann et al. (8) (Fig. 1). The well-defined acceptor (liquid or semisolid) ensures the optical contact with the ATR crystal and enables the calibration of the drug content in the acceptor medium separately. The advantages of this cell are that acceptor and donor and the initial and boundary conditions are well defined, which is of particular importance for the mathematical model describing the underlying process and estimating the associated diffusion coefficient.

An interesting option of ATR spectroscopy, in particular for in vivo studies, is the use of a silver halide fiber probe, also named fiber optic evanescent wave Fourier transform IR spectroscopy (FEW-FTIR, FEWS). In this version, the IRE sensor section is usually a U-shaped probe with a radius of 4 mm (9,10) or the fiber itself (11–13).

Photoacoustic Spectroscopy

In PAS, intensity modulated or pulsed radiation impinges on the sample is absorbed and generates heat waves within the sample. In turn, after propagation

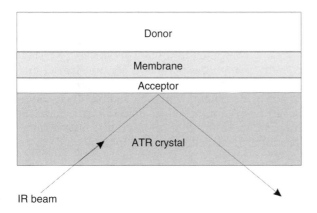

FIGURE 1 Schematic of the FTIR-ATR diffusion cell. A Franz-type diffusion cell is adapted to the ATR technique permitting an intimate optical contact between the acceptor and the ATR crystal. The penetrated drug in the acceptor can be calibrated separately. *Abbreviation*: FTIR-ATR, Fourier transform infrared-attenuated total reflection.

to the sample surface, these thermal waves generate pressure modulation (i.e., sound) in the surrounding transfer gas, usually helium. A sensitive microphone coupled to the acoustic chamber detects the sound signal that provides information about the properties of the sample.

In the case of pulsed PAS (PPAS), laser with different wavelengths (1.064 μm, 532 nm, 354 nm) are used as a radiation source. Otherwise, the interferogram available in a FTIR spectrometer is applied for modulated PAS. Due to the acoustic detection, both optical and thermal properties of the sample determine the PA signal. The modulation frequencies determine the sampling depth of the IR beam (from several μm to 100 μm) and enable a controllable depth profiling of the sample. Hence, applying a sequence of several modulation frequencies in repeated manner, it is possible to acquire data from various probing depths in the course of the penetration process (14–16).

Thermal Emission Decay-Fourier Transformed Infrared Spectroscopy

In thermal emission decay-Fourier transformed infrared spectroscopy (TED-FTIR) a pulsed laser (e.g., wavelength 2.94 μm) is employed as an excitation source to momentarily raise the sample surface temperature with a small increment. A time–domain measurement technique is used to discriminate between transient thermal emission emanated from the heated layer only and steady-state black-body-like emission derived from the bulk of the skin. The entire nonequilibrium MIR emission spectrum is analyzed by a purpose-designed Michelson interferometer. TED-FTIR can acquire in vivo near-surface depth-resolved spectra of the skin (17,18).

Vibrational Microspectroscopy

The collection of vibrational spectra through microscope optics and the visualization of the spectral data by imaging represent a technique that uses spectral features as a native intrinsic contrast mechanism. Hence, the distribution of molecular species within a matrix can be determined quickly and at high lateral resolution. There are two strategies of visualization, namely mapping and imaging. In the mapping mode of operation, spectra are sequentially (in time) collected by point-to-point measurements with a computer-controlled motorized XY-stage attached to the microscope. Generally, mapping experiments are time consuming. In the imaging mode of operation, thousands of spatially resolved spectra may be collected simultaneously from analyses distributed within the sample. The imaging is performed using focal-plane arrays as multichannel detectors. It should be emphasized that the successful application of vibrational spectroscopic imaging requires the combination of spectral analysis, chemometric analysis, and digital imaging analysis (19,20).

Confocal Raman spectroscopy can be applied to obtain information regarding the molecular composition of the skin down to several hundred micrometers below the skin surface with an axial resolution of about 3 to 5 μm. Raman spectra can be obtain from different XY and Z positions. Hence, a three-dimensional profiling of the sample is possible. It permits studies of skin without physical dissection of the sample. However, it should be noted that in vivo Raman spectroscopic measurements must fulfill the laser-safety legislation (21,22).

PENETRATION OF SUBSTANCES INTO SKIN

Vibrational spectroscopic methods enable the simultaneous detection of several compounds within a mixture. FTIR-ATR spectroscopy has emerged as one of the standard techniques used to study the uptake of various substances in natural membranes and hence it's use in dermal/transdermal bioavailability and dermal risk assessment. Information from the deeper regions of the SC can be obtained in conjunction with other analytical methods or by sequential tape stripping, where successive layers of the SC are progressively removed and analyzed. Naik and Guy (23) have given an excellent review on this topic.

Alberti et al. evaluated the SC bioavailability of terbinafine (TB), following topical treatment with four different formulations, using FTIR-ATR measurements of SC tape strips from human skin. For the validation of this spectroscopic method, the amount of TB extracted from the tape strips was determined by high performance liquid chromatography (HPLC). The concentration profiles of TB were fitted to the appropriate solution of Fick's second law of diffusion, thereby enabling the determination of the characteristic diffusion and partitioning parameters of the permeating drug. These studies showed that FTIR-ATR in conjunction with HPLC allows the estimation of drug bioavailability in the SC and may be useful in the critical evaluation of bioequivalence of topical formulations. However, the disadvantage of this approach is the tape-stripping technique itself (24).

The model permeant 4-cyanophenol (CP) is a favored molecule for diffusion studies because it exhibits the nitrile group (C≡N) absorption at 2230 cm^{-1} well separated from IR bands of the SC. Pellett et al. (25,26) studied the permeation of CP through both artificial (silicone) membrane and human SC by FTIR-ATR spectroscopy. Using silicone membranes, a good correlation between permeability coefficients measured with a standard Franz-type diffusion cell and FTIR-ATR spectroscopy was demonstrated. On the other hand, it could be shown that the morphological differences between the inner and outer region of the SC were reflected in variations in permeability, and that the diffusion route through the fully hydrated human SC may be indeed via a direct pathway. The results implied that, depending on the permeant's lipophilicity, lateral molecular diffusion either within the head groups or the lipid tails of the SC bilayers may be a relatively rapid process.

Other groups investigated the dermal absorption of pesticides and other pollutants. Carden et al. compared the absorption of captan and azinphos-methyl after occlusion by FTIR-ATR spectroscopy with multivariate data analysis in conjunction with wipe-sampling, extraction, and gas chromatography (27). Fenske's group quantified the absorption of *O,O*-dimethyl phosphorodithionate and chlorpyros (28).

Silicone derivatives are used as dermal protectants and several groups have characterized the protection effect and possible dermal absorption of these substances. Evaluating the IR band of water at 2100 cm^{-1}, Branagan et al. (29) directly determined the water content in skin after application of a transparent adhesive silicone gel having low water permeability, and a hydrophilic polyurethane membrane coated with acrylic emulsion exhibiting high water permeability. Silicone dressings increased the level of hydration during the experimental time, whereas polyurethane dressings did not increase the hydration level after two hours. FTIR-ATR spectroscopy was also utilized to determine the distribution of silicon in the SC as a function of time. Silicone bands at 790 and 1260 cm^{-1} could be detected after three hours. The content of silicone in SC decreased with depth.

Klimisch et al. (30) compared the permeability of dimethicone derivatives with different molecular masses. Polydimethylsiloxane fluids were applied on the skin. The dimethicone content in the skin increased with increasing molecular mass.

Multiple O/W/O emulsions containing triterpenic compounds as model drugs were studied by Laugel et al. (31). They investigated the influence of different dimethicones on the penetration and the structure of the residual film on the skin by FTIR-ATR and differential scanning calorimetry (DSC). The penetration and distribution of the triterpenes correlated with the silicone structure.

Williams et al. (32) determined the barrier properties of cyclodextrins (CD), in cream formulations, against toluene exposure by studying phase solubility and permeation and by performing thermal analysis. It was found that β-CD retarded toluene permeation. They also evaluated β- and 2-hydroxypropyl-β-cyclodextrine loaded with model drugs (5-fluorouracil and estradiol) as possible penetration enhancers. There was no flux enhancement of the drugs (hydrophilic or lipophilic) when the CDs were used.

Knutson et al. (33) analyzed the influence of water and temperature on the permeability of lipophilic drugs in human skin by DSC and FTIR-ATR spectroscopy. Perhaps not surprisingly, if the fluidity of the hydrophobic lipid matrix increased, the diffusion resistance decreased.

A review on skin integrity after iontophoresis, studied using different methods including IR spectroscopy, is given by Curdy, Kalia, and Guy (34).

Hartmann et al. estimated the diffusion coefficients of urea through isolated SC and bovine hoof membrane using a mathematical model with dynamic boundary conditions. Spectroscopic data were acquired using a specially designed FTIR-ATR diffusion cell. Figure 2 shows the ATR spectra of urea uptake into the acceptor compartment. The calculated intensity of the urea band and the appropriate fit are presented in Figure 3 (8,35).

Ring et al. (36) studied the lipid and water content of lip skin following the application of lip-care products using ATR spectroscopy with silver halide fiber probes. Changes in the lipid content of lip skin and increasing water content were observed in the absorption spectra after treatment with water-free lip-care products. Skin-care products (O/W emulsions with different concentrations of glycerol) caused an increase of polyalcohol and ester vibrations and an increase of the amount of glycerol, water, and lipids on skin surface.

Another approach for ATR spectroscopy using silver halide fiber probes was demonstrated by Heise and colleagues (9,10). After tape stripping they quantified keratin on the adhesive tape surfaces, performed a microscopic inspection of the keratinocyte distribution on the tape. IR microscopy and atomic force microscopy were also used.

Spielvogel et al. examined the diffusion of topically applied Dermoxin® (clobetasol-17-propionate; GlaxoSmithKline, Munich, Germany) and Neribas® (difluorcortolon-21-valerate; Intendis, Berlin, Germany) through human and pig skin using FEWS (11). Diffusion constants for the drugs and water (in case of Neribas) were calculated from these data. Nonconstant environmental conditions resulted in the drying of the skin during the measurement. Raichlin et al. determined the diffusion of UV sunscreen lotions through the skin in vivo by FEWS (12). An interesting review from Afanasyeva, Bruch, and Katzir gives detailed information on the possible applications of FEWS (37).

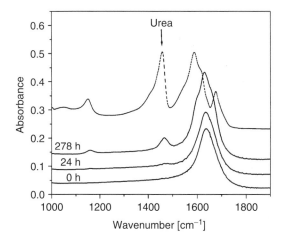

FIGURE 2 FTIR-ATR spectra of the acceptor fluid recorded at different times in a diffusion experiment. An aqueous solution of 10% (w/w) urea acted as donor, water as acceptor, and isolated human SC as membrane. For comparison, the spectrum of crystalline urea is also depicted. The arrow indicates the urea band. *Abbreviation*: FTIR-ATR, Fourier transform infrared-attenuated total reflection.

Applying step scan FTIR-PAS with phase modulation techniques, Hanh et al. studied the penetration of 1-cyanodecane (CyD) into isolated human SC (38). Figure 4 shows the difference FTIR-PA spectra $Sp(t) - Sp(t = 5$ minutes) in the spectral range from 1200 to 1500 cm^{-1} for the SC/Vaseline-CyD system registered with a phase modulation frequency of 13.5 Hz at given times t of the experiment.

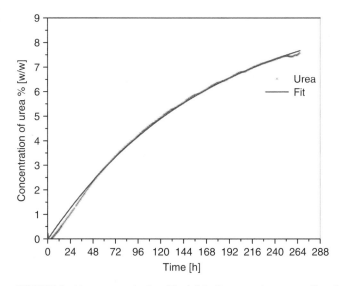

FIGURE 3 Urea concentration (%w/w) in the acceptor versus time for the diffusion experiment: aqueous urea solution/SC/water. The fitting curve with $D = 6.68 \times 10^{-10}$ cm^2 s^{-1} was obtained using a mathematical model with dynamic boundary conditions. *Source*: From Ref. 8.

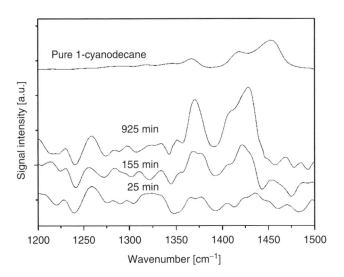

FIGURE 4 Difference in FTIR photoacoustic spectra Sp(t) − Sp(t=5 minutes) (spectral range from 1200 to 1500 cm^{-1}) for a SC/Vaseline-1-cyanodecane system at various times in a penetration experiment. These spectra were registered using step-scan technique with a phase modulation frequency of 13.5 Hz. For comparison, the photoacoustic spectrum of 1-cyanodecane is also shown.

It is obvious that several alterations in the spectra appeared during the course of the penetration. The uptake of CyD in the SC was quantified by monitoring the alterations between 1348 and 1467 cm^{-1} using multivariate analysis. The experiments showed that the effective diffusion coefficient for CyD in SC is depth dependent; in the inner region of the SC, this coefficient is approximately 1.6-fold that measured in the outer region. This finding is not unexpected and can be explained by the inherent, nonuniform homogeneous structure of the SC. The evaluation of the spectroscopic data was based on the assumption that the SC can be considered as an optical and thermal homogeneous medium with a layered structure only with respect to the diffusion behavior. Certainly, this is a rough approximation and an improved model should take into consideration the optical absorption and thermal propagation in a layered structure.

PPAS has been used for the determination of sunscreen emulsions effects in skin. If a topically applied cream diffuses into the bulk of the SC, the thickness of the SC decreases and the time needed for main heat emission to diffuse from the inside of the layer of the cream to the interface with the gas buffer is reduced (39).

Sennhenn et al. employed different spectroscopic methods to evaluate the penetration of UV-filter substances; PPAS was used for depth profiling (40).

The penetration of propylene glycol (PG) through human skin as a function of time and depth was studied by Nothinger and Imhof using TED-FTIR (41). This method is limited by the long time required for each measurement (∼15 minutes). Spectra were collected every 25 minutes over three hours. The maximum depth reached by PG was 6 to 7 μm.

The first attempt to apply IR imaging and mapping methods was reported by Mendelssohn, Rerek, and Moore (42). Jiang et al. employed FTIR imaging to analyze the penetration of hyperosmotic agents (dimethyl sulfoxide and glycerol) into skin (43).

Mendentorp et al. (44) reported the first application of NIR spectroscopy for determining the diffusion of CP and econazole nitrate in vitro through hairless guinea pig skin. They compared pure substances, solutions of the drugs in water or PG and topical creams (1% econazole nitrate), and skin samples after different exposure times with multivariate analysis versus HPLC quantification.

There were also attempts to employ electron paramagnetic resonance spectroscopy (EPR) for in vivo imaging of distribution and metabolism of nitroxide radicals in human skin (45). However, EPR imaging of biological objects requires a large sample volume and low frequency (1.4 GHz or less) to avoid the strong attenuation of the EPR signals because of the absorption of the microwave power by the water molecules at higher (X-band) frequency. The imaging depth is on the order of only a few millimeters and the spatial resolution is limited to 0.2 mm at a frequency of about 1.2 GHz. Thus, using this method, only paramagnetic radicals like nitroxide spin probes and not real drugs or non-paramagnetic molecules can be detected. Nonetheless, the layer where the radicals are enriched and the kinetic of their clearance can be investigated. Because of the unknown attenuation of the EPR signals with increasing skin depth the results can only be interpreted in a semiquantitative way. Different hydrophilic and lipophilic ^{15}N enriched and deuterated spin probes give the opportunity to investigate the influence of skin water content on penetration, enrichment, and clearance.

EFFECTS OF PENETRATION MODIFIERS ON THE PROPERTIES OF SKIN AND SC

The ordered nature of the SC renders it well suited for vibrational spectroscopic studies. Lipid conformations may be quantitatively evaluated without the use of probe molecules. The methylene stretching, scissoring, and wagging modes of acyl chains are extremely sensitive to changes in the chain order and packing. There are many publications reporting the influence of various penetration enhancers on the SC barrier function as studied by FTIR-ATR (46–59). Quantification of penetration enhancement has been reviewed by Moser et al. (60).

Smyth et al. (61) reported the effect of iontophoresis and permeation enhancer on the transdermal delivery of a model peptide through the human epidermal membranes ex vivo. Structural changes in the SC membrane were monitored by FTIR-ATR and other methods. They observed shifts in the wave number positions of the asymmetric and symmetric methylene stretching vibration in the order of a few cm^{-1}. Because of the complex nature of the SC and the fact that ATR probes only the superficial layer of the membrane, these findings should be interpreted with caution.

The effect of different types of liposomes on SC alkyl chain conformation and the percutaneous absorption of sodium fluorescein (Na-Fl) were studied by Coderch and co-workers (62). Phosphatidylcholine liposomes showed the highest penetration rate for Na-Fl and increased the SC lipid disorder. On the other hand, liposomes consisting of SC lipids exhibited a higher affinity to the SC and increased the lipid order. It was postulated that the SC represented a reservoir for Na-Fl, if the amount of the substance was higher in the SC than in other skin layers.

Alcohol–water mixtures were evaluated as penetration enhancers, using sodium salicylate as a model drug. Since ethanol–water mixtures extract SC lipids, SC was rehydrated in water or D_2O and put in ethanol–water or ethanol–D_2O solutions. For estimating the effect of ethanol, the amide I band of the deuterated samples was examined. Concentrations above 0.25% (v/v) ethanol resulted in shoulders on the sides of the amide I band, caused by extended chains disordering the protein domains. The vacuum dried water-prepared samples were evaluated with transmission FTIR. The intensity ratio of the N–H band at 3320 cm^{-1} and the asymmetric CH_2-streching band at 2917 cm^{-1} decreased due to lipid extraction (63).

Different enhancing mechanisms were postulated for Azone® (Whitlay Research, Inc., Richmond, Virginia, U.S.A.) and Transcutol®(Gattefossé, Saint-Priest Cedex, France). Whereas Azone reduced the diffusional resistance, Transcutol increased the solubility of the penetrant in the barrier (64).

Mak et al. (51,52) investigated the influence of PG and oleic acid (OA) on the penetration of CP. After application, the skin was cleaned and ATR spectra were recorded for about nine hours after application. The band intensities of the C≡N vibration of the CP and the C–O stretching vibration of PG at 1040 cm^{-1} related to the SC absorbance at 1741 cm^{-1} were calculated. It was shown that CP was eliminated from the upper SC under first-order kinetics. A change of the band position of the asymmetric CH stretching mode at 2920 cm^{-1} was observed for samples treated with OA, indicating a higher fluidity of the membrane. Reference measurements with excised porcine skin (Franz-type diffusion cell, ^{14}C-CP) confirmed the enhancer effect of OA on CP flux through the skin.

Higo et al. (55) used tape stripping in conjunction with ATR spectroscopy and liquid scintillation counting (LSC) to study the influence of PG and OA on the penetration of CP and ^{14}C-CP. The ATR data were correlated to the amounts of labeled drug determined by LSC. Different mixtures consisting of 10% (w/v) CP in pure PG or PG with 5% (v/v) OA were applied on the skin. After three hours, SC integrity decreased when OA was used and a higher amount of CP was observed in deeper SC regions.

Grewal et al. estimated the flux and the pathlength normalized diffusion coefficient for the following systems: CP in water, PG, or PG +5% 12-azido oleic acid or oleic acid. The SC was directly in contact with the ATR crystal (65). ATR and tape-stripping technique in conjunction with external quantification of radiolabeled drug by LSC and accelerator mass spectrometry enabled the estimation of concentration profiles and generation of a non-steady-state diffusion equation (58).

An increase of the transepidermal water loss (TEWL) following application of OA in PG under occlusion was related to spectral changes in the region 1710 to 1740 cm^{-1}. Both substances acted synergistically in enhancing skin permeation (66).

Terpenes in PG increased the in vitro permeation of haloperidol. Carvacrol showed the highest increase in solubility, linalool in flux, and permeability. Different enhancing mechanisms were discussed. For example, linalool influenced molecular orientation in the horny layer. Furthermore, therapeutic plasma concentrations and therapeutic daily amounts of haloperidol could only be achieved by adding this particular terpene to the formulation. The other terpenes were found to align within the bilayer. There were no changes in the keratin secondary structure, but a different dehydration rate of the SC was observed. The extraction of SC lipids by terpenes or terpene–PG mixtures was less than by pure PG (67,68).

DETERMINATION OF WATER CONTENT AND NATURAL MOISTURIZING FACTOR IN SKIN

The influence of substances on skin lipids can also induce variations in TEWL. When TEWL increases, the barrier function of the skin, especially the SC lipid barrier, is disturbed and structural changes, such as increasing fluidity in the lipid matrix, can appear. Moreover, the water content or the hydration state of the SC influences transdermal delivery of drugs from aqueous solutions. The hydration state or the NMF content can also correlate to some skin diseases (69,70).

Puppels and colleagues combined FTIR-ATR and Raman spectroscopy to obtain a depth profiling of the water content and water profiles in the skin (71,72). Limited by the sampling depth of 1 to 2 μm using the ATR technique, water content can only be determined in the upper SC. However, Raman spectroscopy accesses information from the epidermis (sampling depth up to 80 μm). Confocal methods also offer the possibility of epidermal water depth profiling. Figure 5 shows Raman spectra of the SC obtained at different sampling depths.

The content and the composition of NMF can also be examined by Raman spectroscopic methods. Using laser excitations at various operating wavelengths (730 and 850 nm), the spectral ranges 2000 to 4000 cm^{-1} (730 nm) and 400 to 1850 cm^{-1} (850 nm) can be detected with confocal Raman spectroscopy. A qualitative analysis of NMF content was performed using the water–protein intensity ratio $I(3390 \text{ cm}^{-1})/I(2935 \text{ cm}^{-1})$. For semiquantitative predictions, the relative signal contribution of NMF and keratin between two locations in the skin was used. Since the amide I band showed a high variability, all calculations were estimated without this region (21,22,73).

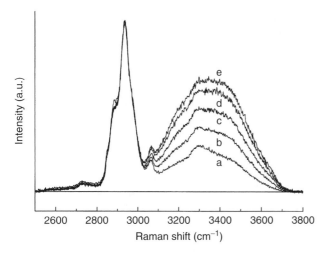

FIGURE 5 In vivo Raman spectra of the SC in the spectral interval from 2500 to 3800 cm^{-1} illustrating the spectral changes due to differences in water content. The spectra were obtained at the tenar, at different depths below the skin surface. Distance to skin surface (a) 0, (b) 75, (c) 80, (d) 85, and (e) 90 μm. The spectra were normalized to the intensity of the protein signal (2910–2965 cm^{-1}). The signal collection time for each spectrum was three seconds, the excitation wavelength 730 nm, and the laser power on the skin 100 mW. *Source*: From Ref. 22.

The correlation between the NIR absorbance and the water content in skin was used to evaluate skin moisture using a new portable NIR system. The relative water content of the SC determined by a capacitance method provided a basis for a partial least squares regression to predict skin moisture (74,75).

Arimoto and Egawa (76) reported that the sampling depth strongly depends on water absorption in the spectral range from 4000 to 8000 cm^{-1}. They measured the water content in vivo and in vitro, and compared these data with the water content determined by a capacitance method. Various statistical equations were used to fit the spectroscopic data: a multivariate analysis for quantification and Monte Carlo simulation for the sampling depth. It was shown that NIR spectroscopy monitors water from deeper regions than the capacitance method. The regional differences in the water content and the influence of probing depth were also determined in vivo. For calibration, in vitro prepared SC was equilibrated at different humidities and the water bands integrated at 5260 and 6900 cm^{-1} were used as a measure for contact and noncontact conditions simulating different penetration depths. Regional differences of the water content were calculated from the comparison of the intensity of the water band at 5260 cm^{-1} and the amide band at 4600 cm^{-1}. These data were compared to Monte Carlo simulation. It was shown that the regional differences depended on sampling depths, differences in the reflection at the skin surface as well as the thickness of SC (77).

The influence of drying agents and moisturizers in dependence on the wavelength was also examined and the distribution of skin moisture was determined as a function of location. For this purpose, NIR bands at long wavelengths showed a better correlation to the water content than short wavelengths (78).

Martin and Curtis differentiated between four types of water in skin: water associated with lipid bilayers, primary and secondary water of hydration on protein, and free bulk water. They determined the water content in different skin layers and the influence of moisturizers in vivo by NIR reflectance spectroscopy (79). It is important to appreciate that, although NIR spectroscopy seems to be a useful method to estimate water content in skin, there are some difficulties. The sampling depth of the NIR beam depends on both the radiation frequencies and the water content in the sample itself. Therefore, some basic work to determine the correlation between NIR frequencies or water content and the sampling depth are necessary, if NIR spectroscopy is to become a versatile tool for the determination of water content in skin. Martin has prepared a critical review on IR and Raman studies of skin and hair (80).

IR imaging and Raman microspectroscopy studies showed that the amount of NMF in corneocytes is twice as much in deeper than in upper skin regions (70). Furthermore, the influence of cosmetics and pharmaceuticals on the hydration state of the skin was investigated. As the following examples demonstrate, ATR spectroscopy—with and without tape stripping for depth profiling—is an often-utilized method in this field.

Sviridov et al. estimated the water and protein content in subsurface layers of treated skin (81,82). The mechanisms of various water donors such as liquid crystalline creams and phospholipid liposomes have been studied by different groups (83,84).

FTIR-ATR in conjunction with gravimetry was applied to investigate the effect of occlusion due to hydrocolloid adhesives. Dressings with high in vitro water vapor uptake exhibited a significantly higher in vivo water uptake and lower skin hydration than those with low in vitro water vapor uptake (85). Brancaleon et al. combined ATR spectroscopy with conductivity experiments to study the hydration level of the skin after application of self-adhesive patches (86).

CONCLUSION

It has been shown that the techniques of MIR and Raman spectroscopy are versatile tools to investigate skin absorption processes both in vitro and in vivo. Both the absorption of substances and their influence on the molecular structure of the SC or skin can be studied using these methods. First attempts to apply NIR and EPR spectroscopy for penetration studies have been reported, but it seems that the results obtained are not so promising.

Owing to the enormous technical improvement in vibrational microspectroscopy in the last few years, this unique technique offers completely new possibilities to study lateral diffusion of drugs in the SC. However, its application is so far limited to in vitro investigations.

Confocal Raman microspectroscopy and TED-FTIR show potential for acquiring depth profiling and time-resolved data of drug penetration.

REFERENCES

1. Chalmers J, Griffiths PR, eds. Handbook of Vibrational Spectroscopy. Vols. 1–5. Chichester: Wiley, 2001.
2. Colthup NB, Daly LH, Wiberley SE. Introduction to Infrared and Raman Spectroscopy. 3rd ed. San Diego: Academic Press, 1990.
3. Günzler H, Heise HM, Gremlich HU. IR Spectroscopy. Weinheim: WILEY-VCH, 2002.
4. Gremlich HU, Yan B, eds. Infrared and Raman Spectroscopy of Biological Materials. New York: Marcel Dekker, 2001:231–58.
5. Lin-Vien D, Colthup NB, Fateley WG, et al. The Handbook of Infrared and Raman Characteristic Frequencies of Organic Molecules. Boston: Academic Press, 1991.
6. Schrader B, ed. Infrared and Raman Spectroscopy. Methods and Applications. Weinheim: VCH, 1995:63–188.
7. Siesler HW, Ozaki Y, Kawata S, et al. Near-Infrared Spectroscopy. Principles, Instruments, Applications. Weinheim: Wiley-VCH, 2001.
8. Hartmann M, Hanh BD, Podhaisky M, et al. A new FTIR-ATR diffusion cell for drug diffusion studies. Analyst 2004; 129:902–5.
9. Heise HM, Kupper L, Butvina LN. Mid-infrared attenuated total reflection spectroscopy of human stratum corneum using a silver halide fiber probe of square cross-section and adhesive tape stripping. J Mol Struct 2003; 661–662:381–9.
10. Heise HM, Kupper L, Pittermann W, et al. Epidermal in vivo and in vitro studies by attenuated total reflection mid-infrared spectroscopy using flexible silver halide fiber-probes. J Mol Struct 2003; 651–653:127–32.
11. Spielvogel J, Reuter S, Hibst R, et al. Monitoring the diffusion of topically applied drugs through human and pig skin using fiber evanescent wave spectroscopy (FEWS). In: Proceedings of SPIE—The International Society for Optical Engineering, Vol. 3596, 1999:99–107.
12. Raichlin Y, Golderg I, Brenner S, et al. Infrared fiber optic evanescent wave spectroscopy for the study of diffusion in the human skin. In: Proceedings of SPIE—The International Society for Optical Engineering, Vol. 4614, 2002:101–8.
13. Brooks A, Afanasyeva NI, Makhine V, et al. New method for investigations of normal human skin surfaces in vivo using fiber-optic evanescent wave Fourier transform infrared spectroscopy (FEW-FTIR). Surf Interface Anal 1999; 27(4):221–9.
14. Rosencwaig A, Gersho A. Theory of the photoacoustic effect with solids. J Appl Phys 1976; 47:64–9.

15. Rosencwaig A. Photoacoustics and Photoacoustic Spectroscopy. New York: Wiley, 1980.
16. Mandelis A, Royce BSH. Time-domain photoacoustic spectroscopy of solids. J Appl Phys 1979; 50:4330–8.
17. Notingher I, Xiao P, Imhof RE, et al. New instrument for FT-Thermal emission decay spectroscopy. Anal Sci 2001; 17:486–9.
18. Notingher I, Imhof RE, Xiao P, et al. Spectral depth-profiling of arbitrary surfaces by thermal emission decay Fourier transform infrared spectroscopy. Appl Spectrosc 2003; 57:1494–501.
19. Sommer AJ. Mid-infrared transmission microscopy. In: Chalmers J, Griffiths PR, eds. Handbook of Vibrational Spectroscopy. Vol. 2. Chichester: Wiley, 2001:1369–85.
20. Dhamelincourt P. Raman microscopy. In: Chalmers J, Griffiths PR, eds. Handbook of Vibrational Spectroscopy. Vol. 2. Chichester: Wiley, 2001:1418–28.
21. Caspers PJ, Lucassen GW, Wolthuis R, et al. In vitro and in vivo Raman spectroscopy of human skin. Biospectroscopy 1998; 4:31–9.
22. Caspers PJ, Lucassen GW, Carter EA, et al. In vivo confocal Raman microspectroscopy of the skin: noninvasive determination of molecular concentration profiles. J Invest Dermatol 2001; 116(3):434–42.
23. Naik A, Guy RH. Infrared spectroscopic and differential scanning calorimetry investigations of the stratum corneum barrier function. In: Potts RP, Guy RH, eds. Mechanisms of Transdermal Drug Delivery. New York: Marcel Dekker, 1997:87–162.
24. Alberti I, Kalia YN, Naik A, et al. In vivo assessment of enhanced topical delivery of terbinafine to human stratum corneum. J Control Release 2001; 71:319–27.
25. Pellett MA, Watkinson AC, Hadgraft J, et al. Comparison of permeability data from traditional diffusion cell and ATR-FTIR spectroscopy. Part I. Synthetic membranes. J Control Release 1997; 154:205–15.
26. Pellett MA, Watkinson AC, Hadgraft J, et al. Comparison of permeability data from traditional diffusion cell and ATR-FTIR spectroscopy. Part II. Determination of diffusional pathlengths in synthetic membranes and human stratum corneum. J Control Release 1997; 154:217–27.
27. Carden A, Yost MG, Fenske RA. Noninvasive method for the assessment of dermal uptake of pesticides using attenuated total reflectance infrared spectroscopy. Appl Spectrosc 2005; 59(3):293–9.
28. Doran EM, Yost MG, Fenske RA. Measuring dermal exposure to pesticide residues with attenuated total reflectance Fourier transform infrared spectroscopy. Bull Environ Contam Toxicol 2000; 64:666–72.
29. Branagan M, Chenery DH, Nicholson S. Use of attenuated total reflectance for the in vivo measurement of hydration level and silicone distribution in the stratum corneum following skin coverage by polymeric dressing. Skin Pharmacol Appl Skin Physiol 2000; 13(3-4):157–64.
30. Klimisch HM, Chandra G. Use of Fourier transform infrared spectroscopy with attenuated total reflectance for in vivo quantification of polydimethylsiloxane on human skin. J Soc Cosmet Chem 1986; 36(2):73–87.
31. Laugel C, Rafidison P, Potard G, et al. Modulated release of triterpenic compounds from an O/W/O multiple emulsion formulated with dimethicones: infrared spectrophotometric and differential calorimetric approaches. J Control Release 2000; 63(1-2):7–17.
32. Williams AC, Shatri SR, Barry BW. Transdermal permeation modulation by cyclodextrins: a mechanistic study. Pharm Dev Technol 1998; 3(3):283–96.
33. Knutson K, Potts RO, Guzek DB, et al. Macro- and molecular physical–chemical consideration in understanding drug transport in the stratum corneum. J Control Release 1985; 2:67–87.
34. Curdy C, Kalia Y, Guy RH. Non-invasive assessment of the effects of iontophoresis on human skin in-vivo. J Pharm Pharmacol 2001; 53(6):769–77.
35. Günther U, Hartmann M, Wartewig S, et al. Diffusion of urea through membranes. Diffusion Fundamentals 2006; 4(1):1–5 (http://www.uni-leipzig.de/diffusion/journal/pdf/volume 4/diff_fund_4(2006)4.pdf).
36. Ring A, Schreiner V, Wenck H, et al. Mid-infrared spectroscopy on skin using a silver halide fibre probe in vivo. Skin Res Technol 2006; 12(1):18–23.

37. Afanasyeva N, Bruch RF, Katzir A. Infrared fiber optic evanescent wave spectroscopy: applications in biology and medicine. In: Proceedings of SPIE—The International Society for Optical Engineering, Vol. 3596, 1999:152–64.
38. Hanh BD, Neubert RHH, Wartewig S, et al. Penetration of compounds through human stratum corneum as studied by Fourier transform infrared photoacoustic spectroscopy. J Control Release 2001; 70(3):393–8.
39. Lahjomri F, Benamar N, Chatri E, et al. Study of the diffusion of some emulsions in the human skin by pulsed photoacoustic spectroscopy. Phys Med Biol 2003; 48(16):2729–38.
40. Sennhenn B, Giese K, Plamann K, et al. In vivo evaluation of the penetration of topically applied drugs into human skin by spectroscopic methods. Skin Pharmacol 1993; 6:152–60.
41. Nothinger I, Imhof RE. In vivo study of penetration of propylene glycol in human SC using depth resolved TED-FTIR spectroscopy. Skin Res Technol 2004; 10(2):113–21.
42. Mendelssohn R, Rerek ME, Moore DJ. Infrared spectroscopy and microscopic imaging of stratum corneum models and skin. Phys Chem 2000; 2(20):4651–7.
43. Jiang J, Boese M, Tunner P, et al. Investigation on dynamic optical clearing effect of skin tissue under topical application of hyperosmotic agents studied with FTIR imaging as an analytical tool. In: Proceedings of SPIE—The International Society of Optical Engineering, Vol. 6085, 2006:60850O/1–9.
44. Medentorp J, Yedluri J, Hammell DC, et al. Near-infrared spectroscopy for the quantification of dermal absorption of ecanozole nitrate and 4-cyanophenol. Pharm Res 2006; 34(4):835–43.
45. He G, Samouilov A, Kuppusami P, et al. In vivo EPR imaging of the distribution and metabolism of nitroxide radicals in human skin. J Magn Reson 2001; 148:155–64.
46. Puttnam NA, Baxter BH. Spectroscopic studies of skin in situ by attenuated total reflectance. J Soc Cosmet Chem 1962; 18:469–72.
47. Comaish S. Infrared studies of human skin by multiple internal reflection. Br J Dermatol 1968; 80:522–8.
48. Puttnam NA. Attenuated total reflectance studies of the skin. J Soc Cosmet Chem 1972; 23:209–26.
49. Baier RE. Noninvasive, rapid characterization of human skin chemistry in situ. J Soc Cosmet Chem 1978; 29:283–306.
50. Potts RO, Guzek DB, Harris PR, et al. A non-invasive, in vivo technique to quantitatively measure water concentration in the stratum corneum using attenuated total reflectance infrared spectroscopy. Arch Dermatol Res 1985; 277:489–95.
51. Mak VHW, Potts RO, Guy RH. Oleic acid concentration and effect in human stratum corneum: non-invasive determination by ATR infrared spectroscopy in vivo. J Control Release 1990; 12(1):67–75.
52. Mak VHW, Potts RO, Guy RH. Percutaneous penetration enhancement in vivo measured by attenuated total reflectance. Pharm Res 1990; 7:835–41.
53. Bommannan D, Potts RO, Guy RH. Examination of stratum corneum barrier function in vivo by infrared spectroscopy. J Invest Dermatol 1990; 95:403–8.
54. Potts RO, Golden GM, Francoeur ML, et al. Mechanism and enhancement of solute transport across the stratum corneum. J Control Release 1991; 15:249–60.
55. Higo N, Naik A, Bommannan DB, et al. Validation of reflectance infrared spectroscopy as a quantitative method to measure percutaneous absorption in vivo. Pharm Res 1993; 10:1500–6.
56. Takeuchi Y, Yasukawa H, Yamaoka Y, et al. Effect of oleic acid/propylene glycol on rat abdominal stratum corneum: lipid extraction and appearance of propylene glycol in the dermis measured by FTIR-ATR spectroscopy. Chem Pharm Bull 1993; 41:1434–7.
57. Clancy MJ, Corish J, Corrigan OI. A comparison of the effects of electrical current and penetration enhancers on the properties of human skin using spectroscopic FTIR and calorimetric DSC methods. Int J Pharm 1994; 105:47–56.
58. Pirot F, Kalia YN, Stinchcomb AL, et al. Characterization of the permeability barrier of human skin in vivo. Proc Natl Acad Sci USA 1997; 94(4):1562–7.

59. Brand RM, Singh P, Aspe-Carranza E, et al. Acute effect of iontophoresis on human skin in vivo: cutaneous blood flow and transepidermal water loss measurements. Eur J Pharm Biopharm 1997; 43:133–8.

60. Moser K, Kriwet K, Naik A, et al. Passive skin penetration enhancement and its quantification in vitro. Eur J Pharm Biopharm 2001; 52(2):102–12.

61. Smyth HDC, Becket G, Mehta S. Effect of permeation enhancer pretreatment on the iontophoresis of luteinizing hormone releasing hormone (LHRH) through human epidermal membrane (HEM). J Pharm Sci 2002; 91:1296–307.

62. Coderch L, de Pera M, Perez-Cullell N, et al. The effect of liposomes on skin barrier structure. Skin Pharmacol Appl Skin Physiol 1999; 12:235–46.

63. Kurihara-Bergstrom T, Knutson K, DeNoble LJ, et al. Percutaneous absorption enhancement of an ionic molecule by ethanol–water systems in human skin. Pharm Res 1990; 7(7):762–6.

64. Harrison JE, Watkinson AC, Green DM, et al. The relative effect of Azone and Transcutol on permeant diffusivity and solubility in human stratum corneum. Pharm Res 1996; 13(4):542–6.

65. Grewal B, Naik A, Irwin WJ. Drug, vehicle and enhancer interactions in percutaneous transport: simultaneous analysis by ATR-IR spectroscopy. In: Proceedings of the International Symposium of Controlled Release Bioactive Materials, Vol. 25, Las Vegas, U.S.A., 1998:569–70.

66. Tanojo H, Junginger HE, Bodde HE. In vivo human skin permeability enhancement by oleic acid. Transepidermal water loss and Fourier transform infrared spectroscopy studies. J Control Release 1997; 47(1):31–9.

67. Vaddi HK, Ho PC, Chan SY. Terpenes in propylene glycol as skin-penetration enhancers: permeation and partition of haloperidol, Fourier transform infrared spectroscopy and differential scanning calorimetry. J Pharm Sci 2002; 91(7):1639–51.

68. Vaddi HK, Ho PC, Chan SY, et al. Terpenes in ethanol: haloperidol permeation and partition through human skin and stratum corneum changes. J Control Release 2002; 81:121–33.

69. Eikje NS, Ozaki Y, Aizawa K, et al. Fiber optic near-infrared Raman spectroscopy for clinical noninvasive determination of water content in diseased skin and assessment of cutaneous edema. J Biomed Opt 2005; 10(1):14013.

70. Zhang G, Moore DK, Mendelsohn R, et al. Vibrational spectroscopy and imaging the molecular composition and structure during human corneocyte maturation. J Invest Dermatol 2006; 126:1088–94.

71. Lucassen GW, Caspers PJ, Puppels GJ. Water content and water profiles in skin measured by FTIR and Raman spectroscopy. In: Proceedings of the SPIE—The International Society for Optical Engineering, Vol. 4162, 2000:39–45.

72. Caspers PJ, Lucassen GW, Bruining HA, et al. Automated depth-scanning confocal Raman microspectrometer for rapid in vivo determination of water concentration profiles in human skin. J Raman Spectrosc 2000; 31:813–8.

73. Caspers PJ, Lucassen GW, Puppels GJ. Combined in vivo confocal Raman spectroscopy and confocal microscopy of human skin. Biophys J 2003; 85(1):572–80.

74. Suh EJ, Woo YA, Kim HJ. Determination of water content in skin by using FT near infrared spectrometer. Arch Pharm Res 2005; 28(4):458–62.

75. Woo YA, Ahn JW, Chun IK, et al. Development of a method for the determination of human skin moisture using a portable near-infrared system. Anal Chem 2001; 73:4964–71.

76. Arimoto H, Egawa A. Non-contact skin moisture measurement based on near-infrared spectroscopy. Appl Spectrosc 2004; 58(12):1439–46.

77. Egawa M, Arimoto H, Hirao T, et al. Regional difference of water content in human skin studied by diffuse-reflectance near-infrared spectroscopy: consideration of measurement depth. Appl Spectrosc 2006; 60(1):24–8.

78. Attas EM, Sowa MG, Posthumus TB, et al. Near-IR spectroscopic imaging for skin hydration: the long and the short of it. Biopolymers 2002; 67(2):96–106.

79. Martin K, Curtis H. In vivo measurement of water in skin by near-infrared reflectance. Appl Spectrosc 1998; 52(7):1001–7.

80. Martin K. IR and Raman studies of skin and hair: a review of cosmetic spectroscopy. Internet J Vibr Spectrosc 1999; 3(2) (http://www.ijvs.com/volume3/edition2/section2.htm).

81. Sviridov AP, Zimnyakov DA, Sinichkin YP, et al. Attenuated total reflection Fourier transform infrared and polarization spectroscopy of in vivo skin ablated layer by layer by erbium:YAG laser. J Biomed Opt 2004; 9(4):820–7.

82. Sviridov AP, Zimnyakov DA, Sinichkin YP, et al. IR Fourier spectroscopy in vivo of human skin during its ablation on exposure to YAG:erbium laser radiation and polarization of the light scattered by the integument. J Appl Spectrosc 2002; 69(4):560–5.

83. De Haan FHN, Hekimogl S, Pechthold LARM, et al. Liquid crystalline creams for controlled skin moisturization; use of ATR-FTIR for studying underlying mechanisms. In: Proceedings of the International Symposium of Controlled Release Bioactive Materials, Vol. 18, 1991:527–8.

84. Bodde HE, Pechthold LARM, Subnel MTA, et al. Monitoring in vivo skin hydration by liposomes using infrared spectroscopy in conjunction with tape stripping. Liposome Dermatics—Griesbach Conference, 1992:137–49.

85. Edwardson PAD, Walker M, Breheny C. Quantitative FTIR determination of skin hydration following occlusion with hydrocolloid containing adhesive dressings. Int J Pharm 1993; 91(1):51–7.

86. Brancaleon L, Bamberg MP, Sakamaki T, et al. Attenuated total reflection-Fourier transform infrared spectroscopy as a possible method to investigate biophysical parameters of stratum corneum in vivo. J Invest Dermatol 2001; 116(3):380–6.

11 Physiologically Based Pharmacokinetics and Pharmacodynamics of Skin

Yuri Dancik, Owen G. Jepps, and Michael S. Roberts

Department of Medicine, Princess Alexandra Hospital, University of Queensland, Woolloongabba, Queensland, Australia

INTRODUCTION

The study of the percutaneous absorption and penetration of exogenous compounds through human skin is relevant to transdermal drug delivery and risk assessment of toxic chemicals. Around 40% of drugs under clinical evaluation are related to delivery to or through the skin (1). The transdermal mode of delivery offers the possibility of eliminating the pain and possible infection associated with injections. It also enables the drug to bypass the hepatic first pass associated with oral delivery, and can provide sustained release of the drug for up to seven days (2). An earlier review of transdermal delivery was provided by Roberts et al. (3).

The advantages of transdermal drug delivery over oral delivery do not mean, however, that the full amount of the topically applied chemical diffuses unhindered to the targeted site in the skin or elsewhere in the body (henceforth called the site of action). A topically applied solute must pass through the formidable stratum corneum (SC) barrier (Fig. 1A), and, if it does so, is likely to penetrate after a lag time. The solute is then subjected to accumulation in reservoirs within the SC. In the viable skin layers the solute is subjected to physiological phenomena which cause a further decrease in the amount of solute reaching the site of action. These phenomena are absorption (A), distribution in the skin (D), metabolism in the skin (M), and elimination by the blood flow (E) occurring in the skin (S). In this chapter we refer to these phenomena by the acronym ADME(S). The ADME(S) phenomena define the solute concentration in the plasma and at the site of action. Physiologically based pharmacokinetics of the skin [PBPK(S)] relates these concentration–time profiles to the underlying physiology in the skin or in the body. Skin pharmacodynamics deals with the steady-state effect, either therapeutic or toxic, of a drug at a particular site in the skin.

The physiologically based pharmacokinetic and pharmacodynamic approach is commonly used in pharmaceutical science but is less developed in the literature pertaining to percutaneous absorption and penetration. The focus, most often, is on the determination of the drug steady-state permeability coefficient needed to overcome the barrier property of the SC. We have termed this approach "traditional SC penetration kinetics." Our goal in writing this chapter is to provide the reader with a basic understanding of the physiological phenomena which affect the transfer kinetics of a given chemical through human skin in terms of PBPK(S).

We begin with the traditional SC penetration kinetics approach and summarize the simple mathematical models used to calculate the flux and the permeability

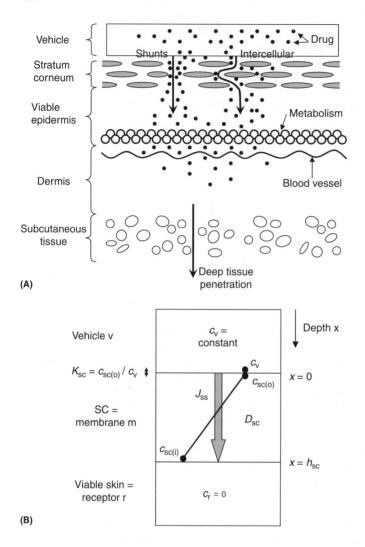

(A)

(B)

FIGURE 1 (**A**) Diagrammatic overview of penetration into the viable skin layers through the stratum corneum (SC) (intercellular) and the shunt pathways. (**B**) Solute concentrations in the skin and physicochemical parameters used in the calculation of the steady-state flux J_{ss} across the SC membrane [equation (1)]. (**C**) Solute amount versus time profile obtained from the exact solution to the diffusion equation [equation (12)] (*solid line*) and steady-state flux J_{ss} (*dashed line*). The lag time and the slope J_{ss} are equal to 1. (**D**) Example of skin compartmental models. (*C and D on facing page.*)

coefficient of solutes through the SC. We then develop physiologically based pharmacokinetics of skin, beginning with the fundamental physical concepts of input rate to the site of action, extent of exposure, and clearance and their relation to the ADME(S) properties. We introduce pharmacodynamics and focus on steady-state relationships between the drug effect at the site of action and the drug

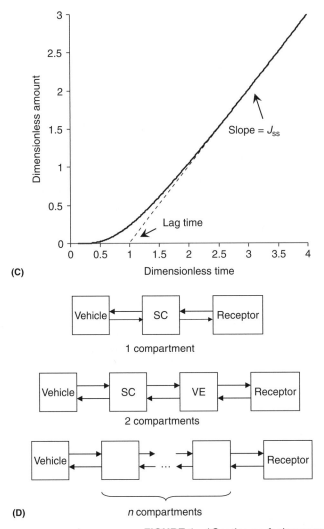

FIGURE 1 (*Caption on facing page.*)

plasma concentration. We extend this discussion to time dependences using pharmacokinetic/pharmacodynamic (PK/PD) models. PK/PD models yield the time dependency of the drug effect at the site of action. To date most experimental work in percutaneous absorption is done in vitro. It is important to correlate in a reliable way the in vitro results to what happens in vivo. We present regression analyses of in vitro and in vivo data obtained from the literature.

TRADITIONAL SC PENETRATION KINETICS

In traditional percutaneous penetration kinetics, the SC is designated as the rate-determining barrier to penetration into the viable skin for most exogenous chemicals, including topically applied drugs. Transport through the SC is then generally described assuming a diffusion process through a homogeneous membrane, devoid of its biological complexity. Typically, topically applied solutes are administered in a formulation consisting of the solute itself and a vehicle usually chosen to dissolve the solute and maximize its penetration. The three parameters most often used to characterize percutaneous penetration are the steady-state flux J_{ss}, the permeability coefficient k_p, and the lag time t_{lag}. J_{ss} represents the rate of penetration at steady state of an amount of permeant after application over a given area of the SC. The permeability coefficient reflects the speed with which a chemical penetrates across the SC. The lag time reflects the time taken for the drug to cross the SC after topical application. The permeability coefficient and the steady-state flux depend not only on the nature of the drug and the state of the SC, but also on the vehicle used to deliver the solute. A more useful parameter describing percutaneous penetration is the maximum flux of solute across the SC, J_{max} (4,5). This parameter is vehicle-independent when the vehicle does not affect the skin. Below we present a simple mathematical model describing penetration of a compound across the SC and show how the model yields the parameters J_{ss}, J_{max}, k_p, and t_{lag}.

A Simple Diffusion Model
Commonly Used Parameters: The Steady-State Flux and Permeability Coefficient
The model presented here is a simple steady-state model based on Fick's first law of diffusion. It yields the permeability coefficient and the lag time through the SC for drug penetration into the skin. This model does not take into account the physiological complexities of the SC, nor does it consider various possible vehicle and exposure conditions. However, it is the model most widely used in evaluating in vitro studies of SC drug penetration.

The steady-state approximation for the rate of penetration per unit area A, or diffusive flux J_{ss}, of the amount Q (mass or number of moles) of a chemical absorbed across the SC, for an exposure time t, is related to the compound's diffusivity D_{sc} in the SC, the thickness of the SC h_{sc}, and the difference in permeant concentration $\Delta c_{sc} = c_{sc(o)} - c_{sc(i)}$ across the SC, i.e., from immediately below the vehicle–SC boundary to immediately above the SC–receptor boundary (Fig. 1B):

$$J_{ss} = \frac{Q}{A\left(t - t_{lag}\right)} = \frac{D_{sc}\Delta c_{sc}}{h_{sc}} \tag{1}$$

Generally, perfect sink conditions are assumed to hold in the receptor phase, such that $\Delta c_{sc} \approx c_{sc(o)}$. The permeant concentration in the vehicle, c_v, can be related to $c_{sc(o)}$ by a partition coefficient K_{sc}, i.e., $c_{sc(o)} = K_{sc}c_v$, so that the steady-state flux across the SC given in equation (1) can be expressed as

$$J_{ss} = \frac{K_{sc}D_{sc}c_v}{h_{sc}} \tag{2}$$

or, by defining a steady-state permeability coefficient k_p as $k_p = K_{sc}D_{sc}/h_{sc}$ as,

$$J_{ss} = k_p c_v \tag{3}$$

A More Useful Parameter: The Maximum Flux

Although the permeability coefficient is widely used in percutaneous absorption studies as a measure of solute penetration into the skin, it is an impractical parameter because, for a given solute, the value of k_p depends on the vehicle used to deliver the solute (5). The most useful parameter is the maximum solute flux J_{max}, i.e., the flux attained at the solubility S_v of the solute in the vehicle

$$J_{max} = \frac{D_{sc}K_{sc}}{h_{sc}}S_v = \frac{D_{sc}}{h_{sc}}S_{sc} \tag{4}$$

where S_{sc} is the solute solubility in the SC.

The Lag Time

A mathematical expression for the lag time is obtained by considering the diffusion equation, which relates the change in permeant concentration over time (non-steady state) with the change in the concentration with depth x

$$\frac{\partial c_{sc}}{\partial t} = D_{sc}\frac{\partial^2 c_{sc}}{\partial x^2} \tag{5}$$

The simplest solution to equation (5) is obtained from the initial and boundary conditions expressing (Fig. 1B)

1. a lack of drug initially in the SC: $c_{sc}(x,t=0)=0$;
2. a constant drug concentration in the vehicle in partition equilibrium with the concentration in the SC at the vehicle/SC boundary: $c_{sc}(x=0,t)=K_{sc}c_v$; and
3. a perfect sink below the SC: $c_{sc}(x=h_{sc},t)=0$.

At steady state the amount of solute $Q_{ss}(t)$ at a given time t calculated from equation (5) and the initial and boundary conditions approximate a straight line (asymptote) given by

$$Q_{ss}(t) = K_{sc}Ac_v h_{sc}\left(\frac{D_{sc}t}{h_{sc}^2} - \frac{1}{6}\right) \tag{6}$$

or, in terms of the familiar parameter J_{ss},

$$Q_{ss}(t) = J_{ss}A(t-t_{lag}) = \frac{K_{sc}D_{sc}c_v}{h_{sc}}A(t-t_{lag}) = k_p c_v A(t-t_{lag}) \tag{7}$$

The lag time is

$$t_{lag} = h_{sc}^2/6D_{sc} \tag{8}$$

Figure 1C shows the $Q(t)$ profile predicted by the diffusion equation (5). The lag time t_{lag} can be obtained by extrapolating the linear part of the curve to the t axis. Equation (7) states that the exposure (i.e., the total amount absorbed) depends on the area of application A, the duration of application t, the solute concentration in the vehicle c_v, and the SC permeability coefficient k_p. Table 1 shows the percentage difference between the actual amount $Q(t)$ attained per multiple of lag time and the amount $Q_{ss}(t)$ predicted by equation (7). As seen in Figure 1C, the steady-state approximation begins at $t=t_{lag}=1$. Thus the percentage difference reported in Table 1 would be negative for $t/t_{lag}<1$.

From Table 1 it is evident that equations (6) and (7) only give accurate estimates of the actual amount $Q(t)$ at steady state (i.e., less than 10% error) when

TABLE 1 Percent Difference Between the Steady-State Amount $Q_{ss}(t)$ [Equation (7)] and the Actual Amount $Q(t)$ with t/t_{lag}

t/t_{lag}	% Difference $= [1-(Q_{ss}(t))/Q(t)] \times 100$
1	100
1.5	17.1
1.7	9.9
2.0	4.3
3.0	0.4
4.0	0.1

t is about 1.7 times the lag time t_{lag}. Of practical value is the actual flux $J(t)$ at any time t, defined by

$$J = \frac{\Delta Q}{A \Delta t} \qquad (9)$$

where ΔQ is the change in amount over a very small time Δt.

More complex models are discussed in greater detail by Roberts and Anissimov (5). These models highlight the effect of the size of the vehicle or donor compartment on the amount of drug absorbed systemically and compare the results obtained for various external skin exposure conditions.

Compartmental Models

Compartmental models represent the skin and the receptor as well-stirred compartments, with transfer between compartments described by first-order rate constants. These models yield the average permeant concentration within each compartment (6). The use of compartmental models has been reviewed by Roberts and Anissimov (5). Figure 1D shows examples of compartmental models with the skin modeled as: one compartment representing the SC; two compartments representing the SC; and the viable epidermis and more than two compartments.

Non-Sink Conditions

As explained later, the solute concentration in the viable skin may also depend on clearance, which itself is a function of dermal blood flow, lymphatic flow, shunt transport, and solute binding. Therefore it cannot be assumed that a perfect sink condition always applies in vivo.

Anissimov and Roberts (7,8) have developed a diffusion model which accounts for non-sink conditions, that is, $c_{sc}(x=h_{sc},t) > 0$. In these papers the receptor clearance was introduced as a parameter describing the removal rate of solute from the receptor phase. This parameter is the same one that would describe dermal clearance of solutes from the viable epidermis in vivo. A removal permeability coefficient $k_{p,r}$ was defined in terms of the receptor clearance Cl_r, the partition coefficient between the receptor phase and the vehicle K_r, and the area of application A: $k_{p,r} = Cl_r K_r / A$. A decrease in the receptor phase clearance will result in a reduced penetration of solute through the skin, i.e., a lower steady-state flux, J_{ss}.

In reality, there are a series of barriers that may affect transport of a solute through the skin and which can be represented in terms of permeability coefficients. These are, in addition to the SC permeability coefficient [$k_{p,sc}$ in equation (10)], the viable epidermis and vehicle–SC interfacial layer permeability coefficients ($k_{p,ve}$ and $k_{p,v}$). The steady-state flux J_{ss} through the SC with a constant vehicle concentration c_v was obtained as

$$J_{ss} = c_v \left(\frac{1}{k_{p,sc}} + \frac{1}{k_{p,ve}} + \frac{1}{k_{p,v}} + \frac{1}{k_{p,r}} \right)^{-1} = k_p'' c_v \tag{10}$$

The permeability coefficient k_p in equation (3) is thus replaced by an "effective" permeability coefficient k_p'' that encompasses the SC and viable epidermis permeability coefficients, the receptor removal permeability coefficient, and vehicle–SC interfacial layer permeability coefficient. The corresponding maximum flux through the SC is given by

$$J_{max} = S_v \left(\frac{1}{k_{p,sc}} + \frac{1}{k_{p,ve}} + \frac{1}{k_{p,v}} + \frac{1}{k_{p,r}} \right)^{-1} = k_p'' S_v \tag{11}$$

This expression is more useful than equation (10) and is a simplified form that, from equation (9), can be expressed as a sum of exponentials using the exact solution $Q(t)$ to the diffusion equation

$$Q(t) = c_v K_{sc} h_{sc} \left(\frac{D_{sc} t}{h_{sc}^2} - \frac{1}{6} - \frac{2}{\pi^2} \sum_{n=1}^{\infty} \frac{-1^n}{n^2} \exp \left(\frac{-n^2 \pi^2 D_{sc} t}{h_{sc}^2} \right) \right) \tag{12}$$

Siddiqui et al. (9) fit equation (12) to in vitro penetration data of steroids to get more precise values for $K_{sc} h_{sc}$ and D_{sc}/h_{sc}^2, which can be used to obtain k_p and t_{lag}.

Effect of Vehicle Volume

Anissimov and Roberts also considered the effect of vehicle volume on skin absorption (8). A decrease in the vehicle volume yields lower cumulative amounts of solute in the skin which plateau at earlier times. Finite vehicle volumes yield asymmetric bell-shaped flux–time profiles. The maximum flux and the time at which maximum flux is reached increase with vehicle volume (Fig. 2A).

Cross and Roberts have shown that infinite and finite doses of a sunscreen benzophenone-3 yield opposite trends in the epidermal flux as the viscosity of the formulation increases (10). An increase in formulation viscosity decreases the flux from an infinite dose. Penetration into the skin is limited by diffusion inside the formulation (Fig. 2B). In the case of a finite dose, the epidermal flux increases with increasing formulation viscosity. The thicker formulation decreases water evaporation from the skin and therefore enhances penetration. These results serve to show that caution must be taken in using infinite dose data to infer real, "in use," results. To obtain in use results, finite dose experiments need to be conducted.

In the models presented thus far, the effect of metabolism and excretion on solute concentration has not been explicitly taken into account. Anissimov and Roberts underlined the fact that in the case of "perfect" receptor sink conditions and no epidermal resistance, the steady-state flux J_{ss} and amount absorbed $Q(t)$ would be reduced by a fraction representing the amount of solute lost due to metabolism and excretion (7). As distinct from traditional SC penetration kinetics, which focuses on the barrier property of the SC (or of SC and the viable epidermis), physiological skin pharmacokinetic models incorporate the physiologically relevant processes of solute absorption, distribution, metabolism, and elimination.

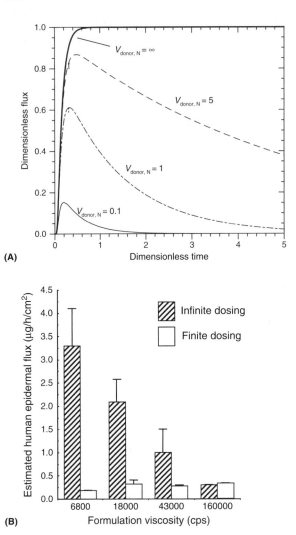

FIGURE 2 (**A**) Effect of the vehicle (donor) volume number $V_{donor,N}$ ($= V_{donor}/V_m K_m$) on the flux–time profile, where V_{donor} = donor volume, V_m = stratum corneum (SC) membrane volume, K_m = SC-donor partitioning coefficient at steady state. *Source*: Adapted from Ref. 8. (**B**) Effect of formulation viscosity on the epidermal flux of benzophenone-3. Shaded histogram represents the infinite dose donor and light histogram represents the finite dose donor. *Source*: Adapted from Ref. 10.

PHYSIOLOGICALLY BASED PHARMACOKINETICS OF SKIN
Overview

Physiologically based pharmacokinetic models of the skin take into account the physiological processes of drug absorption, distribution, metabolism, elimination in the skin, summarized by the term "ADME(S) properties" (Fig. 3A). The issue of toxicity (ADMET(S) properties) is discussed in the context of pharmacodynamics (see the section Skin Pharmacodynamics and PK/PD Models). Absorption designates the process by which the drug proceeds from the site of administration to the site of measurement. Distribution refers to the reversible transfer of drug to and from the site of measurement. Metabolism describes the enzymatic transformation of exogenous substances into other, potentially toxic products. The main sites of metabolism are the liver, the gut wall, and the skin. Elimination refers to the irreversible loss of drug from the site of measurement, both by metabolism and excretion, in which a fraction of the unchanged drug is irreversibly lost. For details on ADME properties, see Ref. 11.

The goal of PBPK(S) models is to calculate the drug concentration–time profile at the site of action after topical application $c^*(t)$. The term "site of action" designates the location in the body at which the drug must be delivered in order to have the desired therapeutic effect. The site of action may be: cutaneous (i.e., in the skin or the skin appendages) as is the case for corticosteroids for the treatment of inflammation; systemic, as for example in the case of β-blockers to treat arterial tension; or in an organ (Fig. 3A). In this last case, the concentration is measured in the plasma, because of the practical difficulty of measuring a drug concentration in an organ other than the skin.

Equations are given below for the concentration at the systemic and cutaneous sites of action in the steady state. The quantities that determine the steady-state concentration at the site of action, c_{ss}^*, are the input flux J_{ss} to the site of action, the fraction of absorbed dose reaching the site of action (the availability), $F_{available}$, and the clearance Cl^* from the site of action

$$c_{ss}^* = \frac{\text{Steady state input flux} \times \text{Availability} \times \text{Area of application}}{\text{Clearance from site of action}}$$

$$= \frac{J_{ss} F_{available} A}{Cl^*} \tag{13}$$

Goal: Concentration in the Systemic Circulation After Topical Application
The Plasma Concentration–Time Profile

The rate and extent of input and the clearance determine the important features of the plasma concentration–time profile. Key parameters are the fraction absorbed f_a, the absorption and elimination rate constants k_a and k_e, and the absorption time $t_{0.5,a}$ (the time necessary for half of the amount of drug in the vehicle to be absorbed into the plasma) and the elimination half-life $t_{0.5,e}$ (the time necessary for half of the amount of drug present in the plasma to be eliminated), the maximum drug plasma concentration c_{max} and the time t_{max} at which it occurs. c_{max} is the plasma concentration at which the rate of absorption equals the rate of elimination. Figure 3B shows the maximum nicotine concentrations following a single transdermal patch application to the upper arm, the back, and the abdomen of volunteers (12). The values of c_{max}, t_{max}, and the $t_{0.5,a}$ obtained after application at each site in this study are reported in Table 2. The authors posit skin blood flow, lipid content, and hydration of the SC causing a different input flux, as possible reasons for the differences in these pharmacokinetic parameters.

The elimination half-life for nicotine after intravenous dosing is shorter, i.e., 2 to 2.5 hours (12). In general, if the terminal elimination phase half-life after topical

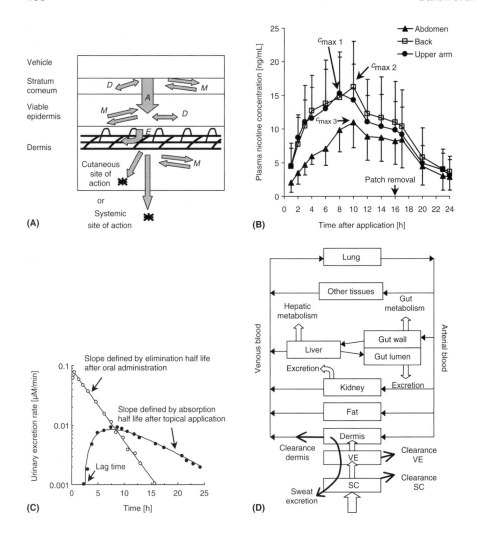

FIGURE 3 (**A**) Schematic of solute absorption (*A*), distribution (*D*), metabolism (*M*), and elimination (*E*) in the skin. (**B**) Plasma nicotine concentration–time profile and maximum nicotine concentrations following a single transdermal patch application to the upper arm, the back, and the abdomen of volunteers. *Source*: Adapted from Ref. 12. (**C**) Excretion rate following oral (*open circle*) and topical (*closed circle*) application of norephedrine HCl. *Source*: Adapted from Ref. 39 (cited in Ref. 3). (**D**) Schematic of a whole-body physiological pharmacokinetic model. *Source*: Adapted from Ref. 13. (**E**) Mean serum concentration–time profile of fentanyl obtained after IV injection. (**F**) Mean serum concentration–time profile of fentanyl obtained from transdermal delivery. *Source*: Adapted from Ref. 17. (**G**) Schematic of the amounts of solute in the skin, the body organs, and recovered in the urine upon topical application and IV administration, based on the fraction of solute absorbed into the skin (f_a) and the fraction lost due to metabolism in the skin ($f_{m,skin}$), and in body organs ($f_{m,body}$). (**H**) Schematic of the skin and body as compartments for the derivation of the effect clearance from the skite of action [equation (29)]. (**E** through **H** on facing page.)

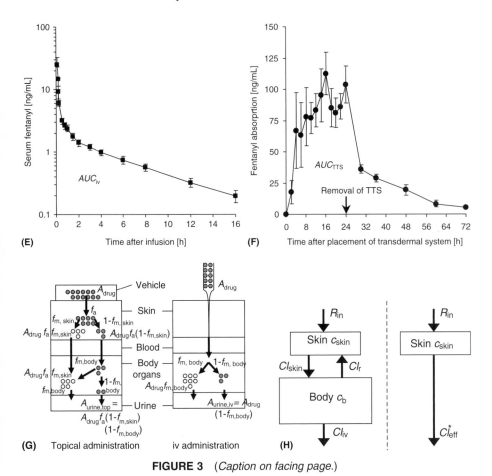

FIGURE 3 (*Caption on facing page.*)

elimination is much longer than that after other modes of administration, "flip-flop" kinetics (explained below) exist. Roberts et al. showed such a relationship for norephedrine (Fig. 3C) (3).

For most orally administered drugs, $t_{0.5,a}$ is shorter than $t_{0.5,e}$, that is, most of the drug has been absorbed and little has been eliminated by the time maximum concentration c_{max} is reached (13). The rate of decrease in plasma concentration following c_{max} is limited primarily by the rate of elimination k_e. In other words, the half-life of drug loss from the body depends on the elimination half-life. A decrease

TABLE 2   Mean c_{max}, t_{max}, and $t_{0.5,e}$ Values Obtained from the Transdermal Application of Nicotine to 3 Body Sites

Site of administration	c_{max} (ng/mL)	t_{max} (h)	$t_{0.5,e}$ (h)
Upper arm	15.45±5.42	8.7±1.0	5.10±2.42
Back	16.64±6.62	8.9±2.0	5.10±2.42
Abdomen	11.51±3.78	10.1±2.9	4.97±1.67

Source: From Ref. 12.

in the rate of absorption yields an increase in t_{max} and a lower peak plasma concentration c_{max}.

In contrast, for topically applied drugs, the absorption half-life $t_{0.5,a}$ is usually longer than the elimination half-life. In this regime absorption is so slow that it is eliminated from the body as soon as it enters the systemic circulation. The rate of elimination equals the rate of absorption, which now determines the rate of drug loss from the body. In other words, the half-life represents the rate of input to the systemic circulation rather than the clearance from it (14). Since the roles of absorption and elimination are swapped, one speaks of "flip-flop kinetics." Tozer and Rowland point out that in this case, the terms "absorption phase" and "elimination phase" with respect to the plasma concentration–time profile are "misleading" (13). Lefèvre et al. have recently described the pharmacokinetics of a rivastigmine transdermal patch applied to various body sites of volunteers (15). The elimination half-life of 3.2 to 3.9 hours was found to be longer to the elimination half-life of intravenously administered rivastigmine [1.39 ± 0.37 hours, (16) cited in (15)]. These data are consistent with flip-flop kinetics. The longer elimination half-life is due to slow rivastigmine absorption into the systemic circulation.

The rate of input is determined by the lag time t_{lag} of penetration into the skin and the steady-state flux J_{ss} discussed above.

The extent of absorption is characterized in skin by the first-pass availability $F_{available}$ (3,13). $F_{available}$ is the fraction of topically applied permeant that reaches the systemic circulation unchanged by metabolism in the skin.

The clearance of a drug from the systemic circulation can be calculated from the input flux, the area of application, and the systemic (plasma) concentration following an intravenously administered dose, $c_{ss,p}$. In the case of IV administration, the availability is unity. The clearance is thus

$$Cl_{iv} = \frac{J_{ss}A}{c_{ss,p}} \tag{14}$$

In the case of an IV bolus injection, the clearance is obtained from the total administered dose D_{iv} and the area under the plasma concentration–time curve, AUC_{iv}^{∞}, a measure of the total systemic exposure to the drug (13)

$$Cl_{iv} = \frac{D_{iv}}{AUC_{iv}^{\infty}} \tag{15}$$

Steady-State Plasma Concentration

Under steady-state conditions the plasma concentration upon topical application is

$$c_{ss,p} = \frac{J_{skin}A}{Cl_{iv}} = \frac{J_{ss}F_{available}A}{Cl_{iv}} \tag{16}$$

where the flux through the skin J_{skin} is expressed as the fraction $F_{available}$ of the flux through the skin at steady state, J_{ss}. The body clearance is the drug clearance measured from IV administration, Cl_{iv}. Equation (16) can be used to calculate the skin first-pass availability $F_{available}$ for an infinite topical dose.

If the site of action is an organ in the body other than the skin itself, the operative concentration at that site depends on blood flow to other organs, and hepatic, renal, and gut clearance in addition to clearance from the skin (Fig. 3D).

Goal: Concentration at the Cutaneous Site of Action

The total steady-state concentration of solute reaching the cutaneous site of action depends on the rate of input to the site of action and the effective clearance from it [equation (13)]. The concentration actually measured is the steady-state concentration of unbound solute, c_u^*. It is related to the total steady-state concentration at the site of action by the fraction of unbound solute f_u

$$c_u^* = f_u c_{total}^* = f_u \frac{\text{Rate of input to site of action (g/h)}}{\text{Effective clearance from site of action (cm}^3\text{/h)}} \qquad (17)$$

The rate of input depends on the flux to the cutaneous site of action, J_{skin}^* [amount/(area × time)] and the area of topical application A[area]. As previously shown, when a compound is applied to the skin continuously over a surface area A, there is a steady-state flux J_{ss} of permeant given by equation (2). J_{ss} is the flux at the skin surface resulting from exposure. It depends only on the physicochemical parameters of the permeating compound and the vehicle used to deliver the active compound, and on the thickness of the SC which is approximated as a homogeneous membrane. For a very small finite dose, J_{ss} will also depend on the external exposure conditions, that is, on inclusion or exclusion of donor removal, wash off, evaporation. The flux of drug that actually reaches a cutaneous site of action is a fraction F_{cut} of J_{ss} because some of the permeant will be eliminated in the skin due to metabolism,

$$J_{skin}^* = F_{cut} J_{ss} \qquad (18)$$

F_{cut} is the cutaneous availability. It depends on the fraction of solute absorbed from the vehicle into the skin and the fraction of absorbed drug subsequently metabolized in the skin.

The steady-state unbound concentration at the cutaneous site of action is thus

$$c_u^* = f_u c_{total}^* = f_u \frac{J_{skin}^* A}{Cl_{eff}^*} = f_u \frac{J_{ss} A F_{cut}}{Cl_{eff}^*} \qquad (19)$$

where Cl_{eff}^* is the effective clearance from a cutaneous site of action. In the section Estimation of Skin First-Pass Availability from Excretion Data, we show the dependency of the cutaneous availability on the fraction of solute absorbed into the skin, f_a, and the fraction of solute metabolized in the skin, f_m. In the section Effective Clearance from Cutaneous Site of Action, we give an explanation of the components of the effective clearance Cl_{eff}^*.

Estimation of Skin First-Pass Availability Based on Plasma Concentration Data

Equation (13) applies to the steady-state situation, represented by an extended constant rate of absorption. Rearranging for $F_{available}$ gives

$$F_{available} = \frac{c_{ss}^* Cl^*}{J_{ss}}. \qquad (20)$$

Equation (20) can be used if the steady-state flux J_{ss} is known, for example, from in vitro skin studies.

A more reliable estimate for $F_{available}$ after topical administration is provided by the area under the plasma concentration–time curve following topical application, $AUC_{topical}^{\infty}$

$$F_{available} = \frac{AUC_{topical}^{\infty} \, Cl_{iv}}{D_{topical}}. \tag{21}$$

Where $D_{topical}$ is the amount of solute absorbed through the skin as, for example, determined as the amount of solute lost from a patch after topical administration. Recognizing that the clearance from the plasma Cl_p is obtained from an IV bolus injection [equation (15)], equation (21) becomes

$$F_{available} = \frac{AUC_{topical}^{\infty}}{D_{topical}} \frac{D_{iv}}{AUC_{iv}^{\infty}}. \tag{22}$$

Varvel et al. used equation (22) with dose-normalized areas under the curve to calculate the systemic availability of the opioid fentanyl following transdermal absorption (17). $D_{topical}$ was estimated by residual analysis as the amount of fentanyl lost from the transdermal delivery system after removal of the system at 24 hours. Figure 3E and F show the mean serum concentration–time profiles obtained after IV injection, used to calculate the clearance of fentanyl from equation (15), and the mean serum concentration–time profile obtained from transdermal delivery. The areas under the curve AUC_{iv}^{∞} and $AUC_{topical}^{\infty}$ were obtained by adding the AUCs of Figure 3E and F to AUCs extrapolated from the final point of these curves to infinity. The mean availability obtained was 0.92 ± 0.33. This high value indicates that little fentanyl is eliminated by cutaneous metabolism or degradation (17).

Estimation of Skin First-Pass Availability from Excretion Data

In the usual situation in which there is no saturation in absorption, metabolism, or elimination (i.e., linear kinetics), it is also possible to calculate $F_{available}$ from other measured quantities. The availability can be calculated directly from the ratio of amounts excreted (A_e) by different routes i and metabolized (A_m) to the applied topical dose

$$F_{available} = \frac{\sum_i A_{e,i} + A_m}{D_{topical}}. \tag{23}$$

The ratio of the amounts of drug excreted in the urine following a topical and an intravenous dose can also be used to determine $F_{available}$

$$F_{available} = \frac{\text{urinary excretion of unchanged drug, topical}}{\text{urinary excretion of unchanged drug}}$$

$$= \frac{A_{urine,topical}}{A_{urine,iv}}. \tag{24}$$

To see why equation (24) is valid, consider Figure 3G. The fraction of topically applied solute that penetrates into the skin and is subsequently metabolized is f_a $f_{m,skin}$. The fraction of permeant absorbed into the skin which remains unaffected by skin metabolism (the cutaneous availability) is

$$F_{cut} = f_a(1 - f_{m,skin}) \tag{25}$$

After the solute has penetrated into the systemic circulation, it is subjected to metabolism in various organs of the body. A fraction $f_{m,body}$ of the solute is eliminated from the body organs (in particular the liver and the gut) and through excretion via the feces. The fraction $F_{skin,syst}$ of unchanged topically applied solute remaining in the body is

$$F_{skin,syst} = f_a(1 - f_{m,skin})(1 - f_{m,body})$$ (26)

Equation (26) gives the fraction of topically administered drug which is excreted from the body to the urine. Upon IV administration the fraction of unchanged drug excreted from the body into the urine is

$$F_{iv,syst} = 1 - f_{m,body}$$ (27)

Dividing equation (26) by equation (27) yields the fraction of permeant applied topically present in the systemic circulation—the skin first-pass availability

$$F_{available} = \frac{F_{skin,syst}}{F_{iv,syst}} = f_a(1 - f_{m,skin})$$ (28)

Roberts et al. calculated the skin bioavailability of methyl salicylate in various commercial products from urinary amounts (18). The values obtained for $F_{available}$ are low, ranging from 0.12 to 0.20. The usefulness of the methyl salicylate formulations is thus limited to local cutaneous effects. The authors suggest using other drugs, such as nitroglycerin or hyoscine, to achieve greater systemic levels from topical administration. Table 3 shows in vivo availabilities calculated from urinary excretion data for topically applied estradiol (19) and diclofenac (20).

It is important to note that the *percentage urinary excretion from IV dose* is not the percentage of permeant that *enters* the systemic circulation upon IV administration, but rather the percentage of IV administered drug that remains unchanged in the systemic circulation over time [$F_{iv,syst}$, equation (27)]. $F_{skin,syst}$ determines the total amount of unchanged drug over time in the systemic circulation, given by AUC_{iv}^{∞}. Upon entry into the systemic circulation, a permeant is subjected to metabolism in the blood and elsewhere in the body, therefore the values for the *percentage urinary excretion from IV dose* in Table 2 are not 100%.

Factors Affecting Skin First-Pass Availability

The nature of the skin (vascularization, metabolism, presence of shunt pathways) varies from one body site to another and it should be expected that $F_{available}$ will vary depending on the site of topical application. Table 2 shows the difference in the parameters c_{max} and t_{max} obtained by Sobue et al. (12) from the transdermal

TABLE 3 In Vivo Availabilities of Topically Applied Estradiol (Protected Dose Site) and Diclofenac

	Estradiol	Diclofenac
% Urinary excretion from topical dose	3.9 ± 2.1	4.03
% Urinary excretion from IV dose	51.6	61
$F_{available}$ (%)	7.5 ± 4.1	6.6

Source: From Refs. 19,20.

TABLE 4 Cumulative Urinary Salicylate Recovery from Different Sites of Application

Region of topical application	Cumulative urinary salicylate recovery after 48 hours (mg)
Abdomen	210
Forearm	180
Instep	88
Heel	56
Plantar	41

Source: From Ref. 18.

delivery of nicotine to different sites of the body. Roberts et al. obtained different cumulative urinary amounts of excreted salicylate 48 hours after topical application to different body sites (Table 4) (18). The significant difference between these cumulative amounts is likely due to a thicker SC and fewer hair follicles acting as shunts in the regions of the foot.

The factors that affect the absorption of permeant into the skin (f_a) are blood flow, binding, the reservoir effect in the skin (discussed in the section The Reservoir Effect), deeper tissue penetration, shunt transport and lymphatic flow, as well as skin physiological changes due to age, gender, and disease (see Ref. 21 for more details).

Other Interpretations of Availability

In the percutaneous absorption literature one also finds calculations of availabilities characterizing only the concentration of drug found in the SC. Kalia et al. (22) and Alberti et al. (23) define topical (bio)availability as the total solute concentration measured in the stratum corneum following exposure. They measured an "external bioavailability" which addresses the input into the skin from the vehicle but not physiological processes occurring within it.

Different drug administration methods or vehicles are often compared using *relative* availabilities. In Krishnaiah et al. (24), the delivery of nicarpidine hydrochloride from a transdermal therapeutic system is compared to the delivery from an immediate release capsule dosage form by means of a relative availability, defined as the ratio of the AUCs obtained from plasma concentration profiles. Järvinen et al. compared the absorption of estradiol from a transdermal, a tablet, and a patch using relative availabilities computed as the ratios of AUCs (25).

Effective Clearance from Cutaneous Site of Action

The Problem

In this section we give an expression for the effective drug clearance from the cutaneous site of action [Cl_{eff}^*, equation (19)]. Figure 3H shows the parameters of importance for the calculation of the effective clearance. The rate of drug input to the skin site of action is given by R_{in}. The drug concentration in the skin is c_{skin}. The drug is cleared into the body with clearance Cl_{skin}; however, there is also a return clearance, Cl_r. The drug concentration in the body is represented by the plasma concentration c_p. The drug is cleared from the body with clearance Cl_{iv}. The effective clearance from the cutaneous site of action (Fig. 3H) is a function of the clearance from the skin to the body, the return clearance from the body to the skin, and the body clearance

$$Cl^*_{eff} = \frac{Cl_{skin}Cl_{iv}}{Cl_{iv} + Cl_r} \tag{29}$$

The mass balance for drug in the skin, i.e., "the amount entering the skin equals the amount exiting it," is

$$R_{in} = c_{skin}Cl^*_{eff} \tag{30}$$

Limiting Cases

We now consider the implications of our solution [equation (29)] for two limiting cases: (*i*) when the body clearance is much *greater* than the return clearance ($Cl_{iv} \gg Cl_r$) and (*ii*) when the body clearance is much *less* than the return clearance ($Cl_{iv} \ll Cl_r$).

In the first case, we find that $Cl^*_{eff} \approx Cl_{skin}$—the effective clearance is just the clearance from the skin site of action. In this limit, the return clearance has a negligible effect on the drug kinetics; the effective clearance is essentially what we would observe if the return clearance was altogether absent. This can be clearly seen from our model once we realize that this limiting case is equivalent to assuming that $c_p Cl_r \ll c_p Cl_{iv} = R_{in}$. In this context, equation (29) becomes $R_{in} \approx c_{skin} Cl_{skin}$ and the return clearance plays no effective role.

In the second case, we find that $Cl^*_{eff} \approx Cl_{skin} c_p / Cl_r \ll Cl_{skin}$. Furthermore, we note that $c_p Cl_r \gg c_p Cl_{iv} = R_{in}$, implying that the return clearance provides a much greater source of drug than the applied dose. The steady state [equation (30)] implies that all the drug is returned to the body, so that the exchange between skin and body is much greater than input at the site of action (and output via body clearance). This limit is the limit of the closed system, where $R_{in}/(Cl_{skin} c_{skin}) \to 0$ and equation (30) becomes $c_{skin} Cl_{skin} = c_p Cl_r$, consistent with the partitioning observed for a closed system.

Prodrugs and Soft Drugs

Far from being considered only as a physiological process causing irreversible drug loss, skin metabolism is also exploited in order to improve drug transport through the skin. The pro- and soft drug approaches are drug design paradigms that take advantage of skin metabolism.

Figure 4A illustrates the mechanisms of pro-, soft, and pro–soft drugs. The prodrug method consists of attaching a promoiety to a parent drug rendering it pharmacologically inactive, with the goal of improving its cutaneous bioavailability F_{cut} [equation (18)] and the skin first pass bioavailability $F_{available}$ [equation (20)]. The promoiety improves the parent drug's water solubility, or circumvents an elimination, or formulation problem (26), thereby increasing the compound's absorption into the skin. Table 5 compares the in vitro steady-state fluxes of several parent drugs and prodrugs as an indicator of increased throughput across the SC. The flux of the active compound to the site of action, i.e., the internal exposure flux $J^*_{act,int}$, can be expressed in terms of the cutaneous bioavailability and the external exposure flux of the inactive parent drug ($J_{inact,ext}$) as follows:

$$J^*_{act,int} = (1 - F_{cut})J_{inact,ext} \tag{31}$$

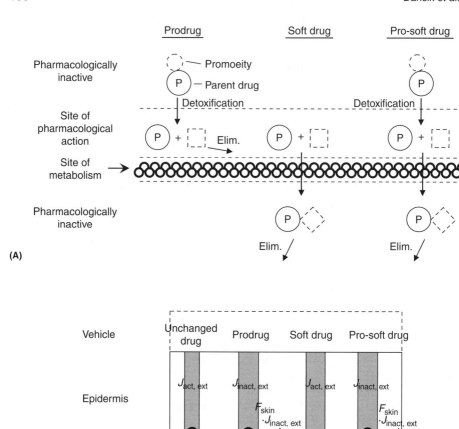

FIGURE 4 (**A**) Schematic of the pro-, soft, and pro–soft drug mechanisms. (**B**) Illustration of the mechanism of topically applied pro-, soft, and pro–soft drugs. $J_{act,int}$ designates the internal (subscript "int") exposure flux of the pharmacologically active (subscript "act") compound, i.e., the flux reaching the site of action. Subscript "inact" designates the pharmacologically inactive drug. Subscript "ext" designates the external exposure flux, the flux of drug to which the site of action is not exposed.

The soft drug mechanism consists of utilizing skin metabolism to deactivate pharmacologically active compounds to nontoxic products (26) after the pharmacological effect has been attained at the site of action. This approach is the opposite of the prodrug approach.

A pro–soft drug is the inactive prodrug of a soft drug. A pro–soft drug is converted enzymatically to the active soft drug upon penetration into the skin, then deactivated enzymatically following the pharmacological action (26). Figure 4B

TABLE 5 Comparison of the Steady-State Flux of Selected Parent Drugs and a Prodrug Obtained from the Literature

Parent drug/prodrug	Skin model	Flux (nmol/cm² per hour)	Ref.
N/N decanoate	Mouse skin, in vitro	1.40/51.6	27
5-FU/1,3 bisacetyl-5-FU	Mouse skin, in vitro	240/2200	28
NTX/NTX-3-acetate	Human skin, in vitro	2.50/15.6	29
K/1-propyl ester K	Rat skin, in vitro	3.86/46.6	30

Abbreviations: FU, fluorouracil; K, ketorolac; N, Nalbuphine; NTX, naltrexone.

illustrates the difference between pro-, soft, and pro–soft drugs in terms of the external exposure and internal exposure fluxes.

The Reservoir Effect

Effect on Diffusion into the Skin

Roberts and coworkers have recently published a comprehensive analysis of the skin reservoir effect (31). In this section we review the most important points of their publication. The term "skin reservoir effect" designates the sequestration of solutes in the SC or the viable skin tissue and the formation of pools of solute within these skin layers. Upon provocation a given amount of solute may be released from the reservoir and diffuse to the cutaneous or systemic site of action, resulting in a delayed pharmacological effect. The formation of reservoirs within the skin thus affects the flux of solute to the site of action and the extent of absorption. The capacity for a drug to form a reservoir depends on the diffusion coefficient of the drug in the SC, the amount of drug in the SC, and the clearance from the viable epidermis.

Slow diffusion or a short topical application time compared to the diffusion time will not yield enough drug in the SC for a reservoir to form. Diffusion into the SC and reservoir formation may be enhanced by occlusion, which hydrates the SC. Roberts et al. have developed a compartmental model that includes three compartments representing the SC, the viable epidermis, and the systemic circulation to study the corticosteroid reservoir effect in the SC. During the first 120 hours of diffusion into the skin, the amount of corticosteroid decreases by about 15%. A 20-fold increase in SC diffusivity as a result of occlusion at the 120-hour mark yields an exponential decrease in the amount of corticosteroid; over the next 120 hours nearly 100% of the amount remaining in the SC is lost. The amount in the viable epidermis on the other hand increases about 20-fold at the 120 hours time point. Pellanda et al. have recently compared the effect of pre-occlusion to post-occlusion in the penetration of the corticosteroid triamcinolone acetonide (TACA) into the SC (32). Contrary to pre-occlusion, post-occlusion increased the retention of TACA in the SC and delayed its release, indicating the formation of a reservoir in the SC.

The amount of drug in the SC depends on the drug's affinity for the SC. This depends on the drug's lipophilicity, quantified by the octanol–water partitioning coefficient, and on the vehicle. Figure 5A shows the partitioning of various hydrocortisone-21-esters into the SC from water increases with the octanol–water partitioning coefficient $K_{o/w}$. A lipophilic compound will partition more readily into the SC than a hydrophilic solute and is expected to show a greater reservoir effect. Figure 5B shows that increasing the affinity of a drug for the SC increases

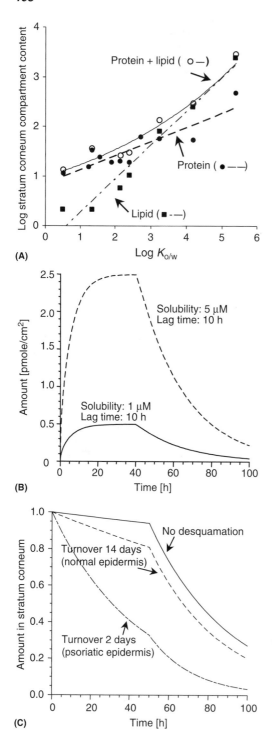

FIGURE 5 (**A**) Log apparent stratum corneum (SC) (protein and lipid)–water partitioning coefficient versus log octanol–water partitioning coefficient (log $K_{o/w}$) for various hydrocortisone-21-esters, ratio of 0.85 protein to 0.15 lipid. Also shown is the contribution of the SC protein domain (0.85 protein) and the SC lipid domain (0.15 lipid) to the SC-water partitioning coefficient. *Source*: Data abstracted from Ref. 53. (**B**) Amount in the SC versus time for two solutes of varying SC solubilities, based on a diffusion model developed by Roberts et al. (31). *Source*: Adapted from Ref. 31. (**C**) Amount of cortisone remaining in the SC with no desquamation, a normal epidermal turnover time of 14 days, and a psoriatic epidermal turnover time of two days, obtained by Roberts et al. using a hydrated epidermal lag time of 16.5 hours in a model described in Ref. 31.

the amount in the SC. The time needed to reach the maximum amount and the fractional rate of reservoir depletion, however, remain unchanged. The location of the reservoir in the SC also depends on the solute's lipophilicity. Data reviewed in (31) show that lipophilic steroids have a higher affinity for the SC lipid domain whereas more polar steroids partition preferentially into the protein domain of the SC.

The nature of the vehicle in which the solute is dissolved also influences reservoir formation. A polar vehicle will increase the affinity of a lipophilic solute for the SC compared to a lipophilic vehicle. Solute clearance from the viable epidermis will also affect the amount of time a solute remains in a SC reservoir. Low clearance from the viable epidermis may yield a higher reservoir effect due to slower flux across the SC. Low partitioning from the SC into the viable epidermis will also retain the solute in the SC for longer periods of time.

The Effect of Desquamation on SC Permeability

Roberts et al. included a rate constant for desquamation (epidermal turnover) in their model. Results show that desquamation decreases the amount of corticosterone remaining in the SC upon penetration (Fig. 5C) (31). With high clearance rate from the viable skin, the effect of desquamation is important when the desquamation rate is equal or higher than the SC permeability. The effect of desquamation is increased in the case of diseased skin with a faster epidermal turnover rate, with the steroid reservoir effect decreasing. Reddy et al. (33) used a convection-diffusion model to describe effect of desquamation on the SC reservoir effect. Desquamation was found to be important if the turnover time is small relative to the diffusional SC lag time, for example in the case of diseased hyperproliferative skin. The epidermal turnover reduces the fraction absorbed in the epidermis only for large MW and large log $K_{o/w}$ drugs.

SKIN PHARMACODYNAMICS AND PK/PD MODELS
Pharmacodynamic Models

While physiologically based skin pharmacokinetics describes transdermal delivery to the site of action, skin pharmacodynamics measures the steady-state clinical effect of a drug once the site of action is reached. Typically, the effect (e.g., change in blood pressure) is considered as a function of the steady-state plasma concentration. Simple mathematical models are used to fit these functional relations using the maximum effect E_{max} and the dose required to achieve 50% of the maximum, E_{50}, as model parameters. The models are the E_{max} model [equation (32), Fig. 6A] and the sigmoidal E_{max} model [equation (33), Fig. 6A],

$$E = E_0 \pm \frac{E_{max} \, c_p}{E_{50} + c_p} \tag{32}$$

$$E = E_0 \pm \frac{E_{max} \, c_p^\gamma}{E_{50}^\gamma + c_p^\gamma} \tag{33}$$

The term E_0 is a baseline value (34), from which the effect E either increases, resulting in effect *stimulation* [+ sign in equations (32) and (33)], or decreases, resulting in effect *inhibition* [− sign in equations (32) and (33)]. The difference between equations (32) and (33) is the inclusion of the shape or sigmoidicity factor γ, which is used to obtain a better fit to the AUC data. Equations (32) and (33)

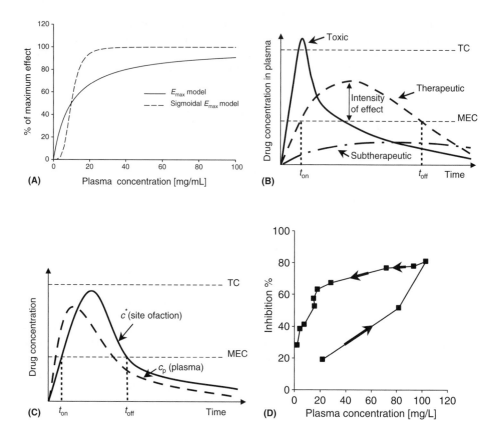

FIGURE 6 (A) Percentage of maximum effect (E_{max}) reached as a function of concentration obtained from the E_{max} model [equation (34)] and the sigmoidal E_{max} model [equation (35)]. Parameter values: $E_{max} = 100$ mg/mL, $E_{50} = 10$ mg/mL, $E_0 = 0$ mg/mL, $\gamma = 4$. (B) Schematic of toxic, therapeutic, and subtherapeutic drugs concentration in plasma versus time profiles. The therapeutic window is the range of concentration lying between the minimum effect concentration (MEC) and the toxicity concentration (TC). t_{on} is the time of onset, at which the MEC at the site of action, which is in the plasma, is first achieved and t_{off} is the time of offset, at which the drug becomes therapeutically inactive. (C) Schematic illustrating the time delay between drug concentration–time profiles in plasma (c_p) and at a different site of action (c^*), where t_{on} and t_{off} relate to the site of action. (D) Percentage effect (angiotensin II AT_1 receptors inhibition) versus plasma concentration for orally administered telmisartan. *Source*: Adapted from Ref. 38.

are models for the steady-state effect, calculated from steady-state plasma concentrations.

The extent of the effect over a given period of time can be modeled by expressing the effect in time of the topically applied dose $D_{topical}$,

$$E = E_0 \pm \frac{E_{max} \, D_{topical}}{ED_{topical,50} + D_{topical}} \tag{34}$$

$$E = E_0 \pm \frac{E_{max} \, D_{topical}^{\gamma}}{ED_{topical,50}^{\gamma} + D_{topical}^{\gamma}} \tag{35}$$

where $ED_{topical,50}^{\gamma}$ is the dose required to reach 50% of the maximum effect. Singh et al. (35) and Tsai et al. (36) have used the dose-based E_{max} model [equation (34)] to successfully fit population AUC data sets for the topical penetration of corticosteroids from various creams and ointments.

Pharmacokinetics/Pharmacodynamic Models

Whereas pharmacodynamic models consider the relation between applied dose and effect of a drug at the (cutaneous or systemic) site of action, PK/PD models yield information on the time dependency of the clinical effect. This is achieved by plotting the effect against the time-dependent drug plasma concentration.

Figure 6B shows a plasma concentration and site of action concentration–time profiles in the context of the drug's therapeutic window. The therapeutic window is the range of concentrations at the site of action within which the drug is therapeutically active. Its bounds are the minimum effect concentration (MEC), below which the drug is therapeutically inactive, and the toxicity concentration, above which the drug is toxic. The time of onset t_{on} is the time at which the MEC at the site of action is first achieved; the time of offset t_{off} is the time at which the drug becomes therapeutically inactive. The time delay between the plasma concentration and site of action concentration (Fig. 6C) may be due to delayed distribution to the site of action, or, in the case of a prodrug, delayed enzymatic conversion of the metabolite into the active drug (37,38). It sholud be noted that the concentrations at the site of action do not correspond to the plasma concentrations.

The time delay is evident when the effect E is plotted against the plasma concentration c_p. The resulting curve is a hysteresis, in which the response (the effect) follows a different path when the plasma concentration decreases to when it increases (37). To date PK/PD models have only been developed for drugs administered either intravenously or orally. Stangier et al. (38) investigated the effect of the orally administered drug telmisartan on the inhibition of the angiotensin II AT_1 receptors, which stimulates an increase in blood pressure. The percentage inhibition was found to vary with telmisartan plasma concentration according to a counterclockwise hysteresis loop (Fig. 6D). The authors suggest this behavior could be explained by tight binding of the drug molecules to the AT_1 receptors and subsequent slow dissociation. An alternative explanation is that of a telmisartan reservoir effect in the smooth muscle. In this case the drug concentration would remain high to the receptor even as it drops in the plasma.

Beckett et al. have compared the oral and percutaneous route of norephedrine administration from the viewpoint of the urinary excretion rate. They showed the time to peak urinary excretion rate was longer and the peak excretion less in the case of topical absorption (39). Orally administered ephedrine has been studied by Persky et al. using the PK/PD approach (40). These authors obtained a hysteretic profile for the systolic blood pressure as a function of the plasma concentration. A comparison of this study with a PK/PD study of topically applied ephedrine would yield valuable information.

IN VITRO–IN VIVO (CLASSICAL/PHYSIOLOGICAL PK/PD)

Excised human skin and animal skin models are approximations of viable human skin as they do not take into account blood flow or skin metabolism. Phosphate buffered saline (PBS) (41) and commercial media followed by incubation in CO_2 (42) have been used to keep excised human skin viable, but it is unclear from the literature how effective these techniques are in mimicking in vivo conditions.

The skin models most often used are excised human and rat skin. We have taken data from published studies (43–51) comparing in vitro and in vivo penetration results for solutes applied in equivalent doses and from the same formulations to excised human and rat skin. Figure 7A and B show in vitro versus in vivo data for excised human skin and rat skin, respectively. The in vitro data obtained from Refs. 43–51 (except Ref. 50) are the percentage of the applied dose

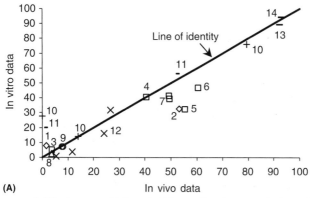

(A)

1: Nitrobenzene [43]; 2: 2,4-Dinitrochlorobenzene [43]; 3: Caffeine in water gel [44]; 4: Caffeine in petrolatum [44]; 5: Caffeine in ethylene glycol gel [44]; 6: Caffeine in benzoic acid [44]; 7: Testosterone [44]; 8: Isofenphos [45]; 9: Chloroform [46]; 10: Lindane [47]; 11: Chlorpyrifos [48,49]; 12: *ortho*-Phenylphenol [50]; 13: Methylene bis-benzotriazoyl tetramethylbutylphenol (MBBT) [51]; 14: Titanium dioxide [51].

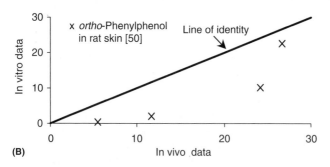

(B)

FIGURE 7 Comparison of published in vitro and in vivo percutaneous absorption data. In vitro data are obtained from **(A)** full-thickness excised human skin and **(B)** excised rat skin. (*Solid line*, line of identity.)

absorbed in the receptor compartment of a diffusion cell and the in vivo data are the percentage of the applied dose measured in the urine. The data from Ref. 50 are the amount systemically available 4 to 48 hours after application. It is included in Figure 7A as the percentage of the applied dose systemically available. The line of identity represents equal percentage values from the in vitro and in vivo experiments.

While the in vitro and in vivo data correlate linearly reasonably well (Fig. 7A), a number of in vitro data points underpredict the in vivo results. Bronaugh and Franz (44) explain the low in vitro data values (nos. 5, 6, 7 in Fig. 7A) by the fact that the abdominal skin temperature in vitro is lower than that in vivo, where it is covered by clothing. A further error could be due to the IV correction in the in vivo study. Cnubben et al. conducted their in vitro experiments with viable full-thickness abdominal skin (50). They explain their low in vitro results (no. 12 in Fig. 7A) by the fact that at early time points (4, 8, and 24 hours), part of the absorbed *ortho*-phenylphenol was not excreted with the urine. At the final time point of 48 hours, however, the in vitro and in vivo data are comparable. Cnubben et al. found that the potentially absorbed dose (the applied dose minus the dose "dislodged" from the applied dose after 4 hours of exposure) obtained in vitro most accurately predicted in vivo percutaneous absorption (50).

Dick et al. (47) and Griffin et al. (48,49) (nos. 10 and 11 in Fig. 7A, respectively) obtained an overprediction of the in vivo results from in vitro experiments. Both groups attributed this finding to the inability of the in vitro setup to mimic the SC reservoir effect. Dick et al. obtained comparable in vitro and in vivo results for the percentage of the applied dose of lindane recovered on a swab and in the SC 6 hours after application, but the results differed markedly at 24 hours after application. Some of the lindane present in the reservoir was recovered externally due to contact or to desquamation. Occlusion in the in vivo case may also have caused lindane in the reservoir to penetrate deeper into the skin. Griffin et al. obtained similar in vitro and in vivo amounts of chlorpyrifos from skin washing. The in vitro percentage of the applied dose recovered in the receptor fluid solution, however, was much larger than the percentage recovered in the urine in vivo. Griffin et al. speculate that chlorpyrifos may have partitioned into the subcutaneous fat tissue and slowly released, resulting in amounts in the urine below the level of detection. The ethanol/water receptor fluid may have also altered the SC, resulting in an over-prediction in vivo (49).

Cnubben et al. also compared viable full-thickness rat skin as an in vitro model to their in vivo results (50). Figure 7B shows that the in vitro results significantly underpredict the in vivo results. A possible reason is that viable rat skin metabolizes *ortho*-phenylphenol to a greater extent than human skin.

The results presented in this section show that excised human skin is a better in vitro model for in vivo percutaneous penetration than excised rat skin. However, design parameters of in vitro experiments need to be improved in order to correctly predict in vivo results. Temperature in the diffusion cell appears to be an important parameter to control. The potential effect of components of the donor solution in vitro on the structure of the SC needs to be taken into account when interpreting in vitro results. In vitro experiments do not take into account reservoir effects or metabolism in the skin. The outlier's testosterone and 2,4-dinitrochlorobenzene in Figure 7A are likely subject to skin metabolism in vivo. Kao et al. showed that the viable epidermis can act as a metabolic barrier to the permeation of testosterone (52).

CONCLUSION

The emphasis in the percutaneous absorption literature has largely been on traditional SC penetration kinetics; that is, how to bypass the SC barrier by optimizing the formulation and/or modifying the SC itself. The solute kinetic parameters most often reported in the literature are its permeability coefficient and/or steady-state flux across the SC. Greater emphasis should be placed on the solute maximum flux across the SC, which is generally independent of the nature of the vehicle.

The traditional approach to skin penetration kinetics, however, does not permit an accurate evaluation of the concentration at the site of pharmacological action (cutaneous or systemic) upon topical application. This concentration depends on the combined effects of the cutaneous physiological processes of absorption into the skin, distribution within the skin tissue and the rest of the body, metabolism in the skin and other organs (liver, gut, etc.), and elimination from the skin or other organs. This paradigm forms the basis of physiologically based pharmacokinetics of skin [PBPK(S)]. The parameters that determine the solute concentration at the site of action are solute flux to the site of action, solute availability, and solute clearance from the site of action.

To assess the validity of PBPK(S) models, in vivo experiments need to be conducted to the extent that they are feasible. In vitro experiments need to predict in vivo results as accurately as possible. We have shown that a reasonable linear correlation exists between published in vitro results obtained with full-thickness excised human skin and corresponding in vivo results. It is evident, however, that the in vitro experiments do not take into account physiological processes occurring in the skin, such as the reservoir effect and cutaneous metabolism.

In PK/PD modeling, time-dependent pharmacokinetic data (in general solute plasma concentration values as a function of time) are combined with pharmacodynamic (steady-state clinical effect vs. applied dose data) to obtain the time dependency of the clinical effect. So far the application of PK/PD modeling to topical drugs has been lacking in the percutaneous absorption literature. A comparison of Persky et al.'s PK/PD for orally administered ephedrine (40) with a PK/PD study of topically applied ephedrine would yield valuable information.

ACKNOWLEDGMENT

We thank the National Health and Medical Research Council (NHMRC) and Australian Research Council (ARC) for support of this work.

REFERENCES

1. Cross SE, Roberts MS. Physical enhancement of transdermal drug application: is delivery technology keeping up with pharmaceutical development? Curr Drug Deliv 2004; 1(1):81–92.
2. Joshi A, Raje J. Sonicated transdermal drug transport. J Control Release 2002; 83(1):13–22.
3. Roberts M, Cross S, Pellett M. Skin transport. In: Walters KA, ed. Dermatological and Transdermal Formulations. New York: Marcel Dekker, 2002.
4. Magnusson BM, Anissimov YG, Cross SE, Roberts MS. Molecular size as the main determinant of solute maximum flux across the skin. J Invest Dermatol 2004; 122(4):993–9.
5. Roberts M, Anissimov Y. Mathematical models in percutaneous absorption. In: Bronaugh R, Maibach H, eds. Percutaneous Absorption. Boca Raton: CRC Taylor & Francis, 2005.

6. McCarley KD, Bunge AL. Physiologically relevant one-compartment pharmacokinetic models for skin. 1. Development of models. J Pharm Sci 1998; 87(10):1264.

7. Anissimov YG, Roberts MS. Diffusion modeling of percutaneous absorption kinetics. 1. Effects of flow rate, receptor sampling rate, and viable epidermal resistance for a constant donor concentration. J Pharm Sci 1999; 88(11):1201–9.

8. Anissimov YG, Roberts MS. Diffusion modeling of percutaneous absorption kinetics: 2. Finite vehicle volume and solvent deposited solids. J Pharm Sci 2001; 90(4):504–20.

9. Siddiqui O, Roberts MS, Polack AE. Percutaneous absorption of steroids: relative contributions of epidermal penetration and dermal clearance. J Pharmacokinet Biopharm 1989; 17(4):405–24.

10. Cross SE, Jiang R, Benson HAE, Roberts MS. Can increasing the viscosity of formulations be used to reduce the human skin penetration of the sunscreen oxybenzone? J Invest Dermatol 2001; 117(1):147–50.

11. Gola J, Obrezanova O, Champness E, Segall M. ADMET property prediction: the state of the art and current challenges. Qsar Comb Sci 2006; 25(12):1172–80.

12. Sobue S, Sekiguchi K, Kikkawa H, Irie S. Effect of application sites and multiple doses on nicotine pharmacokinetics in healthy male Japanese smokers following application of the transdermal nicotine patch. J Clin Pharmacol 2005; 45(12):1391–9.

13. Tozer TN, Rowland M. Introduction to Pharmacokinetics and Pharmacodynamics: The Quantitative Basis of Drug Therapy. Baltimore: Lippincott Williams & Wilkins, 2006:326.

14. Oliyai R, Stella VJ. Prodrugs of peptides and proteins for improved formulation and delivery. Annu Rev Pharmacol Toxicol 1993; 33:521–44.

15. Lefèvre G, Sędek G, Huang HLA, et al. Pharmacokinetics of a rivastigmine transdermal patch formulation in healthy volunteers: relative effects of body site application. J Clin Pharmacol 2007; 47(4):471–8.

16. Hossain M, Jhee SS, Shiovitz T, et al. Estimation of the absolute bioavailability of rivastigmine in patients with mild to moderate dementia of the Alzheimer's type. Clin Pharmacokinet 2002; 41(3):225–34.

17. Varvel JR, Shafer SL, Hwang SS, Coen PA, Stanski DR. Absorption characteristics of transdermally administered fentanyl. Anesthesiology 1989; 70(6):928–34.

18. Roberts MS, Favretto WA, Meyer A, Reckmann M, Wongseelashote T. Topical bioavailability of methyl salicylate. Aust N Z J Med 1982; 12(3):303–5.

19. Wester RC, Hui X, Maibach HI. In vivo human transfer of topical bioactive drug between individuals: estradiol. J Invest Dermatol 2006; 126(10):2190–3.

20. Hui X, Hewitt PG, Poblete N, Maibach HI, Shainhouse JZ, Wester RC. In vivo bioavailability and metabolism of topical diclofenac lotion in human volunteers. Pharm Res 1998; 15(10):1589–95.

21. Cross SE, Roberts MS. Effects of dermal blood flow, lymphatics, and binding as determinants of topical absorption, clearance and distribution. In: Riviere JE, ed. Dermal Absorption Models in Toxicology and Pharmacology. Boca Raton: CRC Taylor & Francis, 2006:251–81.

22. Kalia YN, Alberti I, Naik A, Guy RH. Assessment of topical bioavailability in vivo: the importance of stratum corneum thickness. Skin Pharmacol Appl Skin Physiol 2001; 14(Suppl. 1):82–6.

23. Alberti I, Kalia YN, Naik A, Guy RH. Assessment and prediction of the cutaneous bioavailability of topical terbinafine, in vivo, in man. Pharm Res 2001; 18(10):1472–5.

24. Krishnaiah YS, Satyanarayana V, Bhaskar P. Influence of limonene on the bioavailability of nicardipine hydrochloride from membrane-moderated transdermal therapeutic systems in human volunteers. Int J Pharm 2002; 247(1–2):91–102.

25. Jarvinen A, Nykanen S, Paasiniemi L. Absorption and bioavailability of oestradiol from a gel, a patch and a tablet. Maturitas 1999; 32(2):103–13.

26. Bodor N, Buchwald P. Soft drug design: general principles and recent applications. Med Res Rev 2000; 20(1):58–101.

27. Sung KC, Fang JY, Hu OY. Delivery of nalbuphine and its prodrugs across skin by passive diffusion and iontophoresis. J Control Release 2000; 67(1):1–8.

28. Beall HD, Sloan KB. Topical delivery of 5-fluorouracil (5-FU) by 1,3-bisalkylcarbonyl-5-FU prodrugs. Int J Pharm 2002; 231(1):43–9.

29. Stinchcomb AL, Swaan PW, Ekabo O, et al. Straight-chain naltrexone ester prodrugs: diffusion and concurrent esterase biotransformation in human skin. J Pharm Sci 2002; 91(12):2571–8.

30. Doh HJ, Cho WJ, Yong CS, et al. Synthesis and evaluation of Ketorolac ester prodrugs for transdermal delivery. J Pharm Sci 2003; 92(5):1008–17.

31. Roberts MS, Cross SE, Anissimov YG. The skin reservoir for topically applied solutes. In: Bronaugh RL, Maibach HI, eds. Percutaneous Absorption: Drugs, Cosmetics, Mechanisms, Methodology. Boca Raton: Taylor & Francis, 2005:213–34.

32. Pellanda C, Strub C, Figueiredo V, Rufli T, Imanidis G, Surber C. Topical bioavailability of triamcinolone acetonide: effect of occlusion. Skin Pharmacol Physiol 2007; 20(1):50–6.

33. Reddy MB, Guy RH, Bunge AL. Does epidermal turnover reduce percutaneous penetration? Pharm Res 2000; 17(11):1414–9.

34. Meibohm B, Derendorf H. Basic concepts of pharmacokinetic/pharmacodynamic (PK/PD) modelling. Int J Clin Pharmacol Ther 1997; 35(10):401–13.

35. Singh GJP, Adams WP, Lesko LJ, et al. Development of in vivo bioequivalence methodology for dermatologic corticosteroids based on pharmacodynamic modeling. Clin Pharmacol Ther 1999; 66(4):346–57.

36. Tsai JC, Cheng CL, Tsai YF, Sheu HM, Chou CH. Evaluation of in vivo bioequivalence methodology for topical clobetasol 17-propionate based on pharmacodynamic modeling using Chinese skin. J Pharm Sci 2004; 93(1):207–17.

37. Tozer TN, Rowland M. Introduction to Pharmacokinetics and Pharmacodynamics. Baltimore: Lippincott Williams & Wilkins, 2006.

38. Stangier J, Su CAPF, Van Heiningen PNM, et al. Inhibitory effect of telmisartan on the blood pressure response to angiotensin II challenge. J Cardiovasc Pharmacol 2001; 38(5):672–85.

39. Beckett AH, Gorrod JW, Taylor DC. Comparison of oral and percutaneous routes in man for the systemic administration of 'ephedrines'. J Pharm Pharmacol 1972; 24(Suppl.):65P–70.

40. Persky AM, Berry NS, Pollack GM, Brouwer KLR. Modelling the cardiovascular effects of ephedrine. Br J Clin Pharmacol 2004; 57(5):552–62.

41. Liu P, Higuchi WI, Ghanem AH, Good WR. Transport of beta-estradiol in freshly excised human skin in vitro: diffusion and metabolism in each skin layer. Pharm Res 1994; 11(12):1777–84.

42. Mavon A, Raufast V, Redoules D. Skin absorption and metabolism of a new vitamin E prodrug, delta-tocopherol-glucoside: in vitro evaluation in human skin models. J Control Release 2004; 100(2):221–31.

43. Bronaugh RL, Maibach HI. Percutaneous-absorption of nitroaromatic compounds— in vivo and in vitro studies in the human and monkey. J Invest Dermatol 1985; 84(3):180–3.

44. Bronaugh RL, Franz TJ. Vehicle effects on percutaneous absorption: in vivo and in vitro comparisons with human skin. Br J Dermatol 1986; 115(1):1–11.

45. Wester RC, Maibach HI, Melendres J, Sedik L, Knaak J, Wang R. In vivo and in vitro percutaneous-absorption and skin evaporation of isofenphos in man. Fundam Appl Toxicol 1992; 19(4):521–6.

46. Dick D, Ng KME, Sauder DN, Chu I. In vitro and in vivo percutaneous-absorption of C-14 chloroform in humans. Hum Exp Toxicol 1995; 14(3):260–5.

47. Dick IP, Blain PG, Williams FM. The percutaneous absorption and skin distribution of lindane in man. II. In vitro studies. Hum Exp Toxicol 1997; 16(11):652–7.

48. Griffin P, Mason H, Heywood K, Cocker J. Oral and dermal absorption of chlorpyrifos: a human volunteer study. Occup Environ Med 1999; 56(1):10–11.

49. Griffin P, Payne M, Mason H, Freedlander E, Curran AD, Cocker J. The in vitro percutaneous penetration of chlorpyrifos. Hum Exp Toxicol 2000; 19(2):104–7.

50. Cnubben NHP, Elliott GR, Hakkert BC, Meuling WJA, Van De Sandt JJM. Comparative in vitro–in vivo percutaneous penetration of the fungicide *ortho*-phenylphenol. Regul Toxicol Pharmacol 2002; 35(2):198–208.

51. Mavon A, Miquel C, Lejeune O, Payre B, Moretto P. In vitro percutaneous absorption and in vivo stratum corneum distribution of an organic and a mineral sunscreen. Skin Pharmacol Physiol 2007; 20(1):10–20.
52. Kao J, Patterson FK, Hall J. Skin penetration and metabolism of topically applied chemicals in six mammalian species, including man: an in vitro study with benzo[a]-pyrene and testosterone. Toxicol Appl Pharmacol 1985; 81(3 Pt 1):502–16.
53. Anderson BD, Higuchi WI, Raykar PV. Heterogeneity effects on permeability-partition coefficient relationships in human stratum corneum. Pharm Res 1988; 5(9):566–73.

12 Beyond Stratum Corneum

Yuri Dancik, Owen G. Jepps, and Michael S. Roberts
Department of Medicine, Princess Alexandra Hospital, University of Queensland, Woolloongabba, Queensland, Australia

INTRODUCTION

The stratum corneum is seen as the main physical barrier that prevents the entry of solutes into the skin and manages the egress of water and endogenous molecules from the body. It is the thin outermost layer of the skin consisting of corneocytes (flattened, closely packed, and interdigitated "dead" cells packed with keratin) embedded in a highly organized, dense lipid intercellular space (1,2). The skin also has other barrier and support properties including immunological, metabolic, cushioning, sensing, and temperature control. In addition, the blood and lymphatics in the skin enable the removal of absorbed and skin metabolized solutes into the systemic circulation for further detoxification and excretion. The other distinct skin layers involved in providing these functions are the viable epidermis, dermis, and hypodermis. In this chapter, we first review the morphology of the viable skin layers and the skin appendages. We then examine the role the substructures below the stratum corneum may play in the physical and metabolic barrier properties of the skin and in the removal of solutes absorbed into the skin.

MORPHOLOGY OF THE VIABLE SKIN
Viable Epidermis
The viable epidermis consists of a number of distinct layers and cell types with different functional roles. The viable epidermis is avascular and can be viewed as a composite medium (3), containing about 40% protein, 40% water, and 15% to 20% lipids (4). Diffusion of solutes through the viable epidermis is thus akin to hindered diffusion in an aqueous medium punctured by cell membrane crossings. The major cell of the viable epidermis is the keratinocyte (2). Keratinocytes migrate from the epidermal–dermal junction through the epidermis forming distinct cell layers. These are, in succession, the stratum basale, stratum spinosum, stratum granulosum and stratum corneum. As keratinocytes migrate toward the stratum corneum they flatten and, in the stratum granulosum, shed their lipidic content into the intercellular space from lipid granules lining the cells' membrane (1,2), thereby supplying the intercellular space of the stratum corneum. One of the features of the epidermis is that it is in a continual state of regeneration from cells at the epidermal–dermal interface that are formed and are transformed in a defined progression toward eventual desquamated corneocytes. This turnover can vary with the nature of the skin condition (5). The undulating epidermal–dermal junction consists of papillae which project from the epidermis into the dermis (2). Basal keratinocytes are the most important structural and functional link to the dermis (6).

Dermis and Hypodermis

The bulk of the skin is the dermis, a 300- to 4000-μm-thick vascularized skin layer located below the viable epidermis (Fig. 1A). The dermis comprises the papillary dermis, a thin, 100 to 200 μm layer, and the reticular dermis, which forms the bulk of this skin layer. The papillary dermis consists of thin collagen bundles, elastic fibers, fibrocytes, and ground substance [consisting mainly of water, electrolytes, plasma proteins, and polysaccharides–polypeptide complexes (6)]. The reticular dermis contains predominantly thick collagen bundles and coarse elastic fibers (6). The dermis is the locus of blood vessels, nerves, lymphatics, and supports the skin appendages (4).

The hypodermis, or subcutaneous fat tissue, is located below the reticular dermis and may be up to several millimeters thick (4). The hypodermis consists of fat microlobules separated by fibrous strands consisting mainly of collagen and housing blood vessels, lymphatics, and nerves (6). The main functions of the hypodermis are energy storage, mechanical, and thermal insulation, and the facilitation of skin mobility over underlying structures (4,6,8).

Hair Follicles

The term "pilosebaceous unit" incorporates the hair follicle and the associated sebaceous gland (Fig. 1B). Two types of hair follicles exist: the vellus and the terminal hair follicle. Terminal hairs are wider, longer, and extend more deeply (at least 3 mm) into the skin tissue. Hair follicles are found on all parts of the human body except the soles of the feet, the palms of the hands, the red portion of the lips, and some parts of the genital organs (9). The density of hair follicles correlates with

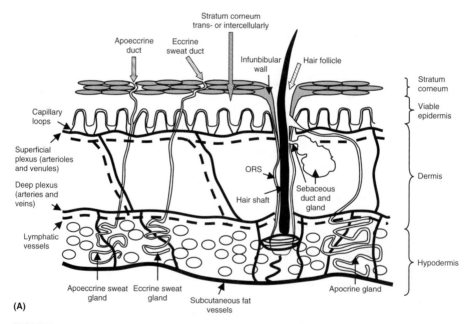

FIGURE 1 (**A**) Overview of skin layers, skin appendages, and pathways of percutaneous penetration. (*Continued*)

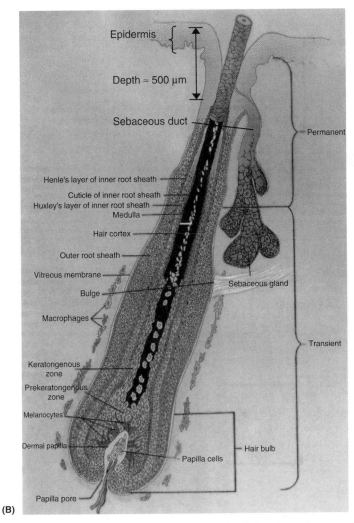

Epidermis {

Depth ≈ 500 μm

Sebaceous duct

Permanent

Henle's layer of inner root sheath

Cuticle of inner root sheath

Huxley's layer of inner root sheath

Medulla

Hair cortex

Outer root sheath

Vitreous membrane

Sebaceous gland

Bulge

Macrophages

Transient

Keratongenous zone

Prekeratongenous zone

Melanocytes

Dermal papilla

Hair bulb

Papilla cells

Papilla pore

(B)

FIGURE 1 (B) Schematic of a terminal human hair follicle and its sebaceous gland. *Source*: Adapted from Ref. 7. (*Continued*)

the thickness of the stratum corneum. Table 1 shows that the thickness of the stratum corneum decreases with increasing hair follicle density.

The terminal hair follicle is an elongated invagination of the epidermis, open to the surface of the skin, and extending through the skin tissue into the hypodermis (Fig. 1B). The conical upper part of the follicle, from the skin surface to a depth of about 500 μm, is the infundibulum. It is filled with sebum, an oily substance produced in the sebaceous gland, which is attached to the follicle by the sebaceous duct at a depth of about 500 μm (8,15). Within the infundibulum the hair shaft moves freely, unattached to the infundibular wall (8). The stratum corneum layer at the outer surface of the skin is continuous with the epithelial wall of the infundibulum, but becomes thinner with increasing depth (8,16).

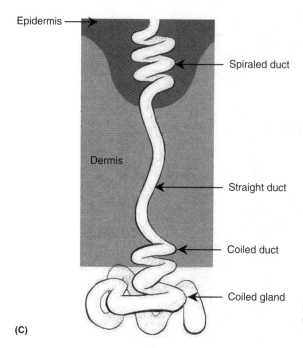

Epidermis

Spiraled duct

Dermis

Straight duct

Coiled duct

Coiled gland

(C)

FIGURE 1 (*Continued*) (**C**) Diagram of an eccrine sweat gland. *Source*: From Ref. 6.

Below the sebaceous duct, the hair follicle consists of a number of tightly packed, concentric cell layers. These are, proceeding from the outermost to the innermost layer: an acellular (vitreous) membrane; the outer root sheath (ORS) cell layer, which is continuous with the viable epidermis (6,17,18); and the inner root sheath (IRS), which includes the Henle layer, the Huxley layer, and the cuticle of the IRS. The IRS is in direct contact with the hair shaft, which is made up of an outer cell

TABLE 1 Literature Values Showing the Correlation Between Hair Follicle Density and Stratum Corneum Thickness

| | Hair follicle density | | Stratum corneum thickness | | |
| | Otberg et al. (10) (no. per cm²) | Pagnoni et al. (11) (no. per cm²) | Holbrook and Odland (12) | | Ya-Xian et al. (13) (no. cell layers) |
			No. cell layers	μm	
Forehead	292	455	—	—	9
Nose	—	1112	—	—	10
Periauricular region	—	499	—	—	10
Back	29	—	~16	~9	13
Abdomen	6ᵃ	—	18	~8	14
Upper arm	32	—	—	—	13–14
Forearm	18	—	~22	~13	16
Thigh	17	—	~19	~11	16

ᵃ From Ref. 14.

layer, the cuticle, the hair cortex and the medulla, the central part of the shaft (8). Above the sebaceous duct, the cells of the ORS are keratinized and similar to those of the epidermis (8). Below the duct they lack keratin, providing protection to the hair shaft and enabling it to mold. The ORS also contains melanocytes, Langerhans, and Merkel cells, which repopulate the epidermis after injury (19). The cells of the IRS are keratinized deeper than in the ORS. The bulge area of the hair follicle consists of highly proliferative cells (9). It has also been speculated that ORS cells in the bulge area serve as a reservoir for the epidermis and the sebaceous gland (19). The hair bulb is the site of the dermal papilla, which play a critical role in the growth of the hair follicle (19).

Sebaceous Glands

Sebaceous glands are multiacinar, holocrine-secreting glands. They are either associated with a hair follicle, and connected to it via the sebaceous duct at a depth of about 500 μm (8,15) (Fig. 1B) or found independently, mainly in facial skin (9). On the face and the scalp there are 400 to 900 sebaceous glands/cm^2, elsewhere on the body, excluding palms, soles, and the lower lip, their density is less than 100 sebaceous glands/cm^2 (20). The diameter of sebaceous glands is 200 to 2000 μm (21).

Sebaceous glands produce sebum, a lipophilic substance formed by the disintegration of sebocytes (sebaceous gland cells) and consisting in decreasing order of importance of triglycerides, wax esters, squalene, cholesterol esters, and cholesterol. Free fatty acids are produced by the breakdown of the triglycerides by enzymes in the follicular infundibulum (6). Some of the purposes of sebum are to protect the body against bacteria, of which the infundibulum contains a variety (6), to transport antioxidants to the skin surface (22), and to express pro- and anti-inflammatory properties. In addition, sebum is known to provide a hydrophobic coat to protect the skin from overwetting, to provide heat insulation, and to contribute via its lipid fraction to the integrity of the skin (23). The lag time between its discharge from the sebaceous duct and appearance on the surface of the skin is eight hours (24).

Eccrine Sweat Glands

Eccrine sweat glands respond to thermal stress by producing sweat, which flows to the surface of the skin and cools the body by evaporation (6). Sweat also improves the grip and sensitivity of skin by keeping it damp (4,7). Over 3 million sweat glands (7) are located all over the body, except in mucosal tissue (8). The greatest densities are found on the palms, the sole, the axillae, and the forehead (8). The components of the eccrine sweat gland are: a hollow coiled secretory gland in its proximal portion, about 100 μm in diameter (25,26) and located in the lower dermis or hypodermis (21,25), a coiled duct leading upwards from the secretory gland to a straight duct rising through the dermis, leading in turn to a spiraled intraepidermal duct opening to the surface of the skin (Fig. 1C) (6). The reabsorption of water, salts, and electrolytes through the walls of the sweat gland duct maintains the body's homeostasis during excessive perspiration (7).

Apocrine and Apoeccrine Glands

Similarly to the eccrine sweat glands, apocrine glands are coiled secretory glands located in the lower part of the dermis or the hypodermis (Fig. 1A) (6). But, while the former occur all over the body and independently of the hair follicle, in adults apocrine glands are found only in the axillae and perineal areas and are connected to hair follicles by a straight duct that empties into the infundibulum, just above the entrance of the sebaceous duct (6). The composition of the product of apocrine glands is not precisely known, as it mixes with the product of eccrine sweat glands and sebaceous glands in the infundibulum. Apocrine glands in humans do not contribute to the thermal regulation of the body and their precise function is unknown (6,8).

Sato et al. and later Wilke et al. provided evidence for the existence of a third type of gland, the apoeccrine gland, by dissection and immunofluorescence studies, respectively (27,28). While distinct from the eccrine and apocrine glands, the apoeccrine gland displays features common to both. Its cells are of the same kind as those found in both glands. Its duct shows segmental dilatation as that of the apocrine duct, but, like the eccrine duct, opens up to the skin surface. Apoeccrine glands are found only in the axillae and develop during adolescence, while the eccrine and apocrine glands are present at birth (27).

Skin Vascularization and Lymphatics

The papillary dermis contains a dense plexus of arterioles and venules running along the epidermal–dermal junction and inside the papilla of the junction. These vessels supply nutrients to the avascular epidermis (Fig. 1A). This plexus is connected to a second, deep, less dense plexus located in the reticular dermis by communicating vessels (6). Arterioles and venules connecting the two plexuses give rise to lateral tributaries that supply the skin appendages. Most of the microvasculature is contained in the papillary dermis (1–2 mm) below the epidermal surface (29). Braverman and coworkers have described in detail the "umbrella" organization of blood vessels in the reticular and papillary dermis (Fig. 2A) (29,30).

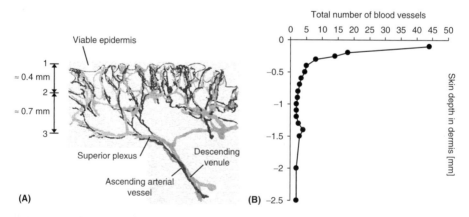

FIGURE 2 (**A**) Computer reconstruction of cutaneous blood vessels in the dermis showing their "umbrella" microorganization. Capillary loops are seen in zone 1–2, and vessels of the superior horizontal plexus in zone 2–3. (**B**) Total number of blood vessels in skin (arterioles plus venules) as a function of skin depth in the dermis. *Source*: From Refs. 29–31.

Cevc and Vierl have used Braverman's results to calculate the number of blood capillaries, arterioles, and venules, as a function of depth into the skin (Fig. 2B) as well as the inner and outer diameter of the blood vessels at each depth (31). The total number of blood vessels decreases about eightfold from a depth of 0.1 mm, corresponding to the top of the papillary dermis (epidermis–dermis junction) to a depth of 0.4 mm within the reticular dermis, and more than 20-fold to a depth of 1.0 mm. From these results, the authors derived profiles for the differential as well as the integral blood vessel surface area as a function of skin depth. This area increases steeply from the epidermis–dermis junction to a depth of about 0.15 mm, corresponding to the capillaries in the papillary dermis. At greater depths the blood vessel surface area decreases in a quasi-exponential fashion.

The hair follicle is heavily vascularized. The lower third (hair bulb) is surrounded by parallel blood vessels running along the long axis of the follicle and interconnected by "cross-shunts" (32). The upper two-thirds of the follicle is surrounded by parallel vessels, which form a continuous network with those enveloping the sebaceous glands. The acini of the sebaceous gland are wrapped in blood vessels. In bald scalp skin, the sebaceous glands are larger and more richly vascularized (32). The eccrine sweat gland is well vascularized at the level of the secretory gland and the coiled, straight, and spiraled portions of the duct (26,32). Similarly, the apocrine glands are surrounded by an intricate network of blood vessels (32).

The network of lymphatic vessels runs roughly parallel to the blood vessels (Fig. 1A) (6). In a similar way, cutaneous lymphatic vessels consist of a superficial plexus in the dermis, a deeper plexus near the subcutaneous tissue and connecting vessels (33).

PENETRATION PATHWAYS PARALLEL TO AND BEYOND THE STRATUM CORNEUM
Overview of Transport Pathways Through Human Skin
The routes of penetration into the skin for exogenous chemical substances are the transcellular and intercellular route through the stratum corneum, the follicular route, and the eccrine sweat gland route (34,35) (Fig. 1A). Much work has been done on characterizing the stratum corneum barrier to penetration, but less information is available on the nature of the transport pathways within the viable skin layers and the skin appendages.

Relatively little theoretical work on the barrier property of the viable epidermis has been published to date. Several groups, however, have observed a dependency of solute binding and sequestration in the viable epidermis on solute lipophilicity. Solute metabolism in the viable epidermis has been shown to occur primarily in the basal layer of the epidermis. Work on active transport in the viable epidermis has been largely focused on identifying transport proteins expressed in human epidermal keratinocytes. Little is known on the mechanisms by which transport proteins may act as active biochemical barriers to the penetration of topically applied drugs into the viable epidermis. Studies on the kinetics of uptake of drugs by transport proteins have yet to appear.

Solute diffusion through the dermis is comparable to hindered diffusion through aqueous tissue, with the important differences being that the dermis is primarily acellular and can bind a number of solutes. The dermis is the locus of blood and lymphatic vessels (4). The role of the dermal vasculature in the distribution and elimination of solutes has been studied extensively with vasoactive drugs. The importance of the fraction of solute unbound and of blood flow is described later. Several groups have also shown the importance of lymphatic transport for the clearance of large molecules. While transport proteins are expressed in epidermal keratinocytes, Schmuth et al. have shown fatty acid transport proteins (FATP) to be expressed in a follicular distribution within the dermis. However, to our knowledge, no other study has shown transporters to be expressed in the dermis.

Due to the lipophilic nature of sebum, the hair follicle has the potential of being an effective conduit for the diffusion of lipophilic compounds as well as a barrier to the diffusion of hydrophilic substances (8). Topically applied compounds may partition from the applied vehicle into the sebum and diffuse into the deeper follicular layers, or from the follicle into the surrounding epidermal and dermal tissues, potentially via the sebaceous gland. Although a number of groups have provided visual evidence for the importance of the follicular pathway beyond the initial stages of transdermal diffusion, a mechanistic understanding of the contribution of sebum, the infundibulum, the hair shaft, the sebaceous duct and gland, and the deeper cell layers (IRS, ORS) of the hair follicle to transdermal penetration and permeation is necessary. Recent studies have established the potential for solute transport via the eccrine and apocrine glands.

In the following sections, we discuss how the structural features of the viable skin layers and appendages may promote solute transport beyond the stratum corneum or constitute barriers to penetration beyond the stratum corneum.

Contribution of Skin Layers to Skin Transport

The principles associated with the contribution made by the skin appendages and the skin layers below the stratum corneum were elucidated in the 1970s. Scheuplein and Blank approximated the skin as a finite membrane encompassing the epidermis and papillary dermis pierced by hair follicles and sweat glands (15,36). The tissue and appendageal pathways were described macroscopically by effective diffusion coefficients. Penetration via the shunt pathway, characterized by higher nominal diffusion coefficients for the hair follicles and sweat glands than for bulk skin, was shown to be greater at early times of the diffusion process, whereas at steady state, penetration occurred predominantly across bulk skin (Fig. 3). This worked allowed Scheuplein and Blank to explain experimental data, which showed one or the other pathway as being the predominant one, depending on the time scale considered.

Scheuplein and Blank recognized the contribution of the viable epidermis and the dermis to the overall permeability resistance of skin. The total skin resistance $1/k_{p,skin}$, in the absence of shunts such as hair follicles and sweat ducts, is given by the sum of the resistances (R_i) in series due to the stratum corneum membrane (sc), the viable epidermis (ve), and the dermis (d) (15):

$$\frac{1}{k_{p,skin}} = \sum_{i=1}^{3} R_i = R_{sc} + R_{ve} + R_d = \frac{h_{sc}}{D_{sc}K_{sc}} + \frac{h_{ve}}{D_{ve}K_{ve}} + \frac{h_d}{D_d K_d} \qquad (1)$$

where the h, D and K are the layer thickness, diffusivity, and vehicle-layer partition coefficient, respectively. Figure 4 (15) compares the resistance due to whole epidermis (stratum corneum plus viable epidermis) and whole dermis as a function of the number of the carbon chain length of alcohols. The whole-epidermis

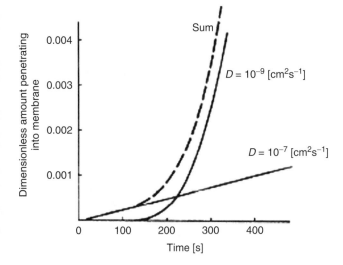

FIGURE 3 Amount of solute penetrating into membranes of different diffusion coefficients versus time calculated by Scheuplein and Blank from an approximation of the skin as a finite membrane. *Source*: From Ref. 15, 36.

resistance is essentially equal to the resistance due to the stratum corneum after removal of the viable cells by trypsination. It decreases with increasing carbon chain length n. For $n > 6$, the resistance due to the epidermis is comparable to that due to the dermis.

Flynn and Yalkowsky (37) and Roberts et al. (38) described the total resistance to diffusion through the whole epidermis $1/k_{p,\text{epid}}$ in a similar way. The overall resistance was the sum of resistances in series due to the stratum corneum and an

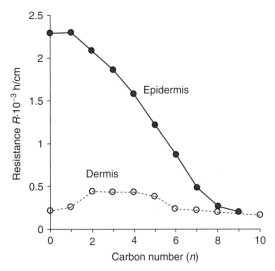

FIGURE 4 Diffusional resistances R in full-thickness epidermis and dermis versus carbon chain length n for alcohols applied in aqueous solution. *Source*: From Ref. 15.

underlying aqueous boundary layer (aq) due to the viable epidermis

$$\frac{1}{k_{p,epid}} = \frac{2h_{aq}}{D_{aq}} + \frac{h_{sc}}{D_{sc}K_{sc}}. \tag{2}$$

In reality, the shunts do contribute as a parallel pathway of penetration, so that one equation for the total resistance to skin permeability is

$$k_{p,skin} = \frac{1}{R_{sc} + R_{ve} + R_d} + \frac{1}{R_{shunts}} = \left(\frac{1}{k_{p,sc}} + \frac{1}{k_{p,ve}} + \frac{1}{k_{p,d}}\right)^{-1} + k_{p,shunts} \tag{3}$$

As discussed by Anissimov and Roberts (39), clearance from the epidermis also affects penetration through the skin. The various physiological factors determining $k_{p,skin}$ in the viable skin are described in the following sections: transport in the viable epidermis, transport in the dermis, and transport in the skin appendages.

TRANSPORT IN THE VIABLE EPIDERMIS
Contribution of the Viable Epidermis Permeability to the Overall Skin Permeability

The relative contribution of viable epidermal resistance and clearance on solute penetration has been described using a resistance-in-series mathematical model by Anissimov and Roberts (39). In the simplest analysis, the viable epidermis is modeled as an unstirred aqueous diffusion layer between the stratum corneum membrane and a receptor phase. The simulation results show a decrease in the amount of solute and an increase in the diffusional lag time as the resistance to diffusion in the viable epidermis increases relative to resistance in the stratum corneum (Fig. 5). When the viable epidermis has a large resistance, the amount penetrated is not greatly affected by variations in receptor clearance (representing sampling rate or flow rate in vitro, and removal by blood flow or transport into deeper tissue in vivo).

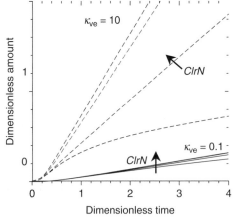

FIGURE 5   Effect of the epidermal resistance, described by the ratio $\kappa_{ve} = k_{p,ve}/k_{p,sc}$ (where $k_{p,ve}$, permeability coefficient in the viable epidermis and $k_{p,sc}$, permeability coefficient in the stratum corneum) on the dimensionless solute amount versus exposure dimensionless time (dashed lines, $\kappa_{ve} = 10$; solid lines, $\kappa_{ve} = 0.1$). The dimensionless parameter ClrN measures the magnitude of the removal rate from the receptor phase. Source: From Ref. 39.

Wenkers and Lippold have examined whether epidermal transport of nonsteroidal anti-inflammatory drugs (NSAIDs) from a lipophilic vehicle was best described by one of three models for the skin resistance (40): the stratum corneum alone provides resistance; the viable epidermis alone provides resistance; or both skin layers are decisive. They suggested that, based on correlations between skin permeability and octanol-vehicle and the phosphate-buffered saline (PBS)-vehicle partition coefficients, the viable epidermis provides a decisive barrier to the penetration of NSAIDs from a lipophilic vehicle.

Transport in the viable epidermis is also affected by hindered transport due to the large amount of proteins and cellular barriers; metabolism in the viable epidermis; keratinocyte; and other cell transporter activity; and protein facilitated transport of solutes within cells as may occur, for example, in the transport of fatty acids by fatty acid-binding proteins within liver cells (41). In general, these mechanisms are not well defined.

Limited work has been done on characterizing the precise contribution of the viable epidermis in hindering the transport of solutes, or on quantifying this hindrance. Cleek and Bunge have compared three models for dermal absorption, yielding a normalized solute amount absorbed into the stratum corneum as a function of time (42). These models are a single-finite membrane representing the stratum corneum; a semi-infinite stratum corneum and a two-membrane composite model representing the stratum corneum and the viable epidermis. While such models have been used before, this study introduces and validates algebraic expressions for the normalized solute amount in stratum corneum, and uses them to explain the role of the viable epidermis. The algebraic expressions are derived from the exact solution to the diffusion equation applied to each model. The contribution of the viable epidermis is taken into account in the third, two-membrane model, through the ratio $B = k_{p,sc}/k_{p,ve}$, i.e., the steady-state permeability from a vehicle v across the stratum corneum ($k_{p,sc}$) divided by that across the viable epidermis ($k_{p,ve}$), and the ratio of lag times $G = L_{sc}^2 D_{ve}/L_{ve}^2 D_{sc}$. The parameter B also relates the resistance through stratum corneum–viable epidermis composite membrane ($1/k_{p,epid}$) to the resistance through the stratum corneum ($1/k_{p,sc}$) (42,43),

$$\frac{1}{k_{p,epid}} = \frac{1}{k_{p,sc}}(1 + B) \tag{4}$$

and equation (4) is identical to equation (2) stated by Flynn and Yalkowsky (37) and Roberts et al. (38). In the case of rate-limiting diffusion in the stratum corneum, that is, for $B \ll 1$, equation (4) yields $k_{p,epid} = k_{p,sc}$. This is the case of the permeability in the whole epidermis being entirely described by the stratum corneum permeability. In terms of the steady-state flux across the stratum corneum,

$$J_{ss} = \frac{K_{sc} D_{sc}}{h_{sc}} c_v = k_{p,sc} c_v \tag{5}$$

Cleek and Bunge's models assume a constant concentration during the exposure event, i.e., no solute depletion due to absorption or evaporation from the vehicle. The parameter B is independent of the vehicle provided the vehicle does not alter the physicochemical properties of the stratum corneum or the viable epidermis. The two-membrane composite model assumes equilibrium partitioning at the stratum corneum/viable epidermis interface.

A comparison of the single membrane and semi-infinite medium models shows that the normalized cumulative amount entering the stratum corneum during the unsteady-state period is well described by the computationally simpler semi-infinite model. This is also verified by the two-membrane model, which shows the normalized cumulative mass to be independent of B and G at early exposure times. Within this period the solute has not yet penetrated into the viable epidermis, and thus mass absorbed depends on the stratum corneum permeability. Beyond the unsteady-state period, the two-membrane model shows absorption into the stratum corneum to be dependent on the value of B, that is, on solute lipophilicity (Fig. 6). For highly hydrophilic chemicals ($B \leq 0.01$), the steady-state mass–time profile is linear, its slope approaching 1 as $B \to 0$. This profile is similar to that obtained by the single membrane model at steady state, and shows that for these compounds, absorption into the skin is limited only by the stratum corneum permeability. As the lipophilicity of the chemical increases (increasing B), the mass–time profile given by the two-membrane model (Fig. 6) decreases and its slope tends to 0 as $B \to \infty$. The effect of the aqueous viable epidermis is to "choke" the flux of lipophilic chemicals from the stratum corneum. This conclusion agrees with Wenkers and Lippold's (40). The degree of lipophilicity (given by B) also determines the transition time t^* from the unsteady-state to the steady-state regime. For $B \geq 0.6$, the mass–time profiles obtained by the semi-infinite stratum corneum and the two-membrane models intersected; the time of intersection was taken as t^* and depends on B as shown in Table 2. For $B < 0.6$, the mass–time profiles did not intersect, but the minimum error between the profiles occurred at $t^* = 0.4\, L_{sc}^2/D_{sc}$. As noted by Cleek and Bunge, this value is close to the value for the onset of the steady-state regime in a single membrane given by Crank (44).

In a second study, Bunge and Cleek (43) described four methods of calculating the parameter B, summarized in Tables 3A and 3B. Method 4, utilizing the stratum corneum and viable epidermis permeabilities, was used to calculate B in the first study (42). The value of B, and thus the contribution of the permeability of the viable epidermis relative to the stratum corneum, will affect the cumulative

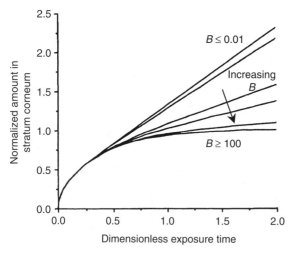

FIGURE 6 Normalized cumulative amount in the stratum corneum as a function of dimensionless exposure time, calculated from a stratum corneum–viable epidermis composite model of the skin. *Source*: From Ref. 42.

TABLE 2 Calculation of the Time t^* Marking the Transition Between the Unsteady and Steady-State Regimes in the Absorption of Chemicals Though a Stratum Corneum–Viable Epidermis Composite Membrane, as a Function of Parameter B [Equation (4)]

$B<0.6$	$B\geq0.6$		
$t^* = \dfrac{0.4L_{sc}^2}{D_{sc}}$	$t^* = \dfrac{(b-\sqrt{b^2-c^2})L_{sc}^2}{D_{sc}},$	$b = \dfrac{2(1+B^2)}{\pi} - c$	$c = \dfrac{1+3B+3B^2}{3(1+B)}$

Source: From Ref. 42.

mass absorbed only when the exposure time is larger than the approximate time to reach steady state (t^*) and for $B\geq0.1$.

Khalil et al. have calculated the permeability of glucose in the viable epidermis by fitting a two layer (viable epidermis and dermis) model to tape-stripped split thickness skin penetration data (46). Glucose permeability was calculated to be 38% of that in dermis. However, this result depends on the efficiency of the tape-stripping technique. The authors report a permeability equivalent to 30% of the dermal value, obtained from a side-by-side diffusion cell experiment on human epidermal membrane, as being more reliable.

TABLE 3A Estimation of Parameter B from Contributing Physicochemical Parameters of Solute in the Stratum Corneum (SC) and the Viable Epidermis (VE) and the Octanol/Water (O/W) Partitioning Coefficient $K_{o/w}$

Method 1: $B = \dfrac{K_{sc/ve}D_{sc}L_{ve}}{D_{ve}L_{sc}} = \dfrac{K_{o/w}}{1150}$	Method 2: $B = \dfrac{K_{sc/ve}D_{sc}L_{ve}}{D_{ve}L_{sc}} = \dfrac{K_{o/w}^{0.74}}{230}$

Equal dependence on MW for permeability of stratum corneum and viable epidermis

$D_{sc}/L_{sc} = 4.4 \times 10^{-7}$ cm/sec (from Potts & Guy correlation for small molecules)

$L_{ve} = 10^{-2}$ cm^2/sec, $\quad D_{ve} = 10^{-6}$ cm^2/sec

$K_{sc/ve} = K_{o/w}/5$, based on (45)	$K_{sc/ve} = K_{o/w}^{0.74}$, epidermis assumed as water phase

TABLE 3B Estimation of Parameter B from the Steady-State Permeabilities of Stratum Corneum (SC) and Viable Epidermis (VE) from Water (W)

Method 3: $B = \dfrac{k_{p,sc}}{k_{p,ve}} = \dfrac{k_{p,sc/w}}{k_{p,ve/w}} = \dfrac{k_{p,sc/w}}{0.36 \text{ cm/hr}}$	Method 4: $B = \dfrac{k_{p,sc}}{k_{p,ve}} = \dfrac{k_{p,sc/w}}{k_{p,ve/w}} = \dfrac{k_{p,sc/w}\sqrt{MW}}{2.6 \text{ cm/hr}}$
MW dependency is $e^{-\beta MW}$ for SC	MW dependency is $e^{-\beta MW}$ for SC
No MW dependency for VE	MW dependency is $1/\sqrt{MW}$ for VE

Log$_{10}$ $k_{p,sc/w}$ given by Potts & Guy correlation

$k_{p,ve/w} = K_{ve/w}D_{ve}/L_{ve}$

$K_{ve/w}=1$, assumes ve behaves as water

$L_{ve} = 10^{-2}$ cm^2/sec, $\quad D_{ve} = 10^{-6}$ cm^2/sec	$L_{ve} = 10^{-2}$ cm^2/sec, $\quad D_{ve} = 7.1 \times 10^{-6}/\sqrt{MW}$ cm^2/sec $\quad D_{ve} = 10^{-6}$ cm^2/sec for MW $= 50$

Source: From Ref. 43.

Sequestration in the Viable Epidermis

Solute sequestration in the skin can be an important effect that must be taken into consideration in the determination of a compound's bioavailability in the skin and the systemic circulation. Baker et al. showed early on evidence for the preferential binding of topical glucocorticoids to rat epidermal tissue (47). Yourick et al. discussed the importance of determining the fate of chemicals retained in the skin. This study quantified the amounts of dihydroxyacetone (DHA, applied from water and oil-in-water emulsion vehicles), 7-(2H-naphtho[1,2-d]triazol-2-yl)-3-phenylcoumarin (7NTPC, applied from chloroform), and disperse blue 1 (DB1, from ethanol and a semi-permeant formulation vehicle) remaining in the stratum corneum and viable skin layers after an in vitro human skin absorption study (48). After 24 hours, 10% of the applied DHA dose remained in the stratum corneum and 12% remained in the viable epidermis and the dermis (for both vehicle types). After 24 hours, 14.7% of the applied dose of 7NTPC was found in the whole epidermis and dermis, including around hair. Approximately 11% of the DB1 applied in an ethanol vehicle was found in the stratum corneum after 24 hours. In the case of DHA and DB1, the percentage of applied dose remaining in the skin was significantly higher than that recovered in the receptor fluid.

Solute lipophilicity and binding to cellular components have been identified as important parameters for the sequestration of solutes in the viable epidermis. Siddiqui et al. have compared the steady-state concentration of lipophilic solutes with and without steroid accumulation in the viable epidermis (49). In the absence of accumulation in the viable epidermis, the steady-state dermal concentration is obtained from the rate of permeation through the epidermis and the clearance into the dermis:

$$c_{ss} = \frac{k_{p,sc} c_v F_{available} A}{Cl} = \frac{J_{ss} F_{available} A}{Cl} \tag{6}$$

where $F_{available}$ is the availability of the pharmacologically active solute at the site of action. Accumulation into the viable epidermis was taken to reduce the steady-state flux, such that $J_{ss} = k_{p,sc} (c_v - c_{ss})$ (49). In this case, the steady-state dermal concentration can be calculated as follows:

$$c_{ss} = \frac{k_{p,sc} c_v F_{available} A}{Cl + k_{p,sc} F_{available} A} \tag{7}$$

Using equations (6) and (7) Siddiqui et al. calculated up to 30% increase in the steady-state dermal concentration of steroids as a result of solute sequestration in the viable epidermis.

Walter and Kurz obtained a correlation between drug lipophilicity and binding in the viable epidermis and dermis. Experiments with lipid-depleted tissue indicated that the lipids do not play a role in binding (50). Instead, solute molecules would bind to other components such as skin protein. Yagi et al. studied the residence of beta-blocking agents of varying lipophilicity in viable skin in vivo and in vitro (51). The elimination rate constants of β-blockers in viable skin correlated inversely with binding to cytosol components of the viable epidermis, but not with lipophilicity. Binding may be an important parameter in the determination of the residence/reservoir effect (see Chapter 11). Cross et al. showed that the distribution of homologous alcohols in the viable epidermis of full-thickness skin (expressed as the fraction of the amount of each alcohol recovered in the tissue) increases with the number of carbons and thus with lipophilicity (52). This trend was also obtained for epidermal membranes for each chemical except decanol (the longest chain of the set). Magnusson et al. investigated the distribution of steroids of varying lipophilicity in skin (53). Distribution in the viable epidermis was greatest for the most lipophilic steroid, progesterone, but that was not the case for distribution in dermis. Binding to tissue components also plays a role in accumulation.

The extent of solute sequestration in the viable epidermis may also depend on metabolism (54). Epidermal metabolizing enzymes are localized is the basal layer of the epidermis.

Metabolism in the Viable Epidermis

In general, metabolism reduces transport of an active compound by detoxification, reducing the availability of the active compound in the viable epidermis and penetrating through to the dermis. The in vivo flux at the cutaneous site of action, J_{skin}^*, is a fraction of the steady-state flux J_{ss},

$$J_{skin}^* = F_{cut}J_{ss} \tag{8}$$

The fraction F_{cut} depends on the fractions of solute absorbed (f_a) and metabolized ($f_{m,skin}$) in the skin:

$$F_{cut} = f_a(1 - f_{m,skin}) \tag{9}$$

where $1 - f_{m,skin}$ is the fraction of solute which remains unaffected by skin metabolism.

Several studies have been performed in order to locate the sites of metabolism within the viable epidermis. Liu et al. have analyzed experimental data for β-estradiol in ethanol through hairless mouse skin using several different enzyme distribution models (55). They concluded that the conversion of β-estradiol to estrone, and inhibition of this reaction due to the presence of ethanol, occur in the basal layer of the viable epidermis.

Hikima et al.'s results agree with those of Liu et al. They presented results showing the enzymatic activity responsible for metabolism of β-estradiol 17-acetate to be present in the basal layer of the viable epidermis (80–120 μm depth), just above the papillary plexus (56).

Sugibayashi et al. (57) measured the distribution of the enzyme esterase [which transforms ethyl nicotinate (EN) to nicotinic acid (NA)] in skin by fluorescence (Fig. 7A). Highest fluorescence intensity was observed throughout the viable epidermis and near hair follicles in the dermis, with low intensity in dermal tissue. The authors conducted skin penetration experiments and simulated simultaneous diffusion and metabolism of EN in skin using Fick's second law of diffusion with a reaction rate term given by the Michaelis–Menten equation. Figure 7B shows their experimentally determined steady-state fluxes as a function of initial donor concentration, and the validation of their model. The concave and convex shapes of the curves suggest that metabolic saturation occurs are higher EN concentration. Various enzyme distribution models were investigated: even enzyme distribution; enzymes located in the upper half, one-third and one-tenth of the viable epidermis. The fluxes of EN and NA were not affected by enzyme distribution. Concentration-depth profiles of EN and NA in viable skin were affected with a low applied EN concentration (50 μmol/mL). NA concentration

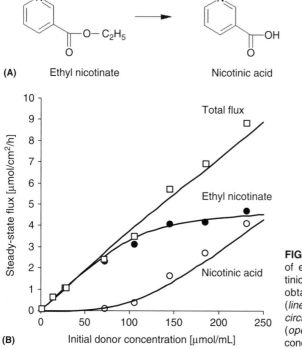

(A)   Ethyl nicotinate   Nicotinic acid

(B)   Initial donor concentration [μmol/mL]

FIGURE 7 (**A**) Chemical structures of ethyl nicotinate (EN) and nicotinic acid (NA). (**B**) Experimentally obtained (*points*) and calculated (*lines*) steady-state flux of EN (*filled circle*), NA (*open circle*) and total flux (*open square*) versus applied EN concentration. *Source*: From Ref. 57.

exceeded EN concentration in the whole skin, and the most partial distribution (one-tenth of the viable epidermis) yielded the largest NA concentration. With an applied EN saturation concentration of 300 μmol/mL, the EN concentration in the skin exceeded that of NA, but the profiles were nearly identical for each enzyme distribution model. The authors suggest that enzyme distribution had little effect on the flux of EN and NA, but greatly influences their concentration gradients.

Boderke et al. (58) conducted experiments of L-Ala-4-methoxy-2-naphthy-lamide (Ala-MNA) permeation into human stripped skin and HaCaT cell culture sheets and simulated the process using a diffusion–metabolism model. They show the influence of the diffusion and partition coefficients, the metabolic rate V_{max}, and the tissue thickness on substrate permeation. A ratio of residence time in the tissue to the metabolic half-life is derived from the model equations. The ratio is an order of magnitude smaller for the HaCaT cell culture sheets when compared with a 40 μm thick epidermal membrane, indicating that intact Ala-MNA would permeate through the former but not the latter. This model does, however, assume a homogeneous distribution of enzymes in the epidermis, which is an oversimplification.

Active Transport in the Viable Epidermis

Protein transporters in the skin have become an important topic in recent years, but little has been done on characterizing their effect on the permeability of solute through the viable epidermis. Most work to date has focused on the nature of the transporters expressed in the skin.

Bleasby et al. have compiled a comprehensive set of carrier-mediated transporters in various tissue of the human body, including the skin (59). The superfamilies of transporters involved in xenobiotic transport in various tissues in the human body are the adenosine-triphosphate-binding cassette (ABC), solute carrier (SLC) and organic anion transporting polypeptide (OATP). The ABC families of transporters identified in the skin are the Multi Drug Resistance Proteins (MDR) i.e., MDR1 and MDR3 and the Multi Drug Resistance-associated Proteins (MRP) i.e., MRP1, MRP3, and MRP5 through MRP9. The SLC transporters expressed in human skin are the peptide and monocarboxylate transporters PEPT1 and MCT1, the organic cation transporters OCT1, OCT3, OCTN1, and OCTN2, the organic anion transporters OAT2, OATP-B, OATP-D, OATP-E, and OATP-H, the concentrative nucleoside transporters CNT1 through CNT3, the equilibrative nucleoside transporters ENT1, ENT2, and ENT4, and the archaeal/bacterial and prostaglandin transporters ABT(0+) and PGT.

MDR1 is an efflux pump, transporting chemotherapeutic drugs such as etoposide and vincristine from the intracellular milieu to the extracellular space (60). MRP1 is one of the highest expressed xenobiotic transporters in the skin (61,62), responsible for the efflux of grepafloxacin in mouse skin (62). The MDR and MRP probably work synergistically with cytochrome P450 enzymes to protect the cells against xenobiotics (63). The MRP1, MRP3, MRP5, and MRP6 are xenobiotic transporters expressed in keratinocytes. The MRP1 and MRP3, for example, mediate the transport and confer resistance to methotrexate (64). The MRP1 and MRP2 mediate the transport of glutathione conjugates (65). Methotrexate is also transported by the reduced folate carrier RFC1, expressed in human skin (66).

The OATP-B, OATP-D, and OATP-E are also found in keratinocytes. They transport various organic anions (including drugs such as pravastatine and benzylpenicillin), conjugated metabolites, steroids, such as estradiol 17b-glucuronide and estrone-3-sulfate, thyroid hormones, peptides, leukotriene C4/E4, prostaglandine E2, and bile acids (67).

The cationic amino acid transporter is also expressed in keratinocytes. It transports L-arginine, which is essential for both inducible nitric oxide synthase and arginase enzyme activities (68).

Li et al. (69) showed that the penetration of two NSAIDs, ^{3}H-labeled flurbiprofen and ^{14}C-labeled indomethacin, is governed by pH- and adenosine triphosphate (ATP)-dependent saturable kinetics. Passive diffusion and reversible kinetics alone cannot account for this, and the authors cite the possible involvement of certain transporters. In the same study, reverse transcription-polymerase chain reaction results show the existence of MRP, MCT, OATP, and OCTN xenobiotic transporters, implying the possible role of these in the transport of flurbiprofen and indomethacin.

Fatty acid transporters FATP are also present in the skin, helping to maintain the barrier function of the skin by taking up the lipids that the keratinocytes do not synthesize (70). FATP1 and FATP3 are expressed mainly by keratinocytes, FATP4 is strongly expressed by sebaceous gland cells, and FATP6 by hair follicle epithelia.

Water in human skin is transported by the membrane proteins aquaporines (71). Some of these are also permeable to glycerol. Aquaporines may be important as a transdermal penetration pathway, as glycerol in used in numerous pharmaceutical and cosmetic formulations.

TRANSPORT IN THE DERMIS AND SUBCUTANEOUS TISSUE
Contribution of the Dermis to Overall Skin Permeability
In the 1970s, Scheuplein and Blank studied the diffusional resistance of various alcohols in the full epidermis and full-thickness dermis, recognizing that the resistance of the full epidermis is mainly due to the stratum corneum, and that the dermis, as a primarily aqueous layer, would have a much lower resistance (15). While for ethanol delivered from an aqueous vehicle, the diffusional resistance in epidermis was about 20 times greater than in dermis, the former decreased sharply while the latter remained very low and approximately constant with an increasing number of carbon atoms n, that is, with increasing lipophilicity (Fig. 4). For $n > 6$, the dermis contributed about as much to the overall skin resistance as the epidermis. For larger or more polar molecules, the relative effect of the permeability resistance due to the stratum corneum will be greater, as these molecules generally have smaller stratum corneum diffusion and partitioning coefficients (15).

These studies compared the resistance offered by bulk dermis to various alcoholic molecules. There are, however, significant physiological differences between the reticular and papillary dermis, the chief among them being the size, density, and orientation of the blood vessels found in either layer. In the following sections, we review studies focusing on the effect of blood and lymphatic flow on dermal transport.

Blood Flow and Tissue Distribution Volume
In general, transport in the dermis is defined by solute diffusion, tissue binding, sequestration, uptake, and transport (redistribution or clearance) by the vasculature, together with uptake and transport in the lymphatic system.

Roberts and Cross have shown the dependency of the solute distribution volume and retention half-life in skin layers such as the dermis or deeper tissue on the fractions of unbound solute in the tissue and the plasma and the plasma flow rate (72,73). Compartmental models represent the site of application and skin layers as well-stirred compartments, that is, the solute concentration in each compartment is homogeneous throughout the whole compartment. Figure 8A shows a two-compartment model of absorption from a finite site of application. Absorption into the tissue and subsequent elimination are characterized by absorption and elimination rate constants k_a and k_e, respectively. Tissue perfusion is described by the perfusate flow rate Q_p into the tissue and the blood flow out of it, Q_t. Assuming exponential absorption kinetics, the amount of solute in the tissue, $M_t(t)$, is

$$M_t(t) = \frac{k_a M_0}{k_a - k_e}(e^{-k_e t} - e^{-k_a t}) \tag{10}$$

where M_0 is in the initial solute amount applied to the dermis. The cumulative amount eluted is

$$Q(t) = M_0 \left(1 + \frac{k_a}{k_a - k_e} e^{-k_e t} - \frac{k_e}{k_e - k_a} e^{-k_a t} \right) \tag{11}$$

When the unbound solute concentrations in the vascular space and the dermal tissue (fu_p and fu_t, respectively) are in distribution equilibrium, the apparent dermal volume of distribution of the solute, V_D, may be obtained from the volume of the vascular space, V_p, and the volume of the tissue extravascular space, V_{te}. Analogously to the whole-body apparent volume of distribution

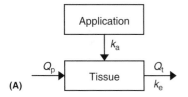

(A)

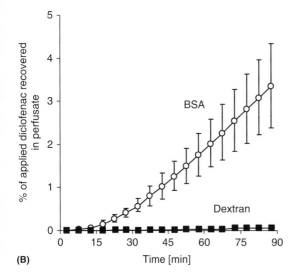

(B)

FIGURE 8 **(A)** Two-compartmental model used by Cross and Roberts to describe the efflux of solutes from tissues after dermal absorption into a perfused limb preparation. k_a, absorption rate constant; k_e, elimination rate constant, Q_p, plasma flow rate; Q_t, flow rate out of tissue. *Source*: Adapted from Ref. 73. **(B)** Cumulative fraction of diclofenac recovered in perfusate for 4% bovine serum albumin and 2.5% dextran. *Source*: From Ref. 72.

described by Tozer and Rowland (72,74), V_D is obtained from:

$$V_D = V_p + \frac{fu_p}{fu_t} V_{te} \tag{12}$$

The elimination rate constant is $k_e = Q_p / V_D$. Equation (12) yields k_e in terms of the perfusate flow rate and the fractions of unbound solute (72):

$$k_e = \frac{Q_p}{V_p + \frac{fu_p}{fu_t} V_{te}} = \frac{Q_p}{\left[\frac{V_p}{V_{te}} + \frac{fu_p}{fu_t}\right] V_{te}} \tag{13}$$

An important parameter in the clinical setting is the sequestration of solute molecules in skin tissues. Tissue blood flow and the binding of solute molecules to cellular components of the dermis can determine the extent of a dermal reservoir. The fraction F_t of solute remaining in the tissue after absorption has ceased is given by $F_t = e^{-k_e t}$ (72). For $fu_p / fu_t > V_p / V_{te}$, this fraction is

$$\ln F_t \approx -\frac{fu_t Q_p}{fu_p V_{te}} t \tag{14}$$

Solute retention may also be characterized by the retention half-life $t_{0.5,e} = (\ln 2) / k_e$. With the above approximation, the half-life is a function of the ratio of

TABLE 4 Experimentally Determined Values of the Fraction Unbound in Bovine Serum Albumin Containing Perfusate and Predicted Values of the Fraction Unbound in the Tissue of Various Solutes

Drug	Fraction unbound in BSA	Fraction unbound in tissue
Water	1	1
Salicylate	0.1	0.12
Lidocaine	0.43	0.25
Diazepram	0.14	0.012
Diclofenac	0.025	0.0027

Abbreviation: BSA, bovine serum albumin.
Source: From Ref. 72.

fractions of unbound solute and the perfusate flow:

$$t_{0.5,e} = \frac{\ln 2 \, V_D}{Q_p} \approx \frac{\ln 2 \, fu_p V_{te}}{fu_t Q_p} \tag{15}$$

Table 4 shows experimentally determined values of the fraction of unbound solutes in plasma perfusate containing bovine serum albumin (BSA) and the predicted values for the fractions unbound in the tissue. The two-compartment model presented above was validated in the case of dermal absorption of diclofenac into underlying tissue (Fig. 8B).

Compartmental models such as the one presented above are approximations of continuum models which represent the skin as a membrane (75). Cevc and Vierl (31) have recently published a membrane model that incorporates diffusion and blood-flow driven clearance of a permeant in skin, including deep tissue. The concentration as function of depth into the skin depends on a permeability sink profile $P(d)$:

$$\frac{\partial c(d,t)}{\partial t} = D(d) \frac{\partial^2 c(d,t)}{\partial d^2} - k_d P(d) c(d,t) \tag{16}$$

where the diffusivity D and the permeability P are a function of the distance d from the viable epidermis–dermis interface and k_d is the rate of clearance from the dermis. Figure 9A shows a convex concentration versus depth profile for an amphiphatic drug obtained by the authors using equation (16). Simple passive diffusion yields a concave curve. Cevc and Vierl used equation (16) to fit experimental concentration-depth profiles in human and rat dermis (Fig. 9B) (31).

Vasoconstriction can prolong solute concentration in the skin by decreasing the amount taken up by the systemic circulation (78)—in other words, decreasing the clearance effect of the blood vessels. Studies on the effect of vasoactive compounds are reviewed in the next section.

Role of Vasculature on Dermal Pharmacokinetics Demonstrated with Use of Vasoactive Drugs

Vasoconstricting and vasodilating compounds have been used in a number of studies to show the role played by blood flow on the penetration of solutes into the dermis and deeper tissue following topical application. In general, changes in cutaneous blood flow modify the cutaneous drug concentration and the extent of solute sequestration in the skin. The effect of vasoconstricting compounds is to increase solute concentration and distribution in the dermis and underlying layers.

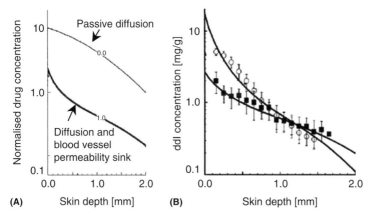

FIGURE 9 (**A**) Normalized concentration-depth profiles obtained for an amphiphatic drug from the diffusion–clearance model [equation (16)]. A clearance adjustment factor is multiplied to the permeability term $k_d P(d)$. The curve labeled "0.0" was obtained for a clearance factor equal to 0, equivalent to passive diffusion, whereas the curve labeled "1.0" was obtained with a clearance factor equal to 1. (**B**) Validation of Cevc and Vierl's model [equation (16)]: (*filled square*, dermis concentration-depth profile of dideoxyinosine (ddI) solution in skin at $t=6$ hours obtained by Morgan et al. by microdialysis (76); *open circle*, ddI dermis concentration-depth profile obtained in rats by Gao et al. (77), and *solid line*, model predictions). The lower thick curve is the same as that labeled "1.0" in Figure 9A. *Source*: From Ref. 31.

As reviewed by Cross and Roberts (73), Riviere et al. (79) have used the vasodilator tolazoline and the vasoconstrictor norepinephrine. In this study, the authors showed that tolazoline marginally decreased the flux of lidocaine delivered by iontophoresis in vitro, but significantly increased it in the isolated perfused porcine skin flap (IPPSF) model and in pigs in vivo. Norepinephrine, on the other hand, decreased the flux of lidocaine in the IPPSF and in vivo. In a second study, Riviere et al. showed that tolazoline yielded decreased concentration of lidocaine when compared with the drug administered alone. Norepinephrine yielded increased lidocaine concentrations to a depth of 3 mm. These decreased to the levels obtained from lidocaine applied alone after a four-hour washout. Thus coadministered vasodilating or vasoconstricting compounds alter the percutaneous delivery of lidocaine, in part by changing the reservoir properties of skin (80).

Singh and Roberts applied salicylic acid (SA), lidocaine, and water along with the vasoconstrictor phenylephrine to the dermis of anesthetized and/or sacrificed rats (78). For each solute, an increase in phenylephrine concentration decreased the solute dermal clearance and increased the concentration in the underlying skin tissues (Fig. 10A,B). The concentration-depth profiles for each solute were well described by Singh and Roberts' pharmacokinetic model (see the section Effect of Lymphatic Flow on Clearance). Sugibayashi et al.'s results with flurbiprofen in the presence of the vasoconstrictor epinephrine (81) and Higaki et al.'s results with phenylephrine and antipyrine (82) support these results.

Cross et al. compared absorption profiles of the vasodilator methylsalicylate (MeSA) and triethanolamine salicylate (TSA) in vitro in diffusion cells and in vivo over a six-hour period in anesthetized rats (83). The in vivo studies yielded higher salicylate concentrations in the dermis and in the underlying tissues following

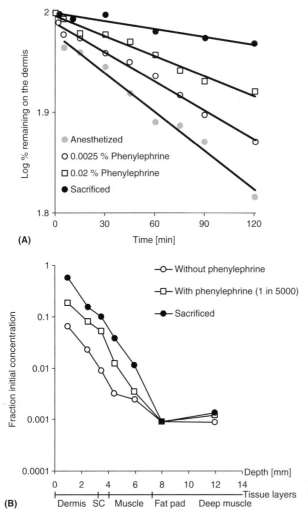

FIGURE 10 (**A**) Percentage of the initial amount of salicylic acid (SA) applied to rat dermis as a function of the degree of vasoconstriction and time. Postmortem conditions in sacrificed rats represent an extreme case of vasoconstriction (78). "Anesthetized" designates. the control group. (**B**) Corresponding tissue concentration-depth profiles for SA two hours after dermal application. Figures adapted from Cross and Roberts. *Source:* From Ref. 73.

the application of MeSA, when compared with the application of TSA, than predicted by the in vitro experiments. Furthermore, a rapid increase in salicylate concentration in the treated and contralateral tissues within 0.5 to 1 hours corresponded to an increase in the blood flow rate occurring within 0.5 hours following MeSA administration.

The change in blood flow rate due to phenylephrine and its influence on the delivery of antipyrine to the muscular layer was recently investigated by Higaki et al. (84). Phenylephrine decreased the local blood flow and led to an increase in the distribution of antipyrine, but to a decrease in the fraction of dose absorbed, the plasma concentration and the concentrations in the viable tissue and in the muscle at the contralateral site. Phenylephrine reduced blood flow below the site of application, but not at the contralateral site. The effect of vasoconstriction due to phenylephrine on the absorption of SA and diclofenac was compared with that of antipyrine. The increase in penetration was the lowest for antipyrine, which has the highest fraction unbound in the viable skin (fu_{vs}) and, consequently, the greatest distribution in the muscular layer (82). The increase in distribution into the muscular layer due to vasoconstriction was the highest for diclofenac, which has the lowest fu_{vs} value. It is suggested that vasoconstriction could be most effective for drugs with poor muscular distribution.

Jacobi et al. studied in vivo the effect of the vasodilator benzyl nicotinate (BN) by applying it to the forearm, the forehead, and the calf of volunteers, and measuring blood flow, cutaneous temperature, and redness due to blood flow at these three sites (85). The basal levels of these parameters are highest on the forehead, suggesting the important role played by the dense vasculature surrounding hair follicles. At each site, the blood flow in the superficial capillaries is greater than that in the deeper plexus. The application of BN causes a significant increase in blood flow at each site. Blood flows were again highest in the forehead and, for each measured parameter, the time to reach half its maximal value was lowest in the forehead. While in the forearm and the calf, the application of BN yielded an increase in the ratio superficial blood flow/deeper blood flow, in the forehead this ratio decreased. This result may be due to penetration into the dermis via the hair follicles of the forehead. Overall, this work demonstrates the importance of the vasculature surrounding the hair follicles, particularly in follicle-dense regions of the body. The fact that the stratum corneum is thinner in these regions may also contribute to the increased penetration.

Other recent studies have used cutaneous microdialysis to assess the effect of blood flow on skin solute concentration, distribution, and clearance, by studying the effect of vasoconstriction and vasodilation on these parameters (76,86–89). Wilson et al. (88) investigated the effect of age on the cutaneous response to vasoconstriction induced in patients 18 to 75 years old. Under conditions of antagonized release of endogenous norepinephrine, they observed decreased vasoconstrictor responsiveness in older patients.

Effect of Blood Vessel Orientation

Several studies suggest that in addition to passive diffusion and distribution via the local systemic circulation, the orientation of blood vessels also plays a role in deep tissue delivery of topically applied solutes (90). McNeill et al. (91) studied the in vivo penetration of piroxicam into dosed and non-dosed sides of rat muscles. Whereas after IV administration one maximum in concentration is observed at 12 hours, after topical administration two maxima, at 4 and 12 hours, are observed in dose and non-dose side muscle. Tissue-plasma level ratios measured in dose side muscles are constant following IV administration, but increase with the time of dosing in the case of topical application. These results indicate that piroxicam is delivered to muscle on the dose side via a process other than systemic delivery. The authors suggest that the cutaneous microvasculature provides a "convective physiological force" for transport into the muscle tissue, distinct from transport via the systemic circulation.

Monteiro-Riviere et al. studied the in vivo penetration of piroxicam in deep tissue of pigs (92) in order to assess the role of systemic absorption. In remote, non-dose sites, only background concentrations of piroxicam were measured, indicating that the systemic circulation did not play a critical role in the penetration. Greater penetration was measured in the cranial sites, which are supplied by musculocutaneous arteries, than in the caudal sites, which are supplied by direct cutaneous arteries. Whereas most of the solute entering the systemic circulation was eliminated, the musculocutaneous arteries retained a greater fraction of solute within the deeper tissues. The orientation of the musculocutaneous arteries is such that piroxicam absorption into the cranial sites is greater than into the caudal sites. This study supports the notion of a "convective physiological force" for solute absorption into deeper tissues, represented by the musculocutaneous vasculature. In vitro studies confirmed that the difference in penetration into the cranial and caudal sites of the pigs was not due to skin permeability differences.

Further results supporting the importance of blood vessel orientation were provided by Cross et al. (93), who studied the distribution of dermally applied solutes to the perfused rat hindlimb. Concentrations of diazepram in a BSA perfusate measured in contralateral skin samples were comparable to those measured in deep tissue sites. The blood vessels may pass directly through the deep tissue on the dose side to the contralateral skin sites and shunt the solute to these sites, or run through the skin below the application site (93).

Effect of Pathological Conditions on Cutaneous Blood Flow

A number of clinical conditions cause changes in blood flow, which may need to be taken into account when considering the possible effects of cutaneous blood flow on solute permeation in the skin layers and the subcutaneous tissue (73).

In addition to reducing the barrier to penetration in the stratum corneum due to an increase in keratinocyte proliferation, psoriasis affects cutaneous blood flow. Cutaneous microvessels are elongated, widened, and tortuous, blood flow, and capillary mass are increased (94,95) and vasoconstriction and vasodilation are altered in magnitude (94,96). Hern et al. have compared laser Doppler measurements of blood flow after laser treatment of psoriatic skin with results from studies on port wine stain skin. Their results suggested that capillary expansion alone is not sufficient to increase blood flow in plaque skin (96). The authors hypothesize that the number of resistance vessels (arterioles) is also increased in psoriatic skin, and/or that there is a chronic widening of arterioles in reticular dermis.

Green et al. have investigated the blood flow response to environmental heating in patients suffering from chronic heart failure (HF) (97). The cutaneous vascular conductance response to heating (calculated from skin blood flow measurements) was significantly lower in HF patients than in the control group. The response is due to a decrease in cutaneous vasodilation.

The human cutaneous blood circulation system is controlled by sympathetic adrenergic vasoconstrictor nerves and sympathetic vasodilator nerves (98). Heat and cold stress may alter deep tissue pharmacokinetics by altering the cutaneous blood flow pattern. Heat stress causes cutaneous vasodilation mediated by neural mechanisms and local cutaneous effects, while cold stress causes arteriolar vasoconstriction and a decrease in skin blood flow (99). Hot flashes during menopause are an example of thermoregulatory dysfunction (98) which increases skin blood flow. Estrogens promote cutaneous vasodilation and thus heat dissipation, whereas progesterone is thought to inhibit this effect.

Type 2 diabetes inhibits cutaneous vasodilation under increased environmental heat exposure. Several studies show impaired sympathetic neural control of sweating and blood pressure in patients with Type 2 diabetes, as well as the possibility of damaged sympathetic vasodilator function (98).

Raynaud's phenomenon is characterized by excessive vasoconstriction in the fingers and toes accompanied by pain, as a response to cold or emotional stimuli. Patients suffering from this disease experience lower blood flow in the fingers, a longer rewarming response following cooling when compared with healthy patients, and a greater drop in body temperature following cold stress (100). Endothelium-dependent vasoconstriction is severely impaired (101).

Erythromelalgia is characterized by intermittent erythema in acral skin accompanied by the sensation of burning pain (98). Studies have shown that erythromelalgia patients have lower baseline skin perfusion and decreased sympathetic as well as local (at the extremities) vasoconstrictor responses (98,102).

Effect of Lymphatic Flow on Clearance

In general, macromolecules such as proteins and large sugars that reach the dermis or subcutaneous tissue, will not be cleared through the blood vessels due to low permeability through the capillary endothelium and restricted movement within the capillaries. Lymphatic vessels are the preferred clearance route for these molecules (73). Cross and Roberts presented evidence for clearance by the lymphatic system by showing that the amount of interferon-g cleared from a subcutaneous absorption cell in an anesthetized rat model was equivalent with and without vasoconstriction by noradrenaline (Fig. 11) (103). The removal of water and lidocaine, two smaller solutes, was compared to that of interferon-g. Lower clearance showed that water was cleared by the local blood supply. Lidocaine was removed by tissue diffusion. Cross and Roberts' conclusions for interferon-g, which has a molecular size of about 17 kDa, agree with Supersaxo et al.'s suggestion that molecules of size greater than 16 kDa are preferentially cleared by the lymphatics which drain the site of administration (33,104). In earlier work, Bocci et al.

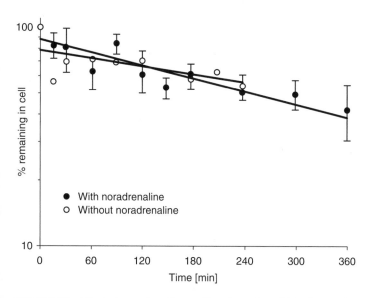

FIGURE 11 Effect of noradrenaline on the absorption of interferon-g into a cell exposed to the subcutaneous abdominal tissue of rats. Experiments were conducted with (*filled circle*) and in the absence of (*open circle*) noradrenaline. *Source*: From Ref. 103.

showed that interferon-2a (molecular size ~ 19 kDa) was preferentially absorbed into the lymphatics following intramuscular or subcutaneous administration, when compared with IV administration (105), and Yoshikawa et al. found the molecular size threshold for blood-lymphatics selectivity in healthy rats to be 10 to 18 kDa (106).

The removal of solutes by the lymphatic system depends on lymphatic flow, which itself increases with heat, massage, inflammation, movement of body parts and increases in hydrostatic pressure within the lumen of lymphatic collecting vessels, and decreases due to cold, lack of movement, and external pressure (107). In addition, lymphatic flow varies from one body site to another (107).

Physiological Pharmacokinetic Models of Deeper Tissue Penetration

It is important to understand whether drugs enter deep (muscle) tissue mainly via direct penetration from the viable skin or from the systemic circulation. Singh and Roberts (108,109) and Higaki et al. (82) have developed compartmental models to predict the contribution of direct solute penetration and delivery from the systemic circulation to subcutaneous tissue and other deep layers of the skin. The parameters determining the solute concentration in each compartment or skin layer are fractions of the unbound solute, clearances, and volumes of distribution.

Singh and Roberts applied SA to the dermis of anesthetized rats and used a physiologically based compartmental model (Fig. 12) to fit the SA concentration values in the dermis, subcutaneous tissue and deep skin layers, from 0 to 16 hours. Figures 13 and 15 A show the concentration–time profiles in the various tissues and in muscle directly below the site of application and in the corresponding contralateral tissues. The results show a maximum in the SA concentration in the dermis and the subcutaneous tissue at two to three hours and in the muscle around four hours. The maximum concentration decreases with increasing tissue layer depth. The concentration maximum in the dermis, subcutaneous tissue and fascia is attributed to direct penetration into these tissues. The maximum, around four hours in the deeper tissues, results from some direct penetration in addition to the predominant delivery from the systemic circulation. A second concentration maximum, obtained at 10 hours, is attributed to delivery from the systemic circulation and some direct penetration. Furthermore, the skin tissue concentrations are always greater than those in the equivalent contralateral site. The degree of difference between the concentrations in various contralateral tissues is less important than that for the overlying tissues. These findings indicate a supply from the systemic circulation to the contralateral sites, whereas the supply to the overlying sites, to a depth of 3 to 4 mm, is predominantly due direct penetration during the first two to three hours.

Higaki et al. developed a six-compartment model (Fig. 14). They fit experimentally obtained concentration–time profiles of six drugs (antipyrine, diclofenac, SA, propanol, ketoprofen (KT), felbinac, and flurbiprofen). Similarly to Singh and Roberts' results, direct drug penetration into the muscle layer below the site of application was significantly more important than systemic delivery during the first two hours of penetration. In the case of felbinac, flurbiprofen, and SA, systemic delivery overtook direct penetration at the 4, 7, and 10 hour time points (Fig. 15B for SA). The clearance from the viable skin to the muscle layer (Cl_{vs-m}) was significantly correlated to the fraction of solute unbound in viable skin (fu_{vs}). The same was the case for the ratio Cl_{vs-m}/Cl_{vs-p}, where Cl_{vs-p} is the clearance from the viable skin to the plasma. As the fraction of unbound drug in the viable skin increases, the proportion of that drug cleared into the muscle layer

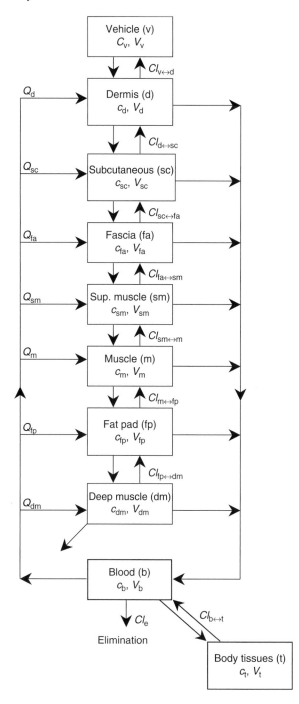

FIGURE 12 Singh et al.'s physiological pharmacokinetic model showing the involvement of individual tissue blood flows and systemic blood recirculation on the tissue concentrations of solutes following topical application in vivo. *Abbreviations*: *c*, concentration; Cl, clearance; *Q*, blood flow rate; *V*, volume. *Source*: From Ref. 109.

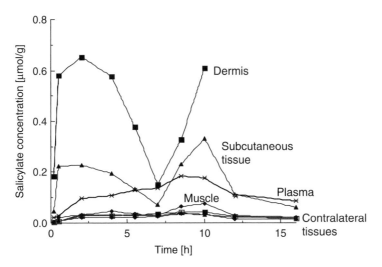

FIGURE 13 Tissue concentration–time profiles of salicylic acid determined in anesthetized rats following dermal application to the abdominal region in their in vivo dermal absorption model. *Source*: From Ref. 78.

(relative to the plasma) increases. Regression analysis for k_{direct}, the rate constant for the penetration from the viable skin into the muscle layer, showed the most important contribution to be from the fraction fu_{vs}. This suggests that a drug with a higher fraction unbound in viable skin can penetrate more into the muscle.

Higaki et al. obtained a greater relative contribution of direct penetration (72%) when compared with systemic delivery (28%) for the delivery of SA to the

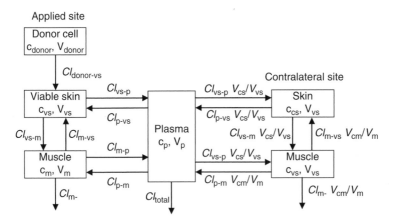

FIGURE 14 Six-compartment model used by Higaki et al. to describe the intradermal kinetics of topically applied antipyrine, diclofenac, salicylic acid, propanol, ketoprofen, felbinac, and flurbiprofen. Cl indicates the clearance between the tissue and tissue or plasma as represented by subscripts, where all clearances, except for Cl_{total}, were calculated as unit of viable skin or muscle mass. *Abbreviations*: c, concentration; V, distribution volume; Cl, clearance; vs, viable skin; m, muscle; p, plasma; cs, contralateral viable skin; cm, contralateral muscle. *Source*: From Ref. 82.

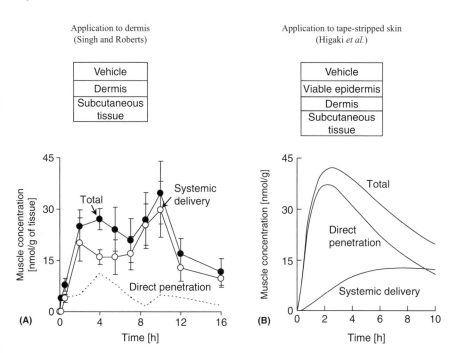

FIGURE 15 (**A**) Salicylic acid concentration in muscle versus time profiles obtained by Singh and Roberts: (*filled circle*, underlying tissue corresponding to total tissue concentration; *open circle*, concentration at contralateral site, corresponding to concentration due to systemic delivery; and *dashed line*, difference corresponding to direct penetration). (**B**) Total salicylic acid concentration in muscle below site of application and concentration due to direct penetration and to systemic delivery measured by Higaki et al. *Source*: From Refs. 82, 108.

muscle layer. Singh and Roberts, on the other hand, showed a greater relative contribution of systemic delivery (Fig. 15A). The total muscle concentration profiles obtained by both groups show a maximum at two to four hours. A second maximum is not visible in Higaki et al.'s results for which the maximum time is 10 hours (Fig. 15B). A longer simulation time could show a second maximum beyond 10 hours, a delay which could be explained by the extra resistance offered by the viable epidermis, which was removed in Singh and Roberts' study.

Questions that have been raised which still remain to be answered in the study of deep tissue penetration include (110): is direct penetration or systemic circulation more important for the delivery of certain drugs to the deep skin tissue; why is the increase in fu_{vs} not important for systemic absorption of certain drugs; and why is systemic delivery more important than direct penetration for diclofenac?

TRANSPORT IN THE SKIN APPENDAGES
Contribution of the Skin Appendages to Overall Skin Permeability
The strong interest in the skin appendages in the study of percutaneous absorption and transdermal drug delivery, stems from the fact that these structures provide punctures through the stratum corneum. In the late 1960s and 1970s Scheuplein

and Blank showed the appendageal pathway to be the dominant one during the early phase of transdermal diffusion, prior to the onset of the steady state. In the steady state, the observed rate of absorption was that through the "unbroken" stratum corneum [Fig. 3, (15,36)]. The authors applied the solution to the problem of diffusion through the stratum corneum approximated as a finite membrane and used nominal values for the diffusion coefficients in the various skin layers and appendages, estimated based on their structural and biological features. The value $D = 1 \times 10^{-7}$ cm^2/sec was estimated for diffusion within a hydrated hair follicle, the value $D = 1 \times 10^{-9}$ cm^2/sec for diffusion within the hydrated stratum corneum. Scheuplein and Blank's analysis explained apparently conflicting data obtained from experiments conducted on different diffusional time scales.

With the constant improvement of imaging techniques and the nanotechnology boom, experimental studies conducted over the past 15 years have provided strong evidence for the contribution of hair follicles to the overall transport of a number of compounds, beyond the initial stages of diffusion. Thus far, eccrine, apocrine, and apoeccrine glands have been the subject of fewer publications on transappendageal transport than hair follicles due to their lower density on the human body. Nonetheless, several studies reviewed below show that they may also constitute transport pathways for exogenous compounds. Conversely, the appendages may potentially retard solute transport through the skin, in particular due to the nature of sebum in the hair follicle and the fluids in the eccrine, apocrine, and apoeccrine glands. Despite the large number of studies on the subject, a clear mechanistic understanding of how the hair follicles and glands promote or retard the transport of chemicals is still lacking. To date little work has been published on the possible contribution of apocrine and apoeccrine glands.

Effect of the Hair Follicle and Sebaceous Gland

Lauer et al. found hairy rat skin to be an efficient barrier for mannitol (hydrophilic) without any permeation enhancer. Liposomal formulations on the other hand yielded greater deposition of mannitol in hairy rat skin (111). The lipophilic nature of sebum has been invoked to explain the facilitated penetration of lipophilic solutes through the hair follicle.

Bernard et al. compared the in vitro and in vivo penetration of an antiandrogen in normal hairless rat skin and scarred hairless rat skin lacking hair follicles and sebaceous glands (112). The vehicles used were an alcoholic solution and a liposomal formulation. The in vitro experiment yielded a higher cumulative percentage of antiandrogen permeated through normal skin than through scarred skin with both vehicles. With the alcoholic solution, permeant accumulation in the stratum corneum and viable epidermis was significantly greater in normal skin, whereas accumulation in the dermis was comparable for both vehicles. With liposomes, accumulation in the stratum corneum and epidermis was similar in both skins, but dermal accumulation was higher in normal skin. In the in vivo experiment, accumulation into the stratum corneum was greater with the alcoholic solution and the liposomes in scarred skin, but it was significantly higher in the viable epidermis and the dermis of the normal skin (Fig. 16). The two types of skin yielded different concentration distribution profiles. Whereas in normal skin most of the permeant was found in the first 500 μm with a sharp decrease in concentration in the deep dermis, in scarred skin the permeant concentration decreased at a depth of

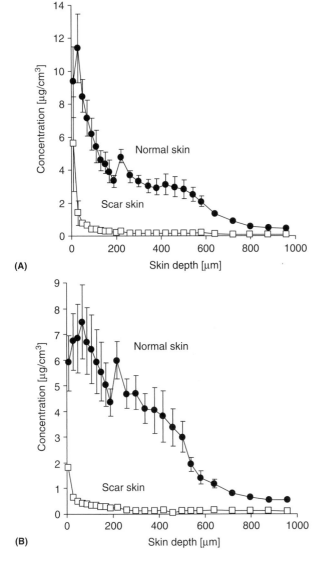

(A)

(B)

FIGURE 16 In vivo results obtained by Bernard et al. for the concentration of the antiandrogen RU 58841 in alcoholic solution (**A**) and liposomes (**B**) in normal and scar (lacking hair follicles and sebaceous glands) hairless rat skin, 24 hours after application. *Source:* From Ref. 112.

40 μm in the epidermis and was negligible in the dermis. The ratio of normal skin concentration to scarred skin concentration was greatest at a depth of 200 to 500 μm, corresponding approximately to the depth at which sebaceous glands are located.

Wu et al. used hairy mouse skin to study the permeation of inulin, a hydrophilic solute, entrapped in a water-in-oil nanoemulsion (113). Nanoemulsions with lower hydrophile–lipophile balance, and therefore more compatible with the lipophilic environment of the hair follicle, yielded greater inulin penetration. Various skin models yielded similar flux values, providing evidence that the transfollicular pathway indeed facilitated penetration into the skin.

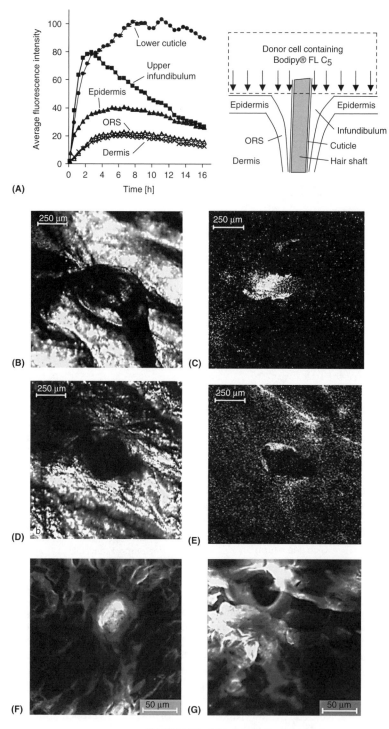

FIGURE 17 (*Caption on facing page.*)

Ogiso and coworkers compared in vitro the transport of the lipophilic drugs melatonin (MT) and KT through human scalp skin and abdominal skin (114). For MT in scalp skin, the steady-state flux was 20 times greater and the lag time nearly half the value compared to abdominal skin. For KT, the flux through scalp skin was 1.5 times larger, and the lag time three times smaller. Ogiso et al. also showed increased penetration for the hydrophilic drugs 5-fluorouracil (5FU) and acyclovir (ACV). The flux of 5FU was 48 times greater through scalp skin than through abdominal skin. The flux values of MT and ACV were used to obtain a linear relationship between the flux and the hair follicle density.

The improvement of microscopy techniques has enabled researchers to determine parts of the hair follicle which contribute significantly to solute deposition into deeper skin layers. Grams et al. visualized the in vitro diffusion of the lipophilic dye Bodipy® FL C_5 (BFL) (Molecular Probes, The Netherlands) into a block of human scalp skin containing a hair follicle (115,116). Their results at early times show intense staining in the infundibulum and the ORS but moderate staining in the viable epidermis, in agreement with Scheuplein et al. (15,36). However, at later times, the staining in the hair follicle remains stronger within the hair follicle than in the surrounding epidermis and dermis. The authors present evidence for the infundibulum as a pathway of BFL diffusion from the surface of the skin into the ORS and the surrounding tissue. An explanation for this result could be the nature of the infundibular wall, which is hydrated stratum corneum becoming thinner with depth into the infundibulum (Fig. 1A), thus providing a weaker barrier for diffusion into the viable epidermis than the stratum corneum at the skin surface (8,115). Figure 17A shows the fluorescence intensity–time profiles in some of the regions of the hair follicle and the viable skin considered by Grams et al.

Lademann and coworkers have surmised that the freely moving hair shaft within the infundibulum acts as a "pump" allowing topically applied nanoparticles to reach the deep parts of the hair follicle (119). In vitro studies with porcine skin showed that a dye in particle form up to about 1400 μm in depth after a massage application, whereas the non-particle form reached a depth of 500 μm. The same experiment performed without massage yielded a lower penetration depth of about 300 μm for both formulations. The authors suggest the cuticle cells of the hair shaft act as a "geared pump," pushing the particles into the follicles as a result of massage. A subsequent in vivo study (85) showed the "geared pump" effect to enable long-term storage (10 days) of the nanoparticles administered with massage compared to the reservoir effect of the stratum corneum (24 hours). While the idea of a pump mechanism makes sense intuitively, further study of this effect is necessary.

FIGURE 17 (**A**) Experimental results for the average fluorescence intensity versus time in various regions of a block of skin containing a hair follicle. The skin regions shown are the upper infundibulum (*filled square*), the upper cuticle (*filled circle*), the outer root sheath (ORS) (*open triangle*), the epidermis (*filled triangle*) and the dermis (*cross*). (**B**) Transmission and (**C**) fluorescence images of cross sections of an "active" hair follicle infundibulum showing the penetration of a 2% curcumin-containing sunscreen emulsion. (**D**) Transmission and (**E**) fluorescence images of cross sections of an "inactive" hair follicle infundibulum showing a lack of curcumin penetration. (**F**) Laser scanning confocal microscope image showing the penetration of a 1% curcumin-containing sunscreen emulsion into an "active" sweat gland. (**G**) Laser scanning confocal microscope image showing the lack of curcumin penetration into an "inactive" sweat gland. *Source*: From Refs. 114, 117, 118.

Lademann et al. (117) have also focused on the role of sebum in follicular penetration. They obtained a correlation between follicular penetration of sunscreen products labeled with 2% curcumin, sebum production and hair follicle growth. Hair follicles exhibiting sebum production and/or growth were termed "active," as they promoted follicular penetration (Fig. 17B,C), whereas the follicles which did not exhibit penetration were termed "inactive" (Fig. 17D,E). The effect of the hair growth cycles and differences/changes in follicle morphology on follicular penetration needs much more precise definition.

The gap between the IRS and the ORS within the isthmus of the follicle appears to be a favorable location for a permeant to diffuse into from the infundibulum. Several groups have visualized permeant at the IRS/ORS junction. Lieb et al. showed that the IRS/ORS junction could be a pathway for the penetration of low and high molecular weight rhodamine-labeled dextrans into the germinal components of the hair follicle and the surrounding epidermis and dermis (120). The same conclusion was reached by Ogiso et al. (114). Both the lipophilic dye nile red and the hydrophilic dye sodium fluorescein were observed in the IRS/ORS junction and, at later times, in the ORS and the surrounding tissue.

The permeability of a solute through the hair follicle is also affected by the binding property of the cuticle of the hair shaft. Grams et al. have shown that the cuticle has a high affinity for BFL present in the infundibulum (Fig. 17A) (115,116). Furthermore, the lipophilic dye remains in the cuticle longer than in the infundibulum, suggesting a reservoir effect. The dye visualized at later times in the inner and ORSs and in the dermis is suggested to have diffused from the cuticle. Cone has suggested that the binding and solute sequestration property of the hair shaft is mainly due to protein and melanin (121). Kelch et al. have visualized the diffusion of the fluorescent dye octadecanoylaminofluorescein into the cuticle and the cortex (the bulk of a human hair shaft) (122).

Further experiments need to be conducted to confirm the presence of a reservoir in the sebaceous gland. Genina et al. (123) have stated that the sebaceous gland acts as a reservoir, but have not provided conclusive data supporting this assertion. Bernard et al.'s (112) results showing sebaceous gland targeted by the antiandrogen liposomal solution indicate that the sebaceous gland could act as a reservoir, but time-dependent measurements are needed to confirm this.

Lademann et al. have stated that the outward flow of sebum does not hinder the penetration of nanoparticles into deeper parts of the hair follicle (124). While the time course of penetration they observed supports this conclusion, experiments establishing the effect of sebum outflow on the permeability of topically applied solutes are still lacking. Similarly, the change in shape and structure of the hair follicle during its growth cycle may have a significant influence on its permeability. We believe in vivo visualization experiments focusing on the diffusion of solutes through hair follicles at different growth stages would be of great value.

In vivo studies on the contribution of the hair follicle and the other skin appendages would be useful since the appendages are surrounding by a dense vascular network. Thus far, no study has been able to assess the diffusion of solutes from the hair follicle to the vascular network or vice-versa. The vascular network surrounding the skin appendages may play an important role in the distribution of solutes within the appendages and the surrounding skin layers, as well as in systemic delivery.

Effect of Eccrine, Apocrine, and Apoeccrine Glands

Based on results for the excretion of four drugs of varying pK_a and partition coefficients in sweat, Johnson and Maibach concluded that the permeability of the sweat gland epithelium is similar to that of other body membranes, in that "lipid solubility is a factor of prime importance in determining the rates of drug passage into sweat" (125). Jackson and Davis developed a one-dimensional mathematical model of diffusion through the sweat duct, which they approximated as a uniform tube (126). This study shows the potential for the sweat duct to act as a reservoir under occlusion and non-sweating conditions.

A number of more recent studies have visually established the potential for eccrine sweat ducts to carry either topically applied substances into the deep skin or intravenously administered drugs to the surface of the skin. Lademann et al. visualized the penetration of curcumin dye into sweat glands and hair follicles (118). They showed some sweat glands could be "active," i.e., allowing penetration (Fig. 17F), whereas others nearby could remain "passive," that is, no dye penetrated (Fig. 17G). Although more studies need to be conducted to validate the concept of "active" and "passive" sweat glands and to determine the criteria of activity, this concept does relate to that of "active" versus "inactive" hair follicles defined by the same group (117) (see the section Contribution of the Skin Appendages to Overall Skin Permeability). Subsequently Lademann et al. visualized the penetration of sodium fluorescein into sweat glands of the forearm to a depth of 60 μm (127). Schmook et al. (128) and Jacobi et al. (129) showed that eccrine sweat glands can transport intravenously administered liposome-encapsulated doxorubicin to the skin surface. After several injections into a patient, the drug was observed deep inside a sweat gland and around its opening in the upper cutaneous layers of the palm, as well as on the skin surface and the uppermost layers of the patient's plantar and palmar areas. These sites exhibit the highest number of eccrine sweat glands (see the section Eccrine Sweat Glands). The authors suggest that the hydrophilic coating of the liposomes allows the sweat to function as a carrier. Taken collectively these studies exhibit not only the shunt nature of the skin appendages, but also the importance of the dense microvasculature surrounding them, which is connected to the dermal vascular plexuses and thus to the body's systemic circulation (see the section Skin Vascularization and Lymphatics). The skin appendages may deliver solutes to the deep layers of the skin as well as to the systemic circulation.

Apocrine (28,129) and apoeccrine glands (28) may also represent pathways of transport for exogenous compounds. Wilke et al. compared the localization of tight-junction-associated proteins occludin, claudin 1, and claudin 4 in the eccrine and apocrine glands, in order to assess their potential as transport pathways or barriers (28). Tight junctions occur in the epidermal layer below the stratum corneum (the stratum granulosum), and are responsible for epidermal permeability and the integrity of the skin barrier (2). The intraepidermal portion of the ducts lacks these tight-junction-associated proteins and possesses a keratinized cell layer (28,130,131). On the other hand, occludin and claudin 4 were co-localized in the secretory coil of the glands and the dermal portion of the ducts (28). This finding, along with the lack of a cornified cell layer, indicates that these sections of the eccrine, apocrine glands could represent transport pathways between the interior of the glands and the surrounding skin tissue (28).

CONCLUSION

In this chapter, we have focused on the components of the viable skin layers and the skin appendages that may influence the permeation of exogenous compounds, and in particular drugs, into the viable skin layers and the underlying tissues. Theoretical and experimental studies show that the ability to make solute molecules reach the viable skin layers and/or the subcutaneous tissue depends not only on a successful crossing or bypassing of the stratum corneum barrier, but also on numerous physical barriers residing below the stratum corneum. Thus, the availability of a drug in pharmacological quantities at a target location below the stratum corneum also depends on one or more of the following parameters: solute binding and sequestration in the viable skin layers, metabolism in the viable epidermis, blood flow, distribution and/or elimination via the systemic circulation, and the contribution of shunt pathways provided by the skin appendages. The identification and role of cutaneous protein transporters and the kinetics of active cutaneous transport processes are emerging areas of interest in transdermal transport. The contribution of cutaneous protein transporters to transdermal transport has yet to be defined in a precise way.

Studies in percutaneous absorption usually focus on one aspect of transport through skin, i.e., the stratum corneum barrier, the use of hair follicles as a means of bypassing this barrier, the effect of dermal blood flow or the effect of metabolism. Some models of cutaneous transport incorporate diffusion and blood flow clearance, or diffusion and metabolism. Physiologically-based pharmacokinetic (PBPK) models seek to incorporate parameters relating to solute absorption into individual tissues, solute redistribution, and clearance through blood flow. The PBPK models have been successful in providing an understanding of the relative importance of direct penetration versus delivery from the systemic circulation, and in identifying parameters critical to permeation to subcutaneous tissue, such as the fraction of solute unbound in viable skin. Thus far, though, PBPK models have not yet taken into account other important structural features such as the pilosebaceous unit. A model that incorporates the contribution of the various skin structures would be beneficial in seeking a global understanding of the penetration of a solute though human skin.

In another paper (132), we argued that the maximum flux is a relevant parameter for the characterization of percutaneous penetration. A maximum flux through the whole skin could be defined taking into account the solute permeabilities through in the stratum corneum, the viable skin layer, the skin appendages, and systemic clearance,

$$J_{max} = \left(\frac{1}{Cl_b/A} + \frac{1}{k_{p,shunts} + \left(\frac{1}{k_{p,sc}} + \frac{1}{k_{p,ve}} + \frac{1}{k_{p,d}} \right)^{-1}} \right)^{-1} S_v = k_p'' S_v,$$

where $k_{p,shunts}$, $k_{p,sc}$, $k_{p,ve}$, and $k_{p,d}$, are the permeability coefficients in the skin appendages, the stratum corneum, the viable epidermis, and the dermis, respectively, Cl_b/A is the rate of removal of solute from the systemic circulation over the area of topical application, k_p'' is an effective permeability coefficient, and S_v is the solute solubility. The challenge lies in defining the permeabilities as functions of the physico-chemical processes affecting solute transport in each skin layer and the skin appendages. The physiological processes described in this chapter are expected to be the key elements determining the values of the permeability coefficients $k_{p,shunts}$, $k_{p,sc}$, $k_{p,ve}$ and $k_{p,d}$ and the clearance Cl_b.

REFERENCES

1. Madison KC. Barrier function of the skin: "La Raison d'Etre" of the epidermis. J Invest Dermatol 2003; 121(2):231–41.
2. McGrath JA, Eady RAJ, Pope FM. Anatomy and organization of human skin. In: Burns T, ed. Rook's Textbook of Dermatology. Oxford: Blackwell Publishers, 2004.
3. Wang TF, Kasting GB, Nitsche JM. A multiphase microscopic diffusion model for stratum corneum permeability. I. Formulation, solution, and illustrative results for representative compounds. J Pharm Sci 2006; 95(3):620–48.
4. Ritschel WA, Hussain AS. The principles of permeation of substances across the skin. Methods Find Exp Clin Pharmacol 1988; 10(1):39–56.
5. Walters KA, Roberts MS. The structure and function of skin. In: Walters KA, ed. Dermatological and Transdermal Formulations. New York: Marcel Dekker, Inc., 2002:1–39.
6. Jakubovic HR, Ackermann AB. Structure and function of skin: development, morphology, and physiology. In: Moschella SL, Hurley HJ, eds. Dermatology. Philadelphia, PA: W.B. Saunders Company, 1992:3–87.
7. Montagna W, Kligman AM, Carlisle KS. Atlas of Normal Human Skin. New York: Springer, 1992.
8. Grams YY, Bouwstra JA. Penetration and distribution in human skin focusing on the hair follicle. In: Bronaugh RL, Maibach HI, eds. Percutaneous Absorption: Drugs–Cosmetics–Mechanisms–Methods. Boca Raton, FL: Taylor & Francis Group, 2005:177–91.
9. Agarwal R, Katare OP, Vyas SP. The pilosebaceous unit: a pivotal route for topical drug delivery. Methods Find Exp Clin Pharmacol 2000; 22(2):129–33.
10. Otberg N, Richter H, Schaefer H, Blume-Peytavi U, Sterry W, Lademann J. Variations of hair follicle size and distribution in different body sites. J Invest Dermatol 2004; 122(1):14–9.
11. Pagnoni A, Kligman AM, el Gammal S, Stoudemayer T. Determination of density of follicles on various regions of the face by cyanoacrylate biopsy: correlation with sebum output. Br J Dermatol 1994; 131(6):862–5.
12. Holbrook KA, Odland GF. Regional differences in the thickness (cell layers) of the human stratum corneum: an ultrastructural analysis. J Invest Dermatol 1974; 62(4):415–22.
13. Ya-Xian Z, Suetake T, Tagami H. Number of cell layers of the stratum corneum in normal skin—relationship to the anatomical location on the body, age, sex and physical parameters. Arch Dermatol Res 1999; 291(10):555–9.
14. Scott RC, Corrigan MA, Smith F, Mason H. The influence of skin structure on permeability: an intersite and interspecies comparison with hydrophilic penetrants. J Invest Dermatol 1991; 96(6):921–5.
15. Scheuplein RJ, Blank IH. Permeability of the skin. Physiol Rev 1971; 51(4):702–47.
16. Schaefer H, Lademann J. The role of follicular penetration. A differential view. Skin Pharmacol Appl Skin Physiol 2001; 14(Suppl. 1):23–7.
17. Odland GF. Structure of the skin. In: Goldsmith LA, ed. Physiology, Morphology and Molecular Biology of the Skin. New York: Oxford University Press, 1991:3–110.
18. Lauer AC. Percutaneous drug delivery to the hair follicle. In: Bronaugh RL, Maibach HI, eds. Percutaneous Absorption: Drugs–Cosmetics–Mechanisms–Methods. Boca Raton, FL: Taylor & Francis, 2005:411–28.
19. Paus R, Cotsarelis G. The biology of hair follicles. N Engl J Med 1999; 341(7):491–7.
20. Montagna W. The sebaceous gland in man. In: Montagna W, Ellis RA, eds. Advances in Biology of Skin. New York: Pergamn Press, Inc., 1961:19–31.
21. Fawcett DW, Raviola E. Bloom and Fawcett: A Textbook of Histology. 12th ed. New York: Chapman and Hall, 1994.

22. Zouboulis CC. Sebaceous gland in human skin—the fantastic future of a skin appendage. J Invest Dermatol 2003; 120(6)xiv–v.
23. Zouboulis CC. Acne and sebaceous gland function. Clin Dermatol 2004; 22(5):360–6.
24. Meidan VM, Bonner MC, Michniak BB. Transfollicular drug delivery—is it a reality? Int J Pharm 2005; 306(1–2):1–14.
25. Cross SE, Anderson C, Roberts MS. Topical penetration of commercial salicylate esters and salts using human isolated skin and clinical microdialysis studies. Br J Clin Pharmacol 1998; 46(1):29–35.
26. Hurley HJ. The eccrine sweat glands: structure and function. In: Freinkel RK, Woodley DT, eds. The Biology of the Skin. New York: Parthenon Publishing Group, 2001:47–76.
27. Sato K, Leidal R, Sato F. Morphology and development of an apoeccrine sweat gland in human axillae. Am J Physiol 1987; 252(1 Pt 2):R166–80.
28. Wilke K, Wepf R, Keil FJ, Wittern K-P, Wenck H, Biel SS. Are sweat glands an alternate penetration pathway? Understanding the morphological complexity of the axillary sweat gland apparatus Skin Pharmacol Physiol 2006; 19(1):38–49.
29. Braverman IM. The cutaneous microcirculation. J Investig Dermatol Symp Proc 2000; 5(1):3–9.
30. Braverman IM, Keh A, Goldminz D. Correlation of laser Doppler wave patterns with underlying microvascular anatomy. J Invest Dermatol 1990; 95(3):283–6.
31. Cevc G, Vierl U. Spatial distribution of cutaneous microvasculature and local drug clearance after drug application on the skin. J Control Release 2007; 118(1):18–26.
32. Ellis RA. Vascular patterns in the skin. In: Montagna W, Ellis RA, eds. Advances in Biology of the Skin. New York: Pergamon Press, Inc., 1961:20–36.
33. O'Driscoll CM. Anatomy and physiology of the lymphatics. In: Charman WN, Stella VJ, eds. Lymphatics Transport of Drugs. Boca Raton, FL: CRC Press, 1992.
34. Barry BW. Novel mechanisms and devices to enable successful transdermal drug delivery. Eur J Pharm Sci 2001; 14(2):101–14.
35. Hadgraft J. Skin, the final frontier. Int J Pharm 2001; 224(1–2):1–18.
36. Scheuplein RJ. Mechanism of percutaneous absorption. II. Transient diffusion and the relative importance of various routes of skin penetration. J Invest Dermatol 1967; 48(1):79–88.
37. Flynn GL, Yalkowsk Sh. Correlation and prediction of mass-transport across membranes. 1. Influence of alkyl chain-length on flux-determining properties of barrier and diffusant. J Pharm Sci 1972; 61(6):838–52.
38. Roberts MS, Anderson RA, Swarbrick J. Percutaneous absorption of phenolic compounds—mechanism of diffusion across stratum-corneum. J Pharm Pharmacol 1978; 30(8):486–90.
39. Anissimov YG, Roberts MS. Diffusion modeling of percutaneous absorption kinetics. 1. Effects of flow rate, receptor sampling rate, and viable epidermal resistance for a constant donor concentration. J Pharm Sci 1999; 88(11):1201–9.
40. Wenkers BP, Lippold BC. Skin penetration of nonsteroidal antiinflammatory drugs out of a lipophilic vehicle: influence of the viable epidermis. J Pharm Sci 1999; 88(12):1326–31.
41. Rajaraman G, Roberts MS, Hung D, Wang GQ, Burczynski FJ. Membrane binding proteins are the major determinants for the hepatocellular transmembrane flux of long-chain fatty acids bound to albumin. Pharm Res 2005; 22(11):1793–804.
42. Cleek RL, Bunge AL. A new method for estimating dermal absorption from chemical exposure. 1. General approach. Pharm Res 1993; 10(4):497–506.
43. Bunge AL, Cleek RL. A new method for estimating dermal absorption from chemical exposure: 2. Effect of molecular weight and octanol–water partitioning. Pharm Res 1995; 12(1):88–95.
44. Crank J. The Mathematics of Diffusion. Oxford: Oxford University Press, 1975.
45. Guy RH, Hadgraft J. Pharmacokinetic interpretation of the plasma levels of clonidine following transdermal delivery. J Pharm Sci 1985; 74(9):1016–8.
46. Khalil E, Kretsos K, Kasting GB. Glucose partition coefficient and diffusivity in the lower skin layers. Pharm Res 2006; 23(6):1227–34.

47. Baker JR, Christian RA, Simpson P, White AM. The binding of topically applied glucocorticoids to rat skin. Br J Dermatol 1977; 96(2):171–8.
48. Yourick JJ, Koenig ML, Yourick DL, Bronaugh RL. Fate of chemicals in skin after dermal application: does the in vitro skin reservoir affect the estimate of systemic absorption? Toxicol Appl Pharmacol 2004; 195(3):309–20.
49. Siddiqui O, Roberts MS, Polack AE. Percutaneous absorption of steroids: relative contributions of epidermal penetration and dermal clearance. J Pharmacokinet Biopharm 1989; 17(4):405–24.
50. Walter K, Kurz H. Binding of drugs to human skin: influencing factors and the role of tissue lipids. J Pharm Pharmacol 1988; 40(10):689–93.
51. Yagi S, Nakayama K, Kurosaki Y, Higaki K, Kimura T. Factors determining drug residence in skin during transdermal absorption: studies on beta-blocking agents. Biol Pharm Bull 1998; 21(11):1195–201.
52. Cross SE, Magnusson BM, Winckle G, Anissimov Y, Roberts MS. Determination of the effect of lipophilicity on the in vitro permeability and tissue reservoir characteristics of topically applied solutes in human skin layers. J Invest Dermatol 2003; 120(5):759–64.
53. Magnusson BM, Cross SE, Winckle G, Roberts MS. Percutaneous absorption of steroids: determination of in vitro permeability and tissue reservoir characteristics in human skin layers. Skin Pharmacol Physiol 2006; 19(6):336–42.
54. Roberts MS, Cross SE, Anissimov YG. The skin reservoir for topically applied solutes. In: Bronaugh RL, Maibach HI, eds. Percutaneous Absorption: Drugs, Cosmetics, Mechanisms, Methodology. Boca Raton, FL: Taylor & Francis, 2005:213–34.
55. Liu P, Higuchi WI, Song WQ, Kurihara-Bergstrom T, Good WR. Quantitative evaluation of ethanol effects on diffusion and metabolism of beta-estradiol in hairless mouse skin. Pharm Res 1991; 8(7):865–72.
56. Hikima T, Yamada K, Kimura T, Maibach HI, Tojo K. Comparison of skin distribution of hydrolytic activity for bioconversion of beta-estradiol 17-acetate between man and several animals in vitro. Eur J Pharm Biopharm 2002; 54(2):155–60.
57. Sugibayashi K, Hayashi T, Morimoto Y. Simultaneous transport and metabolism of ethyl nicotinate in hairless rat skin after its topical application: the effect of enzyme distribution in skin. J Control Release 1999; 62(1–2):201–8.
58. Boderke P, Schittkowski K, Wolf M, Merkle HP. Modeling of diffusion and concurrent metabolism in cutaneous tissue. J Theor Biol 2000; 204(3):393–407.
59. Bleasby K, Castle JC, Roberts CJ, et al. Expression profiles of 50 xenobiotic transporter genes in humans and pre-clinical species: a resource for investigations into drug disposition. Xenobiotica 2006; 36(10–11):963–88.
60. Randolph GJ, Beaulieu S, Pope M, et al. A physiologic function for *p*-glycoprotein (MDR-1) during the migration of dendritic cells from skin via afferent lymphatic vessels. Proc Natl Acad Sci USA 1998; 95(12):6924–9.
61. Smith G, Dawe RS, Clark C, et al. Quantitative real-time reverse transcription-polymerase chain reaction analysis of drug metabolizing and cytoprotective genes in psoriasis and regulation by ultraviolet radiation. J Invest Dermatol 2003; 121(2):390–8.
62. Li Q, Kato Y, Sai Y, Imai T, Tsuji A. Multidrug resistance-associated protein 1 functions as an efflux pump of xenobiotics in the skin. Pharm Res 2005; 22(6):842–6.
63. Baron JM, Holler D, Schiffer R, et al. Expression of multiple cytochrome p450 enzymes and multidrug resistance-associated transport proteins in human skin keratinocytes. J Invest Dermatol 2001; 116(4):541–8.
64. Zeng H, Chen ZS, Belinsky MG, Rea PA, Kruh GD. Transport of methotrexate (MTX) and folates by multidrug resistance protein (MRP) 3 and MRP1: effect of polyglutamylation on MTX transport. Cancer Res 2001; 61(19):7225–32.
65. Keppler D, Leier I, Jedlitschky G. Transport of glutathione conjugates and glucuronides by the multidrug resistance proteins MRP1 and MRP2. Biol Chem 1997; 378(8):787–91.
66. Sprecher E, Bergman R, Sprecher H, et al. Reduced folate carrier (RFC-1) gene expression in normal and psoriatic skin. Arch Dermatol Res 1998; 290(12):656–60.
67. Schiffer R, Neis M, Holler D, et al. Active influx transport is mediated by members of the organic anion transporting polypeptide family in human epidermal keratinocytes. J Invest Dermatol 2003; 120(2):285–91.

68. Schnorr O, Suschek CV, Kolb-Bachofen V. The importance of cationic amino acid transporter expression in human skin. J Invest Dermatol 2003; 120(6):1016–22.
69. Li Q, Tsuji H, Kato Y, Sai Y, Kubo Y, Tsuji A. Characterization of the transdermal transport of flurbiprofen and indomethacin. J Control Release 2006; 110(3):542–56.
70. Schmuth M, Ortegon AM, Mao-Qiang M, Elias PM, Feingold KR, Stahl A. Differential expression of fatty acid transport proteins in epidermis and skin appendages. J Invest Dermatol 2005; 125(6):1174–81.
71. Boury-Jamot M, Sougrat R, Tailhardat M, et al. Expression and function of aquaporins in human skin: is aquaporin-3 just a glycerol transporter? Biochim Biophys Acta 2006; 1758(8)1034–42.
72. Roberts MS, Cross SE. A physiological pharmacokinetic model for solute disposition in tissues below a topical below a topical application site. Pharm Res 1999; 16(9):1392–8.
73. Cross S, Roberts M. Dermal blood flow, lymphatics, and binding as determinants of topical absorption, clearance, and distribution. In: Riviere J, ed. Dermal Absorption Models in Toxicology and Pharmacology. Boca Raton, FL: Taylor & Francis, 2006:251–81.
74. Tozer TN, Rowland M. Introduction to Pharmacokinetics and Pharmacodynamics: the Quantitative Basis of Drug Therapy. Baltimore, MD: Lippincott Williams & Wilkins, 2006; 326.
75. McCarley KD, Bunge AL. Physiologically relevant two-compartment pharmacokinetic models for skin. J Pharm Sci 2000; 89(9):1212–35.
76. Morgan CJ, Renwick AG, Friedmann PS. The role of stratum corneum and dermal microvascular perfusion in penetration and tissue levels of water-soluble drugs investigated by microdialysis. Br J Dermatol 2003; 148(3):434–43.
77. Gao X, Wientjes MG, Au JL. Use of drug kinetics in dermis to predict in vivo blood concentration after topical application. Pharm Res 1995; 12(12):2012–7.
78. Singh P, Roberts MS. Effects of vasoconstriction on dermal pharmacokinetics and local tissue distribution of compounds. J Pharm Sci 1994; 83(6):783–91.
79. Riviere JE, Sage B, Williams PL. Effects of vasoactive drugs on transdermal lidocaine iontophoresis. J Pharm Sci 1991; 80(7):615–20.
80. Riviere JE, Monteiro-Riviere NA, Inman AO. Determination of lidocaine concentrations in skin after transdermal iontophoresis: effects of vasoactive drugs. Pharm Res 1992; 9(2):211–4.
81. Sugibayashi K, Yanagimoto G, Hayashi T, Seki T, Juni K, Morimoto Y. Analysis of skin disposition of flurbiprofen after topical application in hairless rats. J Control Release 1999; 62(1–2):193–200.
82. Higaki K, Asai M, Suyama T, Nakayama K, Ogawara K, Kimura T. Estimation of intradermal disposition kinetics of drugs: II. Factors determining penetration of drugs from viable skin to muscular layer. Int J Pharm 2002; 239(1–2):129–41.
83. Cross SE, Megwa SA, Benson HAE, Roberts MS. Self promotion of deep tissue penetration and distribution of methylsalicylate after topical application. Pharm Res 1999; 16(3):427–33.
84. Higaki K, Nakayama K, Suyama T, Amnuaikit C, Ogawara K, Kimura T. Enhancement of topical delivery of drugs via direct penetration by reducing blood flow rate in skin. Int J Pharm 2005; 288(2):227–33.
85. Jacobi U, Kaiser M, Sterry W, Lademann J. Kinetics of blood flow after topical application of benzyl nicotinate on different anatomic sites. Arch Dermatol Res 2006; 298(6):291–300.
86. Borg N, Götharson E, Benfeldt E, Groth L, Ståhle L. Distribution to the skin of penciclovir after oral famciclovir administration in healthy volunteers: comparison of the suction blister technique and cutaneous microdialysis. Acta Derm Venereol 1999; 79(4):274–7.
87. Boutsiouki P, Thompson JP, Clough GF. Effects of local blood flow on the percutaneous absorption of the organophosphorus compound malathion: a microdialysis study in man. Arch Toxicol 2001; 75(6):321–8.

88. Wilson TE, Monahan KD, Short DS, Ray CA. Effect of age on cutaneous vasoconstrictor responses to norepinephrine in humans. Am J Physiol Regul Integr Comp Physiol 2004; 287(5):R1230–4.
89. Clough GF, Boutsiouki P, Church MK, Michel CC. Effects of blood flow on the in vivo recovery of a small diffusible molecule by microdialysis in human skin. J Pharmacol Exp Ther 2002; 302(2):681–6.
90. Cross SE, Roberts MS. Targeting local tissues by transdermal application: understanding drug physicochemical properties that best exploit protein binding and blood flow effects. Drug Dev Res 1999; 46(3–4):309–15.
91. McNeill SC, Potts RO, Francoeur ML. Local enhanced topical delivery (LETD) of drugs: does it truly exist? Pharm Res 1992; 9(11):1422–7.
92. Monteiro-Riviere NA, Inman AO, Riviere JE, McNeill SC, Francoeur ML. Topical penetration of piroxicam is dependent on the distribution of the local cutaneous vasculature. Pharm Res 1993; 10(9):1326–31.
93. Cross SE, Wu Z, Roberts MS. The effect of protein binding on the deep tissue penetration and efflux of dermally applied salicylic acid, lidocaine and diazepam in the perfused rat hindlimb. J Pharmacol Exp Ther 1996; 277(1):366–74.
94. Hern S, Stanton AW, Mellor R, Levick JR, Mortimer PS. Control of cutaneous blood vessels in psoriatic plaques. J Invest Dermatol 1999; 113(1):127–32.
95. Hern S, Stanton AW, Mellor RH, Harland CC, Levick JR, Mortimer PS. In vivo quantification of the structural abnormalities in psoriatic microvessels before and after pulsed dye laser treatment. Br J Dermatol 2005; 152(3):505–11.
96. Hern S, Stanton AW, Mellor RH, Harland CC, Levick JR, Mortimer PS. Blood flow in psoriatic plaques before and after selective treatment of the superficial capillaries. Br J Dermatol 2005; 152(1):60–5.
97. Green DJ, Maiorana AJ, Siong JH, et al. Impaired skin blood flow response to environmental heating in chronic heart failure. Eur Heart J 2006; 27(3):338–43.
98. Charkoudian N. Skin blood flow in adult human thermoregulation: how it works, when it does not, and why. Mayo Clin Proc 2003; 78(5):603–12.
99. Kellogg DL, Jr. In vivo mechanisms of cutaneous vasodilation and vasoconstriction in humans during thermoregulatory challenges. J Appl Physiol 2006; 100(5):1709–18.
100. Greenstein D, Gupta NK, Martin P, Walker DR, Kester RC. Impaired thermoregulation in Raynaud's phenomenon. Angiology 1995; 46(7):603–11.
101. Khan F, Belch JJ. Skin blood flow in patients with systemic sclerosis and Raynaud's phenomenon: effects of oral 1-arginine supplementation. J Rheumatol 1999; 26(11):2389–94.
102. Littleford RC, Khan F, Belch JJ. Skin perfusion in patients with erythromelalgia. Eur J Clin Invest 1999; 29(7):588–93.
103. Cross SE, Roberts MS. Subcutaneous absorption kinetics and local tissue distribution of interferon and other solutes. J Pharm Pharmacol 1993; 45(7):606–9.
104. Supersaxo A, Hein WR, Steffen H. Effect of molecular weight on the lymphatic absorption of water-soluble compounds following subcutaneous administration. Pharm Res 1990; 7(2):167–9.
105. Bocci V, Pessina GP, Paulesu L, Nicoletti C. The lymphatic route. VI. Distribution of recombinant interferon-alpha 2 in rabbit and pig plasma and lymph. J Biol Response Mod 1988; 7(4):390–400.
106. Yoshikawa H, Takada K, Muranishi S. Molecular weight-dependent lymphatic transfer of exogenous macromolecules from large intestine of renal insufficiency rats. Pharm Res 1992; 9(9):1195–8.
107. Uren RF. Lymphatic drainage of the skin. Ann Surg Oncol 2004; 11(3 Suppl.):179S–85.
108. Singh P, Roberts MS. Dermal and underlying tissue pharmacokinetics of salicylic acid after topical application. J Pharmacokinet Biopharm 1993; 21(4):337–73.
109. Singh P, Maibach HI, Roberts MS. Site of effects. In: Roberts MS, Walters KA, eds. Dermal Absorption and Toxicity Assessment. New York: Marcel Dekker, 1998:353–70.
110. Lee CM, Maibach HI. Deep percutaneous penetration into muscles and joints. J Pharm Sci 2006; 95(7):1405–13.

111. Lauer AC, Elder JT, Weiner ND. Evaluation of the hairless rat as a model for in vivo percutaneous absorption. J Pharm Sci 1997; 86(1):13–8.
112. Bernard E, Dubois JL, Wepierre J. Importance of sebaceous glands in cutaneous penetration of an antiandrogen: target effect of liposomes. J Pharm Sci 1997; 86(5):573–8.
113. Wu H, Ramachandran C, Weiner ND, Roessler BJ. Topical transport of hydrophilic compounds using water-in-oil nanoemulsions. Int J Pharm 2001; 220(1–2):63–75.
114. Ogiso T, Shiraki T, Okajima K, Tanino T, Iwaki M, Wada T. Transfollicular drug delivery: penetration of drugs through human scalp skin and comparison of penetration between scalp and abdominal skins in vitro. J Drug Target 2002; 10(5):369–78.
115. Grams YY, Whitehead L, Cornwell P, Bouwstra JA. Time and depth resolved visualisation of the diffusion of a lipophilic dye into the hair follicle of fresh unfixed human scalp skin. J Control Release 2004; 98(3):367–78.
116. Grams YY, Whitehead L, Cornwell P, Bouwstra JA. On-line diffusion profile of a lipophilic model dye in different depths of a hair follicle in human scalp skin. J Invest Dermatol 2005; 125(4):775–82.
117. Lademann J, Otberg N, Richter H, et al. Investigation of follicular penetration of topically applied substances. Skin Pharmacol Appl Skin Physiol 2001; 14(Suppl. 1):17–22.
118. Lademann J, Otberg N, Richter H, et al. Application of a dermatological laser scanning confocal microscope for investigation in skin physiology. Laser Physics 2003; 13(5):756–60.
119. Lademann J, Richter H, Teichmann A, et al. Nanoparticles—an efficient carrier for drug delivery into the hair follicles. Eur J Pharm Biopharm 2007; 66(2):159–64.
120. Lieb LM, Liimatta AP, Bryan RN, Brown BD, Krueger GG. Description of the intrafollicular delivery of large molecular weight molecules to follicles of human scalp skin in vitro. J Pharm Sci 1997; 86(9):1022–9.
121. Cone EJ. Mechanisms of drug incorporation into hair. Ther Drug Monit 1996; 18(4):438–43.
122. Kelch A, Wessel S, Will T, Hintze U, Wepf R, Wiesendanger R. Penetration pathways of fluorescent dyes in human hair fibres investigated by scanning near-field optical microscopy. J Microsc 2000; 200(Pt 3):179–86.
123. Genina EA, Bashkatov AN, Sinichkin YP, et al. In vitro and in vivo study of dye diffusion into the human skin and hair follicles. J Biomed Opt 2002; 7(3):471–7.
124. Lademann J, Richter H, Schaefer UF, et al. Hair follicles—a long-term reservoir for drug delivery. Skin Pharmacol Physiol 2006; 19(4):232–6.
125. Johnson HL, Maibach HI. Drug excretion in human eccrine sweat. J Invest Dermatol 1971; 56(3):182–8.
126. Jackson RJ, Davis WB. A mathematical approach to the prediction of the rate of penetration of ions in the sweat duct. J Theor Biol 1982; 97(3):481–9.
127. Lademann J, Otberg N, Richter H, et al. Application of optical non-invasive methods in skin physiology: a comparison of laser scanning microscopy and optical coherent tomography with histological analysis. Skin Res Technol 2007; 13(2):119–32.
128. Schmook T, Jacobi U, Lademann J, Worm M, Stockfleth E. Detection of doxorubicin in the horny layer in a patient suffering from palmar–plantar erythrodysaesthesia. Dermatology 2005; 210(3):237–8.
129. Jacobi U, Waibler E, Schulze P, et al. Release of doxorubicin in sweat: first step to induce the palmar–plantar erythrodysesthesia syndrome? Ann Oncol 2005; 16(7):1210–1.
130. Zelickson A. Electron microscopic study of epidermal sweat duct. Arch Dermatol 1961; 83(1):106.
131. Hashimoto K, Gross BG, Lever WF. The ultrastructure of the skin of human embryos. I. The intraepidermal eccrine sweat duct. J Invest Dermatol 1965; 45(3):139–51.
132. Dancik Y, Jepps OG, Roberts MS. Physiologically-based pharmacokinetics and pharmacodynamics of skin. In: Roberts MS, Walters KA, eds. Dermal Absorption and Toxicity Assessment, 2nd ed. New York: Informa Healthcare, Inc. (in press).

13 Biophysical Models for Skin Transport and Absorption

Johannes M. Nitsche
Department of Chemical and Biological Engineering, University at Buffalo,
State University of New York, Buffalo, New York, U.S.A.

Gerald B. Kasting
James L. Winkle College of Pharmacy, University of Cincinnati Academic Health
Center, Cincinnati, Ohio, U.S.A.

INTRODUCTION

Absorption of molecules (applied drugs and chemicals) through the skin proceeds by sequential diffusion steps through the stratum corneum (SC, barrier), viable epidermal, and dermal layers (1–3). Within each of these strata, absorption involves partitioning into and diffusion within several components of an inherently heterogeneous microstructure, and in the dermis it is accompanied by clearance into the systemic circulation via the dermal vasculature. Microscopic theoretical models of these transport processes have evolved to the point where they can often yield mechanistic understanding and reasonable quantitative predictions of transdermal transport rates, subsurface concentration levels, and rates of vascular clearance.

Such models—and the understanding they carry with them—are playing a growing role in the areas of topical and transdermally delivered drug development (4–6) and risk assessment of chemical exposure (7–10). Their importance in the first area is underscored by the facts that "overcoming the skin barrier in a safe and effective way still remains the bottleneck of transdermal and topical therapies" (11), and that "the transdermal route now vies with oral treatment as the most successful innovative research area in drug delivery, with around 40% of drug delivery candidate products under clinical evaluation related to transdermal or dermal systems" (12). Direct relevance of biophysical models to risk assessment is also high because the number of chemicals to which the population is exposed on a daily basis far exceeds the small fraction thereof that could ever be studied experimentally. For the remaining compounds (the vast majority), judicious application of well-conceived mathematical models can make the difference between a plausible and defensible risk analysis and the lack thereof. Both areas furnish strong motivation to understand how microscopic physiological structure and heterogeneity govern penetration.

OVERALL ORGANIZATION OF A PREDICTIVE ABSORPTION MODEL

Figure 1 presents an overall view of and notational scheme for skin structure that is simplified but nevertheless defines an effective framework for quantitative modeling of dermal absorption (13,14). For a given solute (permeant molecule) of interest, each layer α [stratum corneum (α = "sc"), viable epidermis (α = "ed"), and

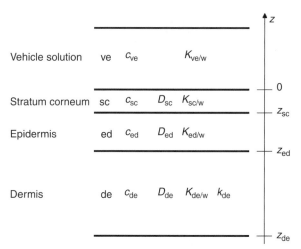

FIGURE 1 Definition sketch for detailed multilayer modeling of dermal penetration.

dermis ($\alpha=$"de")] is characterized in terms of a partition coefficient $K_{\alpha/w}$ quantifying solute affinity for α relative to aqueous reference solution "w" at a prescribed pH, and the diffusion coefficient D_α of the solute in α. [For an ionizable solute, the reference solution is commonly taken to be an aqueous solution in which the solute is completely nonionized (13,14).] The dermis is additionally imbued with a first-order clearance rate coefficient k_{de} defined as the constant of proportionality between the rate of clearance (i.e., rate of decrease of solute concentration by disappearance into dermal capillary loops) and the solute concentration at each locale. The vehicle (donor) solution in contact with the skin surface, from which the solute is absorbed, is denoted as $\alpha=$"ve."

All the tissue layer-specific parameters ($K_{\alpha/w}$ and D_α for $\alpha=$"sc," "ed," and "de," as well as k_{de}) have meaning as average properties of the inherently heterogeneous (and rich) multiphase microstructure of the layer, discussed below. Theory for deriving the macroscopically observable diffusion properties of microscopically heterogeneous media (15) has a distinguished history in mathematical physics and biophysics, and is well established, although its application to a given layer of the skin may be prohibited by mathematical and computational complexity, or by lack of knowledge of requisite microscopic physicochemical parameters. In any case, the average parameters are certainly determinable in principle as phenomenological coefficients by experiment if not by theory. They have meaning on sufficiently long length and time scales such that transdermal diffusion has had a chance to occur over a significant number of cell layers. All the theory outlined here applies to solute concentrations low enough for validity of a linear partitioning equilibrium relationship describable by a constant (concentration-independent) partition coefficient, and Fick's-law diffusion with a concentration-independent dilute-limit diffusivity. The definition of k_{de} additionally applies only as long as the systemic concentration is low enough for the dermal vascular concentration to be negligible.

Within the preceding framework, the ultimate goal of a theoretical calculation is to determine the solute concentration $c_\alpha(z,t)$ as a function of vertical position z and time t within each layer α, which is governed by the transient diffusion equation

$$\frac{\partial c_\alpha}{\partial t} = \frac{\partial}{\partial z}\left(D_\alpha \frac{\partial c_\alpha}{\partial z}\right) - k_\alpha c_\alpha. \tag{1}$$

At present the last term applies only to capillary clearance in the dermis; more generally, it could also represent metabolism or chemical degradation within any of the skin layers. As written, this diffusion equation allows for possible vertical position (z) dependence of the diffusivity, e.g., arising from vertical variations in hydration state within the SC, or from vertical variations in microstructure or physicochemistry in all layers (16,17). Initial conditions [usually $c_\alpha(z,0) = 0$] express the initially solute-free state of layer α. Kasting and Miller (18) formulate a more general initial condition representing initial deposition of a permeant in the uppermost cell layers of the SC. The concentration fields in adjoining strata (α and β, say) are coupled by auxiliary conditions expressing partitioning equilibrium and continuity of solute flux at the interface between them, namely

$$\frac{c_\alpha}{K_{\alpha/w}} = \frac{c_\beta}{K_{\beta/w}}, \tag{2}$$

$$D_\alpha \frac{\partial c_\alpha}{\partial z} = D_\beta \frac{\partial c_\beta}{\partial z}. \tag{3}$$

Similar interfacial conditions link the solute concentration at the top of the SC with that in the vehicle solution ("ve") applied to the skin. In the simplest case of an effectively infinite applied dose, the appropriate mathematical statement is simply

$$\frac{c_{sc}(0, t)}{K_{sc/w}} = \frac{c_{ve}}{K_{ve/w}} \tag{4}$$

with a constant value of c_{ve}. The corresponding mathematical statement is longer in the case of a finite dose (13,19,20), and more so in the case of a volatile solute (14,18). Riley et al. (9) applied a time-dependent set of boundary conditions generalizing equation (4) to model intermittent chemical exposures mimicking, for example, repeated hand contact with a chemically contaminated surface.

Good presentations are available of the complete set of governing equations, including one or more layers α, and of (generally numerical) methods for their solution (9,13,14,17–20).

TISSUE LAYER PROPERTIES AND TRANSPORT MECHANICS

Although many penetration-related properties of the SC, viable epidermis, and dermis present open questions, some of which are under active investigation, sufficient understanding and experience exists to give a thumbnail sketch of the essential attributes of each layer. The ultimate goal is to be able to estimate the parameters $K_{\alpha/w}$ and D_α for each stratum α in terms of solute properties such as molecular weight (MW) and octanol/water partition coefficient ($K_{o/w}$).

Stratum Corneum

Macroscopically the SC is regarded as a tissue layer imbued with average properties $K_{sc/w}$ and D_{sc}, having a typical thickness of ~43.4 or ~13.4 µm in fully hydrated (in vitro) or partially hydrated (in vivo) states, respectively. Wang et al. (cf. Ref. 21, Table 1) give a comprehensive enumeration of microscopic "brick-and-mortar" diffusion models of the permeability of this layer developed

TABLE 1 Equations Giving Effective Properties of the SC, Based on Wang et al.'s Model 2

Fully hydrated SC (in vitro)

$MW_r = MW/100$

$K_{lip/w} = 0.43(K_{o/w})^{0.81}$

$D_{lip} = (1.24 \times 10^{-7}\ cm^2/sec)(MW_r)^{-2.43} + (2.34 \times 10^{-9}\ cm^2/sec)$

$k_{trans} = (0.1884\ cm/sec)\exp[-8.465(MW_r)^{1/3}]$

$(D_{cor})_{free} = (7.736 \times 10^{-6}\ cm^2/sec)(MW_r)^{-0.6404}$

$(K_{cor/w})_{free} = 10^{[-0.0989 - 0.01\ MW_r + 0.000611(MW_r)^2]}$

$R = (7.54513\ cm)k_{trans}/D_{lip}$

$\sigma = D_{lip}K_{lip/w}/[(D_{cor})_{free}(K_{cor/w})_{free}]$

$(P_{sc/w})^{comp} = 1/\{105/(k_{trans}K_{lip/w}) + (0.0042\ cm)/[(D_{cor})_{free}(K_{cor/w})_{free}]\}$ for $R > 100$
                     for $R < 100$ (very rare) see Ref. (37)

$K_{sc/w} = 0.014(K_{o/w})^{0.81} + 0.782 + 1.381(K_{o/w})^{0.27}$

$D_{sc} = (P_{sc/w})^{comp}(0.0043365\ cm)/K_{sc/w}$

Partially hydrated SC (in vivo)

$MW_r = MW/100$

$K_{lip/w} = 0.43(K_{o/w})^{0.81}$

$D_{lip} = [(1.24 \times 10^{-7}\ cm^2/sec)(MW_r)^{-2.43} + (2.34 \times 10^{-9}\ cm^2/sec)]/H_{lat}$ with $H_{lat} = 3$

$k_{trans} = (0.1884\ cm/sec)\exp[-8.465(MW_r)^{1/3}]/H_{trans}$ with $H_{trans} = 3$

$(D_{cor})_{free} = (2.793 \times 10^{-6}\ cm^2/sec)(MW_r)^{-1.011}$

$(K_{cor/w})_{free} = 10^{[-0.444 - 0.0655\ MW_r - 0.00273(MW_r)^2 + 0.000534(MW_r)^3]}$

$R = (7.04642\ cm)k_{trans}/D_{lip}$

$\sigma = D_{lip}K_{lip/w}/[(D_{cor})_{free}(K_{cor/w})_{free}]$

$(P_{sc/w})^{comp} = 1/\{105/(k_{trans}K_{lip/w}) + (0.0012\ cm)/[(D_{cor})_{free}(K_{cor/w})_{free}]\}$ for $R > 100$
                     for $R < 100$ (very rare) see Ref. (37)

$K_{sc/w} = 0.040(K_{o/w})^{0.81} + 0.359 + 4.057(K_{o/w})^{0.27}$

$D_{sc} = (P_{sc/w})^{comp}(0.0013365\ cm)/K_{sc/w}$

Formulas for $(D_{cor})_{free}$ and $(K_{cor/w})_{free}$ are convenient molecular weight-based fits (14), approximating the results of molar volume-based formulas given in Ref. 37.
Values of H_{lat} and with H_{trans} are placeholders for the effects of hydration on lipid-phase mobility, to be defined by future study.
Source: From Ref. 37.

to date. These models offer potential mechanistic explanations of very useful empirical correlations (22–25) of the existing permeability database (25–27). The earliest view, expressed by Yotsuyanagi and Higuchi (28), focused on the overall lamellar microstructure of the SC and emphasized the transcellular pathway, which passes straight through the SC alternating between corneocyte and intercellular lipid layers (Fig. 2). Advocated more recently (27,29,30) has been an alternative picture according to which a penetrating solute does not enter the corneocytes, but rather remains confined to the intercellular lipid and follows its tortuous, zigzag-ging path through the SC. The best arbitrators in this debate are more detailed and rigorous diffusion analyses (21,31–37) that make no a priori assumptions and allow the dominant–flux pathway to emerge as a result of the calculation. Such models have been partly limited in the past by the unrealistic assumption of isotropic diffusion in the lipid phase (31–36). This limitation has been removed in the model developed by Wang et al. (21,37).

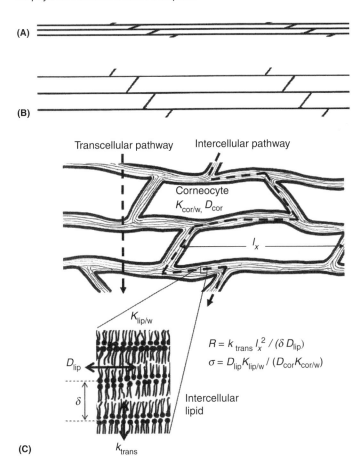

FIGURE 2 Microstructure of the SC and mechanisms of transport through it. (**A,B**) Geometries assumed in the brick-and-mortar model developed by Wang et al. (21,37) for (**A**) partially and (**B**) fully hydrated states. (**C**) Schematic diagram (not to scale) indicating pathways and phase-specific properties. The symbol l_x ($\sim$30 μm) denotes a length approximately equal to the breadth of a corneocyte seen in cross section, and δ ($=13$ nm) denotes the thickness of a lipid bilayer. Transcellular and intercellular pathways are indicated by dashed arrows. The transcellular pathway alternates between diffusion through corneocytes and perpendicular motion through the intercellular lipid by transbilayer hopping, these two processes respectively being characterized by a corneocyte-phase diffusivity D_{cor} and a transbilayer mass transfer coefficient k_{trans}. The intercellular pathway involves zigzagging lateral diffusion within the plane of a bilayer characterized by a lateral diffusivity D_{lip}. The quantities R and σ are dimensionless groups respectively defined as a modified ratio of transbilayer to lateral lipid-phase mobilities, and the ratio of lateral lipid-phase to corneocyte-phase permeabilities.

Several general statements can be made in overall commentary on the preceding developments, according to the authors' understanding, although they are subject to debate and will be contested in some quarters. First, the intercellular lipid pathway can certainly be parametrized to match steady-state SC permeability data, but the lipid-phase diffusion coefficients resulting from such an analysis are so large that the implied lag times for transient penetration are unrealistically short. This is a well-recognized problem associated with the lipid pathway (21,27,36–38).

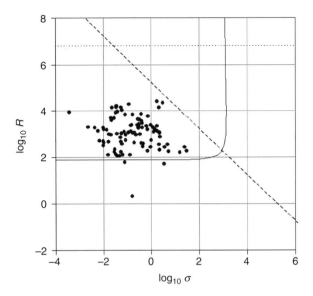

FIGURE 3 Analysis of the ($\log_{10} \sigma$, $\log_{10} R$) parameter space for fully hydrated SC. The solid curve demarcates the boundary between the regions where the transcellular and lipid pathways respectively dominant steady-state solute flux through the SC. Specifically, the transcellular pathway furnishes >50% of the total SC permeability for points above and to the left of this curve. The dashed line refers purely to the transcellular pathway, and represents the dividing line between the regimes where transbilayer transport (to the left) and intracorneocyte diffusion (to the right) respectively constitute the rate-limiting step for this pathway. The dotted line represents the hypothetical case of isotropic lipid-phase diffusion. Points represent the coordinates of all permeants (excepting sucrose) in the permeability database presented by Buchwald and Bodor (25). *Source*: From Ref. 37.

Kasting et al. (38) gave strong evidence for transcellular transport (and concomitant holdup of solute in the corneocyte phase) from considerations of both steady-state permeability and lag time for water. Barbero and Frasch (36) recently came to a similar conclusion based on lag times for a list of 27 hydrophilic compounds. Figures 3 and 4 [adapted from Wang et al. (37), referring to their Model 2] support the same conclusion from both mechanistic considerations of steady-state permeability (Fig. 3) and agreement with lag time data (Fig. 4) generally, regardless of permeant hydro- or lipophilicity. In Figure 3, R and σ denote dimensionless groups respectively defined as a modified ratio of transbilayer to lateral lipid-phase mobilities, and the ratio of lateral lipid-phase to corneocyte-phase permeabilities (21,37) (formulas given in Fig. 2 and Table 1). The solid curve represents a boundary above and to the left of which the transcellular pathway is the dominant contributor to solute flux; all but 3 out of 97 permeant compounds lie above and to the left of this curve.

As discussed elsewhere (39), equilibrium corneocyte-phase holdup of solute comprises free (mobile) solute dissolved in the water hydrating the corneocytes [which has solvent properties essentially identical to those of bulk water (40)], plus solute adsorbed (bound) to keratin (as well as other constituents of the corneocyte phase, e.g., cornified cell envelope proteins and the lipids covalently bonded to them), as depicted schematically in Figure 5. Figure 4 shows that acknowledgment of solute occupancy of at least the aqueous fraction of corneocytes certainly seems

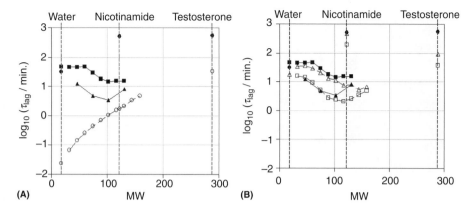

FIGURE 4 Lag times (τ_{lag}) for selected permeants in fully hydrated SC. Water, nicotinamide, and testosterone are indicated explicitly, and alkanols methanol through decanol are distinguishable by their molecular weights (MW). Open symbols represent theoretical values calculated from Wang et al.'s (37) permeability Model 2 (approximated by the equations given in Table 1). (**A**) represents results obtained from an incomplete formula for $K_{sc/w}$ acknowledging only lipid-phase solute holdup. (**B**) presents two views acknowledging corneocyte-phase solute holdup, namely: (*i*) $K_{sc/w}$ including free solute holdup in the water hydrating the corneocytes (open squares) and (*ii*) $K_{sc/w}$ given by the formula listed in Table 1 which includes all (free and bound) solute holdup in the corneocyte phase (open triangles). Filled symbols represent experimentally determined lag times (same data shown in both parts). The MW is used as the abscissa purely as a convenient means of distinguishing the various permeants. Another parameter such as $\log_{10} K_{o/w}$ could have been used instead. *Abbreviation*: MW, molecular weight. *Source*: From Ref. 37.

to be required to explain measured lag times, and that corneocyte-phase binding may often reach equilibrium on a time scale shorter than the lag time for diffusion through the SC. Anderson, Raykar, and coworkers' excellent early papers on SC structure–permeability relationships and partition coefficients (40–42) pioneered this picture of the distribution of solutes within the constituent phases of the SC. As stated well by Raykar et al., experimentally determined SC/water partition coefficients, shown in Figure 6, "reflect… a change in mechanism from protein[corneocyte]-dominated uptake for hydrophilic solutes to lipid-domain dominated uptake for lipophilic solutes" [(40), p. 149]. The scatter evident in the data call for a comprehensive experimental revisitation of this area, and more phase-specific characterizations of the partitioning properties of the lipid and corneocyte phases separately would be particularly valuable. Values of $K_{sc/w}$ for highly lipophilic compounds are particularly sensitive to the lipid content and composition of SC samples, and are therefore subject to high variability and uncertainty; not surprisingly, the data in Figure 6 show an increasing degree of (vertical) spreading with increasing $\log_{10} K_{o/w}$.

One of the open questions contributing to the controversy about pathways through the SC is the permeability (or impermeability) of the cornified cell envelope surrounding each corneocyte. Its attributes of mechanical strength and chemical resistance (43) do not necessarily imply any strong barrier properties. As recognized almost four decades ago [see (1), p. 722] and emphasized recently (38), effective cellular impermeability would imply barrier properties of the cell "wall" (now known as the cornified cell envelope) at exorbitant levels unknown to terrestrial biology. The idea of corneocyte-phase holdup is supported by recent studies

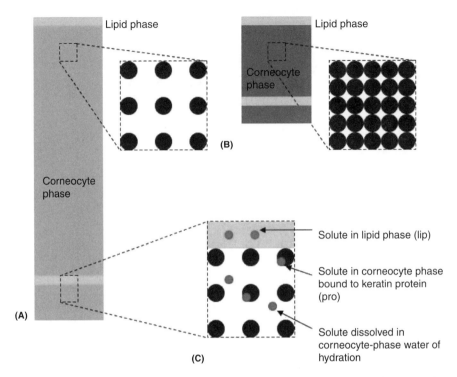

FIGURE 5 Schematic of SC microstructure. (**A**) Fully hydrated state. (**B**) Partially hydrated state. (**C**) Solute distribution among the lipid phase ("lip"), the keratin-bound state ("pro"), and the aqueous part of the corneocyte phase. *Source*: From Ref. 39.

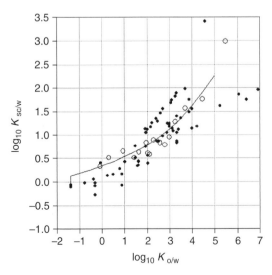

FIGURE 6 Log–log plot showing the dependence of $K_{sc/w}$ upon $K_{o/w}$ for fully hydrated SC. Small filled circles represent available data measured in various laboratories, larger open circles represent the two data sets reported by Raykar et al. (40) and Anderson and Raykar (42), and the curve represents the formula for $K_{sc/w}$ given in Table 1. *Source*: From Ref. 39.

employing two-photon fluorescence measurements in which partial entry of both hydrophilic and hydrophobic substances (44) as well as a pH-sensitive dye (45) into corneocytes was documented, aside from the work of Anderson, Raykar, and coworkers (40–42) cited above. Further experimental studies addressing this question will be extremely valuable in helping to resolve the debate about accessibility of the corneocyte phase.

Besides dominance of the transcellular pathway for almost all permeants, further conclusions can be drawn from Figure 3. As is evident from the positioning of all permeants relative to the diagonal dashed line, the rate-limiting step along the transcellular pathway is passage perpendicularly through the layers of intercellular lipid. Thus, the long-held belief that the lipid phase furnishes the primary barrier of the SC is justified, but this barrier function must usually be attributed to the mass transfer resistance for transbilayer motion, and only rarely to that for lipid-phase lateral diffusion. Also, all compounds lie more than two decades below the hypothetical horizontal dotted line corresponding to isotropic lipid-phase diffusion. Thus, diffusion within the intercellular lipid is highly anisotropic.

If one accepts the notions of solute transport through and holdup within the corneocyte phase, then the equations listed in Table 1 (14,37) can be used to estimate the values of the composite-average partition and diffusion coefficients of the SC, $K_{sc/w}$, and D_{sc}, consistent with both steady-state SC permeability and lag time data. These formulas (or corresponding formulas resulting from any other SC permeability model) may be summarized formally by the placeholders

$$K_{sc/w} = f_1(K_{o/w}), \tag{5}$$

$$D_{sc} = f_2(MW, K_{o/w}) \tag{6}$$

to indicate their purpose within the bigger picture of parametrizing all the skin layers.

An advantage of a mechanistic microscopic model over empirical correlations is that it can be used to relate the values of $K_{sc/w}$ and D_{sc} for the fully hydrated state of the SC in vitro to those for the partially hydrated state applicable to in vivo exposures [Table 1; Fig. 4 of Ref. (39) and Fig. 9 of Ref. (37)]. This comparison is of crucial importance to the practical in vivo application of the large available database on fully hydrated SC permeability.

All the preceding discussion refers to the intrinsic permeability properties of the composite medium represented by defect-free, appendage-free SC. It is well recognized that the permeation of very hydrophilic species such as sugars or inorganic ions involves a second, polar pathway (23,24,46–49). Although this aqueous pathway remains vaguely defined, it is generally associated with defects in SC microstructure (49). Through experiments on passive diffusion of sugar and other molecules and skin electrical resistivity in the papers cited, it has been characterized in terms of effective pore radius [a typical estimate being 15–25 Å (46); cf. similar estimates (48,49)], porosity and tortuosity factors (48,49), and estimates and bounds on the overall permeability contribution (23,24). This pathway may readily be included in a permeability calculation according to the reasonable engineering approximation of additive permeability for parallel pathways (23,24,49). Conceptually, it is important to distinguish this effective aqueous pore pathway from the transcellular aspect of the intrinsic permeability of intact SC.

Skin appendages (primarily hair follicles and sweat ducts) provide distinct additional shunt pathways breaching the SC barrier (1,49–53) about which there is no morphological ambiguity. Dancik (53) formulated and estimated parameters for a diffusion model of fluorescent dye transport around a follicle, and concluded that the permeation pathway may involve solute partitioning and diffusion into sebum in the infundibulum (the conical follicular opening around the hair shaft), and subsequent diffusion through the epithelium lining the infundibulum and/or sebaceous ducts. Jackson and Davis (51) modeled ion motion within an eccrine sweat duct in terms of transient one-dimensional diffusion through an aqueous tube. The inherent difference in pathways (respectively oily and aqueous) presented by these two types of appendages is underscored by the recent probabilistic transient analysis of percutaneous absorption by Ho (52). Macroscopically, these shunt pathways (each characterized by a diffusivity, partition coefficient and skin area fraction) can be incorporated into a transient penetration analysis by superposing their effects on overall solute transport. The conclusion of such analyses (1,50,52) is that the small area fractions of skin associated with these appendageal pathways make them insignificant contributors to steady flux, but their high diffusivities make them the dominant pathway in early phases of transient chemical exposures (Fig. 7).

Dermis

Discussion of the dermis here precedes that of the viable epidermis to streamline the presentation. Dermis is mainly acellular aqueous tissue, typically ~ 2 mm in thickness, comprising, inter alia, ~ 65 wt% water at pH 7.4, ~ 30 wt% collagen, ~ 1 wt% elastin, ~ 1.1 wt% plasma proteins (mainly serum albumin), and a small fraction of lipid (see below) (54–56). A fine herringbone structure of glycosaminoglycans infiltrates much of the aqueous space between the collagen and elastin fibers (56). About 32% of the aqueous volume is accessible to albumin (54), and its concentration in the aqueous volume accessible to it is $\sim 2.7\%$ w/v (56). The dermis is perfused by a vascular plexus located at a depth of ~ 1 mm, from which emanates a system of capillary loops extending nearly to the dermal–epidermal junction. Kretsos et al. (56) have developed a parametric characterization of the dermis of broad scope cast in terms very useful for skin penetration modeling. The discussion here summarizes their presentation.

The partition coefficient $K_{de/w}$ partly reflects volumetric exclusion from the portion of the dermis occupied by its fibrous inclusions, as described by the coefficient

$$(K_{de/w})_{free} = \frac{0.6}{f_{non}}. \tag{7}$$

The numerical value 0.6 represents a slight modification of the water volume fraction (~ 0.7) in dermis made to better fit the experimental dermal partitioning data (56). The symbol f_{non} denotes the fraction of solute nonionized at pH 7.4. For a weak acid or base, f_{non} is given by the well-known formulas $(1 + 10^{7.4-pK_a})^{-1}$ or $(1 + 10^{pK_a-7.4})^{-1}$, respectively. The coefficient $(K_{de/w})_{free}$ denotes the formal partition coefficient for solute distribution between dermal water (at pH 7.4) and an aqueous solution in which the solute is completely nonionized. The latter is used as the reference state for all partition coefficients; clearly $(K_{de/w})_{free} = 0.6$ for nonionizable solutes. The choice of reference states is arbitrary; we chose a pH 7.4 aqueous solution for part of the analysis in a previous report (13). The advantage of choosing a completely nonionized aqueous solution is that solubility data for chemicals in

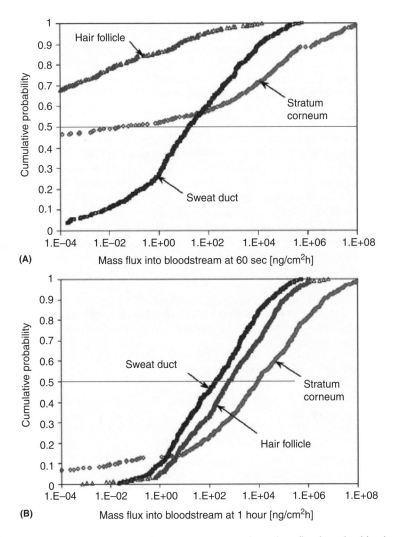

FIGURE 7 Cumulative probability distributions for solute flux into the bloodstream (assuming perfect vascular clearance below the SC) presented by Ho (52). The probability distribution in the computed outcome (solute flux) arises from assumed distributions over specified ranges of 16 compositional, geometrical and physicochemical input parameters characterizing SC structure and the solute. (**A,B**) respectively correspond to times of one minute and one hour after contact with the (infinite) donor solution. Curves are shown for three pathways: diffusion through the bulk of the SC, hair follicles, and sweat ducts. The median solute flux corresponds to an ordinate of 0.5. At an elapsed time of one minute (**A**) the sweat duct pathway provides the greatest median solute flux. At an elapsed time of one hour (**B**) diffusion through the bulk of the SC provides the greatest median solute flux. Although these numerical results are highly dependent upon the assumed ranges and distributions of SC and solute properties, they do effectively illustrate dominance of an appendageal pathway at short times. *Source*: From Ref. 52.

this state are commonly tabulated. The partition coefficient $K_{de/w}$ also reflects noncovalent solute binding (adsorption) to albumin in the albumin-accessible portion of the dermal water, and solute partitioning into dermal lipids. Solute distribution into these additional compartments is described by modifying equation (7) with an effective binding factor [calibrated to provide a reasonable correlation of the experimental dermal partitioning data (56)] as

$$K_{de/w} = (K_{de/w})_{free}[0.68 + (0.32)/f_u + (0.001)f_{non}K_{o/w}]. \tag{8}$$

The symbol f_u denotes the fraction of solute that would be unbound in a 2.7% w/v albumin solution at pH 7.4. If an experimental value of f_u is not available, then it can be estimated from the mathematical model developed by Yamazaki and Kanaoka (57). The symbol f_{non} arises in the last term because only the nonionized form of a (possibly ionizable) solute partitions into the dermal lipid phase, modeled as octanol. The coefficient 0.001 in equation (8) underestimates the true lipid content of dermis [~2.7 wt% (58) as opposed to the assumed value of 0.06 wt%] but this effective value gives the best overall correlation of experimental dermis partitioning data. Equation (8) may overestimate $K_{de/w}$ for highly lipophilic solutes having $\log_{10} K_{o/w}$ values greater than 4. It was calibrated for compounds for which $-3 < \log_{10} K_{o/w} < 4$ and $0.02 < f_u \leq 1$ (56).

Aside from excluding volume, collagen and elastin fibers represent a random network of obstacles hindering free aqueous diffusion of solute through the dermis. Kretsos et al. (56) found that experimentally determined dermis diffusivities are reasonably correlated by the expression

$$(D_{de})_{free} = (7.08 \times 10^{-5} \text{ cm}^2/\text{sec})MW^{-0.655} \tag{9a}$$

over the range $18 \leq MW \leq 477$. To good approximation this result may be recast in the form of the equivalent statement

$$(D_{de})_{free} = \frac{D_{aq}}{3.7} \tag{9b}$$

at the assumed temperature of 37°C, in which D_{aq} is the bulk aqueous diffusivity, which can be estimated using standard correlations such as the Wilke–Chang correlation (59,60) in the absence of an experimental value. The diffusivity given by equations (9a) or (9b) refers to free (mobile, unbound) solute. It is well known (56,61,62) that the effective diffusivity D_{de} describing all (free plus bound) solute is reduced by the solute-binding factor, because solute is immobile in its bound state. Thus,

$$D_{de} = \frac{(D_{de})_{free}}{[0.68 + (0.32)/f_u + (0.001)f_{non}K_{o/w}]}. \tag{10}$$

The product of partitioning and diffusion factors is unaffected by binding, i.e., $K_{de/w}D_{de} = (K_{de/w})_{free}(D_{de})_{free}$. A more refined analysis would allow for albumin mobility, which could provide a significant "piggyback" mobility mechanism for large, highly protein-bound solutes (56).

Capillary clearance occurs as a phenomenon distributed over the volume of the dermis. This volumetric distribution has a dramatic effect on the shape of dermal concentration profiles, which manifests itself already in the simplest context of steady-state diffusion. At steady state, the solution of equation (1) assuming

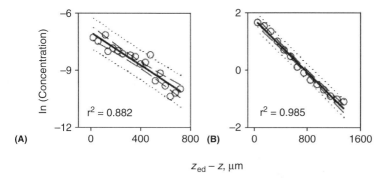

FIGURE 8 Semi-log plots of in vivo skin concentration versus depth profiles determined by cryosectioning of skin biopsies following topical administration of a skin permeant [reproduced from Ref. (56)]. (**A**) hydrocortisone in human skin, mol/L [data from Ref. (64)]; (**B**) didanosine in rat skin, mg/g [data from Ref. (65)]. The lines show linear regressions (*solid*), prediction intervals (*dotted*), and 95% confidence intervals (*dashed*) supporting an exponential decay of concentration with depth. The slope of these lines yields the ratio $(k_{de}/D_{de})^{1/2}$.

spatially uniform dermal clearance (constant k_{de}) is an exponential decay with depth (13,56,63),

$$c_{de} = (c_{de}|_{z=z_{ed}}) \exp[(k_{de}/D_{de})^{1/2}(z-z_{ed})], \tag{11}$$

which differs radically (generally by orders of magnitude) from the linear distribution that is the hallmark of steady one-dimensional diffusion processes in the absence of clearance. Here z_{ed} denotes the value of z at the dermal–epidermal junction (-100 μm) and $c_{de}|_{z=z_{ed}}$ denotes the solute concentration at this depth. Kretsos et al. (56) used this fact to deduce values of $(k_{de}/D_{de})^{1/2}$ and thence k_{de} from semi-log plots of measured dermal concentration profiles reported in the literature for a number of permeants in human and rat skin (Fig. 8). The conclusion of their analysis was to recommend the use of the equation

$$k_{de} = \frac{(k_{de})_{free}}{[0.68 + (0.32)/f_u + (0.001)f_{non}K_{o/w}]} \tag{12}$$

for both species. The denominator of equation (12) is the same binding factor that appears in equations (8) and (10), whereas the numerator is the intrinsic clearance, which is related to blood flow rate and capillary permeability. For small, moderately lipophilic permeants, clearance is likely to be blood flow limited and $(k_{de})_{free} \sim 22 \times 10^{-4}$ sec^{-1}. Kretsos et al. (56) offer remarks about how to generalize this result to allow for capillary permeability limitations on clearance, and Kretsos and Kasting (66) present an extensive review of general dermal capillary clearance. As written, equation (12) applies to free and bound solute; thus, k_{de} is the multiplier of the *total* concentration of solute in the dermis.

Treatment of the dermis as a vertically homogeneous effective continuum characterized by a single value of k_{de} is a simplification of the real situation. Indeed, one might reasonably expect the papillary (upper) dermis to be characterized by a larger value of k_{de} owing to the high concentration of permeable (absorbing) capillary loops there, and the reticular (lower) dermis to be characterized by a lower effective value. Equation (12) represents a collective average representation of both zones. Dancik (53) explicitly incorporated two distinct strata in his parametrization of dermal tissue around a hair follicle.

In principle, capillary transport processes could add a convective dispersion contribution to the effective value of D_{de}. For salicylic acid, Kretsos et al. (13) tentatively concluded that any such contribution seems to be minor, and that solute dispersion in the dermis occurs primarily by molecular diffusion, although further study of this point across a spectrum of permeants is clearly called for.

Viable Epidermis

The viable epidermis is a cellular epithelium sandwiched between the SC and dermis. Its thickness in humans varies between about 50 and 100 μm due to the articulated nature of the dermal–epidermal junction; a nominal thickness of 100 μm may be used for modeling purposes. Less is known about its effective transport properties than about those of the SC or dermis because it is difficult to isolate. Due to its cellular structure (comprising roughly cuboidal keratinocytes with primarily aqueous interiors within cellular membranes, surrounded by extracellular matrix and fluid), it presents a set of obstacles to solute diffusion inherently different than those of the dermis. Transport through it involves a combination of phenomena including: (*i*) hindered permeant diffusion within cytoplasm relative to bulk aqueous diffusion [cf. (67,68)], and permeant binding to cytoplasm [cf. (62,68)], which increases permeant holdup within keratinocytes and further decreases the cytoplasmic diffusivity; (*ii*) cell wall permeation by transbilayer mass transfer (cf. the mass transfer coefficient k_{trans} appearing in Fig. 2 and Table 1) in parallel with intercellular transfer through epidermal gap junctions (69); and (*iii*) diffusion in the interstitial space [cf. (70)], and permeant binding to interstitial plasma proteins [cf. (71,72)]. The precise role played by tight junctions in determining epidermal permeability (73,74) is an open question.

It is worth citing a selection (anecdotal, not exhaustive) of characterizations of viable epidermis. Among other results, Cross et al. (75) reported measured tissue/ buffer (pH 7.4) partition coefficients, approximately equivalent to $K_{ed/w}$, of 0.5 and 14.7 for ethanol and octanol, respectively. As stated by Bunge and Cleek (76), Tojo and Lee (77) reported an average epidermal diffusivity of 9.5×10^{-8} cm^2/sec for drugs with MWs lying between 170 and 490. In view of this result, Bunge and Cleek (76) suggested a hindrance factor of about one order of magnitude relative to bulk aqueous diffusion, as well as the rough estimate $D_{ed} = (7.1 \times 10^{-6}$ cm^2/sec)/(MW)$^{1/2}$. Khalil et al. (78) found the effective diffusivity of glucose in viable epidermis to be between one-eighth and one-two hundredth of the bulk aqueous diffusivity using a combination of desorption and permeability measurements.

Development of a microscopically well-grounded effective medium representation of the epidermis constitutes an important area for future work. It will benefit from more studies comparing the partitioning and permeability properties of isolated SC with those of epidermal membrane or full-thickness skin [cf. (41,75)], as well as experimental and theoretical experience with other cellular tissues (67–69).

Until this area becomes better developed, a reasonable pragmatic approach is to treat the viable epidermis as aqueous tissue roughly equivalent to dermis without any vascular clearance ($k_{ed}=0$) (14). Although it may actually present a greater mass transfer resistance than an equivalent layer of dermis, this approximation has minimal impact for systemic absorption because the resistance of the viable epidermis is low relative to that of the SC. However, it could lead to an underestimation of epidermal concentrations, which are important to the mechanistic understanding of skin sensitization thresholds (79).

PREDICTION OF DERMAL ABSORPTION

In the past, the viable epidermis and dermis have often been treated collectively as a homogeneous aqueous layer extending down as far as the superficial dermal capillaries ($z \sim -200$ µm), where a zero-concentration boundary condition is imposed, implying rapid and absolute clearance through the microcirculation in the upper dermis (23,24,76). This approach has proven to be adequate for many skin permeants (80) and certainly suffices to set upper bounds on solute flux. However, more detailed multilayer models as described here, explicitly representing transient diffusion and volumetrically distributed clearance within the dermis, are crucial in a number of applications. They include cases where strong penetration into deeper tissue occurs [e.g., trandermal drug delivery when the SC barrier has been seriously compromised by a penetration enhancer (81)], and where it is important to quantify actual subsurface concentration levels [e.g., contact sensitization thresholds (79)]. The diffusion framework and tissue parametrizations summarized here are directly useful for the requisite type of more detailed modeling.

   A number of authors (13,14,16–20) have offered good statements of the mathematical formulation and numerical solution of the diffusion problem yielding the solute concentration $c_\alpha(z,t)$ as a function of vertical position z and time t within one or more layers $\alpha =$ "sc," "ed," and "de." As an example of such a calculation, Figure 9 shows predicted levels of salicylic acid at various depths in rat skin applied from a finite dose.

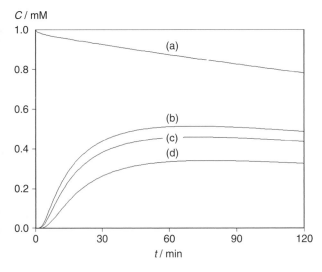

FIGURE 9   Predicted time evolution of concentrations in rat skin resulting from constant contact with a finite (3.9-mm thick) 1 mM dose starting at time $t=0$. The donor solution ("ve") has pH 3. Curves show (a) c_{ve}, (b) c_{ed} halfway into the epidermis, and c_{de} both (c) at and (d) 100 µm below the dermal–epidermal junction. *Source*: From Ref. 13.

Further development of this type of theory rests on progress in a number of areas. Numerical calculations are only as good in applications as the supporting parametrization of physicochemical properties ($K_{\alpha/w}$, D_α) of each tissue layer α. Need exists for more extensive experimental characterization of the partitioning and transport properties of the dermis and epidermis across a broad spectrum of permeants, and a framework of theory to correlate this information in analytical form. A very open area is the characterization of vehicle and/or penetrant effects on the permeability properties of the tissue layers through which the penetrant is diffusing. The transient permeability properties of hair follicles (and possibly also sweat glands) need to be studied by combining experiments isolating follicular penetration (82) with detailed diffusion models in order to characterize this penetration pathway. Many practical applications require extension of the macroscopic theory to cases where the vehicle and/or solute of interest are (is) volatile and evaporates from the surface of the skin. This generalization has been made by Kasting and coworkers (14,18,83) for the case where a single volatile compound evaporates from the surface. Extension of the analysis to multicomponent volatile mixtures applied to the skin represents an important avenue for future study.

ACKNOWLEDGMENTS

The authors gratefully acknowledge support from the U.S. National Institute for Occupational Safety and Health, the U.S. National Science Foundation, COLIPA, and the Procter & Gamble Company's International Program for Animal Alternatives for the development of many of the methods and results summarized here.

REFERENCES

1. Scheuplein RJ, Blank IH. Permeability of the skin. Physiol Rev 1971; 51(4):702–47.
2. Ritschel WA, Hussain AS. The principles of permeation of substances across the skin. Methods Find Exp Clin Pharmacol 1988; 10(1):39–56.
3. Roberts MS, Walters KA. Human skin morphology and dermal absorption. In: Roberts MS, Walters KA, eds. Dermal Absorption and Toxicity Assessment. 2nd ed. New York: Taylor & Francis, 2007.
4. Siddiqui O. Physicochemical, physiological, and mathematical considerations in optimizing percutaneous absorption of drugs. Crit Rev Ther Drug Carrier Syst 1989; 6(1):1–38.
5. Wiechers JW. The barrier function of the skin in relation to percutaneous absorption of drugs. Pharm Weekbl Sci 1989; 11(6):185–98.
6. Wester RC, Maibach HI. Percutaneous absorption of drugs. Clin Pharmacokinet 1992; 23(4):253–66.
7. Poet TS, McDougal JN. Skin absorption and human risk assessment. Chem Biol Interact 2002; 140(1):19–34.
8. Fitzpatrick D, Corish J, Hayes B. Modelling skin permeability in risk assessment—the future. Chemosphere 2004; 55(10):1309–14.
9. Riley WJ, McKone TE, Hubal EAC. Estimating contaminant dose for intermittent dermal contact: model development, testing, and application. Risk Anal 2004; 24(1):73–85.
10. Fitzpatrick D, Corish J. Modelling skin permeability in risk assessment. In: Roberts MS, Walters KA, eds. Dermal Absorption and Toxicity Assessment. 2nd ed. New York: Taylor & Francis, 2007.
11. Karande P, Jain A, Ergun K, et al. Design principles of chemical penetration enhancers for transdermal drug delivery. Proc Natl Acad Sci USA 2005; 102(13):4688–93.

12. Cross SE, Roberts MS. Physical enhancement of transdermal drug application: is delivery technology keeping up with pharmaceutical development? Curr Drug Deliv 2004; 1(1):81–92.
13. Kretsos K, Kasting GB, Nitsche JM. Distributed diffusion–clearance model for transient drug distribution within the skin. J Pharm Sci 2004; 93(11):2820–35.
14. Kasting GB, Miller MA, Nitsche JM. Absorption and evaporation of volatile compounds applied to skin. In: Walters KA, Roberts MS, eds. Dermatological and Cosmeceutical Development: Absorption, Efficacy and Toxicology. New York: Taylor & Francis, 2007.
15. Brenner H, Edwards DA. Macrotransport Processes. Boston: Butterworth-Heinemann, 1993.
16. Mueller B, Anissimov YG, Roberts MS. Unexpected clobetasol propionate profile in human stratum corneum after topical application in vitro. Pharm Res 2003; 20(11):1835–7.
17. Anissimov YG, Roberts MS. Diffusion modeling of percutaneous absorption kinetics: 3. Variable diffusion and partition coefficients, consequences for stratum corneum depth profiles and desorption kinetics. J Pharm Sci 2004; 93(2):470–87.
18. Kasting GB, Miller MA. Kinetics of finite dose absorption through skin 2: volatile compounds. J Pharm Sci 2006; 95(2):268–80.
19. Kasting GB. Kinetics of finite dose absorption through skin 1. Vanillylnonanamide. J Pharm Sci 2001; 90(2):202–12.
20. Anissimov YG, Roberts MS. Diffusion modeling of percutaneous absorption kinetics: 2. Finite vehicle volume and solvent deposited solids. J Pharm Sci 2001; 90(4):504–20.
21. Wang T-F, Kasting GB, Nitsche JM. A multiphase microscopic diffusion model for stratum corneum permeability. I. Formulation, solution, and illustrative results for representative compounds. J Pharm Sci 2006; 95(3):620–48.
22. Potts RO, Guy RH. Predicting skin permeability. Pharm Res 1992; 9(5):663–9.
23. Kasting GB, Smith RL, Anderson BD. Prodrugs for dermal delivery: solubility, molecular size, and functional group effects. In: Sloan KB, ed. Prodrugs: Topical and Ocular Drug Delivery. New York: Marcel Dekker, 1992:117–61.
24. Wilschut A, ten Berge WF, Robinson PJ, et al. Estimating skin permeation. The validation of five mathematical skin permeation models. Chemosphere 1995; 30(7):1275–96.
25. Buchwald P, Bodor N. A simple, predictive, structure-based skin permeability model. J Pharm Pharmacol 2001; 53(8):1087–98.
26. Flynn GL. Physicochemical determinants of skin absorption. In: Gerrity TR, Henry CJ, eds. Principles of Route-to-Route Extrapolation for Risk Assessment. New York: Elsevier, 1990:93–127.
27. Johnson ME, Blankschtein D, Langer R. Evaluation of solute permeation through the stratum corneum: lateral bilayer diffusion as the primary transport mechanism. J Pharm Sci 1997; 86(10):1162–72.
28. Yotsuyanagi T, Higuchi WI. A two phase series model for the transport of steroids across the fully hydrated stratum corneum. J Pharm Pharmacol 1972; 24:934–41.
29. Mitragotri S. A theoretical analysis of permeation of small hydrophobic solutes across the stratum corneum based on scaled particle theory. J Pharm Sci 2002; 91(3):744–52.
30. Frasch HF, Barbero AM. Steady-state flux and lag time in the stratum corneum lipid pathway: results from finite element models. J Pharm Sci 2003; 92(11):2196–207.
31. Tojo K. Random brick model for drug transport across stratum corneum. J Pharm Sci 1987; 76(12):889–91.
32. Heisig M, Lieckfeldt R, Wittum G, et al. Non steady-state descriptions of drug permeation through stratum corneum. I. The biphasic brick-and-mortar model. Pharm Res 1996; 13(3):421–6.
33. Charalambopoulou GCh, Karamertzanis P, Kikkinides ES, et al. A study on structural and diffusion properties of porcine stratum corneum based on very small angle neutron scattering data. Pharm Res 2000; 17(9):1085–91.
34. Frasch HF. A random walk model of skin permeation. Risk Anal 2002; 22(2):265–76.
35. Barbero AM, Frasch HF. Modeling of diffusion with partitioning in stratum corneum using a finite element model. Ann Biomed Eng 2005; 33(9):1281–92.

36. Barbero AM, Frasch HF. Transcellular route of diffusion through stratum corneum: results from finite element models. J Pharm Sci 2006; 95(10):2186–94.

37. Wang T-F, Kasting GB, Nitsche JM. A multiphase microscopic diffusion model for stratum corneum permeability. II. Estimation of physicochemical parameters, and application to a large permeability database. J Pharm Sci 2007; 96(11): 3024–51.

38. Kasting GB, Barai ND, Wang T-F, et al. Mobility of water in human stratum corneum. J Pharm Sci 2003; 92(11):2326–40.

39. Nitsche JM, Wang T-F, Kasting GB. A two-phase analysis of solute partitioning into the stratum corneum. J Pharm Sci 2006; 95(3):649–66.

40. Raykar PV, Fung M-C, Anderson BD. The role of protein and lipid domains in the uptake of solutes by human stratum corneum. Pharm Res 1988; 5(3):140–50.

41. Anderson BD, Higuchi WI, Raykar PV. Heterogeneity effects on permeability–partition coefficient relationships in human stratum corneum. Pharm Res 1988; 5(9):566–73.

42. Anderson BD, Raykar PV. Solute structure–permeability relationships in human stratum corneum. J Invest Dermatol 1989; 93(2):280–6.

43. Nemes Z, Steinert PM. Bricks and mortar of the epidermal barrier. Exp Mol Med 1999; 31(1):5–19.

44. Yu B, Kim KH, So PTC, et al. Visualization of oleic acid-induced transdermal diffusion pathways using two-photon fluorescence miscroscopy. J Invest Dermatol 2003; 120(3): 448–55.

45. Hanson KM, Behne MJ, Barry NP, et al. Two-photon fluorescence lifetime imaging of the skin stratum corneum pH gradient. Biophys J 2002; 83(3):1682–90.

46. Peck KD, Ghanem A-H, Higuchi WI. Hindered diffusion of polar molecules through and effective pore radii estimates of intact and ethanol treated human epidermal membrane. Pharm Res 1994; 11(9):1306–14.

47. Peck KD, Ghanem A-H, Higuchi WI. The effect of temperature upon the permeation of polar and ionic solutes through human epidermal membrane. J Pharm Sci 1995; 84(8):975–82.

48. Tang H, Mitragotri S, Blankschtein D, et al. Theoretical description of transdermal transport of hydrophilic permeants: application to low-frequency sonophoresis. J Pharm Sci 2001; 90(5):545–68.

49. Mitragotri S. Modeling skin permeability to hydrophilic and hydrophobic solutes based on four permeation pathways. J Control Release 2003; 86(1):69–92.

50. Scheuplein RJ. Mechanism of percutaneous absorption II. Transient diffusion and the relative importance of various routes of skin penetration. J Invest Dermatol 1967; 48(1):79–88.

51. Jackson RJ, Davis WB. A mathematical approach to the prediction of the rate of penetration of ions in the sweat duct. J Theor Biol 1982; 97(3):481–9.

52. Ho CK. Probabilistic modeling of percutaneous absorption for risk-based exposure assessments and transdermal drug delivery. Stat Methodol 2004; 1(1–2):47–69.

53. Dancik YH. Mathematical models of diffusion through and near skin appendages: hair follicle and eccrine sweat gland pathways. Ph.D. thesis, University at Buffalo, State University of New York, 2007.

54. Bert JL, Mathieson JM, Pearce RH. The exclusion of human serum albumin by human dermal collagenous fibres and within human dermis. Biochem J 1982; 201(2):395–403.

55. Bert JL, Pearce RH, Mathieson JM. Concentration of plasma albumin in its accessible space in postmortem human dermis. Microvasc Res 1986; 32(2):211–23.

56. Kretsos K, Miller MA, Zamora-Estrada G, et al. Partitioning, diffusivity and clearance of skin permeants in mammalian dermis. Int J Pharmaceut 2007; in press.

57. Yamazaki K, Kanaoka M. Computational prediction of the plasma protein-binding percent of diverse pharmaceutical compounds. J Pharm Sci 2004; 93(6):1480–94.

58. Pearce RH, Grimmer BJ. Age and the chemical constitution of normal human dermis. J Invest Dermatol 1972; 58(6):347–61.

59. Wilke CR, Chang P. Correlation of diffusion coefficients in dilute solutions. Am Inst Chem Eng J 1955; 1(2):264–70.

60. Poling BE, Prausnitz JM, O'Connell JP. The Properties of Gases and Liquids. 5th ed. New York: McGraw-Hill, 2001.

61. Cussler EL. Diffusion: Mass Transfer in Fluid Systems. New York: Cambridge University Press, 1997:32–4.
62. Horowitz SB, Fenichel IR, Hoffman B, et al. The intracellular transport and distribution of cysteamine phosphate derivatives. Biophys J 1970; 10(10):994–1010.
63. Gupta E, Wientjes MG, Au JL-S. Penetration kinetics of 2'-3'-dideoxyinosine in dermis is described by the distributed model. Pharm Res 1995; 12(1):108–12.
64. Zesch A, Schaefer H. Penetrationskinetik von radiomarkiertem hydrocortison aus verschiedenartigen salbengrundlagen in die menschliche haut. Arch Dermatol Res 1975; 252(4):245–56.
65. Gao X, Wientjes MG, Au JL-S. Use of drug kinetics in dermis to predict in vivo blood concentration after topical application. Pharm Res 1995; 12(12):2012–7.
66. Kretsos K, Kasting GB. Dermal capillary clearance: physiology and modeling. Skin Pharmacol Physiol 2005; 18(2):55–74.
67. Mastro AM, Keith AD. Diffusion in the aqueous compartment. J Cell Biol 1984; 99:180s–7s.
68. Nitsche JM. Cellular microtransport processes: intercellular, intracellular, and aggregate behavior. Annu Rev Biomed Eng 1999; 1:463–503.
69. Safranyos RGA, Caveney S, Miller JG, et al. Relative roles of gap junction channels and cytoplasm in cell-to-cell diffusion of fluorescent tracers. Proc Natl Acad Sci USA 1987; 84:2272–6.
70. Schultz JS, Armstrong W. Permeability of interstitial space of muscle (rat diaphragm) to solutes of different molecular weights. J Pharm Sci 1978; 67(5):696–700.
71. Rossing N, Worm A-M. Interstitial fluid: exchange of macromolecules between plasma and skin interstitium. Clin Physiol 1981; 1(3):275–84.
72. Aukland K, Reed RK. Interstitial-lymphatic mechanisms in the control of extracellular fluid volume. Physiol Rev 1993; 73(1):1–78.
73. Furuse M, Hata M, Furuse K, et al. Claudin-based tight junctions are crucial for the mammalian epidermal barrier: a lesson from claudin-1-deficient mice. J Cell Biol 2002; 156(6):1099–111.
74. Bazzoni G, Dejana E. Keratinocyte junctions and the epidermal barrier: how to make a skin-tight dress. J Cell Biol 2002; 156(6):947–9.
75. Cross S, Magnusson BM, Winckle G, et al. Determination of the effect of lipophilicity on the in vitro permeability and tissue reservoir characteristics of topically applied solutes in human skin layers. J Invest Dermatol 2003; 120(5):759–64.
76. Bunge AL, Cleek RL. A new method for estimating dermal absorption from chemical exposure: 2. Effect of molecular weight and octanol–water partitioning. Pharm Res 1995; 12(1):88–95.
77. Tojo K, Lee ARC. Penetration and bioconversion of drugs in the skin. J Chem Eng Jpn 1991; 24(3):297–301.
78. Khalil E, Kosmas K, Kasting GB. Glucose partition coefficient and diffusivity in the lower skin layers. Pharm Res 2006; 23(6):1227–34.
79. Kimber I, Gerberick GF, Basketter DA. Thresholds in contact sensitization: theoretical and practical considerations. Food Chem Toxicol 1999; 37(5):553–60.
80. Scheuplein RJ, Bronaugh RL. Percutaneous absorption. In: Goldsmith LA, ed. Biochemistry and Physiology of the Skin. Vol. 2. New York: Oxford University Press, 1983:1255–95.
81. Bauerova K, Matušová D, Kassai Z. Chemical enhancers for transdermal drug transport. Eur J Drug Metab Pharmacokinet 2001; 26(1–2):85–94.
82. Teichmann A, Otberg N, Jacobi U, et al. Follicular penetration: development of a method to block the follicles selectively against the penetration of topically applied substances. Skin Pharmacol Physiol 2006; 19(4):216–23.
83. Miller MA, Bhatt V, Kasting GB. Dose and air flow dependence of benzyl alcohol disposition on skin. J Pharm Sci 2006; 95(2):281–91.

Mathematical Models for Different Exposure Conditions

Yuri G. Anissimov

School of Biomolecular and Physical Sciences, Griffith University, Nathan, Queensland, Australia

INTRODUCTION

The objective of any mathematical model describing dermal absorption is to represent the processes associated with solute partitioning into and penetration through stratum corneum (SC) accurately, model various experimental data and predict outcomes under varying conditions or, in the context of this chapter, under different exposure scenarios. As mathematical modelling in percutaneous absorption has been described in some detail in Ref. 1, we have concentrated here on elaborating the mathematical approach presented in Ref. 1 to account for different exposure scenarios (Fig. 1). In mathematical modelling, some solutions often suffer from being too complex to be practically useful; therefore, in this work we give priority to simple approximations and consider simplifying assumptions. Solutions in the time domain are presented only when they could be expressed in a simple form. The emphasis in this chapter is on using Laplace domain solutions, which often are presented in simple closed form (no infinite series involved) and allow derivation of equations for some important model outcomes (e.g., total amount of solute absorbed, amount absorbed over long periods of time). The attractiveness of Laplace domain solutions is enhanced by the existence of standard nonlinear regression programs such as MULTI FILT, MINIM, and SCIENTIST, which enable fast analysis of experimental data using Laplace domain solutions directly, and avoid computational complexities associated with infinite series solutions, especially those involving solving transcendental equations. For a complex exposure scenario, analytical solutions, even in the Laplace domain, are often nonattainable or far too complex. In order to deal with such situations, in this chapter we outline a simple numerical approach to computationally model these complex exposure conditions.

DIFFUSION EQUATION

Transport of solutes in the skin is most often modelled by the diffusion equation:

$$\frac{\partial C_m}{\partial t} = D_m \frac{\partial^2 C_m}{\partial x^2} \tag{1}$$

where $C_m(x,t)$ is the concentration in the SC (also referred in this chapter as the membrane) at depth x and time t, and D_m is the diffusion coefficient in the membrane. Equation (1) is generally unaffected by exposure conditions, which are described by the appropriate choice of boundary and initial conditions.

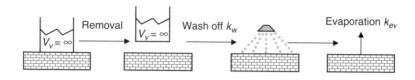

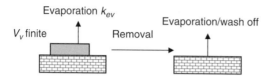

FIGURE 1 Diagrammatic overview of different exposure scenarios.

An initial condition for equation (1) describes concentration in the SC at $t=0$: $C_m(x,0)=C_{t=0}(x)$, where $C_{t=0}(x)$ is the concentration of solute in the membrane at the beginning of exposure (or experiment). For most practical cases, there is no solute present in the membrane in the beginning and the initial condition becomes:

$$C_m(x,0) = 0 \qquad (2)$$

It is the boundary conditions for equation (1) that generate a multitude of solutions to equation (1) when applied to SC solute transport. Usually, two boundary conditions at $x=0$ (outer surface of the SC, which is in contact with the atmosphere or donor compartment) and $x=h_m$ [inner surface of the SC, which is in contact with the viable epidermis (VE) or receptor compartment] are used. In this chapter we will normally consider the simple sink condition for $x=0$:

$$C_m(h_m,t) = 0 \qquad (3)$$

This boundary condition describes very rapid removal of solute from the inner surface of the SC by fast diffusion through the VE and absorption of the solute by blood in the dermis or by a large well stirred receptor compartment. This very rapid removal adequately describes transport kinetics for many solutes and experimental and physiological conditions. The simple boundary condition 3 could be invalid, for example, in the case of a very low solubility of a solute in VE or receptor compartment; these situations are described in detail in Refs. 2 and 3 and are not covered here. As the inner surface boundary condition is unaffected by the exposure scenario, in this chapter we mostly deal with an appropriate choice of the outer surface boundary condition for different exposure conditions.

While in this chapter equation (1) is assumed to adequately model transport of solutes in the SC, it is important to recognize limitations of this equation. It is implicitly assumed in the use of this equation that the SC is described as a homogenous membrane with constant diffusion and partition coefficients. We have recently demonstrated that this assumption is invalid for clobetasol propionate (4) and developed a mathematical approach for the case of spatially variable diffusion and partitioning coefficients (5). As SC permeability is strongly influenced by its water content (6), which could be time dependent, especially in complex exposure scenarios, both diffusion and partitioning coefficients could also be time dependent. While incorporating these complexities coupled with different exposure conditions in an analytical approach is too complex, we will outline a modification of a proposed numerical model due to variable diffusion and partitioning coefficients. Even when diffusion and partitioning coefficients could be assumed constant throughout the SC and in time, the multi-phase nature of the SC, often represented as a brick (corneocytes) and mortar (lipid) model, renders equation (1) at best just a reasonable approximation to solute transport in the SC. This approximate nature of the diffusion equation must be recognized when mathematically modelling SC transport, and especially when developing an appropriate computational model.

SIMPLE EXPOSURE CONDITIONS

By simple exposure conditions, here we mean exposure conditions that do not include washing off or evaporation of the applied solute and result in relatively simple solutions to equation (1) in the Laplace domain. We do not discuss here mathematical complications due to the existence of an unstirred layer in the donor, saturation in the receptor phase, and rate limited transport through the VE into the systemic circulation. Solutions and analysis under these complications can be found in Refs. 2 and 3.

Large Donor Applied for Long Exposure Times
This is the simplest case, commonly encountered in in vitro dermal absorption experiments. Long exposure time here means that the time of dermal exposure (t_{ex}) to solute is greater than at least 3 lag times (lag):

$$t_{ex} \geq 3 \, \text{lag} = \frac{h_m^2}{2D_m} = \frac{t_d}{2} \tag{4}$$

where $t_d(=h_m^2/D_m)$ is the characteristic time of diffusion. The condition of large donor simply represents cases when depletion of the concentration in the donor (vehicle) could be neglected (often referred to as infinite donor), together with the donor being well mixed (fast diffusion or mixing in the vehicle). The outer surface boundary condition in this case is:

$$C_m(0,t) = K_m C_v, \tag{5}$$

where K_m is the dimensionless partition coefficient between the membrane and vehicle, and C_v is the concentration of solute in the vehicle. In the Laplace domain, the solution to equation (1), with initial condition 2, and boundary conditions 3 and 5, is:

$$\hat{C}_m(x,s) = \frac{K_m C_v}{s} \frac{\sinh\left(\sqrt{st_d}(h_m - x)/h_m\right)}{\sinh\left(\sqrt{st_d}\right)} \tag{6}$$

where a circumflex over a function ($\wedge$) denotes the Laplace transform, and s is the Laplace variable. Equation (6) is similar (with different notations and boundary conditions for $x=0$ and $x=h_m$ interchanged) to that presented by Carslaw and Jaeger (7) for the case of heat conduction in solids. The total amount of solute absorbed through the inner surface (Q), which represents systemic absorption of the solute, can be obtained from equation (6) (1):

$$\hat{Q}(s) = -D_m A \frac{1}{s} \frac{\partial \hat{C}_m}{\partial x}\bigg|_{x=h_m} = \frac{K_m D_m A C_v}{h_m s^2} \frac{\sqrt{st_d}}{\sinh\left(\sqrt{st_d}\right)} = \frac{k_p A C_v}{s^2} \frac{\sqrt{st_d}}{\sinh\left(\sqrt{st_d}\right)} \tag{7}$$

where A is an area of exposure to the solute, and $k_p = K_m D_m / h_m$ is the permeability coefficient.

At long exposure times (practically at $t \geq 3$ lag) the analysis of singularities of equation (7) at $s=0$ yields:

$$Q(t) = k_p A C_v (t - \text{lag}) \tag{8}$$

This equation could be used to estimate systemic absorption of solute for the case of large donor and long exposure time ($t \geq 3$ lag $= 0.5 t_d$).

Inversion of equation (7) to the time domain yields infinite series solutions for small ($t \ll t_d$) and large ($t \gg t_d$) times (see for example Ref. 7). We feel that the Laplace domain solution is often more practical than these infinite series solutions, although, using only the first terms in these series solutions a relatively simple closed form solution for $Q(t)$ could be constructed:

$$Q(t) = \begin{cases} k_p A C_v 4 \sqrt{t t_d} \, \text{ierfc}\left(\dfrac{1}{2}\sqrt{\dfrac{t_d}{t}}\right), & t \leq 4.5 t_d \\[4mm] k_p A C_v \left(t - \dfrac{t_d}{6} + \dfrac{2 t_d}{\pi^2}\exp\left(-\dfrac{\pi^2 t}{t_d}\right)\right), & t > 4.5 t_d \end{cases} \tag{9}$$

where

$$\text{ierfc}(x) = \int_x^\infty \text{erfc}(\xi)\,d\xi = \frac{e^{-x^2}}{\sqrt{\pi}} - x\,\text{erfc}(x)$$

$\text{erfc}(x)$ is the complementary error function $[=1-\text{erf}(x)$, where $\text{erf}(x)$ is the error function]. Equation (9) approximates $Q(t)$ with an error of less than 0.16% over an entire range of times and could therefore be considered a precise solution for most practical purposes.

From a practical point of view, any exposure will eventually be terminated. If, at this time of termination, the concentration in the membrane has achieved steady state, that is:

$$C_{ss}(x) = C_m(x, t \to \infty) = \lim_{s \to 0} s\hat{C}_m(x,s) = K_m C_v \frac{(h_m - x)}{h_m} \tag{10}$$

the amount absorbed into the systemic circulation across the skin from the time the dosage form is removed (t_{rem}) could be derived by solving equation (1) with the initial condition:

$$C_m(x,0) = C_{ss}(x) \tag{11}$$

boundary condition 3, and boundary condition describing no solute flux ($J_m(x,t)$) at the outer boundary:

$$J_m(x,t)\Big|_{x=0} = -D_m \frac{\partial}{\partial x} C_m(x,t)\Big|_{x=0} = 0 \tag{12}$$

This solution yields (1):

$$\hat{Q}(s) = \frac{M_\infty}{s^2} \frac{2}{t_d}\left(1 - \frac{1}{\cosh\left(\sqrt{st_d}\right)}\right) \tag{13}$$

where $M_\infty = K_m C_v A h_m / 2 = k_p A C_v t_d / 2$ is the amount of solute present in the skin before removal of the vehicle. Of interest to toxicity assessment is the total amount of solute absorbed, which can be calculated as that absorbed until the time of vehicle removal [equation (8)] plus any solute remaining in the SC at this time:

$$Q_{tot} = M_\infty + k_p A C_v(t_{rem} - \text{lag}) = k_p A C_v(t_{rem} + t_d/3) \qquad (14)$$

Here, and in what follows, mostly equations describing the amount of solute absorbed (Q) are presented. Another important measure of transdermal penetration is the flux of solute (J) through the inner surface of the SC [$J(t) = J_m(t, h_m)$], which could be easily obtained from Q using:

$$J(t) = \frac{1}{A} \frac{d}{dt} Q(t) \qquad (15)$$

or in Laplace domain:

$$\hat{J}(s) = \frac{s}{A} \hat{Q}(s) \qquad (16)$$

Equations (15) and (16) could also be used to express Q if J is defined.

The following is a discussion of another important case arising when donor depletion is not negligible.

Finite Donor Exposure

Two conditions need to be considered in this case: (*i*) whether the donor volume (or rather the capacity for the solute) is still large enough for concentration in the donor to change slowly as compared to the characteristic time of diffusion (t_d); and (*ii*) whether the donor capacity for the solute is comparable to that of skin. Let us first introduce a dimensionless number which represents the ratio of the donor capacity for the solute to that of SC: V_{vN}, to which we will refer as the vehicle volume number. V_{vN} is the dimensionless parameter denoting the relative volume of the donor phase:

$$V_{vN} = \frac{V_v S_v}{V_m S_m} = \frac{V_v}{V_m K_m} \qquad (17)$$

where V_v is the finite volume of the donor, V_m ($= A h_m$) is the volume of the membrane, and S_v and S_m are solubilities of the solute in the vehicle and the membrane, respectively (a simple case of linear relationship between concentration and chemical activity is assumed in equation (17), so that $K_m = S_m/S_v$). Using the vehicle volume number, the first case represents the situation when $V_{vN} \gg 1$, and the second when this condition is not satisfied.

For the first case ($V_{vN} \gg 1$), equations derived for the infinite donor could still be used, but the constant concentration (C_v) has to be replaced with $C_v(t)$, a slow changing function of time. This function could be derived from mass balance in the donor:

$$V_v \frac{dC_v(t)}{dt} = A D_m \frac{\partial C_m(x, t)}{\partial x} \bigg|_{x=0} \qquad (18)$$

As the onset of the steady state is quick compared with the change in concentration in the vehicle, $C_m(x,t)$ in 18 could be replaced with its steady state value [equation (11)], which yields, after some algebra:

$$\frac{dC_v(t)}{dt} = -\frac{1}{V_{vN} t_d} C_v(t) \qquad (19)$$

This equation is readily solvable:

$$C_v(t) = C_{v0}\exp\left(-\frac{t}{V_{vN}t_d}\right) \tag{20}$$

where C_{v0} is the initial concentration in the vehicle. The total amount systemically absorbed therefore will be described at long times $(t \geq t_d/2)$ by:

$$Q(t) = k_p A C_{v0}\exp\left(-\frac{t}{V_{vN}t_d}\right)(t-\text{lag}) \tag{21}$$

For shorter times $(t \leq t_d/2 \ll V_{vN}t_d)$, depletion of solute in the vehicle is negligible, and equation (7) should be used, with C_v replaced by C_{v0}.

The second case $(V_{vN} \sim 1)$ was mathematically described in some detail in Refs. 3 and 8. As for the first case, the boundary condition at the outer surface of the SC should reflect the depletion of donor concentration [equation (18)] together with:

$$C_m(0, t) = K_m C_v(t) \tag{22}$$

These boundary conditions assume a well stirred donor or a situation where diffusion in the vehicle is much faster than diffusion in the SC. Solutions for the case when diffusion in the vehicle is rate limiting are presented in Ref. 9 and more recently discussed in Ref. 1. Solving equation (1) with initial condition 2 and boundary conditions 3, 18, and 22 in Laplace domain yields (3):

$$\hat{Q}(s) = \frac{k_p A C_{v0}}{s^2} \frac{V_{vN}st_d}{\cosh\sqrt{st_d} + V_{vN}\sqrt{st_d}\sinh\sqrt{st_d}}$$

$$= \frac{\text{dose}}{s} \frac{1}{\cosh\sqrt{st_d} + V_{vN}\sqrt{st_d}\sinh\sqrt{st_d}} \tag{23}$$

where dose $(= V_v C_{v0})$ is the total amount of solute applied [it could be seen from equation (23) that: $\lim_{t\to\infty} Q(t) = \lim_{s\to 0} s\hat{Q}(s) = \text{dose}$, so that the total amount of solute absorbed equals the dose applied, which is expected from the conservation of mass principle]. For finite dose applications, the flux of solute is a more important descriptor of the process; therefore, in what follows, we present equations for flux. The approximation of $J(t)$ for short times (practically for $t \leq t_d/2$) can be derived based on equations (23) and (16) (3):

$$J(t) = \frac{\text{dose}}{At_d} f\left(\frac{t}{t_d}, \frac{1}{V_{vN}}\right) \tag{24}$$

where

$$f(\tau, x) = 2x\left[\frac{1}{\sqrt{\pi\tau}}\exp\left(-\frac{1}{4\tau}\right) - x\exp(x^2\tau + x)\text{erfc}\left(x\sqrt{\tau} + \frac{1}{2\sqrt{\tau}}\right)\right] \tag{25}$$

At long times [practically for $t \geq \max(2t_d, 2V_{vN}t_d)$], the approximation of $J(t)$ is (3):

$$J(t) \approx \frac{\text{dose}}{At_d} \frac{2\alpha_1\exp\left(-\alpha_1^2(t/t_d)\right)}{(1 + V_{vN})\sin\alpha_1 + \alpha_1\cos\alpha_1} \tag{26}$$

where α_1 is the smallest positive root of equation $\alpha \tan \alpha = 1/V_{vN}$, which could be approximated by:

$$\alpha_1 \approx \arctan\left(\frac{\sqrt{V_{vN}}}{V_{vN} + \frac{2}{\pi}\sqrt{V_{vN}} + 0.26} + \frac{2}{\pi V_{vN}}\right) \tag{27}$$

Therefore, a log flux versus time profile at long times is linear with a slope of $k = -\alpha_1^2/t_d$ Hence, the terminal half life, $t_{1/2}$ of $J(t)$, in this case is given by: $t_{1/2} = \ln 2/(-k) \approx 0.693 t_d/\alpha_1^2$.

Two important parameters for the analysis of the case of finite donor exposure are the time to reach peak flux (t_{max}) and the maximum flux (J_{max}). These parameters and could be expressed as (3):

$$t_{max} \approx \frac{t_d}{6}\left[1 + \frac{2V_{vN}}{1 + V_{vN}}\right] \tag{28}$$

$$J_{max} \approx \frac{dose}{At_d}f\left(\frac{3V_{vN} + 1}{6(1 + V_{vN})}, \frac{1}{V_{vN}}\right) \tag{29}$$

where $f(\tau,x)$ is defined in equation (25). It is important to note the approximate nature of equations (28) and (29). The expression for t_{max} [equation (28)] has a maximum relative error of less than 6% relative to numerically computed values (3).

Solvent Deposited Solids

An important limiting case of finite donor exposure is solvent deposited solids. In addition to being solvent deposited, the solid must also be absorbed by the SC quickly ($t_{abs} \ll lag$), i.e., the volume of the applied solvent must be sufficiently small, so that $V_{vN} \ll 1$. Although the process of solvent evaporation and underlying change in the concentration of the solid is complex, if both conditions ($t_{abs} \ll lag$, $V_{vN} \ll 1$) are satisfied, the equation for the amount of solid absorbed systemically could be obtained by taking the limit $V_{vN} \rightarrow 0$ in equation (23):

$$\hat{Q}(s) = \frac{dose}{s}\frac{1}{\cosh\sqrt{st_d}} \tag{30}$$

where dose is the dose of solid applied. This equation was first derived in the context of skin absorption by Scheuplein and Ross (10). The approximation of $J(t)$ for short times (practically for $t \leq t_d/2$) could be derived by taking the limit of $V_{vN} \rightarrow 0$ in equation (24):

$$J(t) = \frac{dose}{At_d}\frac{1}{\sqrt{\pi(t/t_d)^3}}\exp\left(-\frac{t_d}{4t}\right) \tag{31}$$

Similarly for long times ($t \geq 2t_d$), taking the limit of $V_{vN} \rightarrow 0$ (which results in $\alpha_1 \rightarrow \pi/2$) in equation (26) yields:

$$J(t) \approx \frac{dose}{At_d}\pi\exp\left(-\frac{\pi^2 t}{4t_d}\right) \tag{32}$$

The time to reach peak flux and the maximum flux for solvent deposited solids could be expressed by taking the limit of $V_{vN} \rightarrow 0$ in equations (28) and (29) (3):

$$t_{max} = \frac{t_d}{6} \tag{33}$$

$$J_{max} = \frac{dose}{At_d} \exp\left(-\frac{3}{2}\right) 6\sqrt{\frac{6}{\pi}} \approx 1.850 \frac{dose}{At_d} \tag{34}$$

EXPOSURES WITH WASH OFF/EVAPORATION
General Approach

A dermal exposure involving wash off and evaporation of both solute and solvent leads to complex time-dependent boundary conditions at $x=0$, with an analytical approach possible only for limited and relatively simple cases. Boundary conditions for evaporation were recently considered in some detail by Kasting and Miller (11), with extensive theoretical considerations and appropriate solutions (numerical and analytical), but, as they noted, "small quantities of volatile chemicals contact the skin many times daily, yet surprisingly little is known about their eventual disposition" and, therefore, more experimental and theoretical work is required in this area. We will formulate the boundary conditions at $x=0$ for a more general exposure scenario (which also includes wash off) and then outline analytical solutions for simpler cases. We note that, for more complex exposures, a numerical solution is usually the only practical approach.

Equation (35) describes the mass balance of solute in the vehicle:

$$\frac{dM_v}{dt} = \frac{d(V_v(t)C_v(t))}{dt} = AD_m\frac{\partial C_m}{\partial x}\bigg|_{x=0} - k_{ev}C_v(t) \tag{35}$$

where M_v is the amount of solute in the vehicle, and k_{ev} is the rate of evaporation of the solute (dimension=volume/time) which depends on surface area of evaporation, solubility of the solute in the vehicle, its vapour pressure, its diffusion coefficient in the air, and the thickness of the unstirred air layer above the vehicle (for more discussion of this coefficient see Refs. 11–13). Equation (22) completes the boundary condition at $x=0$. In equation (35), the volume of the donor ($V_v(t)$) is a function of time due to evaporation of solvent and solute and, in a most general case, is some function of $M_v(t)$ and the amount of solvent in the donor $M_{vs}(t)$: $V_v(t)=f(M_v(t),M_{vs}(t))$. When the concentration of solvent in the vehicle [$C_{vs}(t)$] is much greater than that of the solute ($C_{vs}\gg C_v$) the volume of the donor could be expressed as:

$$V_v(t) = \frac{M_{vs}(t)}{\rho_s} \tag{36}$$

where ρ_s is the density of the solvent, which, for composite solvents, could also be a function of time. If the vehicle is a simple single compound solvent, and $C_{vs}\gg C_v$, the evaporation of the solvent will lead to linear reduction of the vehicle volume:

$$V_v(t) = V_{v0} - k_{evs}t \tag{37}$$

where V_{v0} is the volume of the vehicle at zero time, and k_{evs} is the rate of evaporation of the solvent, which depends on solvent vapour pressure (and therefore on temperature), solvent diffusion coefficient in the air, and the thickness of the unstirred air layer above the vehicle. Equation (37) is only sensible when $V_v(t)>0$ ($t<V_{v0}/k_{evs}$), and care must be taken that the condition $C_{vs}\gg C_v$ is

applicable at all times. This condition could be especially problematic to satisfy when the volume becomes very small ($V_v(t)$ close to zero), as for the case of solvent deposited solids. It is possible that, due to solvent evaporation, the concentration of solute in the donor will increase in time if solute absorption into the skin and evaporation is relatively slow. In this case, an important consideration is the solubility of the solute in the solvent and whether this will result in supersaturated solution (which is not uncommon in transdermal drug delivery formulations Refs. 14–16) or the solute will crystallise into a separate phase. In the latter case, $C_v(t)$ in equation (35) has to be replaced with the solubility of the solute in the vehicle ($C_v(t) = S_v$).

When after some exposure the vehicle is removed, the boundary condition for times after removal ($t > t_{rem}$) will most generally be described by:

$$AD_m\frac{\partial C_m}{\partial x}\bigg|_{x=0} = k_{ev}C_m(0, t)/K_m \tag{38}$$

In the limit of very fast evaporation rate (relatively large k_{ev}), equation (38) has to be replaced by:

$$C_m(0, t) = 0 \tag{39}$$

and for negligible or no evaporation ($k_{ev} \approx 0$) we have:

$$\frac{\partial C_m}{\partial x}\bigg|_{x=0} = 0 \tag{40}$$

When vehicle removal is followed by a washing off of the applied donor, this process has to be reflected in the boundary condition at $x=0$. As with the simple vehicle removal, the process of the washing off could be described by equation (38), with the rate of evaporation (k_{ev}) replaced with the rate of wash off (k_w). This rate will be related to the solubility of the solute in the wash-off solution, its diffusion coefficient in the wash-off solution, and the thickness of the unstirred layer in the wash-off solution. The latter will be determined by the extent of stirring/agitation of the wash-off phase (the more energetic the stirring the thinner will be the unstirred layer which leads to larger k_w). In most practical cases, a wash-off process is designed to maximise the rate of wash off of the solute (for example by selecting the wash-off solution with very high solubility of the solute, or/and by very vigorous agitation during wash off), in this case, k_w could be assumed to be very large, and the washing off will be described by equation (39). After the wash-off period, the boundary conditions at $x=0$ will again be described by equation (38).

Similar to the consideration of finite vehicle volume [equations (17)–(29)], two cases could be considered for the general case of exposure with evaporation of solvent/solute in the vehicle: (*i*) the donor volume number is still large enough throughout the exposure for the concentration in the donor to change slowly as compared to the characteristic time of diffusion (t_d); (*ii*) the donor capacity for the solute is comparable to that of skin, or evaporation of solute/solvent leads to rapid change in the donor concentration, rendering the fist condition invalid. For the first case, the total amount systemically absorbed will be described at long times ($t \geq t_d/2$) by:

$$Q(t) = k_pAC_v(t)(t - \text{lag}) \tag{41}$$

where in a general case $C_v(t)$ will be determined by equation (35). If the variable volume could be represented by equation (37), solving equation (35) yields for $C_v(t)$:

$$C_v(t) = \exp\left[\left(\frac{k_pA + k_{ev}}{k_{evs}} - 1\right)\ln\left(1 - \frac{k_{evs}t}{V_{v0}}\right)\right] \tag{42}$$

For shorter times $(t \leq t_d/2 \ll V_{v0N}t_d)$, depletion of solute in the vehicle is negligible, and equation (7) should be used to determine Q, with C_v replaced by C_{v0}. For the second case, only limited exposure scenarios will be considered analytically in what follows, with numerical analysis being the main approach.

Solute Evaporation

Let us consider the case when only solute evaporates from the finite volume donor phase and there is no change in the donor volume. A similar problem was recently formulated and solved numerically by Kasting and Miller (11). Here we solve this problem in the Laplace domain using notations consistent within this chapter. The boundary conditions at $x=0$ are:

$$V_v\frac{dC_v(t)}{dt} = AD_m\frac{\partial C_m}{\partial x}\bigg|_{x=0} - k_{ev}C_v(t) \tag{43}$$

$$C_m(0,t) = K_m C_v(t), \tag{44}$$

Solving equation (1) with boundary conditions 43, 44, 3, and initial condition 2 in the Laplace domain (similar to solution presented in Ref. 3) yields for the amount absorbed:

$$\hat{Q}(s) = \frac{k_pAC_{v0}V_{vN}t_d}{s\left(\cosh\sqrt{st_d} + \frac{V_{vN}st_d + \kappa_{ev}}{\sqrt{st_d}}\sinh\sqrt{st_d}\right)}$$

$$= \frac{\text{dose}}{s\left(\cosh\sqrt{st_d} + \frac{V_{vN}st_d + \kappa_{ev}}{\sqrt{st_d}}\sinh\sqrt{st_d}\right)} \tag{45}$$

where κ_{ev} is the dimensionless parameter describing the ratio of the rate of evaporation to the rate of absorption:

$$\kappa_{ev} = \frac{k_{ev}}{Ak_p} \tag{46}$$

Using equation (45), the total amount of solute absorbed (Q_∞) can be found:

$$Q_\infty = \lim_{t\to\infty}Q(t) = \lim_{s\to 0}s\hat{Q}(s) = \frac{\text{dose}}{1 + \kappa_{ev}} \tag{47}$$

This equation makes intuitive sense: the total amount absorbed reduces as the rate of evaporation increases relative to the rate of absorption. We note that equation (47) is similar to equation (33) from Ref. 11, with $\kappa_{ev} \leftrightarrow \chi$. The total amount evaporated will be:

$$Q_{ev} = \text{dose} - Q_\infty = \text{dose}\frac{\kappa_{ev}}{1 + \kappa_{ev}} \tag{48}$$

If the rate of evaporation (k_{ev}) is known (for example, using experimental results from evaporation from a non-absorbing surface), and the total amount evaporated is determined from the skin exposure experiment, κ_{ev} could be determined from equation (48) and then, using equation (46), k_p could be determined. This approach is suitable for determining skin permeability in vivo.

For solvent deposited solids/solutes ($t_{abs} \ll \text{lag}$, $V_{vN} \ll 1$) the amount of compound absorbed systemically, when evaporation takes place, could be obtained by taking the limit $V_{vN} \to 0$ in equation (45):

$$\hat{Q}(s) = \frac{\text{dose}}{s\left(\cosh\sqrt{st_d} + (\kappa_{ev}/\sqrt{st_d})\sinh\sqrt{st_d}\right)} \tag{49}$$

The total amount of solute absorbed (Q_∞) and evaporated (Q_{ev}) in this case are still described by equations (47) and (48).

Brief Exposure

Another analytically solvable case is when the duration of exposure to the vehicle is very short compared to the lag time ($t_{ex} \ll \text{lag} = t_d/6$). In this case, after the vehicle is removed, most solute will be distributed only very closely to the surface of the SC. It could be demonstrated that the solution for this brief exposure is identical to that of the solvent-deposited solids [equation (30)]. In equation (30), dose has to be determined by calculating the amount of solute entering SC during exposure (1):

$$\hat{Q}_{in}(s) = -D_m A \frac{1}{s} \left.\frac{\partial \hat{C}_m}{\partial x}\right|_{x=0} = \frac{k_p A C_v}{s^2} \frac{\sqrt{st_d}\cosh\sqrt{st_d}}{\sinh\sqrt{st_d}} \tag{50}$$

For short exposure ($t \ll t_d$), large values of s ($st_d \gg 1$) must be considered in equation (50), so that $\cosh\sqrt{st_d}$ and $\sinh\sqrt{st_d}$ can be replaced by $\exp\sqrt{st_d}$; therefore:

$$\hat{Q}_{in}(s) \approx \frac{k_p A C_v \sqrt{st_d}}{s^2} \tag{51}$$

and inverting equation (51) to time domain yields:

$$Q_{in}(t) \approx 2k_p A C_v \sqrt{\frac{t_d t}{\pi}} \tag{52}$$

The amount systemically absorbed after brief exposure is therefore:

$$\hat{Q}(s) = \frac{2k_p A C_v \sqrt{t_d t_{ex}}}{s\sqrt{\pi}} \frac{1}{\cosh\sqrt{st_d}} \tag{53}$$

We note that approximate equations (31) and (32) could be used in place of equation (53).

If after the removal of the vehicle there is evaporation of the solute from the surface of the SC, equation (49) has to be used in place of equation (30), which yields:

$$\hat{Q}(s) = \frac{2k_p A C_v \sqrt{t_d t_{ex}}}{s\sqrt{\pi}} \frac{1}{\cosh\sqrt{st_d} + \frac{\kappa_{ev}}{\sqrt{st_d}}\sinh\sqrt{st_d}} \tag{54}$$

We note that equation (54) will also apply when wash off takes place instead of evaporation, and κ_{ev} should then be replaced by $\kappa_w = k_w/(Ak_p)$ in equation (54). Equation (54) will then apply until wash off is stopped. The total dose absorbed for the brief exposure with evaporation is:

$$Q_{\infty} = \frac{2k_{p}AC_{v}\sqrt{t_{d}t_{ex}}}{\sqrt{\pi}(1 + \kappa_{ev})} \tag{55}$$

Kasting and Miller (11) presented an infinite series solution to a similar problem (solute is initially uniformly distributed in a superficial part of the SC, for x in $0 < x < h_{dep}$), this problem becomes identical to that represented by equation (54), when $h_{dep} \ll h$.

NUMERICAL APPROACH

The numerical approach in solving equation (1), with appropriate boundary and initial conditions, is usually focused on achieving as much computational precision as practical with current powerful PCs (17–19), which results in introducing hundreds if not thousands of spatial computational nodes. Here we want to present a somewhat simpler (and numerically less demanding) approach that recognises the fact that equation (1) describes SC solute transport only approximately (see discussion in Diffusion Equation section), and this could be used as a simplifying assumption in the computational method. This computational method is not new and was first introduced by Zatz (20), who represented SC as 5 compartments. The exact number of compartments is not essential and could be dictated by experimental conditions (e.g., how many tape-strips are required to remove SC), but should probably not exceed 20 to 25, the number of corneocyte layers in human SC. When more compartments are required (for some reason), the assumed homogeneity of SC is not valid and a different numerical approach has to be used that takes into account the heterogeneous "brick and mortar" structure of the SC (e.g., see Refs. 21 and 22). Here we present the extended n-compartmental computational model of SC solute transport, which also includes the treatment of different exposure scenarios discussed in this chapter.

When SC is replaced by n compartments, with permeability limited "membranes" between them (Fig. 2), the partial differential equation (1) is replaced

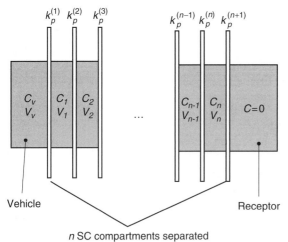

FIGURE 2 Schematic representation of compartmental model.

n SC compartments separated with $n+1$ membranes

by n ordinary differential equations. Equations for the first and last compartments are dependent on boundary conditions at $x=0$ and $x=h_m$, respectively. Equations for compartments 2 to $n-1$ are independent of the boundary conditions and are:

$$V_i \frac{dC_i}{dt} = A\left(k_p^{(i)}C_{i-1} + k_p^{(i+1)}C_{i+1} - k_p^{(i)}C_i - k_p^{(i+1)}C_i\right), \quad i = 2, \ldots, n-1 \tag{56}$$

where C_i is the concentration, V_i is the volume of the i-th compartment, and $k_p^{(i)}$ is the permeability coefficient between compartments i and $i-1$. If necessary, V_i and $k_p^{(i)}$ could be selected so that $k_p^{(i)} \neq k_p^{(j)}$, $V_i \neq V_j$, where $i \neq j$. Such a selection, for example, may describe variable diffusion/partitioning coefficients. In what follows, for simplicity, we assume that $k_p^{(i)} = k_p^{(j)}$ and $V_i = V_j$ for all i and j. In this case $V_i = Ah_m/n$ and, to ensure that permeability of all the compartments together is $k_p = K_m D_m/h_m$, we have to set: $k_p^{(i)} = D_m(n+1)/h_m$. With these parameters, equation (56) could be simplified, which yields:

$$\frac{dC_i}{dt} = \frac{n(n+1)}{t_d}(C_{i-1} + C_{i+1} - 2C_i), \quad i = 2, \ldots, n-1 \tag{57}$$

For the sink boundary condition in the receptor compartment [equation (3)], the equation for the n-th compartment is:

$$\frac{dC_n}{dt} = \frac{n(n+1)}{t_d}(C_{n-1} - 2C_n) \tag{58}$$

The equation for the first compartment will be determined by the exposure scenario and could therefore change in time. When SC is in contact with a vehicle, this equation is:

$$\frac{dC_1}{dt} = \frac{n(n+1)}{t_d}(K_m C_v + C_2 - 2C_1) \tag{59}$$

For the finite vehicle volume with evaporation (this case corresponds to boundary conditions 43 and 44) the concentration in the vehicle (C_v) is the function of time that will be described by equation (60):

$$\frac{dC_v}{dt} = -\frac{1}{V_v N t_d}\left[(n+1)\left(C_v - \frac{C_1}{K_m}\right) + \kappa_{ev}C_v\right] \tag{60}$$

After the removal of the vehicle, equation (59) becomes:

$$\frac{dC_1}{dt} = \frac{n(n+1)}{t_d}\left(C_2 - C_1 - \frac{\kappa_{ev}}{\kappa_{ev} + n + 1}C_1\right) \tag{61}$$

For the case of no evaporation, κ_{ev} has to be set to 0 in equation (61). Equations (57)–(61) fully describe concentrations in all compartments of SC, and the vehicle (if applicable) and could be easily solved numerically, given initial conditions. The initial conditions corresponding to no concentration in the skin originally [equation (2)] and with all solute in the vehicle are:

$$C_i(0) = 0, \quad i = 1, \ldots, n, \qquad C_v(0) = C_{v0} \tag{62}$$

The flux of solute through the inner surface of the SC is related to the concentration in the n-th compartment:

$$J = \frac{D_\mathrm{m}(n+1)}{h_\mathrm{m}} C_n \tag{63}$$

and the amount of solute absorbed can be easily determined from equations (15) and (63). In Figure 3A, a numerical solution for equations (57)–(59) and (62) is presented as the amount of solute absorbed for $n=10$ for the case of no depletion in the vehicle, together with a corresponding solution for the diffusion model

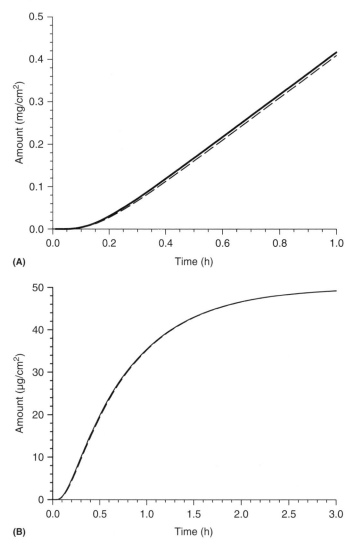

(A)

(B)

FIGURE 3 Amount of solute absorbed for **(A)** an infinitely large vehicle without depletion (parameters: $t_\mathrm{d}=1$ hour, $k_\mathrm{p}=5\times10^{-4}$ cm/hr, $C_\mathrm{v}=1000$ mg/cm^3) and **(B)** for a finite vehicle with depletion and evaporation (parameters: $t_\mathrm{d}=1$ hour, dose$=100$ μg/cm^2, $V_\mathrm{vN}=1$, $\kappa_\mathrm{ev}=1$). The solid line represents the diffusion model, and the dashed line is an approximation using the ten-compartment model.

[equation (7) inverted to time domain numerically]. In Figure 3B, a numerical solution for equations (57)–(60) is presented as the amount of solute absorbed for $n=10$ for the case of depletion and evaporation from the vehicle, together with a corresponding solution for the diffusion model [equation (45) inverted to the time domain numerically]. It can be seen in Figure 3A and B that, for only ten compartments, the compartmental model closely approximates the diffusion model.

For the constant vehicle concentration, equations (57)–(59) and (62) could also be solved in the Laplace domain, yielding:

$$\hat{J} = \frac{D_m K_m C_{v0}}{s h_m}$$

$$\times \frac{(n+1)\sqrt{g^2-4}}{g\left(\left(g+\sqrt{g^2-4}\right)^n - \left(g-\sqrt{g^2-4}\right)^n\right) - 2\left(\left(g+\sqrt{g^2-4}\right)^{n-1} - \left(g-\sqrt{g^2-4}\right)^{n-1}\right)}$$

(64)

where $g=(s t_d/n(n+1))+2$. Using this solution, it is easy to get the steady state flux (J_{ss}) (5):

$$J_{ss} = \lim_{s \to 0} s\hat{J} = \frac{D_m K_m}{h_m} C_{v0} = k_p C_{v0} \tag{65}$$

this $J_{ss} = k_p C_{v0}$ is expected, as the compartmental model was formulated so that the total permeability of all the membranes is $k_p = K_m k_p^{(i)}/(n+1) = D_m K_m/h_m$. The lag time could be determined as a limit as well (5):

$$\text{lag} = \lim_{s \to 0} \left(\frac{1}{s} - \frac{\hat{J}}{J_{ss}}\right) = \frac{t_d}{6}\left(1 + \frac{1}{n+1}\right) \tag{66}$$

Equation (66) gives an idea of how quickly the compartmental model converges to the diffusion model with increase in the number of compartments (e.g., for $n=10$ the compartmental model lag time is about 9% larger than the diffusion model lag time).

We note that the important difference of this model to compartmental models discussed by McCarley and Bunge (23,24) is that more compartments are used, which allows us to relate compartmental parameters more directly to that of the diffusion model. This latter fact makes this compartmental approach essentially an approximate solution of equation (1) with appropriate initial and boundary conditions.

REFERENCES

1. Roberts MS, Anissimov YG. Mathematical models in percutaneous absorption. In: Bronaugh RL, Maibach HI, eds. Percutaneous Absorption: Drugs—Cosmetics—Mechanisms—Methodology. New York: Marcel Dekker, 2005:1–44.
2. Anissimov YG, Roberts MS. Diffusion modeling of percutaneous absorption kinetics: 1. Effects of flow rate, receptor sampling rate and viable epidermal resistance for a constant donor concentration. J Pharm Sci 1999; 88(11):1201–9.
3. Anissimov YG, Roberts MS. Diffusion modeling of percutaneous absorption kinetics: 2. Finite vehicle volume and solvent deposited solids. J Pharm Sci 2001; 90(4):504–20.

4. Mueller B, Anissimov YG, Roberts MS. Unexpected clobetasol propionate profile in human stratum corneum after topical application in vitro. Pharm Res 2003; 20(11):1835–7.
5. Anissimov YG, Roberts MS. Diffusion modeling of percutaneous absorption kinetics: 3. Variable diffusion and partition coefficients, consequences for stratum corneum depth profiles and desorption kinetics. J Pharm Sci 2004; 93(2):470–87.
6. Roberts MS, Walker M. Water—the most natural penetration enhancer. In: Walters KA, Hadgraft J, eds. Skin Penetration Enhancement. New York: Marcel Dekker, 1993:1–30.
7. Carslaw HS, Jaeger JC. Conduction of Heat in Solids. 2nd ed. Oxford: Clarendon Press, 1959.
8. Kasting GB. Kinetics of finite dose absorption through skin. 1. Vanillylnonanamide. J Pharm Sci 2001; 90(2):202–12.
9. Guy RH, Hadgraft J. A theoretical description relating skin penetration to the thickness of the applied medicament. Int J Pharm 1980; 6(3–4):321–32.
10. Scheuplein RJ, Ross LW. Mechanism of percutaneous absorption. V. Percutaneous absorption of solvent deposited solids. J Invest Dermatol 1974; 62(4):353–60.
11. Kasting GB, Miller MA. Kinetics of finite dose absorption through skin. 2. Volatile compounds. J Pharm Sci 2006; 95(2):268–80.
12. Saiyasombati P, Kasting GB. Disposition of benzyl alcohol after topical application to human skin in vitro. J Pharm Sci 2003; 92(10):2128–39.
13. Saiyasombati P, Kasting GB. In vivo evaporation rate of benzyl alcohol from human skin. J Pharm Sci 2004; 93(2):515–20.
14. Nicoli S, Colombo P, Santi P. Release and permeation kinetics of caffeine from bioadhesive transdermal films. AAPS J 2005; 7(1):E218–23.
15. Inoue K, Ogawa K, Okadaa J, Sugibayashic K. Enhancement of skin permeation of ketotifen by supersaturation generated by amorphous form of the drug. J Control Release 2005; 108(2–3):306–18.
16. Kumprakob U, Kawakami J, Adachi I. Permeation enhancement of ketoprofen using a supersaturated system with antinucleant polymers. Biol Pharm Bull 2005; 28(9):1684–8.
17. Manitz R, Lucht W, Strehmel K, Weiner R, Neubert R. On mathematical modeling of dermal and transdermal drug delivery. J Pharm Sci 1998; 87(7):873–9.
18. Boderke P, Schittkowski K, Wolf M, Merkle HP. Modeling of diffusion and concurrent metabolism in cutaneous tissue. J Theor Biol 2000; 204(3):393–407.
19. Twizell EH, Kubota K. Lag time in the dual sorption model for percutaneous-absorption with finite skin-receptor boundary clearance. Math Biosci 1994; 123(1):1–23.
20. Zatz J. Simulation studies of skin permeation. J Soc Cosmet Chem 1992; 43:37–48.
21. Frasch HF. A random walk model of skin permeation. Risk Anal 2002; 22(2):265–76.
22. Frasch HF, Barbero AM. Steady-state flux and lag time in the stratum corneum lipid pathway: results from finite element models. J Pharm Sci 2003; 92(11):2196–207.
23. McCarley KD, Bunge AL. Physiologically relevant two-compartment pharmaco-kinetic models for skin. J Pharm Sci 2000; 89(9):1212–35.
24. McCarley KD, Bunge AL. Physiologically relevant one-compartment pharmaco-kinetic models for skin. 1. Development of models. J Pharm Sci 1998; 87(4):470–81.

15 Modeling Skin Permeability in Risk Assessment

Dara Fitzpatrick
Department of Chemistry, University College Cork, Cork, Ireland

Darach Golden
Centre for High Performance Computing, Trinity College, University of Dublin, Dublin, Ireland

John Corish
School of Chemistry, Trinity College, University of Dublin, Dublin, Ireland

INTRODUCTION

The ability of molecules to pass through human skin is an established and well-studied process in the cosmetic industry and has become increasingly more important to the pharmaceutical industry as it seeks to add to the number of therapeutic agents that can be advantageously administered transdermally. But the most widespread and urgent need to assess dermal penetration will arise in the context of exposures, either occupational or leisure, to chemical substances. The new European Union (EU) REACH legislation (Registration, Evaluation, and Authorization of Chemicals)[a] is effective from June 2007 and requires that such risk assessment be made for a very much greater number of chemical substances than that for which experimental measurements could reasonably be made. The legislation is one of the largest EU texts ever drafted. It runs to more than a thousand pages and its influence will eventually be felt far beyond Europe. The U.S. chemical industry has taken an interest in the progress of the REACH legislation as it may influence federal policy. This legislation together with the desire to limit, or if feasible to eliminate altogether, particularly in vivo experimental measurements has dramatically increased the need to find reliable and widely applicable modeling techniques that can predict the skin penetration properties of molecules for which no relevant experimental measurements have been made. The existence of validated and accepted models for making predictions of toxicity following dermal exposure will allow for the prioritization of chemicals already designated for further investigation or, if confidence in the model is sufficient, for filtering compounds as part of a multi-tiered risk assessment program.

Models for predicting dermal exposure to toxins are divided here into two classes, those involving structure activity relationships, quantitative or otherwise (SARs and QSARs) and differential equation-based models of (usually diffusive) penetration of the skin. SARs typically consist of databases of structural alerts, which identify certain compounds as being potentially hazardous using aspects of their chemical structure (1). QSARs are data-derived statistical mathematical

---

[a] http://europa.eu.int/comm/environment/chemicals/reach.htm.

relationships between the physicochemical properties of a compound and quantities such as its permeability or its maximum chemical flux through skin. In order to validate QSAR models, the Organisation for Economic Cooperation and Development (OECD) established several principles in 2004 to assess models for their use in regulatory chemical safety. The principles state that to be acceptable a model should have a defined output, operate through an unambiguous algorithm, have a defined range of applicability, be appropriately robust, have an acceptable correlation, the ability to predict, and if possible a mechanistic interpretation. Because they are currently the most widely available predictive tool for skin permeation QSARs will be the main focus of this chapter: however, recent progress made with diffusion models will also be considered.

QSARs FOR SKIN PENETRATION

The process by which a molecule penetrates human skin typically combines its passage from a vehicle through the uppermost layer of the skin (the *stratum corneum*) and its subsequent diffusion through the underlying layers (the epidermis and the dermis) until it is absorbed by the blood stream or otherwise metabolized within the skin. It is hardly surprising therefore that the most widely used transport parameter in the prediction of skin penetration is the permeability coefficient of the substance, k_p, which can be defined as:

$$k_p = \frac{J_{ss}}{C_d - C_r}$$ (1)

where J_{ss} is the steady-state flux through the skin, C_d and C_r are the concentrations in the donor and receptor, respectively. For diffusion-based membrane models, k_p, may be expressed as:

$$k_p = \frac{K_{sc/d} D_{sc}}{h_{sc}}$$ (2)

for the stratum corneum. Here D_{sc} is the permeant diffusivity in the membrane; $K_{sc/d}$ is its partition coefficient between the stratum corneum and the vehicle; and h_{sc} is the thickness of the stratum corneum. In many applications, a modified value of the octanol–water partition coefficient, K_{ow}, is utilized to represent $K_{sc/d}$. As is evident from its definition, the permeability is therefore a steady-state quantity. Experiments which measure k_p for compounds must use a dose which is sufficiently large to ensure that steady-state diffusion is closely approximated.

Experimental values of permeabilities have been measured for many years using a variety of techniques. Collections of these data have been used as the bases for QSARs that seek to establish a statistical relationship between k_p and certain physicochemical properties of the penetrant molecules for which the values have been measured. Once established these QSARs can potentially be used in a predictive mode to calculate values of k_p for other molecules for which no experimental penetration experiments have been conducted but for which the values of the physicochemical descriptors on which the QSAR is based are known.

Ideally k_p should be calculated from equation (2) above. This would require knowledge of the diffusion coefficient in the stratum corneum (and of the viable epidermis if it was being considered) as well as knowledge of the effective diffusion length through the stratum corneum. For many more simple molecular systems, it is now feasible to calculate the diffusion barriers faced by molecules and ions from first principles (2,3) and to estimate diffusion rates. However, the complexity of human skin as well as the size and nature of many of the molecules of toxicological interest make it impossible to apply these techniques to the prediction of skin penetration rates. Techniques such as molecular dynamics, in which the molecular forces between the relevant species are represented by interatomic potentials, are also inapplicable. What is possible then is the development of quantitative relationships (QSARs) between the more gross physicochemical descriptors of compounds and their relevant measured permeability parameters such as k_p or maximum flux.

The majority of QSARs for skin penetration, whether developed to encompass large general datasets or confined by virtue of their inclusion of selected specific descriptors to smaller sets of data from homologous compounds, have been constructed by fitting experimental data to functions of physicochemical parameters using linear regression. Many express the permeability k_p as a linear relationship of the form:

$$\log k_p = a(\text{hydrophobicity}) + b(\text{molecular size}) + c \tag{3}$$

The best known of these is the relationship derived by Potts and Guy (4) using the Flynn (5) dataset:

$$\log k_p = 0.71 \log K_{ow} - 0.0061 \, \text{MW} - 6.3 \tag{4}$$

where K_{ow} has been defined previously and MW is the molecular weight of the molecule.

The Potts and Guy QSAR is widely used because of the reasonable correlation obtained when applied to the Flynn dataset ($r^2 = 0.67$ for 93 compounds).

QSARs for skin permeability are not limited to forms such as equation (3) above. A variety of other linear forms have been investigated, including replacement of the simple molecular weight term in equation (4) with some other measure of molecular size. Much research has been devoted to the development of improved linear QSARs by calculating a wide range of molecular descriptors for each compound in a database, including topological and energy-based descriptors as well as the more familiar molecular weight or molecular volume and K_{ow}. A regression is then carried out over as large a dataset as is possible and the number of descriptors is reduced by determining which are the most effective in improving the fitting. A variety of computational techniques is used to eventually determine the most simple and effective model to represent the data. There are numerous examples of this approach (6–10). Another approach, also linear, involves an investigation of the underlying determinants of solubility and partitioning via Linear Solvation Energy Relationships and Linear Free Energy Relationships (11–13).

Nonlinear forms have also been utilized. For example, experimental penetration data from 40 compounds were used to train an artificial neural network which was then used to successfully predict the penetration characteristics of a further 11 molecules (14). More recently, Principal Components Analysis has been used (15,16), as has fuzzy logic (17). Another extensive and successful skin permeation QSAR has been developed to predict maximum fluxes (f_{max}), rather than permeabilities. This is an empirical QSAR and depends principally on the molecular weight of the penetrants (18). Neumann et al. (10) have recently reported a new statistical fully computational data driven model for predicting percutaneous drug absorption. This is based on an ensemble model using k-nearest neighbor models and ridge regression. It contains three purely computational descriptors (molecular weight, calculated K_{ow}, and solvation free energy) and predicts the values for k_p.

QUALITY OF DATA FOR QSARs

It is clear that QSARs built on experimental data when used in the predictive mode cannot have an outcome that is better than the quality of the data from which they are derived. Ideally these data should be purposefully measured in a single laboratory or at least under closely agreed and monitored protocols such as those that are now outlined in OECD Guideline 428. Unfortunately, many of the k_p values that have been and are still now being used in QSARs were determined before the existence of such guidelines and are typically drawn from wherever they became available. Often these data were determined for other purposes, many were measured under conditions that varied widely and, by the nature of their acquisition, some can be expected to vary substantially in quality. It is important to realize that all the QSARs essentially rely on the same datasets although these are, of course, often chosen for specific purposes and combined into a variety of different combinations to give different composite sets. There are therefore significant limitations both in the number and the quality of data currently existing in published values of k_p that can be used to generate QSARs for skin penetration.

The use of the increase in computational power to calculate large numbers of potentially relevant physicochemical descriptors for compounds and to include these in the optimization of the equation for a skin penetration QSAR has already been noted. Unfortunately, however, the very extensive datasets used by some of these authors (7,8,19) contained data for some 60 compounds for which the k_p values had previously been generated (by the Canadian Occupational Safety and Health Administration, or OSHA) (20) using a QSAR of the Potts and Guy form (21). Indeed the results of Fitzpatrick, Corish, and Hayes (19), who found that these large datasets fitted just as well to the Potts and Guy form as the more elaborate QSARs developed, e.g., by Patel et al. (8), is hardly a surprising result as it essentially confirms the conclusions reached earlier by Frasch and Landsittel (21) as to the origin of a sizable fraction of the data included.

A further source of uncertainty in the published QSARs is related to the pH dependence of the partition coefficients, K_{ow} used. Indeed, in this context, Frasch and Landsittel pointed out, in their investigation in the sources of data used in the above QSARs, that their compliance with the Potts and Guy QSAR depended on the choice they made from the different documented partition coefficients for some of the compounds. The potential ionization of a compound has the capacity to alter its physicochemical properties so that it can exhibit a substantially lipophilic nature in its neutral form or become hydrophilic once ionization has occurred. This depends on whether the compound is weakly acidic or basic. This change can affect the transdermal transport of a compound significantly depending on the exposure conditions.

Of the several thousand new compounds for which data are reported each year, a considerable proportion fall into the category of weak acids or bases, which have the potential to ionize. This fact has a significant impact on the risk assessment of exogenous compounds and their transport across human skin. The transport and uptake of ionizable compounds within biological systems has been difficult to predict and they are often classified as outliers in the common predictive linear models (8,19). Of the several factors that determine the transport of ionizable compounds across the skin, those which are most relevant are the pK_a of the compound, its partition coefficient, and the pH of the exposure event which takes place on the skin. Indeed it is necessary to examine each of these factors in detail and the relationships between them to fully understand their role in risk assessment.

Firstly, the partition coefficient is a measure of the degree to which a compound will partition between two immiscible phases; in this case octanol and water. It gives a measure of the lipophilic nature of the compound and this is then in turn related to the partitioning of a compound across the skin from an aqueous vehicle or solvent (4). The partition coefficient, which is one of the primary parameters used in QSAR models, is an experimentally measured parameter and, unlike molecular weight, can contain a degree of error associated with its measurement. However, there are long established and accepted data for the partition coefficients of most compounds and equally there are accurate software packages such as Kowwin (Syracuse Research Corporation/EPA) and ClogP to calculate their values. For this reason, the partition coefficients of, in particular, non-ionizable compounds are often regarded as constants and this has given rise to a degree of complacency in the literature to the point where the ionization potential of a compound has, with few exceptions (13,22–24), been largely ignored. Vecchia and Bunge (25) have used values of K_{ow} corrected for ionization in their assessment of skin permeation data.

International OECD guidelines (OECD 107, 117) stipulate that the partitioning of a compound should be measured in its unionized form. In general, for an acidic compound, this requires the pH adjustment of the compound to a value that is at least 1.8 units below its pK_a value (26). For many weakly acidic compounds, this requirement necessitates the adjustment of the pH in the range of 1 to 3. In practice, however, when an ionizable compound comes in contact with the skin, it encounters an environment of a higher pH range (~ 5.5), in which the partitioning of the compound will be significantly different to that for the same compound at the lower pH. Also, it is highly unlikely that any of the permeability data in the literature were obtained where the vehicle or applied dose to the skin was at a low enough pH value to maintain a weak acid in its non-ionized form, as exposure at this pH would damage the skin. It follows that using a partition coefficient which has been measured in its non-ionized form in a model, can lead to an overprediction of the permeability of that compound as the lipophilic nature of the compound is overstated (13). Conversely, if the pH of the aqueous phase of a partitioning experiment is adjusted upwards to ensure complete ionization, the resulting coefficient when applied to a QSAR will underestimate the permeability of the weak acid. This can lead to significant errors for compounds with pK_a values in the range of ~ 4 to ~ 7.

In order to correctly measure the partitioning of an ionizable compound it is therefore essential to allow the compound to ionize and achieve equilibrium at the pH of the expected exposure event. The ratio of the concentrations of an ionizable compound between two immiscible phases is given the term of distribution coefficient. Recent work by Fitzpatrick and Dullea[b] has shown that employing

---

[b] In course of publication.

distribution coefficients instead of partition coefficients in the Potts and Guy QSAR leads to a significantly better prediction of the passage of ionizable compounds across the skin. Measuring distribution coefficients at a pH close to that of the skin (pH ~ 5.5), results in predicted permeability coefficients that are of the same order of magnitude as those measured experimentally (22). Further information on the importance of measuring partition and distribution coefficients is available (27–29). Vecchia and Bunge (12,25) have extensively reviewed the extant data available for the development of QSARs.

VALIDATION AND ACCEPTANCE OF QSARs

A prerequisite for the use of QSARs as a risk assessment tool is a clear set of guidelines for their validation, possibly targeted within a given domain. The EU, in the form of the European Chemicals Bureau, has recently released a number of documents (1,30,31) and at least one set of guidelines, the Setubal principles which are summarized by Jaworska et al. (32). We are not, however, aware that any QSARs for dermal penetration have thus far been subjected to official testing with respect to any of these criteria. The European Chemicals Agency will handle registration applications and safety data for ~ 30,000 widely used substances as REACH is phased in over an 11-year period to 2018. The legislation will allow the €265 billion European Chemical Industry to continue to use ~ 2000 "substances of high concern" but now requires producers and importers to present an analysis of possible alternatives to hazardous substances. If alternatives are available, applicants must produce "substitution plans" showing how they can phase out the hazardous chemical (33).

MODELING OCCUPATIONAL EXPOSURE

In the majority of real, occupational, and leisure exposure scenarios, the quantity of a chemical substance that enters the systemic system through the stratum corneum will be only a part of the total quantity that may reach that system. However, it is often a very important contributor to the overall risk assessment and must always be estimated and, if relevant, be quantitatively taken into account. It is also necessary to recognize that real-life exposure scenarios typically involve repeated exposures. These are sometimes patterned but can also be random and for the most part they arise from finite sources. They may also entail intermittent cleansing of the skin and the substance may be applied neat rather than in the aqueous solutions often utilized in laboratory experiments. It is clear that useful models will require the flexibility to deal with a variety of potentially complex behavior patterns by those exposed to chemical substances either in the workplace or in their leisure pursuits. It is also clear that the QSARs that have been developed and described above predict steady-state penetration parameters, such as k_p, which, in general, do not apply in real exposure scenarios.

   Ideally therefore effective predictive models for use in accurate risk assessment should cater for non-steady state in addition to steady-state exposure conditions, particularly with reference to occupational exposure. This entails building models of the skin that can encompass the full process of dermal penetration. This process is usually represented as diffusion of the penetrant from a vehicle into the stratum corneum and with its subsequent passage into the viable dermis from where it is incorporated into the systemic blood circulation.

The model should also be capable of correctly treating the early non-steady-state penetration and indeed the exposure may not ever attain a steady state before it is terminated or repeated. The models in question are based on a theory for the selected processes with the resulting equations being solved either analytically or using numerical methods. For percutaneous penetration, the equations first model the partition of the diffusing species between the vehicle and the layers of the skin and then use macroscopic theories for its diffusion through the skin layers. Here we will deal principally with diffusion-based models, but many of the comments will apply to other types of model. Since full, three-dimensional modeling of dermal penetration is generally considered to be prohibitively difficult at this time, due to the demands made by the complexity of the systems involved, all models discussed here are assumed to be simplified one-dimensional models. The models also often ignore other effects such as skin hydration and the presence of appendages, e.g., additional routes may be provided by sweat glands and hair follicles.

It is important to note that non-steady-state models of the type envisaged here can be capable of generating full absorption time courses (such as the cumulative mass into the skin or into a receptor or the systemic blood supply with time) including the early non-steady state. When properly developed in this way they can fulfill the principal purpose of modeling, which is to increase our understanding of the fundamental processes that are involved in dermal penetration. In order to make predictions, such models must give a reasonable representation of the actual processes that occur and reasonable values must also be assigned to their input parameters. Although detailed work has been carried out in developing approximations to model input parameters (34), it is not clear that the parameter values generated by these approximations allow for accurate, general predictions of dermal absorption to be made. Finally, there is, to our knowledge, a lack of sufficient publicly available experimental absorption time course data for use in assessing the ability of a non-steady-state model to make predictions. At this time, therefore, non-steady-state models are less well developed than are QSARs for making predications of dermal absorption based on physicochemical input parameters.

However, some work has been recently carried out on the prediction of (aqueous) finite dose absorption time courses for compounds for which (aqueous) infinite dose absorption measurements (against which the predictions can be checked) have also been made (35). This work made use of two different mathematical models, which were implemented computationally. They were tested against each other and found to be in acceptable agreement, as well as being validated against earlier work. In the first of these models, which was very flexible in terms of modeling occupational exposure scenarios, the diffusion process through the skin was approximated by dividing these layers into multiple sublayers or compartments. The second model was an implementation of earlier models developed by Annisimov and Roberts (36,37) in which a full diffusion equation is utilized over the stratum corneum but not over the viable epidermis. The system of ordinary and partial differential equations was solved numerically using an inverse Laplace transform. Again the outputs are comprehensive and capable of being compared directly with those given by the first model. The approach used in this work partially circumvents the issue of assigning correct input parameters to the models by fitting some of the input parameters to infinite dose data, which was also measured using experimental procedures identical to those used in the finite dose experiments and using standard approximations for others (34). Data were collected for four compounds and the resulting parameters were then used in each case with good success in predicting finite dose absorption results for the same compound. This approach may have some utility in the prediction of relatively simple occupational exposures by representing them as a combination of simple finite dose exposures and the models developed have the facility to do this. In addition, while the approach does not solve the problem posed by the REACH legislation, it requires that only one, infinite dose experimental measurement be made for a given compound, rather than many measurements, each modeling a different type of occupational exposure. It should be emphasized that the work is at an initial stage and will require more validation against additional experimental data before it could be considered valid for use in the above manner.

DISCUSSION

The most often used and perhaps also the most obvious approach to the prediction of the skin permeation of molecules for which no experimental measurements have been made is the use of QSARs. This is reasonable given the quantity of nonproprietary steady-state data that is available in comparison to the availability of non-steady-state time course data. However, there are currently serious limitations on the approach and it is not at all clear that any of the currently published QSARs will be acceptable to regulatory authorities. In the first instance, it is necessary to realize that the vast majority of exposure scenarios most likely relate to finite doses and nonsteady-state absorption whereas the QSARs, in general, have been developed using data measured at steady state from essentially infinite sources. The correct usage of data measured under these conditions to calculate permeation from intermittent exposures to finite sources is very far from trivial. We have already referred to the limited recent progress by Kruse et al. (35) who measured both steady-state and non-steady-state data, in this regard.

Notwithstanding any shortcomings, a large number and variety of linear models and rule sets (16) have been utilized over more than three decades. Early QSARs used a bottom-up approach in which a small number of physicochemical descriptors, often chosen for a series of homologous molecules, was utilized and combinations of these investigated to find that which best fitted the data. More recent QSARs, reflecting the availability of much more computational power, have taken a more brute force approach in which a large number and variety of descriptors are calculated and then searched systematically to determine the optimum subset to best explain the data which is then chosen. It is also instructive to note that the more recent QSARs have tended to use approaches that allow for nonlinear relationships, either explicitly, for example, through the use of neural networks (14), or by using explicitly nonlinear function terms (37). Katritzky et al. (9) have produced both linear and nonlinear QSARs developed with the assistance of exhaustive descriptor searches. All of this work would indicate that the possibility exists that a QSAR may be developed that can adequately predict dermal permeability for a large number of molecules. It is also possible what will emerge is a number of QSARs, each one of which is specific to a particular class of penetrant.

However, there are currently also real limitations on the datasets that have been used to generate the QSAR permeability relationships extant in the literature. These relate to the very varied conditions under which some of the values of k_p have been determined and the uncertainties associated with the pH dependence of the values of K_{ow}. The very detailed analysis of their data, made possible by the fitting to mathematical models, in the recent work of Kruse et al. (35), clearly demonstrated that some of the reported experimental values of k_p may not have been properly determined at steady state. This is because the practice of dividing the steady-state flux by the initially applied concentration of the penetrant can give an incorrect result if the concentration of the penetrant has fallen in bringing the experiment to the steady state. This was shown to be the case and to be especially serious in the case of lipophilic molecules when the penetrant can easily enter the stratum corneum. It is clear that other values of k_p have been measured for commercial and perhaps regulatory and risk assessment purposes. It is now essential that additional reliable datasets be added to the published data currently in use so that confidence can be built to an acceptable level to allow QSARs to be used to estimate the permeabilities of molecules for which no experimental data exist.

CONCLUSIONS

The current general emphasis on risk assessment coupled with the imminent advent of the REACH legislation in the EU has shifted the emphasis in the modeling of percutaneous penetration very firmly to the predictive ability of the models for molecules for which no transdermal data are available. Such predictions now depend on (*i*) QSARs, which are statistical models, and for the most part use a simple set of physicochemical parameters to predict the permeability k_p or, much less frequently, the maximum flux, or (*ii*) on models that represent the penetration by a series of differential or partial differential equations describing the partition of the penetrant between the vehicle and the skin layers and its subsequent transport through each of them.

Both of these approaches are limited. A large number of QSARs, some of which are generic and others that have been developed specifically for particular sets of homologous compounds, exist in the literature. However, it appears likely that only a small number, if any, of those currently available will meet the requirements recently set down by regulatory authorities to provide acceptable calculated parameters for skin penetration by an untested compound. In their present state of development they could, however, provide information for the prioritization of chemicals as a step in a tiered assessment program. It is also possible that more realistic and flexible QSARs based on more extensive and reliable data may be developed using classical regression or some of the multitude of computationally intensive statistical techniques for which implementations are increasingly becoming available. The additional availability of a myriad of molecular descriptors as well as packages for their determination should also facilitate this goal.

The requirement that the dermal penetration process can be modeled under finite dose conditions also requires further investment of effort. A substantial number of mainly one-dimensional differential equation models of skin penetration processes also exist. However, only a very few of these models appear to have been used with experimental data to provide values for the model parameters—thus enabling the models to be used in a predictive capacity. Moreover, these approaches have not been sufficiently validated against a large body of experimental data. Finally, it seems likely that predictive output from such models should not be given in the form of point values, but in the form of distributions indicating the uncertainties in the values of the input parameters to the models.

REFERENCES

1. Worth AP, Bassan A, Gallegos A, et al. The Characterisation of (Quantitative) Structure–Activity Relationships: Preliminary Guidance (EUR 21866 EN), 2006. (Accessed October 2007 at http://ecb.jrc.it/DOCUMENTS/QSAR/)
2. Watson GW, Wells RPK, Willock DJ, Hutchings GJ. A comparison of the adsorption and diffusion of hydrogen on the {111} surfaces of Ni, Pd, and Pt from density functions, l theory calculations. J Phys Chem B 2001; 105:4889–94.
3. Rurali R, Heranadez E, Godignon P, Rebollo J, Ordejon P. First principles studies of vacancy diffusion in SiC. Comput Mater Sci 2003; 27:36–42.
4. Potts RO, Guy RH. Predicting skin permeability. Pharm Res 1992; 9:663–9.
5. Flynn GL. Physicochemical determinants of skin absorption. In: Gerrity TR, Henry CJ, eds. Principles of Route to Route Extrapolation for Risk Assessment. New York: Elsevier, 1990:93–127.
6. Pugh WJ, Hadgraft J. Ab initio prediction of human skin permeability coefficients. Int J Pharm 1994; 103:163–78.
7. Cronin MT, Dearden JC, Moss GP, Murray-Dickson P. Investigation of the mechanism of flux across human skin in vitro by quantitative structure–permeability relationships. Eur J Pharm Sci 1999; 7:325–30.
8. Patel H, ten Berge W, Cronin MTD. Quantitative structure–activity relationships (QSARs) for the prediction of skin permeation of exogenous chemicals. Chemosphere 2002; 48:603–13.
9. Katritzky A, Dobchev DA, Fara DC, et al. Skin permeation rate as a function of chemical structure. J Med Chem 2006; 49:3305–14.
10. Neumann D, Kohlbacher O, Merkwirth C, Lengauer T. A fully computational model for predicting percutaneous drug absorption. J Chem Inf Model 2006; 46:424–9.
11. Roberts MS, Pugh WJ, Hadgraft J, Watkinson AC. Epidermal permeability–penetrant structure relationships: 1. An analysis of methods of predicting penetration of monofunctional solutes from aqueous solutions. Int J Pharm 1995; 126:219–33.
12. Vecchia B, Bunge A. Partitioning of chemicals into skin: results and predictions. In: Guy RH, Hadgraft J, eds. Transdermal Drug Delivery. New York: Marcel Dekker, 2002:143–98.
13. Abraham MH, Martins F. Human skin permeation and partition: general linear free-energy relationship analyses. J Pharm Sci 2004; 93:1508–23.
14. Degim T, Hadgraft J, Albasmi S, Özkan Y. Prediction of skin penetration using artificial neural network (ANN) modeling. J Pharm Sci 2003; 92:656–64.
15. Pugh WJ, Degim IT, Hadgraft J. Epidermal permeability–penetrant structure relationships: 4, QSAR of permeant diffusion across human stratum corneum in terms of molecular weight, H-bonding and electronic charge. Int J Pharm 2000; 197:203–11.
16. Magnusson BM, Pugh WJ, Roberts MS. Simple rules defining the potential of compounds for transdermal delivery or toxicity. Pharm Res 2004; 21:1047–54.
17. Pannier AK, Brand RM, Jones DD. Fuzzy modeling of skin permeability coefficients. Pharm Res 2003; 20:143–8.
18. Magnusson BM, Anissimov YG, Cross SE, Roberts MS. Molecular size as the main determinant of solute maximum flux across the skin. J Invest Dermatol 2004; 122:993–9.
19. Fitzpatrick D, Corish J, Hayes B. Modelling skin permeability in risk assessment—the future. Chemosphere 2004; 55:1309–14.
20. Wittiker C, Walker JD, Gay DA, Neal MW. OSHA chemicals referred to the ISCA Interagency Testing Committee for percutaneous absorption testing and prioritization and analysis of OSHA skin notation criteria. Toxicologist 1993; 13:101.
21. Frasch HF, Landsittel DP. Regarding the sources of data analyzed with quantitative structure–skin permeability relationship methods (commentary on "Investigation of the mechanism of flux across human skin in vitro by quantitative structure–permeability relationships"). Eur J Pharm Sci 2002; 15:399–403.
22. Degim TI, Pugh WJ, Hadgraft J. Skin permeability data: anomalous results. Int J Pharm 1998; 170:129–33.
23. Hadgraft J, du Plessis J, Goosen C. The selection of non-steroidal anti-inflammatory agents for dermal delivery. Int J Pharm 2000; 207:31–7.

24. Gregoire S, Guy RH. Prediction of chemical absorption across the skin under cosmetic/dermatological conditions of use. In: 10th International Conference on Perspectives in Percutaneous Penetration. La Grande Motte, France, 2006.

25. Vecchia B, Bunge A. Skin absorption databases and predictive equations. In: Guy RH, Hadgraft J, eds. Transdermal Drug Delivery. New York: Marcel Dekker, 2002:57–141.

26. Padmanabhan RV, Surnam JM. PCT, WO91/16077, A61K, 74/21, 1991.

27. Sangster J. Octanol–Water Partition Coefficients. Fundamentals and Physical Chemistry. Chichester: Wiley, 1997.

28. Finizio A, Vighi M, Sandroni D. Determination of n-octanol/water partition coefficient of pesticides. Critical review and comparison of methods. Chemosphere 1997; 34:131–61.

29. Valko K. Application of HPLC based measurements of lipophilicity to model biological distribution. J Chromatogr A 2004; 1037:299–310.

30. Gramatica P, Pilutti P. Evaluation of different statistical approaches for the validation of quantitative structure activity relationships, 2006. (Accessed October 2007 at http://ecb.jrc.it/DOCUMENTS/QSAR/)

31. Jaworska J, Nikolova-Jeliazkova N, Aldenberg T. Review of the methods assessing the applicability domains of SARs and QSARs, 2006. (Accessed October 2007 at http://ecb.jrc.it/DOCUMENTS/QSAR/AD_methods.zip)

32. Jaworska JS, Comber M, Auer C, Van Leeuwen CJ. Summary of a workshop on regulatory acceptance of (Q)SARs for human health and environmental endpoints. Environ Health Perspect 2003; 111:1358–60.

33. Milmo S. Ready for REACH? Chemistry World 2007; 4(4):56.

34. Bunge AL, Cleek RL. A new method for estimating dermal absorption from chemical exposure: 2. Effect of molecular weight and octanol-partitioning. Pharm Res 1995; 12:88–95.

35. Kruse J, Golden D, Wilkinson S, Williams F, Kezic S, Corish J. Analysis, interpretation, and extrapolation of dermal permeation data using diffusion-based mathematical models. J Pharm Sci 2007; 96:682–703.

36. Annisimov YG, Roberts MS. Diffusion modeling of percutaneous absorption kinetics: 1. Effects of flow rate, receptor sampling rate, and viable epidermal resistance for a constant donor concentration. J Pharm Sci 1999; 88:1201–9.

37. Annisimov YG, Roberts MS. Diffusion modeling of percutaneous absorption kinetics: 2. Finite vehicle volume and solvent deposited solids. J Pharm Sci 2001; 90:504–20.

38. Wilschut A, ten Berge WF, Robinson PJ, Mckone TE. Estimating skin permeation. The validation of five mathematical skin permeation models. Chemosphere 1995; 30:1275–96.

In Vitro–In Vivo Correlations in Transdermal Drug Delivery

Jonathan Hadgraft and Majella E. Lane

The School of Pharmacy, University of London, London, U.K.

INTRODUCTION

Toward the latter part of the last century, there were considerable expectations for transdermal delivery and a number of very successful products have been developed. However, the number of chemical entities that has been delivered successfully using the transdermal route is very small. There are two major reasons for this. Firstly, the skin is a very good barrier and there is a limitation that only a few milligrams of drug can be delivered daily over a reasonable area. Secondly, many materials can act adversely in the skin and produce irritant or allergic responses. Developing a modern medicine is a very costly process and therefore it is important to determine the feasibility of delivering a candidate using the transdermal route before embarking on a full developmental program. The strategies for this include an examination of the physicochemical properties of the candidate followed by in vitro testing. With this information, a certain amount of confidence is gained before costly development is started. One of the first compounds to be delivered transdermally was nitroglycerin (or glyceryl trinitrate, GTN) and the types of study conducted with it are representative of those that should be considered in a feasibility study.

IN SILICO CALCULATIONS

Before any experimental work is conducted, many compounds can be ruled out on the basis of their daily dose and physicochemical properties. GTN is a very good permeant and the maximum daily dose is 20 mg with the application of two patches. Therefore, drugs that have a higher daily dose than this are unlikely to be successful.

The flux through the skin and hence the daily dose can be estimated from the physicochemical properties. Algorithms have been developed to estimate the skin permeability (k_p). One of the simplest relationships is that described by Potts and Guy (1) which estimates k_p from an aqueous solution

$$\log k_p = -2.7 + 0.71 \log K_{oct} - 0.0061 \, MW \tag{1}$$

where k_p is in cm/hr, K_{oct} is the octanol–water partition coefficient, and MW is the molecular weight.

The maximum flux through the skin will be when a saturated solution is used and therefore

$$J_{max} = k_p c_{sat} \tag{2}$$

where c_{sat} is the aqueous solubility.

The largest reasonable area (A) for a transdermal patch is 50 cm^2. Therefore, a daily dose (D) can be estimated by substitution into

$$D = J_{max} \, A \text{ time} \tag{3}$$

If the clearance kinetics (Cl) are known, it is also possible to calculate the steady-state plasma levels (c_p)

$$c_p = J_{max} \, A/\text{Cl} \tag{4}$$

The utility of this equation will also be seen when actual experimental (in vitro) values for the flux are known.

There are other algorithms that can be used to predict permeability and also neural networks have been developed. However, given the variability in skin permeation, the Potts and Guy equation can be used as a good guide for predicting transdermal absorption. There are some caveats, the equation is used for permeation from an aqueous solution and enhanced uptake may be achieved using nonaqueous vehicles. Many actives are ionized, the equation above applies to the unionized form. In practice, the free base or free acid is used for transdermal delivery (e.g., scopolamine, fentanyl, oxybutynin). Metabolism in the skin is possible and would not be taken into account in the above equations.

IN VITRO EXPERIMENTS

Although it is relatively simple to estimate fluxes from the physicochemical properties of a compound, the next step in the process is to conduct an in vitro human skin permeation study to confirm the values that have been calculated. In the literature, there are many examples where the feasibility of transdermal delivery has been examined using animal skin. It should be noted that animal skin, particularly rodent skin, is more permeable than human skin and therefore fluxes can be overestimated (2,3). It has been suggested that the best animal model to use is pig ear skin but the "gold standard" is clearly to use human tissue. The in vitro experiments should be conducted in an appropriate manner. Many drugs are very lipophilic and have poor water solubility; the conditions in the in vitro evaluation should ensure that there are sink conditions in the receptor medium so that the efficient removal of the drug by the blood supply, as found in vivo, is modeled. This is sometimes achieved by the use of cosolvents in the receptor phase. These can back-diffuse into the skin and it is possible for them to alter the permeability characteristics of the skin thereby overestimating the flux of drug from the device and across the skin. This is less of a problem if the device is the rate-controlling process but in most instances the rate control is from the skin. Because of this, variability in the results should be anticipated in line with the well-documented inter- and intrasubject variability that is found between samples (4–6). For patches designed to last for 24 hours, there should be fewer problems in vitro as the barrier properties of human skin are retained over this time period. However, it may be more problematic to conduct in vitro experiments over a three- or even a seven-day period over which time degradation of the barrier function may be anticipated.

Full-thickness skin can be used if the drug is not too lipophilic in nature and where there are no difficulties with drug binding to components in the deeper layers of the tissue. This is the most robust membrane and there are fewer handling problems. Dermatomed skin (often 200 µm thick) can be used and this thickness is representative of where the dermal blood supply will be located. Heat-separated skin can also be used and finally (and the least robust tissue) stratum corneum can be employed. In general, the membrane of choice for this type of study will be either dermatomed or heat-separated skin.

Another problem that should be considered is possible "edge effects." Matrix patches can be cut down to the size of the skin being used and the supply of the drug to the skin is from an area almost the same size as the diffusional area. For patches that cannot be cut because of their construction (e.g., membrane moderated systems), the area of the patch will be considerably larger than the area available for diffusion. Radial diffusion can occur and spurious results may be obtained (7).

The skin used in this type of in vitro absorption experiment is often stored frozen and will not be viable. If there is significant skin metabolism in vivo, the traditional type of skin permeation study cannot predict the degree of metabolism and there may not be good in vitro–in vivo correlation for this reason.

The diffusion of GTN from four different patches has been studied in vitro across dermatomed skin and the results are presented in Figure 1 (7). The data have been normalized to the total patch area which, as can be seen in Table 1, are significantly different for the four patches. Also, it should be noted that the patches contain different loadings of GTN. The results show that, in vitro, there is no significant difference in the delivery of GTN from these different patches. In vivo these patches all deliver 10 mg GTN per day. Thus, the in vitro amount penetrated after 24 hours is in very good agreement with the in vivo uptake after 24 hours. This means that the flux per day across the skin is the same for all the patches but as the areas are significantly different the flux per day per unit area is different. Therefore, either the thermodynamic activity of the GTN is different or there are components in the patches that alter the barrier function of the skin. Figure 2A,B show the data for NitroDur II and Deponit for five replicates (7). The error bars provide an estimate of the variation in skin permeability. These are larger for NitroDur II; this is a reflection of the relative control from the device and the skin (Table 2).

For regulatory submissions, it has been recommended that 12 replicates are conducted (9). It is comparatively easy to see, with this number of replicates if the skin barrier has been compromised in its preparation, storage, and handling.

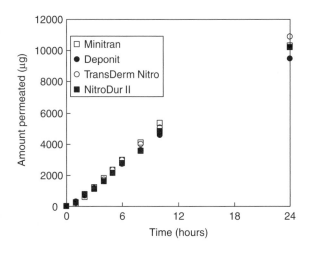

FIGURE 1 A comparison of the in vitro penetration of nitroglycerin through human skin dermatomed to 220 μm.

TABLE 1   Details of the Transdermal Nitroglycerin (GTN) Patches Examined In Vitro

	GTN content (mg)	Area (cm^2)
TransDerm Nitro	50	20
Deponit	32	32
NitroDur II	80	20
Minitran	36	13.3

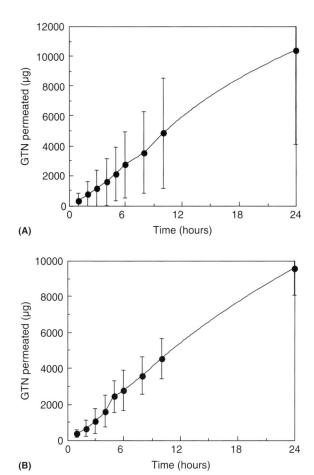

(A)

(B)

FIGURE 2 The amount of nitroglycerin (GTN) penetrated through human skin in vitro from (**A**) NitroDur II and (**B**) Deponit.

TABLE 2   The Relative Control from the Device and the Skin from Different Transdermal Patches

System	Fraction control device	Fraction control skin
TransDerm Nitro	0.45	0.55
NitroDur II	0.13	0.87
Deponit	0.87	0.13
Minitran	0.28	0.72

Source: From Ref. 8.

These will be seen as statistical outliers; however it should be remembered that the permeability follows a log normal rather than a normal distribution (10).

Before considering in vivo experiments, comment should be made concerning in vitro release determinations from the device itself, i.e., where there is no additional diffusional barrier. These can only be used as a quality assurance measure and will not give any indication of in vivo performance (unless the release is slower than permeation across the skin). For example, the release characteristics of the devices given in Table 1 have been measured and are shown in Figure 3 (7).

If there is a homogeneous distribution of drug in a noneroding matrix (e.g., Minitran and NitroDur II), the release kinetics should be linear with the square root of time for <60% release (11). As can be seen for these two devices, the release is rapid with nearly all the payload being released within the first four hours. In the case of TransDerm Nitro, there is a rate-controlling membrane and the release into the receptor phase is zero order. A very similar profile is seen for Deponit. In this particular system, the GTN is not homogeneously dispersed in the polyisobutylene matrix and hence square root of time kinetics is not observed. Figure 4 compares the amount released in vitro in the dissolution test with the claimed in vivo release. There is no correlation apart from Deponit, which exhibited the slowest release profile of the four delivery devices.

The amount released at 24 hours in vitro and delivered through the skin in vivo can be compared to give an indication of the relative control of drug delivery into the body from the device and from the skin (Table 2) (8).

IN VIVO EVALUATION

Since transdermal devices are designed to deliver an active to the blood stream, the most obvious in vivo evaluation is to measure plasma levels of the drug. The levels should be measured during the application time and after removal to determine whether residual drug in the skin continues to supply the systemic circulation. For example, the plasma half-life of fentanyl is longer for transdermal delivery as drug in the skin continues to be absorbed after the patch has been removed (12).

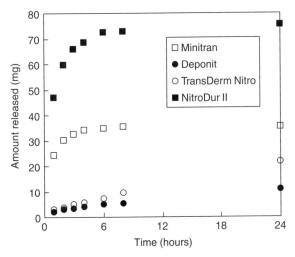

FIGURE 3 In vitro release profiles (determined by the Food and Drug Administration paddle method) for different nitroglycerin devices.

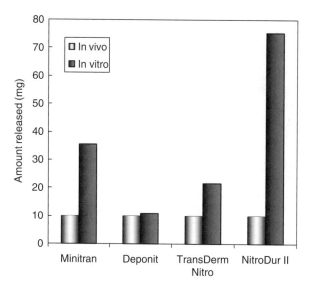

FIGURE 4 A comparison between the in vivo amount delivered and the in vitro intrinsic release (Food and Drug Administration paddle method) over 24 hours for the four patches.

This can also be an issue when patches are replaced and true steady-state plasma levels may not be achieved until after the patches have been removed and replaced several times. This has also been seen in the case of fentanyl where true steady-state levels may not be achieved until two or more patches have been applied and replaced (12). This is not a problem in the case of GTN as the half-life is short and patches may be removed for an interval each day to avoid the induction of tolerance (13).

The systemic levels of GTN are very variable. This is a consequence of the clearance kinetics for this drug. For example, when c_{max} was measured for 18 healthy volunteers during the infusion of GTN (10 mg for 24 hours), the range was 217 to 1900 pg/mL with a median of 716 pg/mL (14). After the application of Deponit (10 mg for 24 hours), c_{max} was 299 ± 184 pg/mL. Therefore, for any pharmacokinetic study and in the evaluation of in vitro–in vivo correlations, a suitable number of subjects have to be selected.

Another way of assessing in vivo performance is to monitor the residual amount of drug in the patch. By difference, it is then possible to calculate the amount that has been absorbed. This can be achieved by removal of the patch at predetermined times to examine if the drug is released at a constant rate. This approach has been used for Deponit and the results are presented in Table 3 (14).

TABLE 3 The Apparent Nitroglycerin Dose from a Deponit Patch as a Function of Time

Time (hr)	Apparent dose (mg)	SD	N
6	3.6	0.6	4
12	5.5	1.4	4
18	7.6	1.2	4
24	8.6	0.5	4
12	5.4	1.2	11

Source: From Ref. 14.

TABLE 4 Apparent GTN Dose (mg/day) from Various Patches Designed to Deliver 5 mg/day

	D	M	MDD	ND	TN
Arithmetic mean	4.5	5.0	6.1	5.0	6.2
Standard deviation	0.2	1.2	1.7	1.7	1.7
N	54	30	31	24	32
Minimum	2.9	2.5	2.8	2.2	3.0
25th percentile	3.9	4.2	4.8	3.6	5.0
Median	4.4	4.9	6.1	4.5	6.3
75th percentile	5.0	5.5	7.4	6.4	7.5
Maximum	6.1	7.6	9.9	8.3	10.0
Coefficient of variation (%)	16	24	28	34	27

Abbreviations: D, Deponit; GTN, nitroglycerin; M, Minitran; MDD, Nitrodisc; ND, NitroDur; TN, TransDerm Nitro.

A comparison was also made between different patches that were designed to deliver 5 mg/day. The study examined the residual amount when the patches were removed at 24 hours (Table 4) (14). Table 4 shows that there is variation in the data and, to an extent, this reflects the difficulty of the studies, particularly for GTN, which has a high vapor pressure. This means that drug can be lost from the patch during dosing, before and during application to the skin site, and after it has been removed and before it is sampled. Appropriate corrections need to be taken into account to allow for the losses during handling.

Residual levels have also been used to estimate the dose delivered from patches that are designed to deliver 10 mg/day (Fig. 4).

Table 2 shows that the control from the skin dominates for NitroDur II. Therefore, if this type of patch is applied to a skin site that is particularly permeable more than 10 mg/day may be delivered. This can clearly be seen in Figure 5. Where more control is with the patch than the skin, the chances of absorbing more than 10 mg/day are reduced. This is seen in the data for Deponit and TransDerm Nitro in Figure 5.

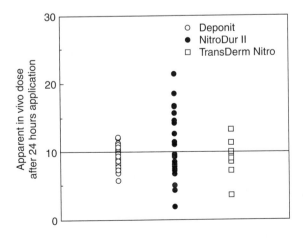

FIGURE 5 The apparent in vivo dose from three nitroglycerin patches designed to deliver 10 mg/day.

Finally, it is possible to measure the pharmacodynamic response after patch application. This can be used if there is a good correlation between the plasma levels of the drug and the biological response. Often these relationships are very variable and this procedure remains the least reliable indicator for in vivo–in vitro correlations.

IN VITRO–IN VIVO CORRELATIONS

In vitro permeation of GTN from Deponit across human skin is shown in Figure 2B and can be compared with the in vivo permeation as determined using the residual GTN found in the patch (Table 3). The comparison is made in Figure 6 and an excellent correlation is seen.

It is also possible to use the in vitro data to estimate the absorption rate into the systemic circulation. This can be equated to the clearance kinetics to give a value for the steady-state plasma levels. The range of anticipated levels, as a result of variation in skin permeability, can be assessed by calculating the maximum and minimum rate of absorption using the upper and lower limits of the error bars in Figure 2A,B. For NitroDur II the mean absorption rate is 443 µg/hr (range 191–694) and for Deponit 405 µg/hr (range 358–451). If a clearance value of 1044 L/hr is used (15) predicted plasma levels are:

NitroDur II 0.42 ng/mL (0.18–0.66)
Deponit   0.39 ng/mL (0.34–0.434)

These values can be compared with $c_{max} \pm SD$ of

NitroDur II 0.42 ± 0.38 ng/mL (16)
Deponit 0.3 ± 0.2 ng/mL (14)

The larger variability for the in vivo levels results from the additional variation in the clearance kinetics.

There have been other reports concerning in vitro–in vivo correlations for transdermal delivery. Examples include propranolol (17), local anesthetics (18,19), ketorolac (20), estradiol (21), and selegiline (22). It is clear that the best in vitro data will be obtained using human tissue but this is not easy to source. Animal skin and

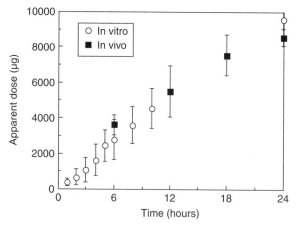

FIGURE 6 A comparison between the apparent dose determined both in vitro and in vivo for a Deponit patch (10 mg/day).

cultured skin models are possibilities but in general these will overestimate the permeation and will give an overestimate of the plasma levels achievable.

The in vitro absorption tests will not be useful in predicting possible problems arising from skin toxicity, although tissue cultured skin can provide indications of potential problems. Also, issues of metabolism of the permeant in the skin may not be addressed.

CONCLUSIONS

Clearly a well thought out and conducted in vitro permeation study can give useful guidance in assessing a transdermal candidate. The process involved in a development program should firstly consider the physicochemical properties of the selected drug. Simple permeation studies should be conducted in vitro in human skin to confirm that the drug flux is of the right order of magnitude to achieve the desired plasma levels. Prototype patches should be made and tested in vitro, if these are successful then a small volunteer study should confirm the possibility of a full development program (23). This type of approach has been reported but the literature is scant in this area.

As our knowledge of skin permeation becomes better with an increased knowledge of what occurs at the molecular level, our ability to predict formulation effects will improve and ultimately in silico–in vivo correlations should prove more reliable.

REFERENCES

1. Potts RO, Guy RH. Predicting skin permeability. Pharm Res 1992; 9:663–9.
2. Scott RC, Ramsey JD. Comparison of the in vivo and in vitro percutaneous absorption of a lipophilic molecule (cypermethrin, a pyrethroid insecticide). J Invest Dermatol 1987; 89:142–6.
3. Barber ED, Teetsel NM, Kolberg KF, et al. A comparative study of the rates of in vitro percutaneous absorption of eight chemicals using rat and human skin. Fundam Appl Toxicol 1992; 19:493–7.
4. Southwell S, Barry BW, Woodford R. Variations in permeability of human skin within and between specimens. Int J Pharm 1984; 18:299–309.
5. Rougier A, Lotte C, Maibach HI. In vivo percutaneous penetration of some organic compounds related to anatomic site in humans: predictive assessment by the stripping method. J Pharm Sci 1987; 76:451–4.
6. Tsai JC, Lin CY, Sheu HM, et al. Non-invasive characterization of regional variation in drug transport into human stratum corneum in vivo. Pharm Res 2003; 20:632–8.
7. Hadgraft J, Lewis D, Beutner D, et al. In vitro assessment of transdermal devices containing nitroglycerin. Int J Pharm 1991; 73:125–30.
8. Guy RH, Hadgraft J. Rate control in transdermal drug delivery. Int J Pharm 1992; 82:R1–6.
9. Skelly JP, Shah VP, Maibach HI, et al. FDA and AAPS report of the workshop on principles and practices of in vitro percutaneous penetration studies—relevance to bioavailability and bioequivalence. Pharm Res 1987; 4:265–7.
10. Williams AC, Cornwell PA, Barry BW. On the non-gaussian distribution of human skin permeabilites. Int J Pharm 1992; 86:69–77.
11. Hadgraft J. Calculations of drug release from controlled release devices. The slab. Int J Pharm 1979; 2:177–94.
12. Physicians' Desk Reference 2007, 61st ed. Montvale, NJ: Thompson Healthcare, 2006.
13. British National Formulary (BNF) 54: September 2007. London: British Medical Journal and Royal Pharmaceutical Society, 2007.

14. Bonn R, Hadgraft J, Wolff HM. Nitroglycerin TTS: biopharmaceutical and pharmacological aspects of transdermal therapy. In: Rezakovic DE, Alpert JS, eds. Nitrate Therapy and Nitrate Tolerance: Current Concepts and Controversies. Basel: Karger, 1993:224–51.

15. Hadgraft J, Beutner D, Wolff HM. In vitro–in vivo comparison in the transdermal delivery of nitroglycerin. Int J Pharm 1993; 89:R1–4.

16. Noonan PK, Gonzalez MA, Ruggirello D, et al. Relative bioavailability of a new transdermal nitroglycerin delivery system. J Pharm Sci 1986; 75:688–91.

17. Verma PR, Iyer SS. Controlled transdermal delivery of propranolol using HPMC matrices: design and in-vitro and in-vivo evaluation. J Pharm Pharmacol 2000; 52:151–6.

18. Padula C, Colombo G, Nicoli S, et al. Bioadhesive film for the transdermal delivery of lidocaine: in vitro and in vivo behavior. J Control Release 2003; 88:277–85.

19. Welin-Berger K, Neelissen JA, Emanuelsson BM, et al. In vitro–in vivo correlation in man of a topically applied local anesthetic agent using numerical convolution and deconvolution. J Pharm Sci 2003; 92:398–406.

20. Roy SD, Manoukian E. Transdermal delivery of ketorolac tromethamine: permeation enhancement, device design, and pharmacokinetics in healthy humans. J Pharm Sci 1995; 84:1190–6.

21. Rohr UD, Saeger-Lorenz K. 17β-estradiol matrix patch removal and reapplication in postmenopausal women: theoretical predictions with an oscillating diffusion coefficient model. J Pharm Sci 2002; 91:822–44.

22. Rohatagi S, Barrett JS, DeWitt KE, et al. Integrated pharmacokinetic and metabolic modeling of selegiline and metabolites after transdermal administration. Biopharm Drug Dispos 1997; 18:567–84.

23. Hadgraft J, Hill S, Humpel M, et al. Investigations on the percutaneous absorption of the antidepressant rolipram in vitro and in vivo. Pharm Res 1990; 7:1307–12.

Estimation of Subsequent Systemic Exposure—Physiological Models

James N. McDougal
*Department of Pharmacology and Toxicology, Boonschoft School of Medicine,
Wright State University, Dayton, Ohio, U.S.A.*

INTRODUCTION

Physiological models are sets of mathematical descriptions of biological processes, which have been shown to be useful for prediction in pharmacology and toxicology. The anatomical, biological, and biochemical basis of these models provide excellent potential for dose, surface area, duration, and species extrapolation. These same strengths furnish a tool to predict efficacy and toxicity as well as a tool for risk assessment. Most of these models use simultaneous differential equations to describe changes in mass of a specific chemical as it undergoes absorption, distribution, elimination, and metabolism in a living system. A physiological model employs a "chemical engineering approach" to describe the animal or human in terms of well-stirred vats connected by flows. In these models, the vats are equivalent to lumped sets of organs that have similar affinity for the chemical and similar blood flows. These lumped compartments have a total volume equal to the sum of the perfused tissues in the organism, and are connected by blood flows equivalent to the sum of the blood flows leaving the heart. Organs are frequently treated separately (rather than being lumped with other organs) when absorption, elimination, or metabolism of the chemical occurs.

The intent of this physiological approach is to mathematically incorporate the simplest principles of thermodynamics, diffusion, fluid dynamics, and interactions with biological systems. A complete set of these dynamic mathematical descriptions is solved over time using an engineering simulation language or a computer language such as FORTRAN or basic. This mass balance approach allows estimation of chemical in blood and tissues, as well as estimation of the amount of chemical absorbed, metabolized, or excreted during the time of interest. Although these models can adequately describe a particular set of data, their strength is that they can be predictive rather than just descriptive. The best physiological models incorporate only parameters that have biological meaning and can be measured or estimated in the laboratory. This restriction maintains the potential for such a model to be predictive of a new situation by changing the physiological, biochemical, and physicochemical parameters to those of the new circumstances—such as smaller exposure concentrations or longer durations. Incorporation of an appropriate absorption coefficient may also allow a physiological model to predict blood or target tissue concentrations from an entirely different exposure route.

Physiological models are also very useful as a tool for hypothesis testing and enhancement of our awareness of toxicological and pharmacological mechanisms involved. This type of model is harder to develop than classical compartmental models, but the biologically meaningful parameters in physiological models facilitate the extrapolation process. Use of these models is limited only by our understanding of the processes involved and our ability to describe them mathematically. They have been applied to pharmacokinetics of chemicals and toxicants in general for over 30 years (1,2). Andersen et al. (3) have recently reviewed these models from a historical perspective. More recently, the use of these models as a tool to predict and understand dermal absorption is becoming established (4). Physiological models applied to dermal exposures can be used to extrapolate from experimental data to realistic human exposure scenarios (5). In conjunction with biomonitoring, physiological models can be used to estimate exposure parameters (6). Appropriate use of these models will allow prediction of absorption when the actual exposure concentrations or duration of exposure is different than the experimental parameters. The physiological and anatomical basis of these models provides a means to accurately extrapolate dermal absorption and effect data for laboratory animals to human exposures (7).

MODEL PARAMETERS

Physiological models (Fig. 1) include physiological, biochemical, and physicochemical variables. The required physiological parameters are organ volumes, blood flows to organs, cardiac output, and respiratory rates (for volatile chemicals). Biochemical parameters such as Michaelis–Menten and first order metabolic rates are needed to describe metabolism of the chemical. Values are also needed for physicochemical variables such as absorption, partition, and binding coefficients. Both biochemical and physicochemical parameters are chemical specific and need

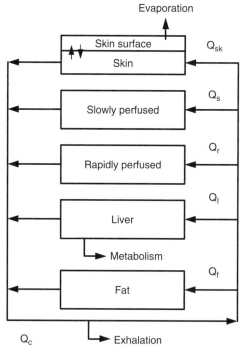

FIGURE 1 Schematic of a simple physiological model that contains five well-stirred compartments (*boxes*), which account for the total perfused body mass, and are connected by the blood flows (*arrows*, Q's), which sum to total cardiac output (Q_c). The physiological model is composed of linked differential equations for mass in each compartment, which are solved simultaneously to maintain a mass balance in the whole system. Initially, all of the chemical is on the skin surface where it can either evaporate or penetrate into the skin. The chemical is carried into the rest of the body by the blood flow, leaving the skin, and is distributed according to affinity for each compartment. In this model, loss of chemical can only occur by evaporation, metabolism, or exhalation.

to be measured in the laboratory or estimated by an appropriate means for each chemical to be modeled. Physiological parameters are generally available in the literature (8–10) and do not usually have to be measured again. Biochemical parameters can be available in the literature but more frequently they need to be determined specifically for the chemical and the physiological model. Often the metabolic parameters can be determined by parameter optimization in the modeling process. Closed chamber studies are used for volatile chemicals (11) and intravenous studies can be used for nonvolatiles (12). Methods have been developed to measure partition coefficients in the laboratory (13–16). Several authors have used parameter optimization to estimate binding coefficients (17) as well as oral (18) and dermal (19) absorption coefficients.

PHYSIOLOGICAL MODELS WITH SKIN COMPARTMENT

A vast majority of the published physiological models do not have skin compartments, but several models have included the skin either as a separate reservoir compartment for the chemical or as a route of chemical entry. Andersen and Keller (20) suggested that a physiological model could be applied to dermal exposures by adding a skin compartment to an inhalation model. McDougal and coworkers (21) modified a physiological model for inhalation exposures to predict blood concentrations in rats after a dermal exposure to organic chemical vapors and later applied physiological models to species extrapolations for eight organic chemical vapors (14). Kedderis and coworkers (22) employed a physiological model to predict tissue concentrations of a dioxin after dermal, inhalation, and oral exposures. Shyr and coworkers (23) used a physiological model that included metabolism in the skin to predict 2-butoxyethanol pharmacokinetics in rats after oral, dermal, and inhalation exposures. Jepson and McDougal (24) applied physiological models to nonsteady state dermal absorption of chemicals in water. Physiological models have been used as an aid to risk assessment when employed with inhalation and dermal exposures in showering and bathing scenarios for chloroform (25,26) and perchloroethylene (27). Models for mixtures of chemicals have been useful to help determine occupational exposure limits and for risk assessments (28,29)

THEORY AND ASSUMPTIONS

Physiological models are mathematical representations of our understanding of the mass transfer processes that occur when a chemical meets a biological system and as such are extremely simplified representations of the processes and organism being modeled. Simplicity is an essential characteristic; otherwise the number of parameters can quickly get too large for measurement. In addition, unnecessary complexity often carries the burden of an increased number of parameters that have to be estimated, thereby increasing the overall uncertainty in the model. The best way to have confidence in the extrapolation process, particularly between species, is to limit the model to biologically meaningful parameters that can be measured in the new species. The key is to find a balance between simplicity and adequate description of all important processes, but generally "the simplest model that works" is the most desirable. A model for predicting body burden of a chemical may have a different form than a model for predicting target tissue dose or a model that is designed to predict a pharmacological or toxicological effect. Simplifying assumptions should always be recognized and evaluated as appropriate for the specific model of interest. Common (major) assumptions are as follows:

1. Organs can be "lumped" into compartments based on their physiological and physicochemical characteristics.
2. Tissues and compartments are homogeneous and well stirred.
3. Concentration of chemical in the compartment, before steady state, is related to the blood flow to the compartment and the concentration difference between the arterial and venous blood.
4. Concentration of chemical in the tissue compartment is in equilibrium with the venous blood leaving the compartment.
5. The venous blood concentration is related to the chemical concentration in blood leaving each compartment and the cardiac output.
6. Passive transport of chemicals across biological membranes in physiological compartments can be described by modifications of Fick's law.

"Lumped" Compartments

One of the primary simplifications is that organs that have similar blood flows and similar affinities for the chemical can be lumped into the same compartment in the model unless there is active binding or elimination of chemical in that organ. Figure 1 shows that two of the five compartments in this model, slowly perfused and rapidly perfused, are "lumped" compartments. Organs combined to form the rapidly perfused compartment, sometimes called vital organs, are stomach, brain, heart, kidney, etc. In a similar manner, the slowly perfused compartment is composed of most of the rest of the body, primarily muscle, and sometimes skin. Skin is a distinct compartment because it is a route of entry. Fat is a separate compartment because it is a large storage depot for chemicals in this model for volatile organic chemicals. Liver is not included in the rapidly perfused compartment, although it would be considered as a vital organ, because the liver is a site of chemical loss (metabolism) and therefore is treated as a separate compartment. Sum of the volumes of the compartments is usually made to be equal to the total perfused body weight of the animal. This excludes tissues which are nonperfused such as hair and parts of teeth and bones.

Homogeneity

Few, if any, organs are composed of tissues that are homogeneous. Consider the complexity of organs like the skin, kidney, and liver, which have amazing functional and structural organization. Most compartments in physiological models are assumed to be homogeneous even though they are composed of different organs containing nonhomogenous tissue. Most physiological models assume that the compartments are well-stirred, that is the concentration is the same throughout the organ group. This assumption will not be valid for some nonlipophilic chemicals and some uses of a model where specific tissue concentrations are required. More complex descriptions of body compartments are available (1,9).

Flows

These physiological models, sometimes called "flow" models are composed of a flow scheme which connects the series of compartments (Fig. 1) in such a way that each compartment receives a realistic proportion of the physiological blood flow. The sum of the flows to each compartment is made to be equal to the cardiac output. This assumption is necessary to preserve mass balance during the simulation. In a simple compartment with no diffusion limitation, binding, or elimination, the differential equation for mass in the compartment would be written as follows:

$$V_i \frac{dC_i}{dt} = Q_i C_b - Q_i C_{vb} \tag{1}$$

where the subscript i denotes a generic compartment, V_i is the volume of the compartment, C_i is the concentration of chemical in the compartment (mass/volume), Q_i is flow to that compartment (volume/time), C_b is arterial blood concentration entering the compartment, and C_{vb} is the concentration of chemical in the venous blood leaving the compartment. The concentration in the compartment at any time is therefore proportional to the difference between the rate that chemical goes in and comes out.

Tissue/Blood Equilibrium

Partition coefficients are an expression of the solubility of the blood or tissues for a chemical. They are defined as the steady-state ratio of chemical concentrations between tissues or blood and tissues,

$$R_{i/b} = \frac{C_i}{C_b} \tag{2}$$

where $R_{i/b}$ is the partition coefficient (unitless). When there is no binding or elimination of chemical in either tissue or blood, this partition coefficient describes the concentration of chemical in the tissue relative to the blood. If we assume venous blood is equilibrated with the tissue concentration,

$$C_{vb} = \frac{C_i}{R_{i/b}} \tag{3}$$

we can substitute equation (3) into equation (1) and rearrange to get

$$V_i \frac{dC_i}{dt} = Q_i \left(C_b - \frac{C_i}{R_{i/b}} \right) \tag{4}$$

The tissue to blood partition coefficient helps determine the mass of chemical in a tissue compartment at all times. If the tissue to blood partition coefficient is high, the partition coefficient in the denominator increases the concentration difference and therefore causes the mass in the tissue to be greater than it would be if the partition coefficient were lower. Equation (4) is the basic equation for mass transfer in a physiological compartment, which has rapid transfer of chemical across the capillary wall into and out of the tissue. In this case, mass transfer is limited by the flow of blood to the organ. For some chemicals, diffusion across the capillary membrane or into tissue cells may be the rate-limiting factor for mass transport into some organs. When necessary, the physiological compartments may contain up to three subcompartments (blood, interstitial space, and tissue) with a transfer coefficient between each subcompartment. For equations for compartments other than the flow-limited ones discussed here, see Gerlowski and Jain (23).

Venous Equilibration

Chemical concentration in venous blood can be expressed as the sum of all the masses of chemical leaving the blood divided by the cardiac output which as follows:

$$C_v = \frac{\sum(Q_i C_i)}{Q_c} \tag{5}$$

where C_v is venous concentration and Q_c is total cardiac output. This equation essentially averages all the blood leaving the compartments, but the model does not contain a blood compartment. This assumption may not be appropriate for chemicals that are very well distributed in the blood or where blood is a target organ. Several physiological models have been developed which have blood compartments.

Fick's Law

Passive diffusion of a chemical across a membrane such as skin can be described as follows:

$$V_{sk} \frac{dC_{sk}}{dt} = Q_{sk}\left(C_b - \frac{C_{sk}}{R_{sk/b}}\right) + P_{sk}A_{sk}\left(C_{sfc} - \frac{C_{sk}}{R_{sk/sfc}}\right) \tag{6}$$

where the subscript sk denotes skin and the subscript sfc denotes surface, P_{sk} is the permeability coefficient of the skin (distance/time), and A_{sk} is the skin surface area exposed. The first term on the right side of the equals sign describes the amount of chemical in the skin, which is due to the blood flow and is analogous to equation (4). The second term on the right side describes the amount of chemical in the skin due to diffusion. It is related to Fick's law for passive diffusion.

$$\text{Flux} = \frac{DK_m}{\delta}(C_{out} - C_{in}) \tag{7}$$

where D is diffusivity (distance^2/time), K_m is membrane partition coefficient (unitless), δ is membrane thickness (distance), C_{out} and C_{in} are concentrations (mass/volume) outside and inside the membranes, respectively. The permeability coefficient is equal to part of the Fick's law equation (30),

$$P_{sk} = \frac{DK_m}{\delta} \tag{8}$$

Figure 2 graphically illustrates equation (6) and makes it clear that in this simplification the permeability coefficient describes the permeability barrier as the interface between the surface compartment and the skin. This assumption may not be valid for chemicals that penetrate slowly because it does not allow for a significant lag time. A more complicated approach to modeling the skin might include subcompartments for the stratum corneum, viable epidermis, dermis, and appendages (31,32).

USE OF ASSUMPTIONS

These major assumptions will, by nature, be inadequate for some uses of physiological models; however they provide the advantage of a place to start. When a specific modeling approach fails because the description is too simple, experiments to determine the appropriate complexity should be designed and accomplished. Riggs (33) provides a wealth of information about mathematical approaches to physiological problems. Advances in the state of our understanding

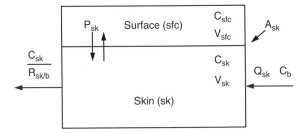

FIGURE 2 Schematic of a simple skin compartment, illustrating the processes that affect the amount of chemical in the skin. The upper compartment represents the chemical in contact with the skin surface. The chemical has a concentration (C_{sfc}) a volume (V_{sfc}) that is spread over a defined surface area (A_{sk}). The skin compartment is represented by a certain volume (V_{sk}) related to the area and depth of the skin. The skin receives the blood flow (Q_{sk}), which contains a known concentration of chemical (C_b). The venous blood leaving the skin is described by the skin concentration (C_{sk}) divided by the partition coefficient between skin and blood ($R_{sk/b}$). Concentration in the skin is solved by a differential equation [equation (6)].

and ability to predict new situations comes from repeating the following sequence of events:

■ Mathematically describe the current state of understanding in a physiological model.
■ Determine where the model simulations fail to describe new laboratory results.
■ Design experiments to increase the understanding of the process occurring well enough for mathematical description.
■ Mathematically incorporate new understanding in the physiological model (as in first step).

PREDICTIONS

Physiological models, by nature, are designed to predict the results of exposures to humans (and sometimes laboratory animals), which have not been or cannot be accomplished. The accuracy and usefulness of these models depend on the care with which they are developed and validated (34). When dermal absorption is a concern, these models have the potential to predict body burden or target tissue dose when absorption coefficients are known. This is a very useful potential for the pharmaceutical and cosmetic industries, toxicologists, regulators, and risk assessors. Appropriate absorption coefficients, primarily permeability coefficient, or diffusivity is essential to accurate the use of these models. Absorption coefficients can be determined either from in vivo or in vitro studies. Usefulness of in vitro diffusion cell studies to predict in vivo absorption is a hotly debated topic that is dealt with elsewhere in this volume. It is enough to say that when using absorption coefficients from in vitro data that one must not ignore the inherent differences between the methods, such as differences in diffusion pathway distance, differences in solubility of the chemical in receptor solution and blood, etc.

Physiological models have two extremely important advantages when used for prediction of chemical absorbed from dermal exposures. First, the concentration of chemical on the surface does not have to be constant. When the amount of chemical on the surface is small relative to the penetration rate, the driving force can decrease with time. Because of the mass balance approach of physiological models, both amount of chemical on the surface as well as absorbed chemical can be accurately predicted. Second, physiological models are designed to handle nonlinear processes such as metabolism and flux. These models do not have to assume that flux is constant during the exposure. Prediction can be accurate throughout an exposure even though flux through the skin is zero at the beginning of an exposure, rises to a maximum and may decrease with time. It does not matter whether the decrease in flux is due to depletion of chemical on the surface or buildup of chemical in the blood and tissues.

Physiological models can also be applied to prediction of the chemical concentration *in* the skin and its various components, when a complex skin compartment is used. These models have substantial potential for predicting efficacy of topically applied preparations and mechanism of action of chemicals that cause skin damage, irritation, or sensitization. Initially applied to nonlinear pharmacokinetic problems, physiological models that address specific mechanisms of action are now being applied in "pharmacodynamic" uses where the effect of the chemical is as important as the pharmacokinetics (35). Some examples and concepts for predictions are as follows.

Exposure Concentrations

Fick's law alone (without a physiological model) gives us the ability to predict how concentration on the surface can affect flux at steady state. Equation (7) shows that if nothing else changes, doubling the concentration on the surface would double the steady-state flux through the skin, but steady state is not the only time in which we are interested. Most actual human exposures never reach steady state. Only a physiological mathematical model of the skin will have the flexibility to accurately predict, throughout the exposure, the impact on the flux of doubling the concentration. A properly developed model would not only be able to describe the absorption rate of a chemical, but also the subsequent distribution, metabolism, and elimination of the chemical in the rest of the body. The simulation results shown in Figure 3 demonstrate the complex shape of the blood concentration curve when a rat was exposed for 24 hours to an aqueous solution of a volatile organic chemical, which also undergoes saturable metabolism and storage in the fat (19).

The ability to accurately predict such complicated pharmacokinetics of parent or metabolite in blood or tissues can be an extremely important therapeutic tool. A similar situation could occur when a therapeutic agent is applied to the skin in an ointment. A physiological model coupled with a skin compartment can predict the effect of nonsteady state dermal exposures in many situations that are important in the pharmaceutical industry and risk assessment.

Surface Areas

The therapeutic or toxicological impact of doubling surface area like doubling exposure concentration is not predictable by Fick's law alone [equation (7)]. Thus, if we double the surface area exposed the flux will double; however the systemic impact of doubling the surface area is not so simple. Table 1 shows the effect of doubling the surface area on some pharmacokinetic parameters when the chemical on the surface is neat dibromomethane. When the surface area is increased by a factor of two, the amount of chemical absorbed doubles, but the peak blood concentration increases by a factor of about 2.7. With the larger surface area

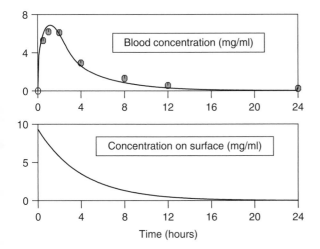

FIGURE 3 Simultaneous simulation of blood and surface concentrations for a dermal exposure to a 100% saturated (initially 9.36 mg/mL) aqueous solution of dibromomethane. Filled circles are measured blood concentrations in one rat drawn from indwelling cannulas. Blood concentration did not peak until one or two hours into the exposure, although by this time the surface concentration had decreased by about 35% to 40%.

exposure, metabolism is already saturated and the peak blood concentration increases by more than would be expected. Doubling the surface area exposed increases the area under the blood curve by more than a factor of three. This simulation illustrates the importance of having a physiological model to predict the impact of different dermal absorption scenarios.

Exposure Durations

Physiological models can also be very useful for estimating absorption from a wide range of exposure times. It has been suggested (36,37) that total absorption from a dermal exposure can be estimated by the following:

$$M = P_{sk}A_{sk}C_{sfc}t \tag{9}$$

where M is total chemical absorbed and t is exposure time. Equation (9) gives a "ballpark" estimate of dermal absorption, particularly for long exposure times (on the order of many hours). However, for chemicals with a long lag time for absorption, the estimate may be very inaccurate. Cleek and Bunge (38) point out that this equation may underestimate the amount of chemical which *enters* the skin if P_{sk} measured at steady state is used, because as the concentration in the skin

TABLE 1 Physiological Simulation of Pharmacokinetic Parameters after Dermal Exposures to Neat Dibromomethane at Two Different Surface Areas Exposed

Surface area (cm²)	Total chemical absorbed (mg)	Peak blood concentration (mg/mL)	Area under the blood concentration curve (mg/hr)
1.75	33.75	42.5	145.9
3.5	67.3	114.0	482.2

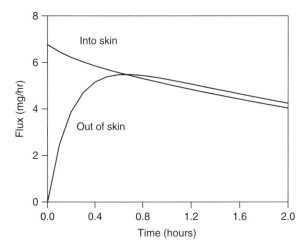

FIGURE 4 Simulation of the flux into and out of the skin during a dermal exposure to aqueous dibromomethane. Flux into the skin is highest at the start of the exposure and decreases as the chemical builds up in the skin. Flux out of the skin starts at zero at the beginning of the exposure and peaks about 0.5 hour and then declines.

builds up with time, the driving force for absorption *into* the skin decreases. From the perspective of what comes *out* of the skin, with a steady state P_{sk}, may overestimate total absorption because the flux out of the skin (into the rest of the body) is zero at the beginning of the exposure and maximum at steady state [equation (9)]. A physiological model accounts for the amount of chemical in the skin and the amount absorbed. Figure 4 illustrates the discrepancy.

The fate of the chemical in the skin after the end of the exposure determines whether the concern about ignoring the amount of chemical in the skin is valid. If the chemical in the skin is eventually lost (evaporation or exfoliated with skin) rather than systemically absorbed, ignoring the amount of chemical in the skin may not be significant. If the skin serves as a good reservoir for the chemical and it is eventually absorbed rather than lost, it might be important to account for it. An appropriately developed physiological model would be able to describe the chemical distribution appropriately and is the best way to avoid inaccuracies.

Species Extrapolation

Humans are almost always the eventual species of interest for dermal absorption studies, yet many studies are accomplished in laboratory animals. Animal skin may be significantly different in form and function when compared to humans (see chap. 2) and these differences can be expected to affect rates of chemical penetration (39,40). Physiological models have been shown to be useful for extrapolating pharmacokinetic information from laboratory animal to humans for styrene (2) and chloroform (41). Extrapolation of dermal absorption coefficients from animals to man based on the anatomy and physiology of the skin would be possible if there were sufficient quantitative understanding of the parameters that impact absorption and penetration. More complete physiological models of the skin, which include anatomical subcompartments and appendages (Fig. 5), could be developed and tested by predicting absorption in a species with anatomical differences (25,26).

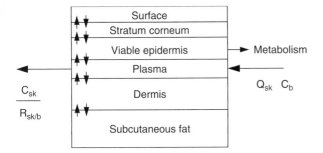

FIGURE 5 Schematic of a complex skin compartment, which shows some of the anatomical detail that may be important to predict dermal absorption between species. The dermis receives the blood flow (Q_{sk}), which contains a known concentration of chemical (C_b). The venous blood leaving the skin is described by the skin concentration (C_{sk}) divided by the partition coefficient between skin and blood ($R_{sk/b}$). In this model, diffusion would control transfer of chemical between the skin layers, and the blood flow to the dermis would carry the chemical to the rest of the body.

Anatomical measurements have been made in several strains and species of laboratory animals (42,43). Species extrapolations based on physiological models that include dermal anatomy have a lot of potential for prediction of human exposures.

CONCLUSIONS

Physiological models are useful tools for prediction of dermal absorption when dose, area exposed, duration, or species is different than experimental. These models are useful because they are based on measurable physiological and anatomical parameters and a mathematical understanding of the fundamental biological processes that occur when a chemical and an organism interact. Physiological models are obvious over simplifications of the systems they represent; it is useful to be aware of both the assumptions and their potential impact on the prediction. Carefully developed and validated models with appropriate skin compartments or subcompartments have the ability to accurately predict the nonlinearities inherent in biological processes. These models also have the potential to predict the efficacy or toxicity of chemicals in the skin or systemically when they are linked with a mathematical understanding of the chemical's mechanism of action. The potential of physiologically based mathematical modeling is only limited by our understanding of the principles involved in biological systems.

REFERENCES

1. Bischoff KB, Dedrick RL, Zaharko DS, et al. Methotrexate pharmacokinetics. J Pharm Sci 1971; 60:1128–33.
2. Ramsey JC, Andersen ME. A physiologically based description of the inhalation pharmacokinetics of styrene in rats and humans. Toxicol Appl Pharmacol 1984; 73:159–75.
3. Andersen ME, Yang RSH, Clewell HJ, et al. Introduction: a historical perspective of the development and applications of PBPK Models. In: Andersen ME, Yang RSH, Clewell HJ, III, Reddy MB, eds. Physiologically Based Pharmacokinetic Modeling: Science and Applications. Hoboken, NJ: Wiley-Interscience, 2005:1–18.

4. McDougal JN, Zheng Y, Zhang Q, et al. Biologically based pharmacokinetic models of the skin. In: Riviere J, ed. Dermal Absorption Models in Toxicology and Pharmacology. Boca Raton, FL: Taylor & Francis, 2006:89–112.
5. Corley RA, Bartels MJ, Carney EW, et al. Development of a physiologically based pharmacokinetic model for ethylene glycol and its metabolite, glycolic acid, in rats and humans. Toxicol Sci 2005; 85:476–90.
6. Tan YM, Liao KH, Conolly RB, et al. Use of a physiologically based pharmacokinetic model to identify exposures consistent with human biomonitoring data for chloroform. J Toxicol Environ Health A 2006; 69:1727–56.
7. Thrall K, Woodstock A. Evaluation of the dermal bioavailability of aqueous xylene in F344 rats and human volunteers. J Toxicol Environ Health A 2003; 66:1267–81.
8. Fiserova-Bergerova V, Hughes HC. Species differences on bioavailability of inhaled vapors and gases. In: Fiserova-Bergerova V, ed. Modeling of Inhalation Exposure to Vapors: Uptake, Distribution and Elimination. Vol. 2. Boca Raton, FL: CRC Press, 1983:97–106.
9. Gerlowski LE, Jain RK. Physiologically based pharmacokinetic modeling: principles and applications. J Pharm Sci 1983; 72:1103–27.
10. Reference Physiological Parameters in Pharmacokinetic Modeling, EPA/600/6-88/004. Washington, DC: U.S. Environmental Protection Agency, Office of Health and Environmental Assessment, Office of Research and Development, 1988.
11. Gargas ML, Andersen ME, Clewell HJ. A physiologically based simulation approach for determining metabolic constants from gas uptake data. Toxicol Appl Pharmacol 1986; 86:341–52.
12. Angelo MJ, Bischoff KB, Pritchard AB, et al. A physiological model for the pharmacokinetics of methylene chloride in B6C3F1 mice following IV administrations. J Pharmacokin Biopharm 1984; 12:413–36.
13. Fiserova-Bergerova V, Diaz ML. Determination and prediction of tissue–gas partition coefficients. Int Arch Occup Environ Health 1986; 58:75–87.
14. Gargas ML, Burgess RJ, Voisard DE, et al. Partition coefficients of low-molecular-weight volatile chemicals in various liquids and tissues. Toxicol Appl Pharmacol 1989; 98:87–99.
15. Jepson GW, Hoover DK, Black RK, et al. A partition coefficient determination method for nonvolatile chemicals in biological tissues. Fundam Appl Toxicol 1994; 22:519–24.
16. Mattie DR, Bates GD, Jepson GW, et al. Determination of skin: air partition coefficients for volatile chemicals: experimental method and applications. Fundam Appl Toxicol 1994; 22:51–7.
17. Gray DG. A physiologically based pharmacokinetic model for methyl mercury in the pregnant rat and fetus. Toxicol Appl Pharmacol 1995; 132:91–102.
18. Frederick CB, Potter DW, Chang-Mateu MI, et al. A physiologically based pharmacokinetic and pharmacodynamic model to describe the oral dosing of rats with ethyl acrylate and its implications for risk assessment. Toxicol Appl Pharmacol 1992; 114:246–60.
19. McDougal JN, Jepson GW, Clewell HJ, et al. Dermal absorption of organic chemical vapors in rats and humans. Fundam Appl Toxicol 1990; 14:299–308.
20. Andersen ME, Keller WC. Toxicokinetic principles in relation to percutaneous absorption and cutaneous toxicity. In: Drill VA, Lazar P, eds. Cutaneous Toxicity. New York: Raven Press, 1984:9–27.
21. McDougal JN, Jepson GW, Clewell HJ, et al. A physiological pharmacokinetic model for dermal absorption of vapors in the rat. Toxicol Appl Pharmacol 1986; 85:286–94.
22. Kedderis LB, Mills JJ, Andersen ME, et al. A physiologically based pharmacokinetic model for 2,3,7,8-tetrabromodibenzo-p-dioxin (TBDD) in the rat: tissue distribution and CYP1A induction. Toxicol Appl Pharmacol 1993; 121:87–98.
23. Shyr LJ, Sabourin PJ, Medinsky MA, et al. Physiologically based modeling of 2-butoxyethanol disposition in rats following different routes of exposure. Environ Res 1993; 63:202–18.
24. Jepson GW, McDougal JN. Physiologically based modeling of nonsteady state dermal absorption of halogenated methanes from an aqueous solution. Toxicol Appl Pharmacol 1997; 144:315–24.

25. Chinery RL, Gleason AK. A compartmental model for the prediction of breath concentration and absorbed dose of chloroform after exposure while showering. Risk Anal 1993; 13:51–62.
26. Corley RA, Gordon SM, Wallace LA. Physiologically based pharmacokinetic modeling of the temperature-dependent dermal absorption of chloroform by humans following bath water exposures. Toxicol Sci 2000; 53:13–23.
27. Rao HV, Brown DR. A physiologically based pharmacokinetic assessment of tetrachloroethylene in groundwater for a bathing and showering determination. Risk Anal 1993; 13:37–49.
28. Dennison JE, Bigelow PL, Andersen ME. Occupational exposure limits in the context of solvent mixtures, consumption of ethanol, and target tissue dose. Toxicol Ind Health 2004; 20:165–75.
29. Maruyama W, Aoki Y. Estimated cancer risk of dioxins to humans using a bioassay and physiologically based pharmacokinetic model. Toxicol Appl Pharmacol 2006; 214:188–98.
30. Flynn GL, Yalkowsky SH, Roseman TJ. Mass transport phenomena and models: theoretical concepts. J Pharm Sci 1974; 63:479–509.
31. McDougal JN. Physiologically-based pharmacokinetic modeling. In: Marzulli FN, Maibach HI, eds. Dermatotoxicology. 5th ed. Washington, DC: Hemisphere Publishing, 1996:353–70.
32. Bookout RL, McDaniel CR, Quinn DW, et al. Multilayered dermal subcompartments for modeling chemical absorption. Environ Res 1996; 5:133–50.
33. Riggs DS. The Mathematical Approach to Physiological Problems: A Critical Primer. Cambridge, MA: MIT Press, 1963.
34. Andersen ME, Clewell HJ, Frederick CB. Applying simulation modeling to problems in toxicology and risk assessment—a short perspective. Toxicol Appl Pharmacol 1995; 133:181–7.
35. Conolly RB, Andersen ME. Biologically based pharmacodynamic models: tools for toxicological research and risk assessment. Annu Rev Pharmacol Toxicol 1991; 31:503–23.
36. Leung HW, Paustenbach DJ. Techniques for estimating the percutaneous absorption of chemicals due to occupational and environmental exposure. Appl Occup Environ Hyg 1994; 9:187–97.
37. Walker JD, Whittaker C, McDougal JN. Role of the TSCA interagency testing committee in meeting the U.S. government data needs: designating chemicals for percutaneous absorption rate testing. In: Marzulli FN, Maibach HI, eds. Dermatotoxicology. 5th ed. Washington, DC: Hemisphere Publishing, 1996:371–81.
38. Cleek RL, Bunge AL. A new method for estimating dermal absorption from chemical exposure. I. General approach. Pharm Res 1993; 10:497–506.
39. Scheuplein RJ, Blank IH. Permeability of the skin. Physiol Rev 1971; 51:702–47.
40. Vinson LJ, Singer EJ, Koehler WR, et al. The nature of the epidermal barrier and some factors influencing skin permeability. Toxicol Appl Pharmacol 1965; 7:7–19.
41. Corley RA, Bormett GA, Ghanayem BI. Physiologically based pharmacokinetics of 2-butoxyethanol and its major metabolite, 2-butoxyacetic acid, in rats and humans. Toxicol Appl Pharmacol 1994; 129:61–79.
42. Monteiro-Riviere N, Bristol DG, Manning TO, et al. Interspecies and interregional analysis of the comparative histologic thickness and laser doppler blood flow measurement of five cutaneous sites in nine species. J Invest Dermatol 1990; 95:582–6.
43. Grabau JH, Dong L, Mattie DR, et al. Comparison of anatomical characteristics of the skin for several laboratory animals, AL/OE-TR-1995-066. Ohio: Armstrong Laboratory, Wright-Patterson AFB, 1995.

RISKOFDERM: Predictions Based on In Vivo Factors

Wim J. A. Meuling
Business Unit Biosciences, TNO Quality of Life, Zeist, The Netherlands

Johannes J. M. van de Sandt and Joop J. van Hemmen
Business Unit Food and Chemical Risk Analysis, TNO Quality of Life, Zeist, The Netherlands

INTRODUCTION

For registration of newly developed chemicals and the reevaluation of existing marketed chemicals, competent authorities need reliable information such as the amount of the chemical used, the various work-related situations in which the chemical will be used, whether the chemical will be used indoors or outdoors, in open or closed situations, and in what way and to what extent workers/consumers may be exposed to the chemicals during their daily practice. With sufficient and reliable data to hand, the registrant and/or the competent authority may predict the occupational risk and the risk for consumers more precisely. However, there are more then 30,000 chemicals on the market. This large number makes it almost impossible to collect these important data for all the substances with respect to the various scenarios whereby these chemicals are being used. The need for a sophisticated method to predict the risks for human in a rather straightforward and easy but sometimes conservative way was the basis for a large project funded by the European Commission (DG Research) in which scientists from 15 institutes of 10 European countries participated to overcome large parts of this problem. The overall outcome and the various items developed within this project, named RISKOFDERM, are outlined in the first part of this chapter. However, a particular substance or a work-related situation may require additional data to predict the risk not only of external exposure but also on the internal exposure combined with the external exposure data. Therefore, knowledge of the various aspects of the dermal absorption process and the kinetics and the influence of various work-related factors on this process is needed. The last part of this chapter gives an overview of such important parameters.

GENERAL INFORMATION ON THE RISKOFDERM PROJECT

In the formal risk assessment for registration of many substances, including agricultural pesticides and biocides, it is essential to assess dermal exposure loading since, in many cases, this forms the major part of the risk related to the chemical at work. In the new Registration, Evaluation, and Authorization of Chemicals (REACH) legislation, dermal exposure needs to be considered before safe use of the substance may be concluded. For agricultural pesticides, this has been known for a long time and the methodology has been developed to optimize the measurement of dermal exposure loading, leading to the development of an Organisation for Economic Cooperation and Development Guidance Document (1). During the work of the Dermal Exposure Network (2), it became clear that there was a need for information on dermal exposure loading to general chemicals. This led to the development of the RISKOFDERM project, which was financed by DG Research of the European Union (QLK4-CT-1999-01197). Many of the results of this project have been published in the *Annals of Occupational Hygiene* (3).

Research Goals

The RISKOFDERM project was intended to help reduce acute and chronic ill health due to dermal exposure to chemicals, and had two *major* operational objectives.

1. Develop a validated predictive model for estimating dermal exposure for use in generic personal exposure risk assessment to chemicals (e.g., under the New and Existing Substances legislation, and its successor in European chemical policy: REACH, as well as the Biocidal Product Directive).
2. Develop a practical dermal exposure risk assessment and management toolkit for use by small- and medium-sized enterprises (SMEs) and others, in actual workplace situations (e.g., under the Chemical Agents Directive).

To achieve these objectives, a research program comprised of four interrelated work parts was carried out.

■ *Work part 1: qualitative dermal exposure survey*
   Main objective: To create an overview of qualitative information about dermal exposure throughout Europe (processes, tasks, populations, and determinants of dermal exposure).
■ *Work part 2: quantitative dermal exposure survey*
   Main objective: Gathering quantitative data on potential (and actual) dermal exposure in selected workplace situations in the Member States, chosen in part from the findings in work part 1.
■ *Work part 3: exposure model set*
   Main objective: To develop an appropriate predictive exposure model (set) for generic assessment of dermal exposure of single chemicals based on actual measurements.
■ *Work part 4: risk assessment and management toolkit*
   Main objective: To develop a risk assessment and management toolkit for exposure and risk assessment (and management) of (specifically) dermal exposure in SMEs.

The four work parts delivered their objectives by employing a close working relationship between the partners in all work parts. This resulted in a large database with information on determinants of dermal exposure for the qualitative survey carried out in various industry sectors throughout Europe (in nine Member States). Two large databases have been created which contain the results of hand and body exposures based on quantitative dermal exposure studies carried out in six Member States under a large series of different use scenarios for chemicals with the best available methodology, as described for pesticides (1). These databases are available for use by policy makers, other researchers, and exposure modelers.

On the basis of these results, the two major products were prepared in accordance with the two main objectives of the project.

■ A predictive dermal exposure model set structured according to the chosen format of six different dermal operation exposure units. A set of adaptations has also been prepared for the Technical Guidance Document Risk Assessment for the new and existing substance regulations (currently being developed into REACH). This set of adaptations can easily be integrated if required by the Commission and Member States.

■ A toolkit for risk assessment and risk management of dermal exposures has been developed and is available on CD-ROM and the Internet, for use by competent authorities, labor inspectorates and SMEs.

The RISKOFDERM Dermal Model

The European Union project RISKOFDERM has gathered a large number of new measurements on dermal exposure to industrial chemicals in various work situations, together with information on possible determinants of exposure. The exposure studies are described in a series of publications that fill a volume of the *Annals of Occupational Hygiene* (volume 48, 2004). These data and information, together with some non-RISKOFDERM data, were used to derive default values for potential dermal exposure of the hands for "Technical Guidance Document (TGD; European Chemicals Bureau website) exposure scenarios." TGD exposure scenarios have similar values for some very important determinant(s) of dermal exposure, such as amount of substance used. They form narrower bands within the so-called RISKOFDERM scenarios, which cluster exposure situations according to the same purpose of use of the products. The RISKOFDERM scenarios in turn are narrower bands within the so-called Dermal Exposure Operation (DEO) units that were defined in the RISKOFDERM project to cluster situations with similar exposure processes and exposure routes. Default values for both reasonable worst-case situations and typical situations were derived, both for single and, where possible, combined datasets that fit the same TGD exposure scenario. These default values are considered useful for estimating exposure for similar substances in similar situations with low uncertainty. Several other default values based on single datasets can also be used, but can lead to estimates with a higher uncertainty, due to their more limited basis. Sufficient analogy in all described parameters of the scenario, including duration, is needed to enable proper use of the default values (4). The default values lead to similar estimates as the RISKOFDERM dermal exposure model, which was based on the same datasets, but uses very different parameters. Both approaches are preferred over older general models, such as Estimation and Assessment of Substances Exposure (EASE) (5), that are not based on data from actual dermal exposure situations.

Warren et al. (6) describe the development of a set of generic task-based models capable of predicting potential dermal exposure to both solids and liquids in a wide range of situations. To facilitate modeling of the wide variety of dermal exposure situations, six separate models were made for the DEO units. These task-based groupings cluster exposure scenarios with regard to the expected routes of dermal exposure and the expected influence of exposure determinants. Within these groupings, linear mixed effect models were used to estimate the influence of various exposure determinants and to estimate components of variance. The models predict median potential dermal exposure rates for the hands and the rest of the body from the values of relevant exposure determinants. These rates are expressed as mg or μL product/min. Using these median potential dermal exposure rates and an accompanying geometric standard deviation allows a range of exposure percentiles to be calculated.

The current model in Excel format, with guidance on use, is available from the coordinator of the project (J. J. van Hemmen). A web-based version with probability assessment features will be soon available on the websites of TNO and the Health and Safety Executive.

Further developments are the integration of the RISKOFDERM data with the Bayesian Exposure Assessment Tool (TNsG, 2002; European Chemicals Bureau website) and the source–receptor model approach (7) into a so-called advanced tool (8), which should cover the needs for the development of worker exposure scenarios under REACH, both for inhalation and dermal exposure. A detailed proposal for the development of the advanced tool is submitted for funding.

The RISKOFDERM Toolkit

Taking into account the methodology of the approaches used for predicting risk from airborne exposure, it was decided to develop a similar scheme for dermal exposure using a number of steps. The toolkit would be built by fitting relevant information into broad categories (scores). After combining these data, the results would also be given in broad bands. It was decided to assess hazard and exposure separately and then combine them to assess the health risk. The toolkit would then advise control actions to the user, with an indication of the remedial efficiency [for a preliminary description see (9)]. In accordance with European law (Chemical Agents at Work Directive 98/24/EEC), the user is encouraged to investigate possible control actions following the STOP hierarchy:

1. Substitution
2. Technical protection
3. Organizational protection
4. Personal protection

If new or additional controls are applied, the toolkit will recommend that the user carry out a new risk assessment. If the control action is shown to be effective, a lower risk should result. This interactive procedure is intended to manage and reduce health risks from occupational dermal exposure.

Hazard

The possible harm to human health in cases of significant exposure is an intrinsic property of a chemical substance or preparation and needs to be assessed as a first step. If two chemicals with very different hazards can be used for a specific working procedure, then the hazard assessment alone can lead to a recommendation of substitution without any exposure assessment, assuming all other relevant variables to be the same. When specific exposure conditions are unknown, or when exposure conditions vary greatly, the selection of alternative products may be based on hazard considerations alone.

Exposure and Risk

The exposure level determines whether a given hazard leads to a significant health risk. Therefore, exposure needs to be estimated and combined with the hazard to estimate the resulting risk. Hazard and exposure are independent of each other, and it may occur that a high hazard chemical at low exposure and a low hazard chemical at high exposure can result in comparable risk levels. Especially, if one considers substituting a hazardous chemical with one of lower toxicity, then it is essential to take into account whether the use pattern of the new substance would result in higher exposures, which would more than offset the benefit of lower toxicity, giving a higher overall risk.

Control

If the assessed hazard, exposure or risk is shown to be unacceptable, then in a next step, control actions are suggested for reducing the hazard (by substitution) or the exposure (by technical, organizational, or personal protection). If these actions are effective, a new and lower risk will be the result of a new hazard and exposure assessment.

Skin Relevant Hazard and Exposure

The skin relevant hazard of a product is assessed separately for local and systemic effects after uptake through the skin. In both cases, the respective intrinsic toxicity is read from toxicological data, such as lethal doses, allergenic potency, skin irritation strength and threshold, and similar data. As this information is not available in the field, the legal labeling and the risk phrases, as required by the European Directive 67/548/EEC, are used as surrogates, possibly complemented by data on acidity and on solubility in skin lipids ($P_{o/w}$), if these can be obtained from a Safety Data Sheet. Details are given by Schuhmacher-Wolz et al. (10).

For the present context only hazardous chemicals that show systemic health effects after uptake are relevant. Intrinsic toxicity scores are based on R-phrases.

The toolkit contains tables for applying the intrinsic toxicity (IT) ranking to dilutions with water. Some suggestions are given for checking the validity of the given information with simple measures, and for adapting the IT scores if additional research indicates this to be necessary, e.g., in the case of low skin permeation coefficients.

Dermal exposure needs to be assessed in three steps, where only two of these are relevant for chemicals with local health effects.

A chemical reaching the outer envelope of the body leads to a *potential exposure*. Potential dermal exposure may occur via three different routes—direct contact to the chemical, contact to contaminated surfaces (e.g., tools, tables, walls), and contact to an aerosol after deposition onto the body.

If the exposed area is not covered, then this potential exposure equals the *actual exposure* because all of the substance approaching the outer envelope of the body will reach the skin. Clothing or protective equipment (e.g., gloves, aprons, helmets) may retain a significant portion of that amount, depending on the percentage of coverage, the thickness of the clothing, and the physical state of the challenge chemical (dust or liquid).

Internal exposure describes the amount that is estimated to be absorbed through the skin. The rate of uptake is not known in many cases. Where it is known, the percutaneous uptake rate is highly variable, depending on the specific exposure conditions, carrier effects, and individual skin properties. Because of this, in many cases a "worst-case" assumption of 100% absorption is used within the toolkit, and the internal exposure then equals the actual exposure or is of the same order of magnitude. But for a limited number of chemicals with low skin penetration, the toolkit considers internal exposure to be lower than actual exposure.

Internal exposure is then related to standard body weight by dividing the internal exposure by the standard weight of an adult person (70 kg)—the unit then is mg/kg.

The basic procedures are handled differently for substances that exhibit mainly local health or systemic effects after percutaneous uptake, respectively.

The exposure situations existing in the field are grouped into the six DEO units, and each of these is subdivided into handling a liquid or solid chemical. The published and experimental data are analyzed for typical potential exposure rates for the whole body and for the hand, and for the corresponding conditions of exposure. An initial assessment of the assigned default potential exposure rates to the DEO units from an analysis of these data is given by Warren et al. (11). In addition, relative contributions were determined for the different routes of exposure (direct contamination, surface contamination, and deposition) for each DEO unit. These default values do not apply to all real situations because the specific exposure conditions may deviate from those conditions that are correlated with the default exposure values. Marquart et al. (12) analyzed how exposure is modified by different exposure conditions, called determinants of exposure. Goede et al. (13) described the magnitude of the effect that these determinants have on exposure. They derived a list of modifying factors (e.g., handling large amounts or small amounts of a chemical) for multiplication of the default exposure. They also showed that the impact of these modifiers on exposure is dependent on the three routes of exposure (direct contact, surface contact, or exposure by deposition). Some determinants, expected to have a certain influence on exposure, are not on the list of modifiers for practical reasons. It was judged impossible to integrate these factors without a measurement or other action that most users of the toolkit will not be able to do. This increases the imprecision of the approach. Nevertheless, the sum of the remaining variables will allow a rough estimate of exposure.

The toolkit then takes the default potential exposure rate for the chosen standard situation (DEO unit), corrects it by multiplication with the modifiers, and generates a potential exposure rate that is specific to the situation under investigation.

Within the toolkit the potential exposure rate and the actual exposure rate of the situation under investigation are determined by selecting a default that then is multiplied with modifying factors. The actual exposure rate was selected as a best estimate of the exposure rate and is assigned to the exposure rate score. This value is modified for chemicals that show low skin penetration. The toolkit will assign low skin penetration if the chemical is among the following categories:

- Solids, dusts
- Gasses
- Substances that show a low solubility in the stratum corneum (SC) (as indicated by a molecular weight > 500 KDa, octanol–water coefficient $P_{o/w} < -1$ or > 5, or permeability $K_p < 0.0010$ cm/hr).

The activity time is handled in a nonlinear manner to reflect the fact that there is a certain threshold before a substance passes through intact skin. On the other hand, skin may become damaged and thus more permeable in many cases when uptake occurs over a long time (hours). Time is ranked and multiplied with the exposure rate score giving the exposure score.

TABLE 1 Health Risk Score for Substances with Systemic Health Effects after Percutaneous Uptake

Internal exposure score (systemic)	Hazard score (systemic)				
	Low (no risk)	Moderate	High	Very high	Extreme
Negligible	1	1	2	5	8
Low	1	2	5	8	10
Moderate	2	3	6	8	10
High	2	4	6	8	10
Very high	3	7	7	9	10
Extreme	7	9	9	9	10

Note: 1, no action; 2, no special measures to be taken, basic skin care; 3, exposure reduction, if easily accomplished; 4, action necessary: primarily exposure reduction to be considered; 5, hazard reduction desirable; 6, action necessary: mixture of measures, priority for detailed analyses; 7, exposure reduction urgent; 8, only exceptionally tolerable, substitute, if possible; 9, reduce exposure drastically, stop working; 10, substitute, stop working.

The toolkit combines the hazard score and the exposure score into a health risk score as given in Table 1. This is not the result of pure science but rather a matter of ethical and political decision as to whether a certain risk is accepted or not. The table was established by agreement between the participants in the process.

Considerations on Risk

Low exposure to very hazardous chemicals may still pose a problem, whereas some exposure to low hazard chemicals may be acceptable. When considering substitution of a hazardous chemical with one of lower toxicity, it is essential to investigate whether the use patterns of the new substance will result in higher exposures, and would that offset the effect of the lower toxicity and give a higher overall risk.

If the resulting risk is sufficiently low, then the risk assessment will not lead to further requirements. If this does not hold, then an application of further control action may reduce the risk to an acceptable level.

The toolkit in its present form is available at (14) and a full description of all aspects of the initial version is available in the *Annals of Occupational Hygiene* (3). Further details are given in the "Deliverables of the RISKOFDERM Project" (obtainable from J. J. van Hemmen). As a further development, the toolkit approach for dermal exposure may be combined with the Stoffenmanager approach [substance manager, (15)] for inhalation exposure at TNO in the Netherlands. This tool is currently being validated with field measurements.

Hazard and Risk Assessment

As indicated above, hazard and exposure are very important components for the risk assessment. For dermal exposure, the degree of absorption is also of key importance for internal exposure assessment and thus for systemic health risks. The RISKOFDERM project has delivered dermal exposure loading data that cover full shifts and differentiate between hand and body exposure. Quantitative data are only produced by the dermal model. The underlying database has, in addition to this, data that are differentiated with respect to body area, i.e., upper arms, forearms, torso, back, and legs (upper and lower). Reviewing the data, it appears that during a wiping scenario (using a cloth) the exposure to the hands generates almost 50% of the total dermal exposure loading. In another scenario (mixing and loading), this is about 10%.

Another important issue of concern is that the exposure loading data cover long periods and does not consider the loading process over time, nor decontamination. The data also cover large body parts and give average figures for that body part, which does not take into account dosage over smaller areas, a fact that is an important determinant of the degree of absorption.

In the toolkit, dermal absorption is treated very conservatively, since the labeling, which is the starting point for the toolkit as far as hazard identification is concerned, do not give information on degree of absorption.

In the current risk assessment approach for pesticides (16), a worst-case value for dermal absorption of 100% is often used when no relevant data are available. This guidance document states that for ongoing evaluations where no measured data are available, a default value of 10% may be used in the risk assessment by the Rapporteur Member State for the purpose of deciding on "one safe use" in accordance with article 5(1) "unless there are clear indications that 10% would be unrealistically low (e.g., based on physical chemical properties of the active substance)."

To qualify for default values of 10%, the following criteria have to be matched:

Molecular weight > 500 and $\log K_{ow} < -1$ or > 4.

It is important to emphasize that this is a conservative cutoff value rather than a quantitative prediction, and that experimental data override these conservative default values for risk assessment purposes. Furthermore, for any type of information on dermal absorption, the data should be related to relevant exposure conditions, since absorption rates can vary considerably depending on the concentrations, amounts, or formulation applied.

Risk Management

Risk management aims to reduce risk. This is best done by reducing the source strength of the exposure and, if necessary, by wearing protective clothing and gloves. In risk assessment, exposure reduction by personal protective measures is done using default reduction factors, which relate to the nature of the material, the quality of the garment ensemble, and the personal hygiene of the worker. Worst-case assumptions are taken. These default values are not consistent between the various national competent authorities involved and proper scientific data to substantiate the selected values are often lacking.

An integral approach to assess the degree of uptake through the skin (and other routes of exposure) uses biomonitoring studies under realistic conditions of work, including the protective measures that are used in the field. Some experience has been obtained for pesticides and biocides (17,18). This approach, however, requires for registration purposes that the biomonitoring data can be interpreted on the basis of human pharmacokinetics, or in special cases (but less accurate) on animal data.

In the above description of the RISKOFDERM project including the developed tools, the toolkit and its approach for the assessment of risk for human exposed to chemicals, it is obvious that this method aims at the establishment of the external exposure risk rather than on internal exposure or systemic absorption.

This approach is certainly not a disadvantage and is more practically related since it is not realistically possible to predict the risk in a more appropriate manner when all relevant data are available. This situation holds for the majority of chemical substances that are on the market. However, it is sometimes necessary to have a more precise indication of risk in terms of internal exposure or systemic absorption which is based on, e.g., work-related situations, skin-related parameters, and physical–chemical properties of the substance under investigation. This requires a more thorough investigation of the various work-related and in vivo factors that may play an important role in uptake via the skin and contribute significantly to the systemic absorption.

IN VIVO FACTORS AND WORK PRACTICE SITUATIONS

Dermal (percutaneous, skin) absorption is a global term that describes transport of chemicals from the outer surface of the skin to the systemic circulation. Dermal absorption can occur after chemical exposure in occupational situations and also after exposure to consumer products or the environment. There are many parameters influencing skin absorption; those dealing with the in vivo situation are discussed below (Table 2).

Species

For regulatory purposes, many dermal absorption studies are performed in experimental animals, most often the rat (19). However, there are obvious and significant differences between the dermal absorption observed in laboratory

TABLE 2 Some Important Considerations in Dermal Absorption

System components	Factors
Test compound	Physical state
	Molecular size
	Lipid–water partition coefficient
	Ionization
	Local skin effects
Skin (sections 3.1–3.3)	Species
	Skin condition
	Temperature and blood flow
	Anatomical site
	Hydration
	Occlusion
	Biotransformation
	Desquamation
Vehicle	Solubility
	Volatility
	Distribution in stratum corneum
	Excipients
	Effect on the stratum corneum
	pH
Application dose	Concentration
	Skin area dose [film thickness, (in)finite dose]
	Total skin area exposed
	Duration of exposure

animals to that in human. For the majority of chemicals, the skin of laboratory animals is considerably more permeable (20,21), and in general the following rank order is observed: rabbit >rat >guinea pig >human. It is also known that data from rat studies generally considerably overestimate human skin absorption (21), a factor of 9 is not unusual, but there are some cases where rat skin is less permeable than that of humans (22). Walters and Roberts (23) reported that differences in the lipid content, structure, and thickness of the SC are important factors explaining these species differences. Furthermore, the skin of laboratory animals has a much greater number of appendageal openings per unit surface area than human skin. This phenomenon may be an additional causative factor for compounds for which appendageal transport may be significant. It is generally accepted that the skin of pigs has similar penetration characteristics to human skin (24).

Skin Condition

Skin condition can have a significant impact on the penetration and permeation of chemicals, especially when the barrier function is disrupted. The permeability of the skin can be increased by physical (e.g., weather, sunlight, occlusion, abrasion), chemical (e.g., solvents detergents, acids, and alkalines), and pathological factors (e.g., mechanical damage, state of disease). Moreover, the skin may be delipidized by mixtures of polar and nonpolar solvents and vehicles such as acetone and ethanol, which result in a substantial reduction of the barrier function of the skin and therefore to a larger skin absorption for many substances. Also, inherited genetic skin diseases with known defects in lipid metabolism producing scaly or ichthyotic skin may dramatically influence the skin absorption process.

Temperature and Blood Flow

Skin temperature can have an impact on the rate of penetration of chemicals in two different ways. Firstly, increasing the temperature of the skin has been shown to increase the rate of penetration by a direct effect on the diffusion within the skin. Temperature can also affect the structure of the SC, particularly of the crystalline structure of lipid bilayers, which can lead to higher permeability. Secondly, temperature may affect blood flow to the skin. However, this will only affect the amount of chemical absorbed if clearance by the blood is rate limiting. Clearance into the blood is only occasionally rate limiting. If the skin is cold, cutaneous blood flow will decrease and the penetration rate through the skin can be larger than the rate of clearance. Otherwise, blood clearance is controlling for chemicals that penetrate the skin rapidly but absorb into the blood slowly. This may be the case for small molecules that are moderately lipophilic.

Effect of Hydration

Normally the SC contains 5% to 15% water, but when the SC is fully hydrated this percentage can be increased up to 50% (25), a situation that can directly affect the permeability of the skin to chemicals. It has been suggested that increasing hydration increases the absorption of all substances that penetrate the skin. However, increasing skin hydration (due to occlusion) does not always increase penetration rates. For example, it has been reported that hydration diminished the penetration rate of hydrophilic compounds such as hydrocortisone (log $K_{ow} = 1.61$).

TABLE 3 Relationship Between Environmental Relative Humidity, Skin Moisture, and Dermal Absorption

Environmental relative humidity (%)	Δ Skin moisture (AU)	% of the dermal dose excreted
50	17	13
70	30	33
90	40	63

In contrast, Wurster and Kramer (26) observed that occlusive coverings that prevented water loss increased the dermal absorption of some hydrophilic compounds. Meuling et al. (27) demonstrated that in dermal absorption studies with the fungicide propoxur under controlled temperature conditions (25°C) with variable controlled relative humidities (50%, 70%, and 90%) in the same subjects, systemic absorption was influenced dramatically. They concluded that environmental humidity directly influenced the skin moisture, which in turn influenced the skin penetration and thus the systemic absorption (Table 3).

Since elevated environmental humidity occurs in various occupational situations (e.g., in greenhouses) and that agricultural workers perform many of their daily tasks bare handed, it was concluded that this phenomenon should be taken into account in the risk assessment procedure for new and existing chemicals.

Occlusion

The normal dermal exposure situation is most accurately simulated using open unoccluded conditions because, in most instances, human skin may be protected but not occluded during exposure. In certain cases, occlusion will be more representative for occupational exposure (e.g., protective gloves). Unoccluded conditions can avoid the skin barrier modulation caused by excessive hydration that, in most cases, increases the penetration rate (28). Experiments performed by Meuling et al. (29) showed that occlusion had a significant effect during skin penetration studies performed with the fungicide propoxur. In these experiments propoxur, which is a relatively hydrophilic compound (log $P_{o/w}$ 1.56) was applied onto the volar aspect of the forearm (100 cm^2) under various conditions: (*i*) open unoccluded (Fig. 1A), (*ii*) the treated area was covered with aluminum foil directly after application of propoxur (Fig. 1B), and (*iii*) aluminum foil plus a protective sleeve of cotton wool (Fig. 1C).

It was reported that occlusion resulted in an approximately 11-fold increase in propoxur absorption (Fig. 2).

In contrast when similar experiments were performed with the fungicide carbendazim, the influence of occlusion was negligible. The latter is not explained by differences in the molecular weight (propoxur=209; carbendazim=191), but predominantly by the fact that carbendazim is a lipophilic substance compared with propoxur, which is more hydrophilic (30).

It is important to appreciate that volatile substances may evaporate during unoccluded testing, and, because of the dosage regimen, infinite dosing experiments with such substances to determine permeability coefficients (K_p) can only be done under occluded conditions (19).

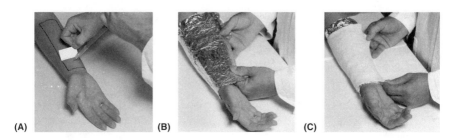

FIGURE 1 Application of a solution onto the forearm to study the effect of maximal occlusion. (A) Example of the non-occluded open situation. (B) Covering the applied area with aluminum foil. (C) Extra protection by a cotton wool sleeve over the aluminum foil.

Occlusive Effects of Clothing and Gloves in Occupational Situations

In occupational scenarios, increased percutaneous absorption rates were seen for 2-butoxyethanol vapors under raised temperature and humidity conditions (31). The mean "baseline" (25°C, 40% relative humidity, shorts, and T-shirts) dermal absorption was 11% (range 9–14%) of the "whole-body" burden. At 30°C, dermal absorption was significantly increased with a mean of 14% (range 12–15%). In a large European Union project (2000), the "Assessment of Operator, Bystander, and Environmental Exposure to Pesticides (SMT4-CT96-2048)," the effect of elevated temperatures (25°C vs. 30°C) and elevated environmental humidity (50% vs. 75%) in a human volunteer study with malathion was investigated. These occupational agricultural conditions are daily common practice in the southern parts of Europe. It was observed that the dermal absorption of malathion under these elevated work-related conditions was increased by a factor of 2.

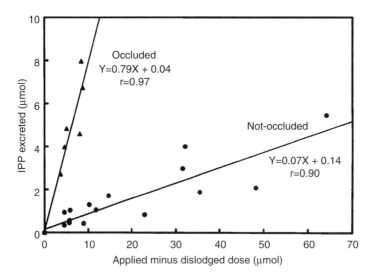

FIGURE 2 Influence of occlusion for the fungicide propoxur. Non-occluded versus occluded results of the excretion of the metabolite 2-isopropoxyphenol (IPP).

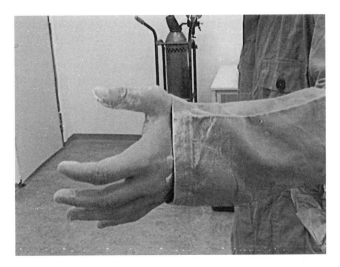

FIGURE 3 Handling dusts (mixing and loading). Note the hand exposure and the dust underneath the sleeve of the overall.

Others have reported that increasing the humidity increased, although not always significantly, the percentage dermal absorption. During the performance of tasks such as handling of dusts, it was observed that after work was terminated the hands of the workers remained contaminated and that the inside of the sleeves of protective overalls was also contaminated (Fig. 3).

This may be denoted as an occlusive situation that may lead to an increased dermal absorption. This study showed that wearing protective gloves during work did not guarantee a lack of skin exposure. Rawson et al. (32) showed that gloves are often internally contaminated and that this contamination may lead to increased dermal absorption due to the partial occlusive effects. This also holds for investigations conducted among agricultural workers in which mixing and loading of chemicals was performed wearing protective gloves (33). This result led to the instruction that gloves should be used only once and discarded after use. In various simulated "industrial" scenarios (20°C, 30°C, 60–65% relative humidity, use of overalls), skin absorption as a percentage of the whole-body burden was significantly increased compared with the baseline dermal study and when compared with any single parameter change. By combining several factors, skin absorption could account for 39% (33–42%) of the total body burden (31,34).

Influence of the Anatomical Site

It has been known for many years that the anatomical site can have a marked effect on the rate and extent of dermal absorption. Feldmann, Maibach, and Wester have reported that percutaneous absorption varied significantly depending on the site of the body (Fig. 4) (35,36) There was also considerable variability at a given site and within and between individuals.

In a human volunteer study, skin exposure of four pesticides (malathion, deltamethrin, captan, *ortho*-phenylphenol) on relevant occupational exposed skin regions (forearm, V-neck, forehead, and lower leg) mimicking the agricultural

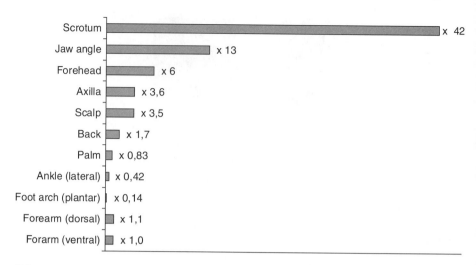

FIGURE 4 Hydrocortisone absorption—effect of anatomic region. *Source*: Adapted from Ref. 35.

working conditions, variable results were obtained relative to the forearm for all four substances and for the different anatomical regions (Table 4) (37).

It is obvious, from these data, that the anatomical site where occupational exposure may occur can have a significant influence on the contribution of the skin penetration process to overall systemic absorption. Therefore, knowledge of the impact of these types of effects is necessary and should be investigated and taken into account in the risk assessment process.

SUMMARIZING FACTS

The approach used to assess the risks for human exposed to chemicals is primarily set up in an easy, but rather conservative way, using various worst-case default values. The strength of the RISKOFDERM method lies in the fact that it can easily be used by trained assessors, gives uniform information on substances, and can be applied to the large number of new and existing chemicals. If additional information on substances is required, e.g., internal exposure data, then specific work-related conditions and the various skin parameters that affect the absorption process have to be taken into account. An integral approach to assess the degree of uptake through the skin in practice uses biomonitoring studies under realistic conditions of work and protective measures. Proper interpretation of these data,

TABLE 4 Influence of Skin Region on the Dermal Absorption of Four Pesticides

Substance	V-neck	Forehead	Lower leg	Forearm
Malathion	0.2	0.9	1	1
Captan	0.3	0.6	0.4	1
o-Phenylphenol	1.1	1.2	0.9	1
Deltamethrin	0.4	0.4	0.3	1

Note: The results are expressed as the ratio relative to the forearm.

however, requires information on potential uptake via other routes of exposure (inhalation, oral) and human pharmacokinetics. Since this information is often lacking and is costly to obtain, most effort should be given to the establishment of more realistic default values for external skin exposure and skin absorption. To bring the field forward, leaders in these fields of expertise should work closely together to develop more realistic default values and more reliable predictive tools.

REFERENCES

1. OECD. Guidance Document for the Conduct of Studies of Occupational Exposure to Pesticides During Agricultural Application. OECD Environmental Health and Safety Publications, Series on Testing and Assessment No. 9, OECD/GD, Paris, France, 1997:14–8.
2. Benford DJ, Cocker J, Sartorelli P, et al. The dermal route in systemic exposure. Scand J Work Environ Health 1999; 25(6):511–20.
3. Annals of Occupational Hygiene 2003, 47, 595–652. 2004, 48, 183–297. 2006, 50, 469–503. Series of publications on results of the RISKOFDERM project.
4. Marquart H, Warren ND, Laitinen J, et al. Default values for the assessment of potential dermal exposure of the hands to industrial chemicals in the scope of regulatory risk assessments. Ann Occup Hyg 2006; 50:469–89.
5. Cherrie JW, Hughson GW. The validity of the EASE expert system for inhalation exposure. Ann Occup Hyg 2005; 49:125–34.
6. Warren ND, Marquart H, Christopher Y, et al. Task-based dermal exposure models for regulatory risk assessment. Ann Occup Hyg 2006; 50:491–503.
7. Cherrie JW, Schneider T. Validation of a new method for structured subjective assessment of past concentrations. Ann Occup Hyg 1999; 43:235–45.
8. Northage C. Easing into the future. Ann Occup Hyg 2005; 49:99–102.
9. Oppl R, Kalberlah F, Evans PG, et al. A toolkit for dermal risk assessment and management: an overview. Ann Occup Hyg 2003; 47:641–52.
10. Schumacher-Wolz U, Kalberlah F, Oppl R, et al. A toolkit for dermal risk assessment: toxicological approach for hazard characterization. Ann Occup Hyg 2003; 47:641–52.
11. Warren N, Goede HA, Tijssen SCHA, et al. Deriving default dermal exposure values for use in a risk assessment toolkit for small and medium-sized enterprises. Ann Occup Hyg 2003; 47:619–27.
12. Marquart H, Brouwer DH, Gijsbers, et al. Determinants of dermal exposure relevant for exposure modelling in regulatory risk assessment. Ann Occup Hyg 2003; 47:599–607.
13. Goede H, Tijssen SCHA, Schipper HJ, et al. Classification of dermal exposure modifiers and assignment of values for a risk assessment toolkit. Ann Occup Hyg 2003; 47:609–18.
14. www.eurofins.com/research_occ_hygiene (Accessed September 2007)
15. www.stoffenmanager.nl (Accessed September 2007)
16. European Commission. Guidance document on dermal absorption, Sanco/222/2000, Rev. 7 2004:1–15.
17. Brouwer DH, Vreede JAF de, Meuling WJA, et al. Determination of the efficiency for pesticide exposure reduction with protective clothing: a field study using biological monitoring in worker exposure to agrichemicals. In: Honeycutt HC, ed. ACS Symposium Series. Baton Rouge, LA: CRC/Lewis Publishers, 2000:65–86.
18. van der Jagt K, Tielemans E, Links I, et al. Effectiveness of personal protective equipment: relevance of dermal and inhalation exposure to chlorpyrifos among pest control operators. J Occup Env Hyg 2004; 1:355–62.
19. OECD. OECD Guideline for the Testing of Chemicals. Skin Absorption: In Vitro Method, Test No. 428. Adopted on April 13, 2004:1–8.
20. Tregear RT. The permeability of skin to molecules of widely differing properties. In: Rook A, Champion RH, eds. Progress in Biological Sciences in Relation to Dermatology. 2nd ed. Cambridge, U.K.: Cambridge University Press, 1964:275–81.
21. ECETOC. Percutaneous absorption. European Centre for Ecotoxicology and Toxicology of Chemicals, Brussels, Monograph 20, 1993:1–80.

22. Hotchkiss SAM, Hewitt P, Caldwell J, et al. Percutaneous absorption of nicotinic acid, phenol, benzoic acid and triclopyr butoxyethyl ester through rat and human skin in vitro: further validation of an in vitro model by comparison with in vivo data. Food Chem Toxicol 1992; 30:891–9.

23. Walters KA, Roberts MS. The structure and function of skin. In: Walters KA, ed. Dermatological and Transdermal Formulations. New York: Marcel Dekker, 2002:1–39.

24. SCCP. Scientific, Committee on Consumer Products. Basic criteria for the in vitro assessment of dermal absorption of cosmetic ingredients. Document. SCCP/0790/06 Adopted by the SCCP on March 28, 2006.

25. Bouwstra JA, Graaff A de, Gooris GS, et al. Water distribution and related morphology in human stratum corneum at different hydration levels. J Invest Dermatol 2003; 120(5):750–8.

26. Wurster DE, Kramer SF. Investigation of some factors influencing percutaneous absorption. J Pharm Sci 1961; 50:288–93.

27. Meuling WJA, Franssen ACh, Brouwer DH, et al. The influence of skin moisture on the dermal absorption of propoxur in human volunteers. A consideration for biological monitoring practices. Sci Total Environ 1997; 199:165–72.

28. Bronaugh RL, Stewart RF. Methods for in vitro percutaneous absorption studies IV: the flow-through diffusion cell. J Pharm Sci 1985; 74:64–7.

29. Meuling WJA, Bragt PC, Leenheers LH, et al. Dose-excretion study with the insecticide propoxur in volunteers. In: Scott RC, Guy RH, Hadgraft J, Boddé HE, eds. Prediction of Percutaneous Penetration. Vol 2.. London: IBC Technical Services Ltd, 1991:13–9.

30. Meuling WJA, Opdam JJG, de Kort WLA. Dose excretion study with the fungicide carbendazim in volunteers. In: Brain KR, James VJ, Walters KA, eds. Prediction of Percutaneous Penetration. Prediction of Percutaneous Penetration. Vol. 3b. London: IBC Technical Services Ltd, 1993:598–603.

31. Jones K, Cocker J. A human exposure study to investigate biological monitoring methods for 2-butoxyethanol. Biomarkers 2003; 8(5):360–70.

32. Rawson BV, Cocker J, Evans PG, et al. Internal contamination of gloves: routes and consequences. Ann Occup Hyg 2005; 49(6):535–41.

33. Brouwer R, van Maarleveld K, Meuling WJA, et al. Dose-excretion study with the pesticide propoxur. Part ll. A field study. Hum Exp Toxicol 1993; 12(1):61.

34. Jones K, Cocker J, Dodd LJ, et al. Factors affecting the extent of dermal absorption of solvent vapours: a human volunteer study. Ann Occup Hyg 2003; 47(2):145–50.

35. Feldman RJ, Maibach HI. Regional variation in percutaneous penetration of ^{14}C cortisol in man. J Invest Dermatol 1967; 48:181–3.

36. Wester RC, Maibach HI. Structure-activity correlations in percutaneous absorption. In: Bronaugh R, Maibach HI, eds. Percutaneous Absorption. New York: Marcel Dekker, 1985:107–23.

37. Meuling WJA, Engel R, Hemmen JJ van. The influence of the skin region on the dermal absorption of four pesticides: a human volunteer study. In: XI Symposium Pesticide Chemistry, Cremona, Italy, 1999.

19 Quantitative Structure–Activity Relationships for Skin Corrosivity and Sensitization

Mark T. D. Cronin, Steven J. Enoch, and Judith C. Madden
School of Pharmacy and Chemistry, Liverpool John Moores University, Liverpool, U.K.

INTRODUCTION

The effect a chemical exerts on a system is dependent on its structure and properties. If one can determine the nature of this dependence, then models may be constructed to allow for extrapolation of this knowledge to other chemicals. Broadly speaking, this is the basis of (quantitative) structure–activity relationships [(Q)SARs] whereby knowledge of a chemical's structure and its properties is related to its effects. When this knowledge is applied to toxicological endpoints, this helps to reduce testing requirements. The science of (Q)SAR in toxicology is now a broad area including SARs, QSARs, expert systems, read across, analogs, and categories. It is variously known as computational toxicology, predictive toxicology, and in silico toxicology, amongst other descriptions. For a more detailed review of the area, the reader is referred to recent volumes edited by Cronin and Livingstone (1) and Helma (2).

At the most fundamental level SARs determine structural features (such as fragments within the molecule) that produce a specific effect. When formalized, for instance into an expert system, fragments identified in a query molecule can assist in the identification of hazardous compounds. It is obvious to say that QSARs are more "quantitative" in nature. This means that they are usually developed for series of compounds and attempt to relate some measure (or estimate) of physico-chemical and/or structural properties of molecule to activity. Within the area of toxicological (Q)SARs there is an immense breadth and diversity of approaches and modeling techniques.

There are clear motivations for developing alternatives to whole animal tests in toxicology, with computational predictions being particularly attractive. Cronin (3) describes a number of such motivations including animal welfare and savings in time and money. In addition, the past few years has seen an increase in interest in predictive toxicology as a response to the requirements of new legislation. In particular in Europe, the Registration, Evaluation and Authorization of Chemicals (REACH) system (4), as well as the Cosmetics Directive(s) (5). The past uses and future possibilities of the use of (Q)SARs to predict toxicity and fate endpoints for regulatory purposes are described by Cronin et al. (6,7) and Cronin (8).

Amongst the human toxicological endpoints for which predictive methods are available, dermal toxicities are well represented. The aim of this chapter is, however, restricted to describe (Q)SARs and computational approaches to predict skin corrosivity and skin sensitization. Other endpoints, for instance skin irritation, are dealt with separately in this volume (see Chapters 29 and 30).

SKIN CORROSIVITY

With regard to modeling any toxicological endpoint, it is always preferable to consider first the mechanism of action. Subsequent (Q)SAR analysis should then try to explicitly include this mechanistic information (9). Chemically induced skin corrosion is associated with the destruction and irreversible alteration of the skin at the site of contact (10). From an extremely simplistic "mechanism of action" point of view, skin corrosion may be thought of as a mechanical or physical destruction of the skin cells. Thus, one would expect models to have some basis in this mechanism. The obvious example would be to identify the structural features associated with strong acids and bases. The reality of modeling skin corrosivity is, however, that it is a complex endpoint, with the possibility of a multitude of mechanisms, some of which will be dependent on the concentration or duration of exposure.

Most skin corrosion data available for modeling are categoric in nature i.e., classification, or positive/negative response data. This has the effect of limiting the number and type of modeling approaches that may be attempted. A further complication is that classifications are usually made according to regulatory guidelines. These may be different between different regulatory authorities, meaning that compilations of data are difficult to achieve. Some data have been brought together by various workers [e.g., Worth (11)].

In terms of modeling, it is trivial to observe that a strong acid or base will be corrosive. Whilst this is true, it can be difficult to define or predict a "strong" acid or base from structure alone (although software to predict pK_a is improving). This has resulted in a number of different approaches to predicting skin corrosivity. First amongst these is the concept of cutoffs for physical properties (a cutoff being an upper or lower limit associated with an activity; the lack of aqueous solubility being an example). Second is the use of structural features associated with corrosion. Finally, there are a small number of "traditional" QSARs relating either to small numbers of related compounds (local QSARs) or larger databases. None of these approaches is ideal to predict skin corrosion in isolation, and an integrated approach would be better (see Chapter 33).

Simple cutoffs for skin corrosivity can be developed on the basis of fundamental physico-chemical properties. These are often simple "if-then" rules, which are easy to computerize. An example is given by Worth (11) who describes the formation of a number of classification models for skin corrosion. The most mechanistically relevant of these is based on the pH of a 10% solution of the chemical:

If pH < 3.9 or pH > 10.5 then predict corrosive, otherwise predict noncorrosive.

The use of pH as a model for corrosion is described by Worth and Cronin (12). Unfortunately, for a structure-based prediction, this usually requires a measurement to be made (thus eliminating some of the advantages of a structure-based assessment). Further cutoff values for skin corrosion are described by Worth (11).

One of the most significant developments in the prediction of dermal toxicity has been decision support system (DSS) for skin irritation and corrosion developed at the German Bundesinstitut für Risikobewertung (BfR) (13–16). The overall system is well described by Gerner (see Chapter 33). The DSS is an automated tool that includes the BfR rulebase. It is designed for regulatory application. The rulebase predicts non-irritation and non-corrosion using physico-chemical cutoff values after defining general rules applicable to all substances and separate rules for special chemical classes of substances. It also predicts corrosion based on the presence of structural alerts in a substance (i.e., fragments associated with corrosive materials). What may be considered to be the training set for development of the (Q)SARs in the BfR DSS contains 1358 chemicals, and is taken from the BfR New Chemicals database called ESTOFF (13–15,17).

Recently Rorije and Hulzebos (18) evaluated the BfR DSS according to the OECD Principles for the Validation of QSARs (19). Their report, on the basis of predictions made for over 200 chemicals not included in the original models, gives a detailed analysis of how the DSS works as well as its strengths and weaknesses.

A further series of papers from Walker, Gerner, Hulzebos, and colleagues describes the development of further (Q)SAR approaches for predicting skin corrosion. These approaches are put in the context of regulatory needs for predictions, such as transparency and potential applicability (20). Based on the analyses of 1833 chemicals, Gerner et al. (13) defined limits for physico-chemical properties to determine whether or not a chemical would have no skin corrosion (or irritation) potential. These physico-chemical properties included melting point, molecular weight, octanol–water partition coefficient, surface tension, vapor pressure, aqueous solubility, and lipid solubility. Structural features known to irritate and corrode skin, in addition to physical properties associated with skin absorption, were described by Hulzebos et al. (21,22). The structural features identified included organic acids and bases, aldehydes, halogenated esters, and chemicals with "reactive" (electrophilic) groups. Finally the Skin Irritation Corrosion Rules Estimation Tool (SICRET) was developed to allow for the estimation of whether chemicals are likely to cause skin corrosion (or irritation) (23). SICRET uses physico-chemical property limits to identify chemicals with no skin corrosion. If a chemical's physico-chemical properties do not meet the prescribed limits to identify chemicals with no skin corrosion or skin irritation potential, then the chemical's structural alerts are applied. If a chemical does not contain structural alerts, suggesting it may have skin corrosion potential, then in vitro skin corrosion is conducted. Positive in vitro data are included in feedback loops for development of new structural alerts. As compared to the efforts to elucidate structural alerts associated with skin corrosion, there have been significantly fewer attempts to derive traditional QSAR analyses. This can be attributed to the fact that this is not an ideal endpoint to model, and that it is probable that the better approach to its modeling is through the application of structural alerts. Examples of QSARs include the work of Barratt (24) who used discriminant analysis to obtain a model to separate corrosive from non-corrosive chemicals on the basis of the logarithm of the octanol–water partition coefficient ($\log P$), molecular volume, and dipole moment of some compounds described as "electrophiles." Whittle et al. (25) used QSAR to assess the corrosive potential of a series of fatty acids. Both studies are of interest as they make successful attempts to model skin corrosivity on the basis of a small number of descriptors selected to be mechanistically interpretable.

There are few performance statistics associated with (Q)SARs for skin corrosivity, although the study by Rorije and Hulzebos (18) does provide some very useful indications. Generally, for all approaches, if a compound is predicted to be skin corrosive then there is a high probability that it will have this effect. If it is not, there is less certainty that it is not corrosive. Integration of this type of knowledge into a tiered or integrated testing strategy [cf. Worth (11)] may not completely replace the information it is possible to obtain from animal models, but it will assist in reducing testing and may allow for classification and labeling (i.e., of corrosive chemicals) with no testing.

SKIN SENSITIZATION

Skin sensitization, or allergic contact dermatitis, is an immunologically mediated cutaneous reaction to a substance usually characterized by occurrences such as erythema and edema (see Chapter 20). There are a number of approaches to the structure-based prediction of skin sensitization. The more rational and transparent of these approaches are based strongly on the mechanistic understanding of the immunogenic response that is skin sensitization. At its most fundamental, the mechanistic comprehension is an appreciation that to elicit a response the chemical must penetrate the skin in sufficient quantity to reach an immunoprotein, there it must react with the protein to initiate the immunological response and the immune system must then be stimulated to form the response.

Of these events, reactivity with a protein and the bioavailability of a compound in the skin are, in theory, most amenable to modeling. Efforts to model skin permeability are described elsewhere in this volume (see Chapter 15), although it can be generally concluded that the prediction of skin bioavailability of compounds is at best challenging, if not impossible due to the physiological complexities and practical complicating factors (for example formulation effects, infinite vs. non-infinite dosing, metabolism etc.) (26).

There are a limited number of reviews in skin sensitization QSARs. In order to comprehend this area it worth noting that there are only three significant data sets for modeling, of these, only the first two data sets (27,28) have received concerted attention. These three data sets comprise:

1. The results for over 250 compounds from maximization tests [mainly guinea pig maximization tests (GPMT)] (27)
2. The results for over 200 compounds from the local lymph node assay (LLNA) (28)
3. The assessment and classification for over 230 compounds from German Federal Institute for Health Protection of Consumers and Veterinary Medicine (BgVV) (29)

At least one study (30) has combined all three data sets for modeling resulting in data for 634 chemicals (there is some overlap between databases). There are smaller quantities of data in other publications (although not modeled), and further data sets have been used in QSAR e.g., a human allergen data set (31), but these are not fully described.

Structure–Activity Relationships

The place of SARs for skin sensitization in predictive toxicology is to predict whether or not a compound has the capability to produce the response (which may be mediated, or ameliorated, by other factors such as formulation which could affect skin whether a compound is bioavailable in the skin). The essence of SARs for skin sensitization is that there is a particular fragment of a molecule that is responsible for causing the effect. The vast majority of these fragments are known to be electrophilic in nature, thus this provides an excellent link to mechanism of action through fundamental organic chemistry. The basis for this work can be traced back to the seminal work by Benezra and Dupuis (32). The process of defining these molecular fragments was initiated by Cronin and Basketter (33) and greatly extended by Payne and Walsh (34) and Barratt et al. (35,36) with reference to the maximization database described by Cronin and Basketter (27). The work by Barratt et al. (35,36) formed much of the basis for the rulebase contained within the DEREK for Windows expert system (see later section). These publications were supplemented by Ashby et al. (37). All of these served to confirm and emphasize the mechanistic basis on which predictions should be made, and the overwhelming role of electrophilicity in eliciting the effect.

Mechanistically Derived QSARs

It is worthwhile to separate mechanistic QSARs from SARs, and also multivariate QSARs (see later section). QSARs, in general, for skin sensitization are, as the name would suggest, quantitative models and generally attempt to predict potency, e.g., the concentration causing a stimulation index of 3 in the LLNA (EC3), or strong, moderate, weak, or non-sensitizer from the GPMT, a smaller number of QSARs also provide models to separate sensitizers from non-sensitizers (38,39). The so-called mechanistically derived QSARs described herein are models that are derived from a knowledge of mechanism of action, rather than an ad hoc selection of descriptors to formulate an algorithm which may, or more commonly may not, have mechanistic interpretation forced upon it at a later stage. It is generally considered that a firm basis on mechanism of action is preferable when developing a model (9).

Quantitative prediction of a skin sensitization response is fraught with difficulties. Notable amongst these is the issue that the skin sensitization data available for modeling were not developed for this purpose, rather they were obtained for risk assessment. As a result, there are a variety of vehicles and solvents used. Currently, the relative effect of different vehicles on the sensitization response has not been quantified and is not fully understood. This, therefore, puts another obstacle in the paths of successful and accurate modeling.

Despite the potential pitfalls, there are a number of excellent examples of "mechanistically" derived QSARs for skin sensitization. Limiting factors for eliciting skin sensitization have been shown to be the ability to reach the active site (penetration) and reactivity once at the active site. The clearest and simplest illustration of this concept was provided by Basketter et al. (40) who studied the LLNA EC3 values for a series of bromoalkanes. Within this series, reactivity is kept constant, but transport is considered to vary with alkyl chain length. For this series of compounds, a parabolic relationship is observed with the logarithm of the octanol–water partition coefficient (log P)

$$pEC3 = 1.61 \log P - 0.09 (\log P)^2 - 7.4 \tag{1}$$

$$n = 9 \quad r = 0.97 \quad s = 0.11 \quad F = 50.0$$

where pEC3, the negative logarithm of the molar concentration of the EC3 value; n, the number of observations; r, the correlation coefficient; s, the standard error of the estimate; F, the Fisher statistic.

Clearly equation (1) has a very restricted structural domain of applicability. However, it can be considered to be representative of the S_N2 (nucleophilic substitution by an electrophile at a reactive carbonyl) reaction domain, and so may be more applicable in that domain. Regardless, it is presented merely to emphasize the role of mechanism in developing QSARs for skin sensitization. Prior to the development of equation (1), a more mechanistically embracing concept of modeling was provided by Roberts and Williams (41), namely the relative alkylation index (RAI) model. The RAI was based on the concept that the degree of sensitization produced at induction, and the magnitude of the sensitization response at challenge, depends on the degree of covalent binding (haptenation) to carrier protein occurring at induction and challenge. The RAI is an index of the relative degree of carrier protein haptenation and was derived from differential equations modeling competition between the carrier haptenation reaction in a hydrophobic environment and removal of the sensitizer through partitioning into polar lymphatic fluid. In its most general form the RAI is expressed as

$$RAI = \log D + a \log k + b \log P \tag{2}$$

where D, the dose of the sensitizer; k, the relative rate constant for the reaction of the sensitizer with a model nucleophile.

Thus, in comparing different sensitization test results with the help of the RAI model, the doses, electrophilic reactivities, and hydrophobicities need to be considered. There have been a number of publications illustrating the applicability of the RAI to historical sensitization data e.g., Goodwin et al. (42); Franot et al. (43,44); Roberts et al. (45). Most relevant is the example provided by Roberts and Basketter (46) who described a QSAR based on the RAI for six alkanesulfonates and alkenesulfonates, for a total of 20 data points (representing different doses). These compounds have the general formula RSO_3R' where the Rs are alkyl or alkenyl; they are also considered to fall within the S_N2 reaction domain. Incorporating all dose–response data gave the following model

$$\log SI = 0.39\ RAI + 0.69 \tag{3}$$

$$n = 20 \quad r^2 = 0.930 \quad s = 0.15 \quad F = 240$$

where SI, the stimulation index, which is the ratio of effect in treated mice as compared to the control; r^2, the square of the correlation coefficient adjusted for degrees of freedom.

Equation (3) can be derived into the more usual form for a QSAR, i.e., one data point per compound,

$$pEC20 = 0.74\ RSP - 0.61 \tag{4}$$

$$n = 6 \quad R^2 = 0.994 \quad s = 0.10 \quad F = 702$$

where EC20, defined as the concentration of test chemical to induce a stimulation index of 20 relative to concurrent vehicle treated controls; RSP, the relative sensitization parameter and is calculated in the same way as the RAI but without the a concentration (or dose) term.

An obvious drawback of the RAI approach is the requirement for measured reactivity data. More "classical" studies using traditional QSAR descriptors have also been performed. Mekenyan et al. (47) reanalyzed data previously studied by Roberts (48) for 20 halo-and pseudohalobenzenes that can be considered to fall within the S_NAr electrophilic domain. The compounds were classified as either sensitizers or non-sensitizers according to the differences between the energy of the lowest unoccupied molecular orbital (E_{LUMO}) of the parent compounds and their Meisenheimer complexes, in combination with the maximum acceptor superdelocalizabilities. Other mechanistically derived models for skin sensitization data (EC3 values) from the LLNA include that of Patlewicz et al. (49,50) for aldehydes.

Further QSAR modeling has been performed, albeit with a reduced mechanistic basis. For example Miller et al. (51) obtained the following QSAR to predict the EC3 in the LLNA:

$$EC3 = 9.16\ \text{FPSA2ESP} + 4.29\ E_{\text{HOMO–LUMO}} - 45.9 \tag{5}$$

$$n = 50 \quad R^2_{\text{adj}} = 0.763 \quad F = 79.9$$

where FPSA2ESP, the fractional positively charged surface area descriptor based on electrostatic potential charge; $E_{\text{HOMO–LUMO}}$, the energy gap between Highest Occupied Molecular Orbital (HOMO) and Lowest Unoccupied Molecular Orbital (LUMO).

Equation (5) does provide a simple method to predict EC3, but is not formulated on a molar basis for EC3 and a large number of outliers were removed to create it. Therefore some caution may be required in its application. Despite potential pitfalls in using equation (5) Kostoryz et al. (52) demonstrated that the QSAR predicted potencies for some siloranes were very useful to determine the doses for experimental studies.

Multivariate QSARs

There are a variety of multivariate QSAR models for skin sensitization. Within such modeling approaches there is always a temptation to over-develop models, i.e., include non-mechanistically relevant descriptors to increase statistical fit, and also overtrain models beyond the limits of the biological data. In addition, many methods are non-transparent and a model may not be provided [e.g., the use of support vector machines (SVM), neural networks etc.]. They therefore have little demonstrable purpose.

An early multivariate QSAR for skin sensitization was reported by Cronin and Basketter (27). Using the maximization database they developed a discriminant analysis model to classify chemicals in the data set as either sensitizing or non-sensitizing. The model was based on 14 parameters of which 12 were structural alerts associated with electrophilic reactivity. The model was able to classify 78% of sensitizing and 88% of non-sensitizing compounds correctly.

These data were later assessed using correspondence analysis by Cronin and Dearden (53). This is a little applied, but very useful technique for relating properties to activities. The latter study confirmed the role of structural fragments, relating to reactivity, in controlling activity.

Similar, multivariate QSAR studies were performed by Magee and co-workers on reduced data sets with good success. Magee et al. (54) developed a classification model for 36 non-allergens and 36 allergens using regression analysis based on descriptors for hydrophobicity and hydrogen bonding [equation (6) was developed after the removal of a single outlier].

$$\text{Class} = 0.00974\,\text{MR} - 0.153\,\text{PL} + 0.0468\,\text{HBA} - 0.154\,\text{HBD} - 0.251\,I_{\text{COOR}}$$
$$+ 0.127\,I_X + 0.215\,I_{\text{OH}} + 0.564\,I_{\text{POS}} + 0.465\,I_{\text{QUIN}} + 0.203 \tag{6}$$
$$n = 71 \quad r^2 = 0.677 \quad r = 0.823 \quad s = 0.307 \quad F = 14.19$$

where MR, the molar refraction; PL, the partial log P of lipophilic substructures; HBA, a count of electron pairs on O and N; HBD, a count of OH and NH bonds; I_{COOR}, a count of ester substructures; I_X, a count of reactive halogens; I_{OH}, a count of metabolizable primary hydroxyls; I_{POS}, the sum of counts for double bonds conjugated to C=O or sulfonyl and any other reactive electrophile; I_{QUIN}, the sum of counts for reactive phenolic and aniline rings.

The applicability of the Magee et al. (54) approach was assessed in further studies (55), in particular for the prediction of the sensitization potential of fragrance allergens which were not included in the original model (56). The model was also extended and evaluated by making predictions for 102 diverse structures (51 human sensitizers and 51 non-sensitizers) (57).

The usefulness of the two-value regression approach was also confirmed by Hatch and Magee (58) by the modeling of a much smaller group of anthraquinone disperse dyes (9 actives and 10 inactives). In their study descriptors for reactivity, namely the summation of the Hammett σ constants for the anthraquinone ring substituents combined with the gap between the computed energies of HOMO and LUMO ($E_{HOMO-LUMO}$) of the radical anion, gave an excellent separation of the two classes.

$$\text{Class} = 0.603\ \Delta\text{RAD} - 0.921\ \text{RNG}\sigma - 2.20 \tag{7}$$

$$n = 16 \quad s = 0.267 \quad r^2 = 0.764 \quad F = 21.06$$

where ΔRAD, $E_{LUMORAD} - E_{HOMORAD}$ ($E_{LUMORAD}$ is the AM1 LUMO energy of the radical anion, $E_{HOMORAD}$, the AM1 HOMO energy of the radical anion); RNGσ, the sum of the Hammett σ constant for each of the ring substitution groups of the most electron donating rings

Li et al. (59) developed a random forest, i.e., collection of decision trees, to predict LLNA activity. This approach forms a number of clusters of compounds; however, little evaluation was performed to determine a possible mechanistic insight. Further analyses using (part of) the LLNA data set include that of Ren et al. (60). These authors have demonstrated that a SVM was better able to classify the LLNA response of 131 compounds than a linear discriminant model.

Other approaches to modeling skin sensitization have attempted to include descriptors derived from molecular topology. Estrada and coworkers (61,62) utilized the topological substructural molecular design (TOPS-MODE) methodology. The TOPS-MODE descriptors used were calculated directly from two-dimensional (2D) structure and are spectral moments of a bond matrix weighted for six different physicochemical properties and raised to a different power. These are complex descriptors to visualize and their meaning is difficult to determine. However, it is argued that analysis of the results reveals structural features that are positively (and negatively) associated with skin sensitization. In addition to the creation of models, extraction of structural information may assist in elucidating fragments associated with, or ameliorating, skin sensitization. Estrada et al. (61) further discuss the use of the TOPS-MODE approach to model the EC3 values from the LLNA for 93 compounds. The EC3 values were categorized into bands of potency with a chemical having an EC3 value less than 1% being defined as strong sensitizer, that with an EC3 between 1% and 10% as moderate, 10% and 30% as weak, 30% and 50% as extremely weak and greater than 50% as non-sensitizing. These classifications were combined into two groups with two QSAR models being developed. The first discriminated strong/moderate sensitizers (EC3 < 10%) from all other chemicals and the second discriminated weak sensitizers (10% < EC3 < 30%) from extremely weak and non-sensitizing chemicals (EC3 > 30%). A positive score in model 1 classes a chemical as a strong/moderate sensitizer. A negative score necessitates the need for model 2 to be used. A positive score in model 2 classes a chemical as a weak sensitizer, a negative score as an extremely weak or non-sensitizing chemical. The algorithm is transparent and easy to use as it takes the form of a regression type equation where class is related to various descriptors weighted by coefficients

$$\text{Class 1 model} = (1.331 \times \mu_1^H) - (0.00598 \times \mu_4^H) + (0.0078 \times \mu_2^{PS})$$

$$- (0.00021366 \times \mu_3^{PS}) + (0.0755 \times \mu_1^{MR}) + (0.0319 \times \mu_2^{MR})$$

$$- (0.0011133 \times \mu_5^{Pol}) - (2.3797 \times \mu_1^{Ch}) + (0.1547 \times \mu_3^{Ch})$$

$$+ (0.00425 \times \mu_6^{Ch}) + (2.0932 \times \mu_1^{vDW}) - (0.8683 \times \mu_2^{vDW})$$

$$+ 0.7954 \tag{8}$$

If the value of this model is greater than zero, the compound is classed as a strong/moderate sensitizer. If it is less than zero, the class 2 model is used to distinguish between weak and very weak/non-sensitizing

$$\text{Class 2 model} = (0.946 \times \mu_1^H) - (0.00468 \times \mu_7^H) - (0.894 \times \mu_1^{PS}) + (0.1004 \times \mu_2^{PS})$$

$$- (0.0024 \times \mu_3^{PS}) + (0.0057 \times \mu_3^{Pol}) - (1.429 \times \mu_1^{Ch})$$

$$+ (0.0053 \times \mu_8^{Ch}) - (0.00111 \times \mu_9^{Ch}) - 5.309 \tag{9}$$

where the superscripts indicate atomic contributions to partition coefficients (H); polar surface (PS); molar refraction (MR); polarizability (Pol); charges (CH); and van der Waals forces (vDW).

Whilst transparent models are developed, the TOPS-MODE approach is not necessarily transparent in terms of mechanistic significance. The descriptors are variously considered to parameterize molecular properties such as lipophilicity, polar surface area, van der Waals radii, atomic charges, and polarizability. These may relate to phenomena such as partitioning and reactivity, but the exact meaning is more difficult to determine. Despite these limitations, the model was used to make predictions for, and thus rank, the sensitization potential for 229 substances related to hair dyes (63). In addition, the authors claim that the TOPS-MODE approach is valuable to relate activity to local bond contributions. Specifically this could lead to the formulation of structural rules highlighting fragments and substructural features. For instance, Estrada et al. (62) describe how the TOPS-MODE classification model for skin sensitization led to the development of structural alerts implemented into the DEREK for Windows software (see section Expert Systems to Predict Skin Sensitization).

Expert Systems to Predict Skin Sensitization

(Q)SARs can be formalized into computational systems, often referred to under the broad term "expert systems." Such systems allow the user to input a chemical structure (usually graphically or by the use of a 2D line entry system) and to obtain a prediction, without the need to reformulate the model. Often other information is provided e.g., supporting information such as data for similar compounds or evidence of the mechanistic basis of an effect. The majority of systems are commercial, with only a small number being freely available. Table 1 provides a summary of the major expert systems and their distributor. The expert systems described in Table 1 represent a variety of different approaches, methodologies, and philosophies. Whilst they are mostly straightforward for a non-expert to use, it is preferred that an expert user applies and interprets the results. The information provided in this section is somewhat cursory and the reader is referred to the software suppliers and the references provided for more information. General reviews of expert systems for toxicity prediction (across a number of endpoints) are given by Greene (69) and Helma (2).

DEREK

The DEREK for Windows software is a knowledge-based expert system for the prediction of toxicological hazard [for an overview the reader is referred to Sanderson and Earnshaw (70); Greene et al. (71); Combes and Rodford (72)]. To make predictions DEREK for Windows uses a knowledge base, which contains alerts describing structure–toxicity relationships, with an emphasis on the understanding of mechanisms of toxicity and metabolism. The software identifies the toxicophore, or substructure associated with toxicity, and highlights this to the user with a brief statement about the hazard it represents. The user can also access additional information concerning the structure–toxicity relationship including literature references and supporting examples. The DEREK for Windows knowledge base is written and maintained by toxicologists who form a collaborative group comprising agrochemical, pharmaceutical, and regulatory organizations. The skin sensitization rulebase within DEREK for Windows is one of the better developed for a toxicological endpoint. It includes over 60 rules for sensitization, the derivation of many is discussed above [Cronin and Basketter (33); Barratt et al. (35,36); Payne and Walsh (34)]. There have also been efforts to validate the skin

TABLE 1   Details of Selected Commercial and Non-Commercial Expert Systems to Predict Skin Sensitization

Software	Supplier	Brief description of model	Reference
DEREK for Windows	LHASA Limited, Leeds, England	Knowledge-based system	64
TOPKAT	Accelrys Ltd, Oxford, England	QSAR based on (atomic) topological, and other descriptors	65
MultiCASE, CASE, CASETOX etc.	MultiCASE Inc., Beachwood, OH, U.S.A.	QSAR developed from molecular fragments	66
TIMES/OASIS	Laboratory of Mathematical Chemistry, University "Prof. Assen Zlatarov," Bourgas, Bulgaria	Rules to predict skin metabolism linked to QSARs for skin sensitization	67
OECD QSAR Application toolbox	OECD, Paris, France	Read across using existing data, categories, and mechanisms	68

Abbreviations: CASE, Computer-Automated Structure Evaluation; MultiCASE, Multiple Computer-Automated Structure Evaluation; OECD, Organisation for Economic Development and Co-operation; QSAR, quantitative structure–activity relationships; TIMES, tissue metabolism simulator.

sensitization of the DEREK rulebase [e.g., Barratt and Langowski (73); Zinke et al. (74)]. Most recently there have been improvements to the rulebase for skin sensitization. These include modifications to the alerts describing the skin sensitization potential of aldehydes, 1,2-diketones, and isothiazolinones and consist of enhancements to the toxicophore definition, the mechanistic classification, and the extent of supporting evidence provided [Langton et al. (75)].

MultiCASE

The Multiple Computer-Automated Structure Evaluation (MultiCASE) methodology predicts toxicity by the creation and detection of structural alerts [for an overview the reader is referred to Klopman (76); Klopman and Rosenkranz (77); and Greene (69)]. To achieve this, the structure of each molecule is divided up into all possible fragments, from two heavy (non-hydrogen) atoms in length to potentially any number of atoms (although, in practice, the use of fragments greater than six atoms is unwieldy). Statistical methods are then used to classify the fragments as biophores or biophobes, according to whether they are associated with the biological activity of interest, or no activity, respectively. The fragments are then combined to give an equation of the following form

$$\text{CASE units} = \text{constant} + a\,[\text{Fragment 1}] + b\,[\text{Fragment 2}] + \cdots \tag{10}$$

To work optimally MultiCASE requires a large and (chemically and mechanistically) heterogeneous database of toxicity data. The MultiCASE approach can produce a quantitative model, even from data which would normally be considered qualitative. In terms of skin sensitization Graham et al. (31) describe the MultiCASE model for skin sensitization. The data base was derived from reports of animal and human studies for 1034 chemicals of which 317 were classified as sensitizers, 22 chemicals had marginal activity, and 695 were inactive. MultiCASE identified 49 biophores with related expanded fragments which accounted for the activity of all active chemicals. The major biophores were predominantly related to electrophilic moieties.

TOPKAT

TOPKAT predicts a number of toxicological endpoints, it contains algorithms that relate structural properties of a series of chemicals to their biological activity [for an overview the reader is referred to Enslein et al. (78) and Greene (69)]. The structural properties are typically calculated from 2D structure and encode information regarding atoms, fragments, and the whole molecule. Many of these indices are calculated from the knowledge of the molecule's topological and electronic environment (e.g., molecular connectivities, electrotopological state indices etc.). The TOPKAT approach has been applied to both quantitative and qualitative toxicological information. Different statistical techniques, regression, and discriminant analyses, are typically applied to the different data to develop the models.

The skin sensitization module of the TOPKAT package is a suite of two modules. In the non-sensitizers versus sensitizers module, a discriminant analysis model calculates the probability of a submitted structure being a sensitizer or a non-sensitizer. The second module is for the discrimination of strong and weak or moderate sensitizers. The models are developed from the results for 335 compounds [mainly taken from Cronin and Basketter (27)] and are described in more detail by Enslein et al. (79).

TIMES-OASIS

The TIMES-OASIS model for the prediction of skin sensitization comprises a number of different programs. The first is a tissue metabolism simulator (TIMES), which uses a heuristic algorithm to generate plausible metabolic maps from a comprehensive library of biotransformations and abiotic reactions and estimates for system-specific transformation probabilities. The transformation probabilities can be calibrated to specific reference conditions using transformation rate information from systematic testing [Mekenyan et al. (80)]. This simulator contains 203 hierarchically ordered spontaneous and enzyme controlled reactions. Phase I and II metabolism were simulated by using 102 and 9 principal transformations, respectively [Mekenyan et al. (81)]. In addition, a QSAR system for estimating skin sensitization has been developed. It incorporates skin metabolism and considers the potential of parent chemicals and/or their activated metabolites to react with skin proteins. The model is based on the results for over 600 chemicals assigned to one of three classes: significant, weak, or non-sensitizing. The covalent interactions of chemicals and their metabolites with skin proteins were described by 83 reactions that fall within 39 alerting groups. For some alerting groups, 3D-QSARs were developed [Dimitrov et al. (30)].

OECD QSAR Application Toolbox

At the time of writing this chapter, a further tool for toxicity prediction is under development. The so-called "QSAR Application Toolbox" is being developed under the auspices of the Organisation for Economic Co-operation and Development. The Toolbox is aimed at the regulatory assessment of chemicals, with a particular emphasis toward the European Union REACH legislation. The Toolbox will make assessments for a variety of endpoints including skin sensitization. These assessments will allow decisions to be made for risk assessment purposes on the basis of the effects of "similar" chemicals and predictive technologies.

Other Strategies to Predict Skin Sensitization Incorporating QSARs and Reactivity

There is considerable interest in the use of in silico systems, not in isolation, but in combination with other approaches. These include the development of integrated testing strategies and other frameworks. Tools such as the forthcoming OECD QSAR Application Toolbox will be invaluable in this regard. Such strategies foresee the combination of various "alternative" techniques into a tiered approach. The most rational and most likely to succeed approaches to predict skin sensitization are based on a firm mechanistic background.

An approach to predict skin sensitizing potential has been provided by Jowsey et al. (82). This approach provides a framework for not only the identification of skin sensitizing chemicals but also the estimation of relative sensitizing potency. As such it attempts to parameterize the various biological, biochemical, and chemical factors that impact on the allergenic properties of chemicals and the elicitation of skin sensitization, and an ability to measure these in vitro. More specifically, Jowsey et al. (82) propose a scheme to calculate an Index of Sensitizing Potency value from the presence or absence of a structural alert (e.g., from the DEREK for Windows software), bioavailability, protein reactivity, dendritic cell maturation, and T-cell proliferation.

In a related approach, many workers [e.g., Jowsey et al. (82)] are now investigating the role of reactivity in skin sensitization. More specifically, the assumption is that the ability of a chemical to react covalently with a skin protein is one of the determining, or rate-limiting, steps in the elicitation of skin sensitization. It is well appreciated that many skin sensitizers are electrophilic in nature [Payne and Walsh (34)], and many efforts have gone into elucidating mechanisms of action. Most mechanisms can be related back to organic chemistry and have been the basis of a number of in silico studies. Magee and coworkers were amongst the pioneers in attempting to model the relative reactivity of chemicals with skin proteins using quantum chemistry. The study of Hatch and Magee (58) for anthraquinone disperse dyes [equation (7)] is one such example. In addition Magee (83) investigated the effect of structural changes on quinone reactivity with protein end-groups. Using AM1 computational heats of reaction at different positions on quinones with simple models of protein end-groups, the entire chemistry of quinone–nucleophile reactions were well predicted and extrapolations made to sensitization potential. This computational approach was extended by Magee (84) to further groups of compounds. More recently Aptula et al. (85) utilized a novel activation energy index (AEI) to interpret the skin sensitization potential of 5-chloro-2-methylisothiazol-3-one and 2-methylisothiazol-3-one. The AEI was calculated from the knowledge of the energy changes in the frontier molecular orbitals as the electrophile (i.e., the sensitizer) is converted to an anionic intermediate.

Other workers have made efforts to rationalize the mechanistic chemistry behind skin sensitization, placing sensitizers into "mechanisms," rather than chemical classes. The basis of this work goes back to the analysis and mechanistic interpretation of LLNA data by Ashby et al. (37). The mechanisms have been refined more recently by Aptula et al. (86). Subsequently the 106 sensitization data originally described by Ashby et al. (37) have been categorized into the following electrophilic mechanisms by Roberts et al. (87):

- Michael acceptor,
- pro-Michael acceptor,
- S_NAr,
- S_N2,
- Schiff base,
- acyl transfer, and
- non-electrophiles (which are assumed to be nonsensitizers).

Classification of compounds in this manner by Roberts et al. (87) enabled sensitizers to be identified in terms of their mechanistic chemistry alone.

The concepts of mechanistic chemistry applied to skin sensitization have been expanded upon to provide mechanistic domains of applicability. These provide useful indications of how the models may be utilized. For instance, Aptula et al. (88) presented rules, with particular emphasis on reactive toxicity, that were based on organic reaction mechanistic principles. Such rules are able to classify reactive toxicants into their appropriate mechanistic applicability domains which are then related to endpoints such as skin sensitization. Within each mechanistic domain, it may be possible to build separate QSARs to predict potency. For instance, Roberts et al. (89) derived the following model, based on the LLNA EC3, for eleven aliphatic aldehydes, one α-ketoester, and four α,β-diketones. All these compounds were considered to be sensitizers due to their ability to bind covalently to skin proteins via Schiff base formation

$$pEC3 = 1.12 \sum \sigma^* + 0.42 \log P - 0.62 \tag{11}$$

$$n = 16 \quad R^2_{adj} = 0.945 \quad s = 0.12 \quad F = 129.6$$

where $\sum \sigma^*$ is the sum of Taft σ^* values for the two groups R and R' in RCOR'.

The modeling, and prediction from, reactive mechanisms of toxicity shows a very great potential for providing transparent models to replace and reduce animal usage for the assessment of skin sensitization. However, it is restricted in terms of quantitative predictions due to the limitations in modeling (and hence estimating) chemical reactivity. More research is required in this particular area. In order to alleviate this bottleneck some workers are extending the role of experimental measurements of reactivity (termed in chemico assessment). For instance, Aptula et al. (90) described attempts to investigate the relationship between LLNA data and a thiol reactivity index based on glutathione in combination with a measure of cytotoxicity to the ciliate *Tetrahymena pyriformis*. When taken together, the thiol and *T. pyriformis* assays predict the sensitization potential of 23 of the 24 compounds correctly. Efforts are currently underway to replace experimental measurement with calculated values. The principles of utilizing measurements (or estimates) of reactivity to predict toxicity have been placed into a framework by Schultz et al. (91). At the heart of this framework is a firm basis of mechanistic reaction chemistry and how this may relate to plausible "molecular initiating events" resulting in toxicity.

CONCLUSIONS

There is a strong motivation to use (Q)SARs to predict skin toxicity, particularly skin corrosivity and sensitization. Recently the computational prediction of skin sensitization has been the center of much interest and development, particularly due to European legislation such as REACH and the Cosmetics Directive. (Q)SARs are well developed in some areas, but they must be applied with caution and expertise to appreciate their strengths and limitations. It is likely that future developments in in silico modeling will provide the basis for integrated strategies for toxicity prediction. Increasingly these will built on a firm mechanistic foundation, to allow confidence in predictions and their applications.

ACKNOWLEDGMENTS

The funding of the European Union 6th Framework CAESAR Specific Targeted Project (SSPI-022674-CAESAR) is gratefully acknowledged. The contributions and occasional helpful comments of Dr. Nora Aptula (Unilever Research), Dr. David Roberts (Liverpool John Moores University) and Prof. Terry Schultz (University of Tennessee) are gratefully appreciated.

REFERENCES

1. Cronin MTD, Livingstone DJ, eds. Predicting Chemical Toxicity and Fate. Boca Raton: CRC Press, 2004:445.
2. Helma C, ed. Predictive Toxicology. Boca Raton: Taylor & Francis, 2005:508.

3. Cronin MTD. Predicting chemical toxicity and fate in humans and the environment—an introduction. In: Cronin MTD, Livingstone DJ, eds. Predicting Chemical Toxicity and Fate. Boca Raton: CRC Press, 2004:3–13.

4. EC. Regulation (EC) No 1907/2006 of the European Parliament and of the Council of 18 December 2006 concerning the Registration, Evaluation, Authorisation and Restriction of Chemicals (REACH), establishing a European Chemicals Agency, amending Directive 1999/45/EC and repealing Council Regulation (EEC) No 793/93 and Commission Regulation (EC) No 1488/94 as well as Council Directive 76/769/EEC and Commission Directives 91/155/EEC, 93/67/EEC, 93/105/EC and 2000/21/EC. Off J Eur Union, L 396/1 of 30.12.2006; 2006.

5. EC. Commission of the European Communities. Directive 2003/15/EC of the European Parliament and of the Council of 27 February 2003 amending Council Directive 76/768/EEC on the approximation of the laws of the Member States relating to cosmetic products. Off J Eur Union, (L 66/26-L 33/35 of 11.3.2003), 2003.

6. Cronin MTD, Jaworska JS, Walker JD, et al. Use of QSARs in international decision-making frameworks to predict health effects of chemical substances. Environ Health Perspect 2003; 111(10):1391–401.

7. Cronin MTD, Walker JD, Jaworska JS, et al. Use of QSARs in international decision-making frameworks to predict ecologic effects and environmental fate of chemical substances. Environ Health Perspect 2003; 111(10):1376–90.

8. Cronin MTD. The use by governmental regulatory agencies of quantitative structure–activity relationships and expert systems to predict toxicity. In: Cronin MTD, Livingstone DJ, eds. Predicting Chemical Toxicity and Fate. Boca Raton: CRC Press, 2004:413–27.

9. Cronin MTD, Schultz TW. Pitfalls in QSAR. J Mol Struct 2003; 622:39–51.

10. Emmett EA. Toxic responses of the skin. In: Klaassen CD, Amdur MO, Doull J, eds. Casarett and Doull's Toxicology. New York: Macmillan, 1986:412–31.

11. Worth AP. The tiered approach to toxicity assessment based on the integrated use of alternative (non-animal) tests. In: Cronin MTD, Livingstone DJ, eds. Predicting Chemical Toxicity and Fate. Boca Raton: CRC Press, 2004:391–412.

12. Worth AP, Cronin MTD. The use of pH measurements to predict the potential of chemicals to cause acute dermal and ocular toxicity. Toxicology 2001; 169(2):119–31.

13. Gerner I, Schlegel K, Walker JD, et al. Use of physicochemical property limits to develop rules for identifying chemical substances with no skin irritation or corrosion potential. QSAR Comb Sci 2004; 23(9):726–33.

14. Gerner I, Zinke S, Graetschel G, et al. Development of a decision support system for the introduction of alternative methods into local irritancy/corrosivity testing strategies. Creation of fundamental rules for a decision support system. ATLA Altern Lab Anim 2000; 28(5):665–98.

15. Gerner L, Graetschel G, Kahl J, et al. Development of a decision support system for the introduction of alternative methods into local irritancy/corrosivity testing strategies. Development of a relational database. ATLA Altern Lab Anim 2000; 28(1):11–28.

16. Zinke S, Gerner I. A computer-based structure–activity relationship method for predicting the toxic effects of organic chemicals from one-dimensional representations of their molecular structures. ATLA Altern Lab Anim 2000; 28(4):609–20.

17. Zinke S, Gerner I, Graetschel G, et al. Local irritation/corrosion testing strategies: Development of a decision support system for the introduction of alternative methods. ATLA Altern Lab Anim 2000; 28(1):29–40.

18. Rorije E, Hulzebos E. Evaluation of (Q)SARs for the Prediction of Skin Irritation/Corrosion Potential: Physico-chemical exclusion rules Report written by the National Institute of Public Health and Environment (RIVM), Bilthoven, The Netherlands, for the European Chemicals Bureau, 2005. (Available electronically from http://ecb.jrc.it/DOCUMENTS/QSAR/Evaluation_of_Skin_Irritation_QSARs.pdf)

19. Worth AP, Bassan A, De Bruijn J, et al. The role of the European Chemicals Bureau in promoting the regulatory use of (Q)SAR methods. SAR QSAR Environ Res 2007; 18(1):111–25.

20. Walker JD, Gerner I, Hulzebos E, et al. (Q)SARs for predicting skin irritation and corrosion: mechanisms, transparency and applicability of predictions. QSAR Comb Sci 2004; 23(9):721–5.

21. Hulzebos E, Walker JD, Gerner I, et al. Use of structural alerts to develop rules for identifying chemical substances with skin irritation or skin corrosion potential. QSAR Comb Sci 2005; 24(3):332–42.

22. Hulzebos EM, Maslankiewicz L, Walker JD. Verification of literature-derived SARs for skin irritation and corrosion. QSAR Comb Sci 2003; 22(3):351–63.

23. Walker JD, Gerner I, Hulzebos E, et al. The Skin Irritation Corrosion Rules Estimation Tool (SICRET). QSAR Comb Sci 2005; 24(3):378–84.

24. Barratt MD. Quantitative structure–activity relationships for skin irritation and corrosivity of neutral and electrophilic organic chemicals. Toxicol In Vitro 1996; 10(4):247–53 (see also Toxicol In Vitro 1996; 10(4): R1).

25. Whittle E, Barratt MD, Carter JA, et al. Skin corrosivity potential of fatty acids: in vitro rat and human skin testing and QSAR studies. Toxicol In Vitro 1996; 10(1):95–100.

26. Basketter D, Pease C, Kasting G, et al. Skin sensitisation and epidermal diposition: the relevance of epidermal diposition for sensitation hazard identification and risk assessment. The report and recommendations of ECUAM workshop 59. ATLA Altern Lab Anim 2007; 35(1):137–54.

27. Cronin MTD, Basketter DA. A multivariate QSAR analysis of a skin sensitization database. SAR QSAR Environ Res 1994; 2:159–79.

28. Gerberick GF, Ryan CA, Kern PS, et al. Compilation of historical local lymph node data for evaluation of skin sensitization alternative methods. Dermatitis 2005; 16(4):157–202.

29. Schlede E, Aberer W, Fuchs I, et al. Chemical substances and contact allergy ranked according to allergenic—244 substances potency. Toxicol 2003; 193:219–59.

30. Dimitrov SD, Low LK, Patlewicz GY, et al. Skin sensitization: modeling based on skin metabolism simulation and formation of protein conjugates. Int J Toxicol 2005; 24(4):189–204.

31. Graham C, Gealy R, Macina OT, et al. QSAR for allergic contact dermatitis. Quant Struct Act Rel 1996; 15(3):224–9.

32. Dupuis G, Benezra C. Allergic Contact Dermatitis to Simple Chemicals: A Molecular Approach. New York: Marcel Dekker, 1982.

33. Cronin MTD, Basketter DA. A QSAR evaluation of an existing contact allergy database. In: Wermuth CG, ed. Trends in QSAR and Molecular Modelling 1992. Leiden: Escom, 1993:297–8.

34. Payne MP, Walsh PT. Structure–activity relationships for skin sensitization potential—development of structural alerts for use in knowledge-based toxicity prediction systems. J Chem Inf Comput Sci 1994; 34(1):154–61.

35. Barratt MD, Basketter DA, Chamberlain M, et al. An expert-system rulebase for identifying contact allergens. Toxicol In Vitro 1994; 8(5):1053–60.

36. Barratt MD, Basketter DA, Chamberlain M, et al. Development of an expert-system rulebase for identifying contact allergens. Toxicol In Vitro 1994; 8(4):837–9.

37. Ashby J, Basketter DA, Paton D, et al. Structure activity relationships in skin sensitization using the murine local lymph node assay. Toxicol 1995; 103(3):177–94.

38. Schultz TW, Cronin MTD, Netzeva TI. The present status of QSAR in toxicology. J Mol Struct 2003; 622(1–2):23–38.

39. Schultz TW, Cronin MTD, Walker JD, et al. Quantitative structure–activity relationships (QSARs) in toxicology: a historical perspective. J Mol Struct 2003; 622(1–2):1–22.

40. Basketter DA, Roberts DW, Cronin M, et al. The value of the local lymph-node assay in quantitative structure–activity investigations. Contact Dermatitis 1992; 27(3):137–42.

41. Roberts DW, Williams DL. The derivation of quantitative correlations between skin sensitization and physio-chemical parameters for alkylating-agents, and their application to experimental-data for sultones. J Theor Biol 1982; 99(4):807–25.

42. Goodwin BFJ, Roberts DW. Structure–activity relationships in allergic contact-dermatitis. Food Chem Toxicol 1986; 24(6–7):795–8.

43. Franot C, Roberts DW, Basketter DA, et al. Structure–activity relationships for contact allergenic potential of gamma,gamma-dimethyl-gamma-butyrolactone derivatives. 2.

Quantitative structure skin sensitization relationships for alpha-substituted-alpha-methyl-gamma,gamma-dimethyl-gamma-butyrolactones. Chem Res Toxicol 1994; 7(3):307–12.

44. Franot C, Roberts DW, Smith RG, et al. Structure–activity relationships for contact allergenic potential of gamma,gamma-dimethyl-gamma-butyrolactone derivatives. 1. Synthesis and electrophilic reactivity studies of alpha-(omega-substituted-alkyl)-gamma,gamma-dimethyl-gamma-butyrolactone s and correlation of skin sensitization potential and cross-sensitization patterns with structure. Chem Res Toxicol 1994; 7(3):297–306.

45. Roberts DW, Goodwin BFJ, Williams DL, et al. Correlations between skin sensitization potential and chemical-reactivity for *para*-nitrobenzyl compounds. Food Chem Toxicol 1983; 21(6):811–3.

46. Roberts DW, Basketter DA. Quantitative structure–activity relationships: sulfonate esters in the local lymph node assay. Contact Dermatitis 2000; 42(3):154–61.

47. Mekenyan O, Roberts DW, Karcher W. Molecular orbital parameters as predictors of skin sensitization potential of halo- and pseudohalobenzenes acting as SNAr electrophiles. Chem Res Toxicol 1997; 10(9):994–1000.

48. Roberts DW. Linear free-energy relationships for reactions of electrophilic halobenzenes and pseudohalobenzenes, and their application in prediction of skin sensitization potential for snar electrophiles. Chem Res Toxicol 1995; 8(4):545–51.

49. Patlewicz G, Basketter DA, Smith CK, et al. Skin-sensitization structure–activity relationships for aldehydes. Contact Dermatitis 2001; 44(6):331–6.

50. Patlewicz GY, Basketter DA, Pease CKS, et al. Further evaluation of quantitative structure–activity relationship models for the prediction of the skin sensitization potency of selected fragrance allergens. Contact Dermatitis 2004; 50(2):91–7.

51. Miller MD, Yourtee DM, Glaros AG, et al. Quantum mechanical structure–activity relationship analyses for skin sensitization. J Chem Inf Model 2005; 45(4):924–9.

52. Kostoryz EL, Zhu Q, Zhao H, et al. Assessment of the relative skin sensitization potency of siloranes using the local lymph node assay and QSAR predicted potency. J Biomed Mater Res A 2006; 79A(3):684–8.

53. Cronin MTD, Dearden JC. Correspondence analysis of the skin sensitization potential of organic chemicals. Quant Struct Act Rel 1997; 16(1):33–7.

54. Magee PS, Hostynek JJ, Maibach HI. A classification model for allergic contact-dermatitis. Quant Struct Act Rel 1994; 13(1):22–33.

55. Hostynek JJ, Maibach HI. Scope and limitation of some approaches to predicting contact hypersensitivity. Toxicol In Vitro 1998; 12(4):445–53.

56. Hostynek JJ, Magee PS. Fragrance allergens: classification and ranking by QSAR. Toxicol In Vitro 1997; 11:377 (see also Toxicol In Vitro 1997; 12(2):AR1).

57. Hostynek JJ, Magee PS. Performance of an SAR-QSAR model predictive of human ACD. In Vitro Mol Toxicol 1999; 12(4):203–11.

58. Hatch KL, Magee PS. A discriminant model for allergic contact dermatitis in anthra-quinone disperse dyes. Quant Struct Act Rel 1998; 17(1):20–6.

59. Li SQ, Fedorowicz A, Singh H, et al. Application of the random forest method in studies of local lymph node assay based skin sensitization data. J Chem Inf Model 2005; 45(4):952–64.

60. Ren YY, Liu HX, Xue CX, et al. Classification study of skin sensitizers based on support vector machine and linear discriminant analysis. Anal Chim Acta 2006; 572(2):272–82.

61. Estrada E, Patlewicz G, Chamberlain M, et al. Computer-aided knowledge generation for understanding skin sensitization mechanisms: The TOPS-MODE approach. Chem Res Toxicol 2003; 16(10):1226–35.

62. Estrada E, Patlewicz G, Gutierrez Y. From knowledge generation to knowledge archive. a general strategy using TOPS-MODE with DEREK to formulate new alerts for skin Sensitization. J Chem Inf Comput Sci 2004; 44(2):688–98.

63. Sosted H, Basketter DA, Estrada E, et al. Ranking of hair dye substances according to predicted sensitization potency: quantitative structure–activity relationships. Contact Dermatitis 2004; 51(5–6):241–54.

64. http://www.lhasalimited.org (Accessed September 3, 2007).

65. http://www.accelrys.com/products/topkat/ (Accessed September 3, 2007).
66. http://www.multicase.com/ (Accessed September 3, 2007).
67. http://oasis-lmc.org/ (Accessed September 3, 2007).
68. http://www.oecd.org (Accessed September 3, 2007).
69. Greene N. Computer systems for the prediction of toxicity: an update. Adv Drug Deliv Rev 2002; 54(3):417–31.
70. Sanderson DM, Earnshaw CG. Computer-prediction of possible toxic action from chemical-structure—the DEREK system. Hum Exp Toxicol 1991; 10(4):261–73.
71. Greene N, Judson PN, Langowski JJ, et al. Knowledge-based expert systems for toxicity and metabolism prediction: DEREK, StAR, and METEOR. SAR QSAR Environ Res 1999; 10:299–313.
72. Combes RD, Rodford RA. The use of expert systems for toxicity prediction: illustrations with reference to the DEREK program. In: Cronin MTD, Livingstone DJ, eds. Predicting Chemical Toxicity and Fate. Florida: CRC Press LLC, 2004:153–204.
73. Barratt MD, Langowski JJ. Validation and subsequent development of the DEREK skin sensitization rulebase by analysis of the BgVV list of contact allergens. J Chem Inf Comput Sci 1999; 39(2):294–8.
74. Zinke S, Gerner I, Schlede E. Evaluation of a rule base for identifying contact allergens by using a regulatory database: comparison of data on chemicals notified in the European Union with "structural alerts" used in the DEREK expert system. ATLA Altern Lab Anim 2002; 30(3):285–98.
75. Langton K, Patlewicz GY, Long A, et al. Structure–activity relationships for skin sensitization: recent improvements to DEREK for Windows. Contact Dermatitis 2006; 55(6):342–7.
76. Klopman G. A Hierarchical computer automated structure evaluation program. Quant Struct Act Rel 1992; 11(2):176–84.
77. Klopman G, Rosenkranz HS. Approaches to SAR in carcinogenesis and mutagenesis—prediction of carcinogenicity/mutagenicity using Multi-CASE. Mutat Res 1994; 305(1):33–46.
78. Enslein K, Gombar VK, Blake BW. Use of SAR in computer-assisted prediction of carcinogenicity and mutagenicity of chemicals by the TOPKAT program. Mutat Res 1994; 305(1):47–61.
79. Enslein K, Gombar VK, Blake BW, et al. A quantitative structure–toxicity relationships model for the dermal sensitization guinea pig maximization assay. Food Chem Toxicol 1997; 35(10–11):1091–8.
80. Mekenyan OG, Dimitrov SD, Pavlov TS, et al. A systematic approach to simulating metabolism in computational toxicology. I. The TIMES heuristic modelling framework. Curr Pharm Des 2004; 10(11):1273–93.
81. Mekenyan O, Dimitrov S, Dimitrova N, et al. Metabolic activation of chemicals: in-silico simulation. SAR QSAR Environ Res 2006; 17(1):107–20.
82. Jowsey IR, Basketter DA, Westmoreland C, et al. A future approach to measuring relative skin sensitising potency: a proposal. J Appl Toxicol 2006; 26(4):341–50.
83. Magee PS. Exploring the chemistry of quinones by computation. Quant Struct Act Rel 2000; 19(1):22–8.
84. Magee PS. Exploring the potential for allergic contact dermatitis via computed heats of reaction of haptens with protein end-groups—Heats of reaction of haptens with protein end-groups by computation. Quant Struct Act Rel 2000; 19(4):356–65.
85. Aptula AO, Roberts DW, Cronin MTD. From experiment to theory: molecular orbital parameters to interpret the skin sensitization potential of 5-chloro-2-methylisothiazol-3-one and 2-methylisothiazol-3-one. Chem Res Toxicol 2005; 18(2):324–9.
86. Aptula AO, Patlewicz G, Roberts DW. Skin sensitization: reaction mechanistic applicability domains for structure–activity relationships. Chem Res Toxicol 2005; 18(9):1420–6.
87. Roberts DW, Aptula AO, Patlewicz G. Electrophilic chemistry related to skin sensitization. Reaction mechanistic applicability domain classification for a published data set of 106 chemicals tested in the mouse local lymph node assay. Chem Res Toxicol 2007; 20(1):44–60.

88. Aptula AO, Roberts DW. Mechanistic applicability domains for nonanimal-based prediction of toxicological end points: general principles and application to reactive toxicity. Chem Res Toxicol 2006; 19(8):1097–105.

89. Roberts DW, Aptula AO, Patlewicz G. Mechanistic applicability domains for non-animal based prediction of toxicological endpoints. QSAR analysis of the Schiff base applicability domain for skin sensitization. Chem Res Toxicol 2006; 19(9):1228–33.

90. Aptula AO, Patlewicz G, Roberts DW, et al. Non-enzymatic glutathione reactivity and in vitro toxicity: a non-animal approach to skin sensitization. Toxicol In Vitro 2006; 20(2):239–47.

91. Schultz TW, Carlson RE, Cronin MTD, et al. A conceptual framework for predicting the toxicity of reactive chemicals: modeling soft electrophilicity. SAR QSAR Environ Res 2006; 17(4):413–28.

Haw-Yueh Thong and Howard I. Maibach
Department of Dermatology, School of Medicine, University of California San Francisco, San Francisco, California, U.S.A.

INTRODUCTION

Allergic contact dermatitis (ACD) is an inflammatory skin disease characterized by erythema, edema, and vesiculation, which appear as delayed skin responses following cutaneous exposure to allergenic chemicals. ACD is widespread, in part because of the introduction of large numbers of new chemicals into the marketplace, some of which ultimately turn out to be allergenic under use conditions. In addition, older allergenic chemicals employed in occupational settings provide a continuing source of ACD and are difficult to eliminate from the environment. Among the documented allergens, medicaments and cosmetics contain preservatives and fragrances (1–3); rubber, plastics, metals, epoxy resins, wood products, metal-working fluids, printing chemicals, and others (4); and culinary and nonedible plants are well-known sources (5).

EPIDEMIOLOGY OF ACD

ACD is a skin disease that affects around 1% to 4% of the global population at considerable cost to society and industry (6,7). Patch testing is the most worthwhile diagnostic tool for the evaluation of patients with suspected ACD. Storrs et al. (8) analyzed the prevalence and relevance of allergic reactions in patients patch tested in North America from 1984 to 1985. The most common sensitizers identified were nickel, p-phenylenediamine, quaternium-15, neomycin, thimerosal, formaldehyde, cinnamic aldehyde, ethylenediamine, potassium dichromate, and thiuram mix. Krob et al. (9) analyzed the prevalence and relevance of contact dermatitis allergens as tested by the Thin-layer Rapid Use Epicutaneous test (TRUE Test) from 1966 to June 2000 using meta-analysis. The meta-analysis showed that nickel (14.7% of tested patients), thimerosal (5.0%), cobalt (4.8%), fragrance mix (3.4%), and balsam of Peru (3.0%) were the most prevalent allergens, and the five least prevalent allergens were paraben mix (0.5%), black rubber mix (0.6%), quaternium-15 (0.6%), quinoline mix (0.7%), and caine mix (0.7%).

The North American Contact Dermatitis Group (NACDG) reported the results of patch testing from January 1, 2001 to December 31, 2002 with an extended screening series of 65 allergens and found that the top 10 allergens were: nickel sulfate (16.7%), neomycin (11.6%), Myroxilon pereirae (balsam of Peru) (11.6%), fragrance mix (10.4%), thimerosal (10.2%), sodium gold thiosulfate (10.2%), quaternium-15 (9.3%), formaldehyde (8.4%), bacitracin (7.9%), and cobalt chloride (7.4%) (10). Mirshahpanah and Maibach (11) calculated a ratio of percent positivity of eczema to random sample population for each allergen to delineate the relationship between the allergic patch test reaction frequency of a random sample versus an eczema population to common allergens, and noted that eczematic skin is more prone to reactivity relative to healthy skin. The authors also suggested that building a greater database of patch test results in both healthy and eczematic skin will lead to better understanding of ACD in man.

TEST METHODS FOR ACD

Regulatory agencies such as the Food and Drug Administration (FDA), U.S. Environmental Protection Agency, and Consumer Product Safety Commission often require that chemicals and untested substances that are to be introduced into the marketplace be evaluated for their potential to cause ACD. Tests for ACD potential must demonstrate that the chemical is capable of producing a more severe subsequent skin effect than was encountered on initial contact, signifying an allergic (immunologic) response rather than an irritant (non-immunologic) response. At present, there are no validated in vitro tests available that allow the identification of a chemical's potential to cause ACD despite legislative and ethical pressure to reduce animal testing (12). Animal tests remain the preferred method to predict human ACD potential. This is a precautionary measure that is undertaken to avoid sensitizing a significant segment of the human population to the test chemical and to a vast array of closely related (cross-reacting) chemicals that will be encountered by the test subject at a later time. Human tests for ACD potential are often needed as a follow-up to animal tests, since the correlation between animal and human test results is not exact (13). Human tests are employed both for predicting ACD potential of new chemicals and for diagnosing ACD in clinical patients that present to dermatologists for evaluation and treatment of contact dermatitis.

Predictive Tests
Quantitative Structure–Activity Relationship
A large database exists involving animals and humans that have been tested with a wide variety of chemicals for skin sensitization potential. These data are available for studying the relationship of chemical structure and potency as skin sensitizers. The chemical properties that appear to be associated with a propensity for skin sensitization have been summarized (14,15). Structure–activity relationships were investigated by Ferguson et al. (16) who targeted electrophilicity as an important factor in a chemical's capacity to sensitize. Hostynek et al. (17) studied fragrance sensitizers by applying quantitative structure–activity relationship. More recently, Langton et al. (18) demonstrated the use of computer prediction models for the analysis of structure–activity relationships and as an important alternative approach for the prediction of skin sensitization as new information from experimental and theoretical studies becomes available.

Human Test Methods
Human test methods for predicting skin sensitization were largely developed and refined between 1941 and 1975. The Draize human repeat insult patch test was presented in 1944 as an attempt to decrease the frequency of ACD (19). The test techniques at that time were just being validated and this experimental design was largely empiric. The principle of the test is as follows:

1. Multiple inductions of the study material at relatively non- or low-irritancy levels for approximately three weeks

2. Approximately a two-week rest period
3. A standard diagnostic challenge of approximately 48 hours and a delayed reading at approximately 96 hours after patch application.

In 1945, Henderson and Riley (20) demonstrated that a test panel sample size of 30,000 subjects would have to be employed to ensure statistically that there would be no more than 0.1% sensitization. Currently, the modified Draize procedure (21) and the modified maximization technique of Kligman and Epstein (22) are methods of choice.

Animal Test Methods

Official regulatory guinea pig methods are available as OECD test Guideline No. 406 (23). Another category of "nonregulatory"/investigative testing strategies is represented by various modifications of the Draize test, the guinea pig maximization test (GPMT), and the split adjuvant test. The common principle of all these methods is to initiate exposure(s) of a test article or its test samples to the same skin site or area (*induction phase*), which after a rest period of at least seven days is followed by a *challenge exposure* of the article or of its test sample(s) to a virgin skin site or area.

Guinea Pig Maximization Test

The GPMT, as described by Magnusson and Kligman (24), is a very sensitive procedure for allergenicity screening of test articles (25–32) but with a tendency to overestimate the potency of many weak, mild, and moderate human sensitizers. The GPMT is strongly recommended as a legislative method despite the fact that its experimental data are less suitable for sensitization hazard calculation related to intended, accidental, or occasional exposure of skin to various environmental allergens. The method, which employs 20 tests and 10 to 20 control guinea pigs, is as follows (24).

Induction Phase

The induction, consisting of two phases, is initiated (day 0) by paired intradermal injections (0.1 mL each) of one complete Freund's adjuvant (CFA) into the clipped and shaved shoulder region of the test animals. For induction, the use of a mildly or moderately irritating test concentration is recommended. When nonirritating test articles are involved, pretreatment of the freshly clipped shoulder region with 10% sodium lauryl sulfate on day 6 is indicated.

Challenge Phase (Day 21)

On the left flank of all animals, a skin site of 4 cm^2 is shaved and the test article is applied in suitable vehicle at primary nonirritating concentration(s) using a 24-hour occlusive "patch unit." The vehicle may be simultaneously tested, if indicated. The challenge reactions are examined 24 and 48 hours after removal of the patch and scored according to a standard rating scale in which allergenic potential is graded from none to extreme. Rechallenge or cross-test may follow at weekly intervals, always on contralateral flanks. Control animals are treated similar to test animals, except that during the induction phase the test article is omitted.

There are drawbacks to the modified GPMT:

1. Intradermal administration is an unnatural exposure route for a contact allergen, often resulting in overestimation of allergenicity of test articles.
2. It is not suitable for testing poorly soluble or insoluble test articles and "end-use" products, since these are not injectible.

Due to limits and deficiencies of this testing strategy, various modifications of the GPMT have been proposed to improve its predictivity (33–37) or to reduce the number of test animals (38,39).

The Modified Draize Test

The aim of all modifications of the Draize test (40) is to enhance the sensitivity of this assay in detecting weaker skin sensitizers by:

1. Increasing the test substance concentration to cause moderate irritant skin responses (41),
2. Including control animals for challenging (25),
3. Replacement of intradermal administration by open application (42),
4. Increased frequency of exposures by rechallenge and/or repetition of the whole study course in the same test animal group (double Draize test), and
5. Shortening the duration of the induction to one-day treatment by administration of four intradermal injections at sites overlying the axillary and inguinal lymph nodes (43).

The modified Draize test (44) consists of two parts and involves two groups, each of 10 guinea pigs, and is described below.

Part I: Induction Phase

Ten test animals are used. On day 0, four intradermal administrations of the test article at a dose of 0.1 mL and at a concentration corresponding to 2.5 times the intradermal challenge concentration (may cause slight but perceptible irritation on guinea pig skin) on the clipped skin site overlying both axillary and inguinal lymph nodes. The resulting 24 hours skin reactions are examined, their intensity graded (erythema and edema), and the average reaction size evaluated based on the measurement of the longitudinal and lateral axes diameters of each of the four skin reactions.

Challenge Phase

On day 14 each of the experimental animals is challenged, using intradermal administration of 0.1 mL of the test articles in suitable solvents at a nonirritant or slightly irritant concentration at maximum on one clipped flank, and open epicutaneously on the opposite clipped flank with 0.1 mL of the test samples at primary nonirritant concentration to a circular test site of about 8 cm^2. The 24-hour reactions are examined, graded, and their size evaluated. Confirmation rechallenge may follow on days 21 and 28. For each rechallenge 10 control animals, which had been treated with CFA for induction solely, are challenged similarly to the test animals.

Part II

If both challenge tests of Part I are negative (no evidence that skin sensitization occurred in test animals), a second set of intradermal injections is administered on day 35. The challenge procedure is similar to the one described for Part I, but confirmation rechallenge is done intradermally and epicutaneously at weekly intervals. New control animals have to be involved.

This technique is suitable for testing of soluble or suspendible chemicals exclusively and is more sensitive than the Draize guinea pig test, though still less sensitive than the GPMT.

Split Adjuvant Technique

In this assay, the test article and CFA are administered separately (45,46), and two groups of 10 to 20 guinea pigs each are involved.

Induction Phase

On day 0, the skin of the suprascapular region is shaved to remove hair and a window dressing is secured over the site. The induction site of 2 cm^2 is exposed to "dry ice" for at least 5 seconds prior to application of 0.2 mL semisolid or 0.1 mL liquid test sample and then covered with filter paper, fixed with adhesive tape, and occluded for 48 hours. This procedure is repeated every other day for a total of four induction treatments. On day 4, prior to topical application of the test sample, two intradermal injections of 0.1 mL CFA are administered into the induction site. On day 9, the dressing is removed.

Challenge Phase

On day 21, challenge is performed by 24-hour occlusive or open patch test application of 0.5 mL semisolid or 0.1 mL liquid test article to a 2-cm^2 virgin clipped skin site on the dorsum. Controls are treated similarly, except that test article administration is omitted during induction phase. Reading and scoring of the skin reactions is done on day 22, 23, and 24. Rechallenge or cross-tests can follow at in intervals of 10 days.

This test protocol is designed to evaluate chemicals and "end-use" products. It is less sensitive than the GPMT. Its performance is rather complicated, and it is stressful for animals due to the use of window dressing during the induction phase.

Local Lymph Node Assay

The acquisition of skin sensitization depends on the initiation of a cell-mediated immune response. It is now clear that epidermal Langerhans cells play an important role in the generation of cutaneous immune responses, the induction of skin sensitization and the transport of antigen, via the afferent lymphatics, to draining lymph nodes. The molecular and cellular mechanisms that result in the induction and elicitation of contact allergy have been reviewed extensively elsewhere (47,48). The ability of chemical allergens to induce the activation of skin draining lymph nodes and to stimulate lymph node cell (LNC) proliferative responses is the event upon which the local lymph node assay (LLNA) is based. Several review articles are available on the LLNA (49–53), which is supplementing and potentially replacing the GPMT (54).

In contrast to the guinea pig methods (in which activity is measured as a function of challenge-induced cutaneous reactions in previously sensitized animals), LLNA focuses on events during the induction phase of skin sensitization, and particularly on changes provoked in lymph nodes draining the site of exposure. Several parameters of lymph node activation could be viewed as legitimate potential correlates of skin sensitization. These include the increase in lymph node weight and cellularity, the appearance of pyroninophilic cells, and the stimulation of LNC turnover (55,56). The ability to measure lymph node hyperplastic responses in situ (57,58) was an important milestone. This adaptation not only provided a more holistic and more sensitive assessment of LNC proliferative activity, it also served to obviate the need for tissue culture. It is this form of the LLNA that was the subject of extensive evaluations and that was subsequently validated.

The basic protocol for the LLNA has been detailed elsewhere (59,60) but in summary: Groups of mice (CBA strain) receive topical applications of various concentrations of the test chemical (or of the relevant vehicle control) daily for three consecutive days. Recommendations regarding suitable test concentrations and vehicle choice are available elsewhere (61–63). Five days following the initiation of exposure, mice receive an intravenous injection of ^{3}H-TdR. Animals are sacrificed five hours later and draining auricular lymph nodes excised. These are either pooled for each experimental group or are pooled on a per animal basis. Single-cell suspensions of LNC are prepared and the cells washed and suspended in trichloroacetic acid (TCA) for at least 12 hours at 4°C. Precipitates are suspended in TCA and transferred to an appropriate scintillation fluid. The incorporation by draining LNC of ^{3}H-TdR is measured by scintillation counting and recorded as mean disintegrations per minute for each experimental group, or for each animal. In instances where it is appropriate to include within the test protocol a positive control it is recommended that hexyl cinnamic aldehyde is used for this purpose (50).

For each concentration of test material, a stimulation index (SI) is calculated using the value derived from the concurrent vehicle control as the comparator. Skin sensitizers are defined as those chemicals that, at one or more test concentrations, are able to induce an SI of 3 (an arbitrary, but appropriate criterion for a positive response (64)) or greater. Despite the proven value of an SI of 3 for hazard identification, some flexibility is appropriate when interpreting LLNA data (61).

CLINICAL ASPECTS
Diagnostic Test

Patch Test

In vivo patch testing in which the skin can process the allergen for presentation remains the "gold standard" for the diagnosis of ACD. Patch testing constitutes the most important tool at present for the study of delayed hypersensitivity and the only "scientific proof" of ACD (5). In diagnostic tests, a preparation is applied to a patient's skin under an occlusive patch for 48 hours and the skin is evaluated for evidence of erythema, edema, or more severe skin changes occurring 24, 48, or 72 hours after removal of the patch. Allergenic materials are thereby identified by producing skin disease on a small scale. The TRUE test, is currently the only allergen patch test that has received marketing approval from the U.S. FDA, has become a global standard and is the only commercially available patch test system currently used within the United States (9). Over 3700 chemicals have been identified as causing ACD of which the TRUE test tests only 23. Krob et al. (9) compared the prevalence of contact dermatitis allergens as tested by the TRUE test with the NACDG data. The comparison with NACDG data suggests that clinically important allergens may be missed by the TRUE test. Thus, the TRUE test is a screening test at best.

The NACDG Standard 65 Allergen Series is another commonly used diagnostic test in the United States. Pratt et al. (10) reported the results of patch testing from January 1, 2001 to December 31, 2002 by the NACDG. Of the 4913 patients tested, 16.7% had a relevant reaction to an allergen not in the NACDG standard series and 5.5% had a relevant reaction to an occupational allergen not in the standard series. The authors concluded that there is a need for a more comprehensive group of diagnostic allergens than those found in the standard screening kits, and the usefulness of patch testing is enhanced when a greater number of allergens are tested, especially nonstandard allergens occupationally encountered.

Recently, investigations have become more specific in discussing patch test frequency data (65). The term *allergic patch test reaction frequency* typically refers to patch test positivity numbers—without attempt to correct for clinical relevance—i.e., the clinical disease of ACD, present or past. The number may include the result of false positives and non-reproducible positives from the excited skin syndrome. *Contact allergy* implies true delayed hypersensitivity (a true allergic patch test response) but does not imply clinical relevance has been established.

The most important aspect in the interpretation of diagnostic test results is an assessment of the relevance of positive patch test findings to the diagnosis. The investigator must establish that positive patch test results are consistent with a history of exposure to a particular chemical in a product and must exclude other possible environmental exposure conditions. Next, the location of the present dermatitis must correspond to the site of contact with the putative offending chemical. Finally, the patch test concentration must be nonirritating, as demonstrated by a dose–response effect when dilution of the putative allergen is employed.

Algorithm for Diagnosis of Clinical ACD in Man

Ale and Maibach (66) have suggested an operational definition of ACD using the following algorithm to establish the relation (causality) between a positive patch test and the likelihood of clinical ACD:

1. History of exposure,
2. Appropriate morphology,
3. Positive patch test to a nonirritating concentration of the putative allergen,
4. Repeat patch test if excited skin syndrome is operative (more than one positive patch test),
5. Employ serial dilution patch testing to distinguish allergen from marginal irritant,
6. Employ use test or open patch test, and
7. Resolution of dermatitis.

Special Considerations
Irritant Versus ACD

Although ACD closely resembles irritant contact dermatitis (ICD) on gross inspection of the skin, ACD has an immunologic etiology that is lacking in irritant dermatitis. On the contrary, contact with external irritating agents such as detergents can result in ICD, a localized non-immunologic condition. ICD ensues when irritant stimuli from either acute or cumulative injury overpower the defense and repair capacities of the skin (67,68), and may involve inflammation or skin necrosis (corrosive). Testing for irritation and the management of ICD are discussed elsewhere (69,70). A number of animal, human, and *in vitro* test methods have been developed, but no one assay is able to accurately portray irritation in its entirety. Preventive measures, including the utilization of proper skin care, the avoidance of harsh soaps, and the use of protective garments such as gloves, will decrease the risk of ICD.

Excited Skin Syndrome

"Angry back," "excited skin," "skin hyperreactivity," and "excited skin syndrome" are terms used to describe a hyperirritable skin condition that occurs when multiple concomitant inflammatory skin conditions prevail (71,72). When this hypersensitive skin condition exists, multiple positive reactions appear in patch testing as a result of strongly positive responses that induce nonspecific reactions in contiguous test sites. Interpretation of these false-positive test results is challenging (73).

Contact Urticaria

Maibach and Johnson (74) defined contact urticaria syndrome (CUS), characterized by skin reactions appearing within minutes to about 1 hour after exposure of the urticariant to the skin, and disappearing within 24 hours of onset, often associated with complaints of a local burning sensation, tingling, itching, swelling, and/or redness (wheal and flare). A variety of compounds, such as foods, preservatives, fragrances, plant and animal products, and metals, have been reported to cause CUS (75). Because the exposure to contact urticariants can be similar to contact irritants (e.g., health care workplaces), vigilance is required to ensure that the patient is properly evaluated and diagnosed because CUS in the setting of hand eczema may be overlooked.

Details of CUS are dealt with elsewhere (76,77). In essence, CUS can be described in two broad categories: non-immunologic contact urticaria (NICU) and immunologic contact urticaria (ICU). The former does not require pre-sensitization of the patient's immune system to an allergen, whereas the latter does.

NICU is more frequent and the symptoms vary depending on the exposure site, the concentration, the vehicle, the mode of exposure, and the substance itself. The mechanism of NICU is incompletely understood. Previously, histamine was assumed to be released from mast cells in response to exposure to an eliciting substance. However, evidence exists that NICU may be mediated by prostaglandins (78).

ICU is less frequent in clinical practice than NICU. ICU is a type 1 hypersensitivity reaction mediated by immunoglobulin E (IgE) antibodies specific to the eliciting substance. Therefore, prior immune (IgE) sensitization is required for this type of contact urticaria. Sensitization can be at the cutaneous level, but it may also be via the mucous membranes, such as in the respiratory or gastrointestinal tracts. The latter two routes of sensitization have frequently been reported among patients with ICU to latex (79–82). ICU reactions may spread beyond the site of contact and progress to generalized urticaria. When more severe, ICU may lead to anaphylactic shock. One such example is ICU from natural rubber latex. While anaphylactic reactions to topical medicaments from immunologic contact urticaria are uncommon, their potentially serious nature warrants attention. Commonly used topical application techniques in both ICU and NICU are the prick test, the chamber prick test, the scratch test, the open test, the chamber test, and the use test (76).

CONCLUSION

ACD is one of the most frequent and vexing dermatologic problems. While the disease has probably plagued humans for millennia, its clinical recognition by patch testing is barely a century old. With the advent of experimental animal models and noninvasive bioengineering methods on human testing, studies concerning the pathophysiology of ACD became possible. The management of ACD lies in identifying its cause correctly and thoroughly instructing the patient to avoid the responsible allergen(s). Unfortunately for patients and physicians, the allergenic component of many materials will almost never be labeled. Increasing awareness is seen among physicians, scientists, legislators, industry, and the general population that it is possible to prevent many allergies and allergy-related diseases. Legislation can be an effective tool in the prevention of contact dermatitis. Occupational safety has a long tradition of setting different types of rules and limitations to prevent hazardous exposure, and some focus on hazardous skin exposure. Recently, increasing awareness to the safety issues has also been seen in the cosmetic industry.

REFERENCES

1. Bandmann HJ, Calnan CD, Cronin E, et al. Dermatitis from applied medicaments. Arch Dermatol 1972; 106:335–7.
2. Marzulli F, Maibach H. Contact allergy: predictive testing of fragrance ingredients in humans by Draize and maximization methods. Environ Pathol Toxicol 1980; 3:235–45.
3. Opdyke DL. Monographs on fragrance raw materials. Food Cosmet Toxicol 1972; 12:807–1016.
4. Maibach H. Occupational and Industrial Dermatology. 2nd ed. Chicago: Year Book Medical, 1987.
5. Fisher AA. Contact Dermatitis. 3rd ed. Philadelphia, PA: Lea and Febiger, 1986.
6. Smith CK, Hotchkiss SAM. Allergic Contact Dermatitis: Chemical and Metabolic Mechanisms. London: Taylor & Francis, 2001.
7. Rietschel RL. Human and economic impact of allergic contact dermatitis and the role of patch testing. J Am Acad Dermatol 1995; 33:812–5.
8. Storrs F, Rosenthal LE, Adams RM, et al. Prevalence and relevance of allergic reactions in patients patch-tested in North America—1984 to 1985. J Am Acad Dermatol 1989; 20:1038–45.
9. Krob HA, Fleischer AB, Jr., D'Agostino R, Jr., et al. Prevalence and relevance of contact dermatitis allergens: a meta-analysis of 15 years of published TRUE test data. J Am Acad Dermatol 2004; 51(3):349–53.
10. Pratt MD, Belsito DV, Deleo VA, et al. North American Contact Dermatitis Group patch-test results, 2001–2002 study period. Dermatitis 2004; 15(4):176–83.
11. Mirshahpanah P, Maibach HI. Relationship of patch test positivity in a general versus an eczema population. Contact Dermatitis 2007; 56(3):125–30.
12. Kimber I, Cumberbatch M, Betts CJ, et al. Dendritic cells and skin sensitisation hazard assessment. Toxicol In Vitro 2004; 18:195–202.
13. Marzulli F, Maguire H. Usefulness and limitations of various guinea-pig test methods in detecting human skin sensitizers—validation of guinea-pig tests for skin hypersensitivity. Food Chem Toxicol 1982; 20:67–74.
14. Benezra C, Sigman C, Maibach H. A systematic search for structure–activity relationships of skin contact sensitization: II. Paraphenylenediamines. Semin Dermatol 1989; 8:88–93.
15. Dupuis A, Benezra C. Allergic Contact Dermatitis to Simple Chemicals: A Molecular Approach. New York: Marcel Dekker, 1983.

16. Ferguson J, Rosenkranz HS, Klopman C, et al. Structural determinants of dermal and respiratory sensitization determined using a computer-assisted structure–activity expert system (multicase). Abstracts of the 33rd annual meeting. Toxicologist 1994; 14(1).
17. Hostynek JJ, Magee PS, Maibach HI. Identication of fragrance sensitizers by QSAR. In: Froasch PJ, Johansen JD, White IR, eds. Fragrances: Benefical and Adverse Effects. Berlin: Springer, 1997:57–65.
18. Langton K, Patlewicz GY, Long A, et al. Structure–activity relationships for skin sensitization: recent improvements to Derek for Windows. Contact Dermatitis 2006; 55(6):342–7.
19. Draize JH, Woodard G, Calvery HD. Methods for the study of irritation and toxicity of substances applied topically to the skin and mucous membranes. J Pharmacol Exp Ther 1944; 83:377–90.
20. Henderson CR, Riley EC. Certain statistical considerations in patch testing. J Invest Dermatol 1945; 6:227–32.
21. Marzulli F, Maibach H. The use of graded concentrations in studying skin sensitizers: experimental contact sensitization in man. Food Cosmet Toxicol 1974; 12:219–27.
22. Kligman AM, Epstein WL. Updating the maximization test for identifying contact allergens. Contact Dermatitis 1975; 1:231–9.
23. Organization for Economic Cooperation and Development. Guidelines for Testing of Chemicals. OECD, Paris, France, 1981, revised 1992.
24. Magnusson B, Kligman AM. The identification of contact allergens by animal assay. The guinea pig maximization test. J Invest Dermatol 1969; 52:268–76.
25. Maurer T, Thomann P, Weirich EG, et al. Predictive evaluation in animals of the contact allergenic potential of medically important substances. I. Comparison of different methods of inducing and measuring cutaneous sensitization. Contact Dermatitis 1978; 4:321–33.
26. Kero M, Hannuksela M. Guinea pig maximization test, open epicutaneous test and chamber test in induction of delayed contact hypersensitivity. Contact Dermatitis 1980; 6:341–4.
27. Stampf JL, Benezra C. The sensitizing capacity of helenin and of two of its main constituents, the sesquiterpene lactones alantolactone and isoalantolactone: a comparison of epicutaneous and intradermal sensitizing methods and of different strains of guinea pigs. Contact Dermatitis 1982; 8:16–24.
28. Andersen KE. Potency evaluation of contact allergens: dose–response studies using the guinea pig maximization test. Nordiske Seminar og Arbejdsrapporter, Copenhagen, 1993.
29. Andersen KE, Boman A, Volund AA, et al. Induction of formaldehyde contact sensitivity: dose–response relationship in the guinea pig maximization test. Acta Dermato-Venereol (Stockh) 1985; 65:472–8.
30. Andersen KE, Maibach HI. Contact allergy predictive tests in guinea pigs. Curr Probl Dermatol 1985; 4:59–61.
31. Andersen KE, Maibach HI. Guinea pig sensitization assays an overview. Curr Probl Dermatol 1985; 14:263–90.
32. Wahlberg JE, Boman A. Guinea pig maximization test. Curr Probl Dermatol 1985; 14:59–106.
33. Rochas H, Guillot JP, Martini MC, et al. Contribution l'etude de l'influence des parfums sur le pouvoir sensibilisant de bases cosmetique. 2e partie: role du parfum sur le pouvoir sensibilisant de bases cosmetique. J Soc Cosmet Chem 1977; 28:367–75.
34. Kozuka T, Morikava F, Ohta S. A modified technique of guinea pig testing to identify delayed hypersensitivity allergens. Contact Dermatitis 1981; 7:225–37.
35. Sato Y, Katsumura Y, Ichikawa H, et al. A modified technique of guinea pig testing to identify delayed hypersensitivity allergens. Contact Dermatitis 1981; 7:225–37.
36. Guillot JP, Gonnet JF. The epiculaneous maximization test. Curr Probl Dermatol 1985; 14:220–47.
37. Maurer T, Hess R. The maximization test for skin sensitization potential—updating the standard protocol and validation of a modified protocol. Food Chem Toxicol 1989; 27(12):807–11.

38. Hofmann T, Diehl K-H, Leist K-H, et al. The feasibility of sensitization studies using fewer test animals. Arch Toxicol 1987; 60:470–1.
39. Shillaker RO, Graham MB, Hodgson IT, et al. Guinea pig maximisation test for skin sensitisation: the use of fewer test animals. Arch Toxicol 1989; 63:281.
40. Draize JH. Dermal toxicity. Food Drug Cosmet Law J 1955; 10:722–32.
41. Voss JG. Skin sensitisation by mercaptans of low molecular weight. J Invest Dermatol 1958; 31:273–9.
42. Prince HN, Prince TG. Comparative guinea pig assays for contact hypersensitivity. Cosmet Toiletries 1977; 92:53–8.
43. Sharp DW. The sensitization potential of some perfume ingredients tested, using a modified Draize procedure. Toxicology 1978; 9:261–71.
44. Johnson AW, Goodwin BFJ. The Draize test and modifications. Curr Probl Dermatol 1985; 14:31–8.
45. Maguire HC, Jr. Estimation of the allergenicity of prospective human contact sensitizers in the guinea pig. In: Maibach H, Lowe NJ, eds. Models in Dermatology. Vol. 2. Basel: Karger, 1985:234–9.
46. Maguire HC, Jr., Cipriano D. Split adjuvant test. Curr Probl Dermatol 1985; 14:107–13.
47. Grabbe S, Schwarz T. Immunoregulatory mechanisms involved in the elicitation of allergic contact dermatitis. Immunol Today 1998; 19:37–44.
48. Kimber I, Dearman RJ. Allergic contact dermatitis: the cellular effectors. Contact Dermatitis 2002; 46:1–5.
49. Kimber I, Dearman RJ, Scholes EW, et al. The local lymph node assay: developments and applications. Toxicology 1994; 93:13–31.
50. Dearman RJ, Wright ZM, Basketter DA, et al. The suitability of hexyl cinnamic aldehyde as a calibrant for the murine local lymph node assay. Contact Dermatitis 2001; 44:357–61.
51. Gerberick GF, Ryan CA, Kimber I, et al. Local lymph node assay: validation assessment for regulatorypurposes. Am J Contact Dermat 2000; 11:3–18.
52. Basketter DA, Kimber I. Predictive testing in contact allergy: facts and future. Allergy 2001; 56:937–43.
53. Basketter DA, Evans P, Fielder RJ, et al. Local lymph node assay—validation, conduct and use in practice. Food Chem Toxicol 2002; 40:593–8.
54. Uter W, Johansen JD, Orton DI, et al. Clinical update on contact allergy. Curr Opin Allergy Clin Immunol 2005; 5(5):429–36.
55. Kimber I, Weisenberger C. A murine local lymph node assay for the identification of contact allergens. Assay development and results of an initial validation study. Arch Toxicol 1989; 63:274–82.
56. Kimber I, Mitchell JA, Griffin AC. Development of a murine local lymph node assay for the determination of sensitizing potential. Food Chem Toxicol 1986; 24:585–6.
57. Kimber I. Aspects of the immune response to contact allergens: opportunities for the development and modification of predictive test methods. Food Chem Toxicol 1989; 27:755–62.
58. Kimber I, Hilton J, Weisenberger C. The murine local lymph node assay for identification of contact allergens: a preliminary evaluation of in situ measurement of lymphocyte proliferation. Contact Dermatitis 1989; 21:215–20.
59. Gerberick GF, House RV, Fletcher ER, et al. Examination of the local lymph node assay for use in contact sensitization risk assessment. Fundam Appl Toxicol 1992; 19:438–45.
60. Kimber I. The local lymph node assay. In: Marzulli FN, Maibach HI, eds. Dermatotoxicology Methods: The Laboratory Worker's Vade Mecum. Washington, DC: Taylor & Francis, 1998:145–52.
61. Kimber I, Basketter DA. The murine local lymph node assay: a commentary on collaborative trials and new directions. Food Chem Toxicol 1992; 30:165–9.
62. Dearman RJ, Basketter DA, Kimber I. Local lymph node assay: use in hazard and risk assessment. J Appl Toxicol 1999; 19:299–306.
63. Basketter DA, Kimber I. Olive oil: suitability for use as a vehicle in the local lymph node assay. Contact Dermatitis 1996; 35:190–1.
64. Basketter DA, Lea LJ, Cooper K, et al. Threshold for classification as a skin sensitizer in the local lymph node assay: a statistical evaluation. Food Chem Toxicol 1999; 37:1167–74.

65. Bruze M, Conde-Salazar L, Goossens A, et al. Thoughts on sensitizers in a standard patch test series. The European Society of Contact Dermatitis. Contact Dermatitis 1999; 41:241–50.

66. Ale SI, Maibach HI. Clinical relevance in allergic contact dermatitis: an algorithmic approach. Dermatosen 1995; 43:119–21.

67. Goldner R, Jackson E. Irritant contact dermatitis. In: Hogan D, ed. Occupational Skin Disorders. New York: Igaku-Shoin Medical Publishers, 1994:23.

68. Walle HVD. Irritant contact dermatitis. In: Menne T, Maibach H, eds. Hand Eczema. New York: CRC Press, 2000:133–9.

69. Ale SI, Maibach HI. Irritant contact dermatitis versus allergic contact dermatitis. In: Zhai H, Maibach HI, eds. Dermatotoxicology. 6th ed. Boca Raton, FL: CRC Press, 2004 (chap. 13).

70. Levin C, Maibach HI. Animal, human and in vitro test methods for predicting skin irritation. In: Zhai H, Maibach HI, eds. Dermatotoxicology. 6th ed. Boca Raton, FL: CRC Press, 2004 (chap. 36).

71. Maibach HI. The E.S.S.: excited skin syndrome (alias the "angry back"). In: Ring J, Burg G, eds. New Trends in Allergy. Berlin/Heidelerg/New York: Springer, 1981:208–21.

72. Mitchell J, Maibach HI. Managing the excited skin syndrome: patch testing hyperirritable skin. Contact Dermatitis 1997; 37:193–9.

73. Bruynzeel D, Maibach HI. Excited skin syndrome and the hypo-reactive state: current status. In: Menne T, Maibach HI, eds. Exogenous Dermatoses: Environmental Dermatitis. Boca Raton, FL: CRC Press, 1991:141–50.

74. Maibach HI, Johnson HL. Contact urticaria syndrome. Contact urticaria to diethyltoluamide (immediate-type hypersensitivity). Arch Dermatol 1975; 111(6):726–30.

75. Warner MR, Taylor JS, Leow YH. Agents causing contact urticaria. Clin Dermatol 1997; 15(4):623–35.

76. Amin S, Lahti A, Maibach HI. Contact urticaria and the contact urticaria syndrome (immediate contact reactions). In: Zhai H, Maibach HI, eds. Dermatotoxicology. 6th ed. Boca Rotan, FL: CRC Press, 2004 (chap. 42).

77. Panaszek B, Bielous-Wilk A. Contact urticaria syndrome. Przegl Lek 2005; 62(12):1480–3.

78. Lahti A, Vaananen A, Kokkonen EL, et al. Acetylsalicylic acid inhibits non-immunologic contact urticaria. Contact Dermatitis 1987; 16(3):133–5.

79. Bourrain JL. Occupational contact urticaria. Clin Rev Allergy Immunol 2006; 30(1):39–46.

80. Turjanmaa K, Reunala T. Contact urticaria from rubber gloves. Dermatol Clin 1988; 6(1):47–51.

81. Valsecchi R, Leghissa P, Cortinovis R, et al. Contact urticaria from latex in healthcare workers. Dermatology 2000; 201(2):127–31.

82. Doutre MS. Occupational contact urticaria and protein contact dermatitis. Eur J Dermatol 2005; 15(6):419–24.

Irritancy of Topical Chemicals in Transdermal Drug Delivery Systems

Heidi P. Chan, Cheryl Y. Levin, and Howard I. Maibach
Department of Dermatology, School of Medicine, University of California San Francisco, San Francisco, California, U.S.A.

INTRODUCTION

The use of transdermal drug delivery systems (TDDS) is widely recognized (1). In 2004, the U.S. market for these patches exceeded $3 billion annually (2). The advantages and disadvantages of transdermal drug delivery are well-known (3,4) and the disadvantages include the potential for contact dermatitis [CD, allergic and irritant contact dermatitis (ACD and ICD)]. Contact urticaria, photoirritation, and photoallergic contact dermatitis are possible but have not yet been identified as a clinical problem. CD literally means "inflammation of the skin" when exposed to certain substances and there are two main types: ACD and ICD (5). Table 1 shows the clinical and histopathological features of ACD and ICD (6). It is evident that there are similarities but, apart from the histological features, the distribution of lesions is widespread for ACD and mostly localized for ICD, and the course of healing, i.e., crescendo phenomenon for ACD and decrescendo phenomenon for ICD are the characteristics that help distinguish one from the other (6).

ACD to chemicals in TDDS is well established (7). In some studies establishing ACD to an active drug, the active patch is compared to the placebo patch (8). Such studies confirm a positive allergic reaction to the active if the active patch is positive and the placebo negative. On the other hand, a positive reaction to the placebo patch suggests irritation or allergy to the patch components (Table 2) (8–29).

The different classes of ICD are defined in Table 3 (30,31). This chapter focuses on the irritancy of the chemicals in TDDS (Table 4) (14,23,24,32–76). Unfortunately, post-marketing surveillance of irritant dermatitis is incomplete, thus limiting validation potential of preclinical assays.

PRECLINICAL SCREENING METHODS FOR PREDICTING SKIN IRRITATION

No one assay is able to accurately predict irritation. This is because ICD may result from acute or cumulative injury and may involve inflammation or necrosis (corrosive). A number of animal, human, and in vitro test methods have been developed, each portraying some but not all aspects of irritation. Each model has its own unique benefits and limitations (77).

Animal Irritation Assays
The Draize Rabbit Test
The Draize rabbit test was developed in 1944 (78) and has since been adapted by the U.S. Federal Hazardous Substance Act and utilized to evaluate primary irritation

TABLE 1 Clinical and Histological Differences Between ICD and ACD

	ICD	ACD
Clinical characteristics	Acute lesions: erythema, edema, oozing sometimes vesicles, and bullae; ulceration, necrosis, and pustules may be seen	Acute lesions: erythema, edema, vesicles, oozing; intense vesiculation increases suspicion of ACD; pustules, necrosis, or ulceration are rarely seen
	Chronic lesions: maybe indistinguishable of ACD, including hyperkeratosis, fissuring, redness, chapping, glazed, or scalded appearance of the skin	Chronic lesions: may be indistinguishable of ICD; vesiculation may not be present
	Lesions are characteristically circumscribed to the contact area; usually there is absence of distant lesions, but sometimes dermatitis may be generalized depending on the nature of exposure	Clinical lesions are stronger in the contact area but their limits are usually ill defined; dissemination of the dermatitis with distant lesions may occur
	Lesions may appear after first exposure (at least with strong irritants)	A phase of induction (sensitization) without clinical sign is required; clinical lesions appear right after subsequent challenges; however, exposure to a strong allergen may serve as both induction and elicitation of contact hypersensitivity
	In acute ICD lesions usually appear rapidly, in minutes to few hours after exposure, and are characterized by the "decrescendo phenomenon": the reaction reaches its peak quickly, and heals; however, delayed on set reactions can be seen (12–24 hours or more after exposure)	Lesions usually appear 24 to 72 hours after the last exposure to the causative agent, but they may develop as early as five hours or as late as seven days after exposure; allergic reactions are characterized by the "crescendo phenomenon"
	Symptoms of acute ICD are burning, stinging, pain, and soreness of the skin (pruritus may be present)	Pruritus is the main symptom of ACD
Histological characteristics	Greater pleomorphism than ACD	Less pleomorphism than ICD
	Moderate spongiosis, intracellular edema (ballooning), exocytosis	Spongiosis with microvesicles predominate
	Diffuse distribution of inflammatory infiltrate in epidermis; occasionally, neutrophil-rich infiltrates	Focal distribution of the inflammatory infiltrate in epidermis
	Pustulation and necrosis may develop	Pustulation and necrosis are rare

Abbreviations: ACD, allergic contact dermatitis; ICD, irritant contact dermatitis.
Source: From Ref. 6.

and corrosion. The test uses two (1 in^2) test sites on the dorsal skin of six albino rabbits. The stratum corneum is damaged on one side (using a hypodermic needle), while the other side remains intact. The undiluted "irritant" (0.5 g for solids or 0.5 mL for liquids) is placed on a patch and applied to the test sites, secured with two layers of surgical gauze and tape. The animal is wrapped in cloth to secure the patches for a 24-hour period. Assessment of erythema and edema, utilizing the scale shown in Table 5 (79) takes place at 24 and 72 hours following patch application. Severe reactions are assessed on days 7 or 14. Radiolabeled tracers or biochemical techniques to monitor skin healing are also utilized and some investigators supplement data with histological evaluation of skin tissue (80,81).

TABLE 2 Contact Dermatitis: Documented Allergic Type of Topical Chemicals in TDDS

Transdermal patch	Studies documented allergic type by patch testing [author(s), year (Ref.)]
Scopolamine patch	Fisher, 1984 (9); Trozak, 1985 (10); Van der Willigen et al. 1988 (11); Gordon et al. 1989 (12)
Clonidine patch	Groth et al. 1983 (13); Horning et al. 1998 (14); Maibach, 1985 (15)
Nitroglycerin patch	Machet et al. 1999 (16); Perez-Calderon et al. 2002 (17)
Estradiol patch	Boehncke and Gall, 1996 (18); Carmichael et al. 1992 (19); Koch, 2001 (20); Panhans-Gross et al. 2000 (21); Lamb and Wilkinson, 2004 (22)
Estrogen-progesterone patch	Not reported
Nicotine patch	Jordan, 1992 (23); Vincenzi et al. 1993 (24); Färm, 1993 (25)
Testosterone patch	Buckley et al. 1998 (26); Shouls et al. 2001 (27)
Fentanyl patch	Stoukides et al. 1992 (28); Mancuso et al. 2001 (29)—*Patch test not done to both studies*
Oxybutynin patch	Needs more studies and patch tests to document patch allergy
Selegiline patch	Needs more studies and patch tests to document patch allergy
Methyphenidate patch	Needs more studies and patch tests to document patch allergy

Abbreviation: TDDS, transdermal drug delivery systems
Source: From Ref. 8.

The Draize test quantifies irritation with a primary irritation index (PII), which averages the erythema and edema scores of each test site and then sums the averages. Materials producing a PII of <2 are considered nonirritating, 2 to 5 mildly irritating, >5 severely irritating, and require precautionary labeling. Subsequent studies have demonstrated that PII is somewhat subjective because the scoring of erythema and edema require clinical judgment (82).

Critics of the Draize test contest: (*i*) the harsh treatment of animals; (*ii*) distinguishing between mild and moderate irritants; (*iii*) the accuracy of the test to predict irritancy as it does not include vesiculation, severe eschar formation, or ulceration; and (*iv*) the reliability of the test (83). Some also question its relevance with regard to human experience (84–86). On the other hand, proponents of the Draize test suggest that it over predicts the severity of induced skin damage and thereby favors consumer safety (87). In spite of its advantages and disadvantages, Draize assays are still recommended by regulatory bodies.

Modified Draize Methods
The Draize test has been modified in response to criticisms over the years (77). Alterations include changing the preferred species, use of fewer animals, testing only on intact skin, and reduction of the exposure period to irritants (77). Table 6 (88) gives a comparison of the modified Draize tests.

Cumulative Irritation Assays
Frequently, ICD is produced through cumulative exposure to a weak irritant. While the Draize test assesses acute exposure to a strong irritant, there have been many assays developed to measure repetitive, cumulative irritation (77).

Repeat animal patch test (89) is method used for epidermal erosion, it is the test used for comparing irritation potential of surfactants. Solutions are applied

TABLE 3 Classification of ICD

Type	Onset	Description	Prognosis
Acute ICD	Acute—often single exposure	Signs: mild erythema, edema, inflammation, and vesiculation to frank epidermal necrosis Symptoms: burning, stinging, and pain e.g., chemical burn	Good
Delayed acute ICD	Delayed—12 to 24 hours or longer	Same as acute ICD	Good
Irritant reaction	Acute—often multiple	Usually chapped skin in first months of exposure Monomorphic (only one parameter is present) e.g., hairdressers	Good
Chronic ICD	Chronic ICD	Dermatitis usually more than six weeks Signs: erythema and increasing xerosis, followed by hyperkeratosis e.g., "housewives' eczema"	Variable
Traumatic ICD	Slowly developing after preceding trauma	Signs: erythema, vesicles, papules, and scaling e.g., trauma: burns and lacerations	Variable
Acneiform ICD	Moderately slowly developing (weeks to months)	Pustular or follicular Pustules usually sterile and transient e.g., acne cosmetica	Variable
Non-erythematous (suberythematous) irritation	Slowly developing	Subtle skin damage may occur without visible damage Objectively registered via cutaneous bioengineering techniques	Variable
Subjective (sensory) irritation	Acute	Lack of clinical manifestation upon exposure to chemical e.g., lactic acid	Excellent
Friction dermatitis	Slowly developing	Pathology: hyperkeratosis and acanthosis e.g., callus	Variable
Asteatotic irritant eczema	Slowly developing	Variant of ICD usually seen in the elderly Occupational setting: repeated exposure chemical insult, etc.	Variable

Abbreviation: ICD, irritant contact dermatitis.
Source: From Ref. 30.

occlusively to the clipped dorsum of albino mice for a 10-minute period. The process is repeated seven times and the skin is subsequently examined microscopically for epidermal erosion.

The repetitive irritation test (RIT) (90) utilizes guinea pigs to determine the protective efficacy of cream against various chemical models. In one study, the irritants sodium hydroxide (NaOH), sodium lauryl sulfate (SLS), and toluene were administered daily for two weeks to shaved dorsal skin. Barrier creams were

TABLE 4 Summary of the Type of Irritant Contact Dermatitis of Topical Chemicals in Transdermal Systems

Transdermal patch	Type of ICD	Supporting studies [author(s), year (Ref.)]
Scopolamine patch	Acute irritant type	Homick et al. 1983 (132)
Clonidine patch	Irritant reaction type	Fillingham et al. 1989 (35); Briedhart et al. 1993 (36)
Nitroglycerin patch	None (ICD only from patch components)	Muller et al. 1982 (37); Vaillant et al. 1990 (40); Kounis et al. 1996 (39); Ramey, et al. 2006 (38)
Estradiol patch	With ICD, but uncertain if it is due to estradiol	Ibarra et al. 2002 (48); Samsioe, 2002 (51); Jarupanich et al. 2003 (49); Toole et al. 2004 (50)
Estrogen-progesterone patch	With ICD, but uncertain if it is due to estrogen-progesterone	Creasy et al. 2001 (53); Zieman et al. 2002 (52); Longsdon et al. 2004 (54)
Nicotine patch	With ICD (ICD type not clearly described)	Campbell et al. 2003 (56); Hasford et al. 2003 (55); Mulligan et al. 1990 (59); Rose et al. 1990 (61); Hurt et al. 1990 (63); Daughton et al. 1991 (65); Jordan et al. 1992 (23); Vincenzi et al. 1993 (24); Kornitzer et al. 1995 (64); Abelin et al. 1989 (60); Eichelberg et al. 1989 (66)
Testosterone patch	With ICD, but uncertain if it is due to testosterone	Meikle et al. 1998 (70); Dobs et al. 1999 (71); Schulthesis et al. 2000 (68); Hameed et al. 2003 (69); Chik et al. 2005 (67)
Fentanyl patch	None	Jeal, Benfield, 1997 (76)
Oxybutynin patch	Needs more studies to establish irritancy potential	
Selegiline patch	Needs more studies to establish irritancy potential	
Methyphenidate patch	Needs more studies to establish irritancy potential	

Abbreviation: ICD, irritant contact dermatitis.

TABLE 5 Draize Scoring System

Erythema	
No erythema	0
Slight erythema	1
Well-defined erythema	2
Moderate or severe erythema	3
Severe erythema or slight eschar formation (injuries in depth)	4
Edema	
No edema	0
Very slight edema	1
Slight edema (well-defined edges)	2
Moderate edema (raised > 1 mm)	3
Severe edema (raised > 1 mm and extending beyond area of exposure)	4

Source: Adapted from Ref. 79.

TABLE 6 Modified Draize Irritation Method

	Draize	FHSA	FIFRA	DOT	OECD
No. of animals	3	6	6	6	6
Abrasion	Yes	Yes	Two of each	No	No
Exposure period (hours)	24	24	4	4	4
Examination (hours)	24, 72	24, 72	0.5, 1, 24, 48, 72	4, 48	0.5, 1, 24, 48, 72
Excluded from testing	—	—	Toxic materials, pH 2 or 11.5	—	Toxic materials, pH 2 or 11.5

Abbreviations: FHSA, Federal Hazardous Substance Act; FIFRA, Federal Insecticide, Fungicide, and Rodenticide Act; DOT, Department of Transportation; OECD, Organization for Economic Cooperation and Development.
Source: Adapted from Ref. 88.

applied two hours prior to and immediately following irritant exposure. Visual scoring, laser Doppler flowmeter (LDF), and transepidermal water loss (TEWL) quantified the resultant erythema. The study found that one barrier cream was effective against SLS and toluene injury, while another showed no efficacy. In general, RIT is most useful in evaluating the efficacy of barrier creams in preventing cumulative irritation.

To rank products for their irritant potential, repeat application patch tests have been developed. Diluted test materials are applied occlusively to the same site for 15 to 21 days. The sensitivity of the test is influenced by both the duration of occlusion and the type of patch used to apply the irritants. In general, a longer occlusive period results in enhanced percutaneous penetration. Similarly, the Draize-type gauze dressing will produce less percutaneous penetration compared with the Duhring metal chambers. In order to facilitate interpretation of the results, a reference material that produces a known effect is incorporated into the tests. Rabbits and guinea pigs are the most commonly used animal species in this type of test. Scoring of the test sites is made in accordance with the following scale: $0 =$ No reaction; $1+ =$ Mild erythema covering the patch area; $2+ =$ Erythema and edema; $3+ =$ Erythema, edema, and vesicles; and $4+ =$ Erythema, edema, and bullae.

One variation of the repeat application patch test involves the measurement of the edema producing capacity of irritants using a guinea pig model. Visual inspection and Harpenden calipers measure skin thickness following application of irritants for 3 to 21 days. This model demonstrates clear dose–response relationships and discriminating power for all irritants, excluding acids and alkalis (91).

Open application assays (92) involve application of irritants onto the backs of rabbits 16 times over a three-week period. Visual scoring of erythema and skin thickness measurements quantify the results. A high correlation has been observed when comparing erythema and skin thickness. In addition, using 60 test substances, rabbit data correlated strongly with cumulative irritation studies in man, suggesting that the model is useful.

A modified open application assay (93) applied test substance once a day for three days to a 1-cm^2 test site on the backs of guinea pigs. Sites were evaluated visually for erythema and edema. In addition, biopsies were taken and the skin samples were evaluated for epidermal thickness and dermal infiltration. Irritants were compared to a standard irritant, 2% SLS, and potency ranked. Extensive processing involved in properly performing this assay may limit its usefulness.

Immersion Assay

Aqueous detergent solutions and other surfactant-based products are evaluated for irritancy using the guinea pig immersion assay (94–96). This assay involves placing 10 guinea pigs in a restraining device that is immersed in a 40°C test solution for four hours daily for a total of three days (97). The restraining apparatus allows the guinea pig's head to be above the solution. Twenty-four hours following the final immersion the flanks are shaved and the skin is evaluated for erythema, edema, and fissures. In one study, the dermatotoxic effects of detergents in guinea pigs (immersion) and humans (patch test) were concomitantly tested (96). Irritation of guinea pig skin led to epidermal erosion and a 40% to 60% increase histamine content. Seven of eight human subjects had a positive patch test to the same irritants, suggesting a good correlation between the guinea pig and the human models.

Mouse Ear Model

The *mouse ear model* is used to evaluate the degree of inflammation associated with shampoos and surfactant-based products. Uttley and Van Abbe (98) applied undiluted shampoos to one ear of mice daily for four days and visually assessed the erythema, vessel dilatation, and edema. However, the anesthetic used to anesthetize the mice in this study may have altered the development of inflammation and confounded the results. Patrick and Maibach (99) measured mouse ear thickness at various times following surfactant application. Pretreatment of the ear with croton oil or 12-*O*-tetradecanoylphorbol 13-acetate 72 hours prior to irritant application increased the sensitivity of the assay. This assay was most useful in testing surfactant-based products and had little efficacy with oily or highly perfumed materials.

Recent Assays

Animal assays continue to be developed to quantify irritant response. Humphrey et al. (100) measured Evan's blue dye recovered from the rat skin after exposure to inflammatory agents. Trush et al. (101) assessed the dermal inflammatory response to numerous irritants by measuring the level of myeloperoxidase enzyme in polymorphonuclear leukocytes in young CD-1 mice.

Human Models

Following the development of patch test, Draize et al. (77) suggested a 24-hour single-application patch test in humans. Human testing facilitates extrapolation of data to the clinical setting. Testing is often performed on non-diseased skin (102) of the dorsal upper arm or the back. The required test area is small and up to 10 materials may be tested simultaneously. A reference irritant is often included to account for variability in test responses. In general, screening of new materials involves open application on the back or dorsal upper arm for a short amount of time (30 minutes to 1 hour) to minimize potential adverse events.

Single-Application Patch Testing

The National Academy of Sciences (103) recommended a four-hour single-application patch test for routine testing of skin irritation in humans. In general, patches are occluded and placed on the dorsal upper arm or back of skin of patients. The degree of occlusion varies according to the type of occlusive device; the Hilltop or

Duhring chambers or an occlusive tape will enhance percutaneous penetration compared to a non-occlusive tape or cotton bandage (104). Potentially volatile materials should always be tested with a non-occlusive tape. Exposure time to the test material varies and is often customized by the investigator. Volatile chemicals are generally applied for 30 minutes to 1 hour, while some chemicals have been applied for more than 24 hours.

Following patch removal the skin is rinsed with water to remove residue. Skin responses are evaluated 30 minutes to 1 hour following patch removal in order to allow hydration and pressure effects of the patch to subside. Another evaluation is performed 24 hours following patch removal. The Draize scale is used to analyze test results (Table 5). The Draize scale does not include papular, vesicular, or bullous responses; other scales have been developed to address these needs. Single-application tests generally heal within one week.

Cumulative Irritation Tests

Utilizing statistical analysis of test data, Kligman and Woodling (104) calculated the IT50 (time to produce irritation in 50% of subjects) and ID50 (dose required to produce irritation in 50% of subjects following a 24-hour exposure). This formed the basis for the 21-day cumulative irritation assay. The "21-day assay" is used to screen new formulations prior to marketing (105). The original assay involved application of a 2.5 cm^2 of Webril saturated with the test material (either liquid or 0.05 g of viscous material) to the skin of undamaged upper back, secured with occlusive tape. Twenty-four hours after patch application, the test site is examined and material is reapplied. The test is repeated for 21 days.

Two modifications of the cumulative irritation test were reported (106). One assay involved Finn chamber application of metalworking fluids onto the midback of volunteers for one day. The sites were evaluated and the fluids were then reapplied for an additional two days. In the other assay, a two-week, six hours per day, RIT (excluding weekends) was utilized. Better discrimination of irritancy and shorter duration was observed with a three-day model.

Chamber Scarification Test

The chamber scarification test assesses the irritancy potential of materials on damaged skin (107). Subjects included in this assay are highly sensitive to 24-hour exposure to 5% SLS (vesicles, severe erythema, and edema post-application). Six to eight 10 mm^2 areas on the volar forearm are scratched 8 to 10 times with a 30-gauge needle. Scarification damages the epidermal layer without drawing blood. Four scratches are parallel and the other four are perpendicular to the test site. A 0.1 g of test material (or 0.1 mL of liquid) is then applied to the scarified area for 24 hours using Duhring chambers. Non-occlusive tape is used to secure the chambers in place.

With fresh specimens, patches are applied daily for three days. A visual scoring scale is used to quantify test results 30 minutes following patch removal. An analogous area of intact skin is also scored, so evaluation is based upon comparison between compromised and intact skin. The visual score of scarified test sites divided by the score of intact test sites, known as the scarification index, allows this comparison to be made.

Immersion Tests

Patch tests often overpredict the irritant potential of some materials. Immersion tests were established to improve irritancy prediction by mimicking consumer use. Kooyman and Snyder developed an arm immersion technique to compare the relative irritancy of two soap or detergent products (97). Soap solutions of up to 3% are prepared and one hand and forearm are immersed in each solution, comparing different products or concentrations. Temperature is maintained at 41°C. The exposure period varies between 10 and 15 minutes per day for a total of five days or until observable irritation is produced on both arms. The antecubital fossa is generally the first area to experience irritation, followed by the hands (89,97).

Variations of this technique have been developed to separately test the antecubital fossa and the hands. Variations incorporated differing dosing regimens and endpoints. Clarys et al. (108). investigated the effects of temperature and anionic character on the degree of irritation caused by detergents. TEWL, erythema (colorimetry), and skin dryness (capacitance) were used to quantify test results. The irritant response was increased at higher temperature and higher anionic content. Utilizing a modified arm immersion technique, it was noticed that once skin was compromised (erythema of 1+ on a visual scale), irritants applied to the forearm and back caused exaggerated responses (109).

Soap Chamber Technique

The "chapping" potential of bar soaps is evaluated with the soap chamber technique (92). While patch testing is useful in predicting erythema, it does not address the dryness, flaking, and fissuring observed with bar soap use. Using this method, 0.1 mL of an 8% soap solution is applied to the forearm via Duhring chambers fitted with Webril pads. Non-occlusive tape is used to secure the chambers. Patches are applied for 24 hours on day 1 and 6 hours on days 2 to 5. Skin responses are evaluated with visual scoring of erythema, scaling, and fissures. The test tends to over predict irritant responses of some materials.

Protective Barrier Assessment

The skin barrier function assay tests the efficacy of protective creams in preventing an irritant response (110). Creams were applied and the skin dosed with either SLS or ammonium hydroxide. Paraffin wax in cetyl alcohol was the most effective in preventing irritation. In another study (106), petrolatum was applied to the backs of 20 subjects who were then exposed to SLS, NaOH, toluene, and lactic acid. Irritation was assessed by the visual scoring, TEWL, and colorimetry. Petrolatum was found to be an effective barrier against SLS, NaOH, and lactic acid and moderately effective against toluene.

Frosch et al. (90) revised the RIT to evaluate the effect of two barrier creams in preventing SLS-induced irritation. The irritant was applied to the ventral forearms of the subjects for 30 minutes daily for two weeks. Visual scoring, LDF, colorimetry, and TEWL were utilized to assess resultant erythema. TEWL was found most useful in quantifying results, while colorimetry was the least beneficial.

In Vitro Tests

In vitro skin irritation assays are of benefit in addressing concerns associated with animal testing. These "alternative" methods may reduce the number of animals needed in irritation testing, or in some cases may fully replace them. Numerous in vitro skin irritation assays have been developed but most have not been validated to determine their usefulness, limitations, and compliance with regulatory testing requirements. Furthermore, dose–response relationships have not been fully explored using in vitro methods.

Studies evaluating in vitro testing indicate usefulness in predicting starting doses for in vivo studies, potentially reducing the number of animals used for such determinations. The U.S. Interagency Coordinating Committee on the Validation of Alternative Toxicological Methods (ICCVAM) and the U.S. National Toxicologic Program Center for the Evaluation of Alternative Toxicological Methods (NICEATM) were established to help develop in vitro irritant testing. In 2004, there were four approved irritation assays: Corrositex® (MB Research Laboratories, Spinnerstown, Pennsylvania, U.S.A.), EpiDerm™ (MatTek Corporation, Ashland, Massachusetts, U.S.A.), EPISKIN® (IMEDEX, Trévoux, Lyon, France), and Rat Skin Transcutaneous Electrical Resistance (TER) Assays (Table 7).

Corrositex is a collagen matrix acting as synthetic skin and is used to assess the dermal corrosivity potential of chemicals. Should a chemical pass through the biobarrier by diffusion and/or destruction, Corrositex elicits a color change in the underlying liquid chemical detection system. Corrositex is currently used by the U.S. Department of Transportation (U.S. DOT) to assign categories of corrosivity for labeling purposes according to the United Nations guidelines. However, its use is limited to specific chemical classes, including acids, acid derivatives, acylhalides, alkylamines, and polyalkylamines, bases, chlorosilanes, metal halides, and oxyhalides, and its value for defining less drastic irritation has not been demonstrated.

A peer review panel—NICEATM and ICCVAM—elucidated some of the advantages of Corrositex, including its possible use in replacing or reducing the numbers of animals required. Positive test results often eliminate the need for animal testing. When further animal testing is necessary, often only one animal is required to confirm a corrosive chemical. The panel also concluded that most of the chemicals identified as negative by Corrositex or nonqualifying in the detection system are unlikely to be corrosive when tested on animals.

EpiDerm (EPI-200) is a three-dimensional human skin model that uses cell viability as a measure of corrosivity. It has been used with several common tests of cytotoxicity and irritancy, including MTT, IL-1a, PGE_2, LDH, and sodium fluorescence permeability.

TABLE 7 In Vitro Assays

Assay	Description	Methodology
Corrositex	Collagen matrix acting as synthetic skin	A color change in the underlying liquid Chemical detection system when irritant passes through matrix
EpiDerm	Three-dimensional matrix Acting as synthetic skin	Cell viability as a measure of corrosivity
EPISKIN	Three-dimensional matrix Acting as synthetic skin	Cell viability as a measure of corrosivity
TER	Skin disks taken from the pelts of humanly killed young rats	Significantly lower inherent transcutaneous electrical resisitance when skin barrier is compromised

Abbreviation: TER, Rat Skin Transcutaneous Electrical Resistance Assay.
Source: Adapted from Ref. 111.

EPISKIN is a three-dimensional human skin model comprised a reconstructed epidermis and a functional stratum corneum. In a study supported by the European Centre for the Validation of Alternative Methods, EPISKIN was useful in testing potential irritants, including organic and inorganic acids, organic and inorganic bases, neutral organics, electrophiles, phenols, and soaps/surfactants. With both EpiDerm and EPISKIN, the test material is topically applied to the skin for up to four hours with subsequent assessment of the effects on cell viability.

In TER assay, irritants will cause a loss of normal stratum corneum integrity and barrier function. A reduced barrier function will give a lower inherent TER. TER assay involves up to 24 hours application of test material to the epidermal surfaces of skin disks taken from young rats. Comparing EpiDerm, EPISKIN, and TER, only EPISKIN was able to significantly distinguish between two particular layers of chemicals. Currently, the ICCVAM recommends that EpiDerm, EPISKIN, and TER are used to assess the dermal corrosivity potential of chemicals in a "weight-of-evidence" approach. In general, positive corrosivity tests will not require further testing, while negative corrosivity will.

ICD AND TDDS

Musel and Warshaw (8) summarized the spectrum of cutaneous reactions to transdermal therapeutic systems, mainly ACD and ICD. Some of these adverse effects lead to poor patient compliance or patch discontinuation (8,112,113). The risk of topical irritation produced by chemicals depends on their ability to penetrate into the skin and their contact with irritated or damaged skin. The penetration of chemicals into the skin depends on the skin condition, anatomic location, chemical characteristics of the permeant, and concentration. Penetration is also influenced by external factors, especially solvents, surface-active agents, alkalies, moisture, temperature, extreme dehydration, and mechanical effects. Hogan and Maibach (113) reported that the duration of skin irritation increased with the duration of skin occlusion. Kahawara and Tojo observed that the chemical ingredient (active pharmaceutical ingredient) in the patch resulted to skin irritation and they recommended that, on removal of the patch, the skin site should be washed (114).

ICD from Scopolamine TDDS

Scopolamine, a belladonna alkaloid, is indicated for nausea and vomiting associated with motion sickness, anesthesia, and surgery (32) and was the first drug approved for transdermal delivery (2). Rarely known to cause ACD (8), transdermal scopolamine was reported to cause ICD to the patch components in isolated cases (3,8).

ICD from Clonidine TDDS

Clonidine is a centrally acting α-agonist used primarily as an antihypertensive agent for mild to moderate hypertension (14). The clonidine patch may cause irritation and/or an allergic reaction (33,34). In long-term treatment (22 months) with transdermal clonidine in mild hypertension in 41 patients, it was reported that the incidence of CD peaked between the 6th and 26th weeks of treatment (35). A total of 13 patients (32%) experienced irritant reactions. Of the 32%, ICD manifested primarily as mild erythema (17%) to moderate (16%) erythema, attributable to the week-long patch occlusion. In the second year of the study, none of the patients experienced ICD (35).

The mild skin reactions were classified as non-immunological transient skin irritations because all reactions subsided and did not reappear despite continued long-term clonidine transdermal treatment (35,36).

ICD from Nitroglycerin TDDS

Nitroglycerin is an organic nitrate used for the prevention and treatment of angina pectoris. Because nitroglycerin causes vasodilation, erythema under the patches is frequent. Rubefaction at the margins of covered skin, noticed with a similar frequency in placebo and active nitrate patches, was indicative of mild irritation (37). Irritant reddening disappeared spontaneously. Transdermal nitroglycerin causes ACD from nitroglycerin and the other patch components (38–40). On the other hand, ICD from nitroglycerin patches are from the patch components only, not the active chemical (38–40).

ICD from Estradiol TDDS

Estradiol transdermal therapeutic systems provide a simpler way of prescribing hormonal replacement therapy that has the potential for long-term use through improved patient compliance (41). Studies involving more than 100 patients reported that the incidence of skin reactions due to estradiol TDDS was between 5% and 35% (42–47). Most skin reactions consisted of mild erythema and/or pruritus at the application site, which generally resolved after removal of the system. Patients tend to transfer the patch from one site to another. Irritation from estradiol TDDS was more common in hot humid climates (48,113). In a six-month study, Jarupanich et al. (49) classified local skin irritations as: erythema, burning sensation, vesicle, and itching from a 12.5-cm^2 matrix patch applied weekly in 50 patients. They recorded the skin irritations in the first, third, and sixth month. Results revealed the overall incidence of skin irritation was 40.3% (49) Studies (48,50,51) suggested that there was an advantage in the use of the newer DOT (delivery optimized thermodynamics) Matrix™ (Novartis Pharamaceuticals, North Ryde, New South Wales, Australia) estradiol patch over the conventional patches, in its efficacy and tolerability, that improving patient compliance.

ICD from Estrogen/Progesterone TDDS

Transdermal contraceptive patches are more convenient to the user and may decrease contraceptive failures associated with incorrect use (52). Creasy et al. (53) reported that a specific brand of contraceptive transdermal patch (Ortho Evra®; Ortho-McNeil, Inc., Raritan, New Jersey, U.S.A.) was not associated with photo-toxicity or photoallergy. Logdon et al. (54) reported that of the 62 patients enrolled in a study, 3 (5%) discontinued treatment because of moderate-to-severe skin irritation.

ICD from Nicotine TDDS

Transdermal nicotine is one of the many forms of nicotine replacement therapy (NRT) for smoking cessation (55,56). Campbell (56) reported NRT success rates in two studies, ~10% with the active (nicotine) patch and ~6% with the placebo patch. In one of these studies, the incidence of local irritant reactions (pruritus and erythema) at the application site was more common with the active patch than the placebo patch (57). Hasford and Fagerstrom (55) reported skin irritation in their study which includes itching, skin rashes, sweating, and dryness of skin from transdermal nicotine.

Smith et al. (58) explained the mechanisms of sudorific (sweating) and rubiform (erythema) responses accompanied by subtle piloerection, hyperalgesia, and pruritus following percutaneous nicotine absorption. They proposed a complex mechanism for the direct nicotine stimulation of sweat glands, piloerection, and vasoconstriction. These reactions were accompanied by secondary activation and release of vasodilator peptides, which produced a predominating vasodilator tone following topical administration, this response masking the direct axon reflex-mediated vasoconstriction.

Musel and Warsaw (8) summarized 10 studies showing irritant reactions to transdermal nicotine with the active patch (compared with the placebo patch) and these were erythema, pruritus, burning, edema, papules, pustules, stinging, soreness, and tingling (14,23,24,59–66).

ICD from Testosterone TDDS

Currently licensed for the treatment of hypogonadism in men, transdermal delivery systems of testosterone include patches and gels (67). These products deliver testosterone concentrations at physiological levels (68,69). Schulthesis et al. (68) found that the patches had more adverse skin reactions than the gel. This may be due to the occlusive property of the patch. Their study also concluded that the gel was easier to apply than the patch.

Hameed et al. (69) discussed the difference between scrotal and non-scrotal patches. Although absorption of testosterone is more rapid through scrotal than non-scrotal skin, adverse skin reactions (e.g., itching, blisters, and erythema) occurred at both sites. Meikle (70) favored the non-scrotal patch but suggested pretreatment of the site with 0.1% triamcinolone acetonide cream as it had been shown to reduce skin irritation and allow continued use of the system (67,71,113).

ICD from Fentanyl TDDS

Fentanyl is a narcotic analgesic used for the management of persistent, moderate-to-severe chronic pain (72). Fentanyl transdermal reservoir patches have been used since 1991 (73). It is a potent opioid analgesic and offers the advantages of simplicity and noninvasive delivery (74). Skin irritations from fentanyl patch include papules, pustules, erythema, and pruritus (8). Radbruch and Elsner (75) reported that 12% of 1005 patients in their study experienced dermatologic adverse effects with fentanyl TDDS. Jeal and Benfield (76) suggested that the transient skin irritation associated with fentanyl patches was due to the plastic patch or the adhesive, rather than the drug.

ICD from Oxybutynin TDDS

Oxybutynin has been the most commonly prescribed treatment for overactive bladder (OAB) syndrome (115). OAB is characterized by urinary urgency with or without urge incontinence, urinary frequency, and nocturia (116). Transdermal oxybutynin delivers oxybutynin continuously and consistently over a three- to four-day interval after application to intact skin (117). Adverse skin irritations associated with the patch application site have been noted and include pruritus and erythema (115–121), burning sensation, pain, and hyperpigmentation (118). All reactions resolved after the patch was removed (118).

ICD from Selegiline TDDS

The transdermal selegiline patch is a treatment for depression (122,123). Amsterdam and Bokin (122) conducted a one-year study, involving 674 patients, and reported that application site reactions were more common in the active patch treatment (5%) than the placebo patch. Twenty-six (3.9%) of the 674 patients who received selegiline patches discontinued as a result of application site reactions.

ICD from Methylphenidate TDDS

Stimulants are the first line therapy for Attention Deficit Hyperactive Disorder (ADHD) (124). Methylphenidate is a short-acting stimulant used for the treatment of ADHD in children. Most children treated with short-acting stimulants need multiple doses for continuous treatment that requires them to take oral medications during school hours (124). In April 2007, FDA approved the first transdermal methylphenidate patch for ADHD (125). There appear to be no data on adverse skin reactions brought about by the active ingredient and patch components.

MANAGEMENT AND GENERAL PREVENTIVE MEASURES FOR ICD FROM TDDS

ICD from TDDS can be managed by pretreating the application site with topical corticoids (71,112,113). Kahawara and Tojo (114) recommend washing the application site upon removal of the patch to prevent development and/or further skin irritation. It is also recommended to change the application site with each new transdermal system (115,116).

PHYSICAL MODES OF SKIN PENETRATION OF DRUGS

Chemical enhancers, used in TDDS for skin penetration, alter the barrier's chemical properties. On the other hand, physical skin penetration enhancement techniques may be used to overcome the limitations of the chemical enhancers, thus promoting an alternate way of drug penetration (126). These techniques include iontophoresis (126,127), electroporation (2,126), phonophoresis (2,128), and magnetophoresis (128,129). Other techniques that should be mentioned for completeness include nanotechnology (128,130), microneedles (131), and pulsed CO_2 lasers (129). Many of these physical methods are discussed elsewhere in this volume. All would benefit from detailed irritation evaluation.

CONCLUSIONS

The skin is an important route of drug delivery (2). Efforts to improve TDDS are focused on the evaluation of the chemical substance in relation to their skin penetration-enhancing properties, to help minimize adverse skin reactions (106). Making diagnostic patch test kits to ascertain if the lesion is ACD or ICD more readily available will greatly refine pharmacovigilance. It was suggested that matrix fentanyl patches produced less skin irritation than reservoir devices (74), and such findings should be taken into account in future patch development.

Further studies involving synergy of chemical and physical penetration enhancers are significant for the future of TDDS. Taken together, current transdermal systems produce sufficient irritation to warrant further investigations to: (*i*) improve the ability to identify irritation potential prior to marketing; (*ii*) identify methods to decrease irritation; and (*iii*) develop a more efficient and reliable post-marketing irritation database, so as to further validate the premarketing irritation assays.

REFERENCES

1. Ranade V V. Drug delivery systems. 6. Transdermal drug delivery. J Clin Pharmacol 1991; 31(5):401–18.
2. Langer R. Transdermal drug delivery: past progress, current status, and future prospects. Adv Drug Deliv Rev 2004; 56:557–8.
3. Levin C, Maibach HI. Transdermal drug delivery system—an overview. In: Zhai H, Maibach HI, eds. Dermatotoxicology. 6th ed. Boca Raton, FL: CRC Press, Taylor & Francis Group, 2004:141–4.
4. Bronaugh R, Maibach HI, eds. Percutaneous Absorption. New York: Marcel Dekker, 1999:419.
5. James WD, Berger TG, Elston DM. Contact dermatitis and drug eruptions. In: Andrew's Diseases of the Skin—Clinical Dermatology. 10th ed. St. Louis, MO: Elsevier Inc., 2006:91.
6. Ale IS, Maibach HI. Irritant contact dermatitis versus allergic contact dermatitis. In: Zhai H, Maibach HI, eds. Dermatotoxicology. 6th ed. Boca Raton, FL: CRC Press, Taylor & Francis Group, 2004:243.
7. Levin C, Maibach HI. Transdermal drug delivery systems: dermatologic and other adverse reactions. In: Zhai H, Maibach HI, eds. Dermatotoxicology. 6th ed. Boca Raton, FL: CRC Press, Taylor & Francis Group, 2004:633.
8. Musel AL, Warshaw EM. Cutaneous reactions to transdermal therapeutic systems. Dermatitis 2006; 17(3):109–22.
9. Fisher AA. Dermatitis due to transdermal therapeutic systems. Cutis 1984; 34:526–31.
10. Trozak DJ. Delayed hypersensitivity to scopolamine delivered by a transdermal device. J Am Acad Dermatol 1985; 13:247–51.
11. van der Willigen AH, Oranje AP, Stoltz E, van Joost T. Delayed hypersensitivity to scopolamine delivered by a transdermal therapeutic system. J Am Acad Dermatol 1988; 18(1 Pt 1):146–7.
12. Gordon CR, Shupak A, Doweck I, Spitzer O. Allergic contact dermatitis caused by transdermal hyoscine. Br Med J 1989; 298:1220–1.
13. Groth H, Vetter H, Knuesel, Vetter W. Allergic skin reactions to transdermal clonidine. Lancet 1983; 2:850–1.
14. Horning JR, Zawada ET, Simmons JL, et al. Efficacy and safety of two-year therapy with transdermal clonidine for essential hypertension. Chest 1998; 93:941–5.
15. Maibach H. Clonidine: irritant and allergic contact dermatitis assays. Contact Dermatitis 1985; 12:192–5.
16. Machet L, Martin L, Toledano C, et al. Allergic contact dermatitis from nitroglycerin contained in 2 transdermal systems. Dermatology 1999; 198:106–7.
17. Perez-Calderon R, Gonzalo-Garijo MA, Rodriguez-Nevado I. Generalized allergic contact dermatitis from nitroglycerin in a transdermal therapeutic system. Contact Dermatitis 2002; 46:303.
18. Boehncke WH, Gall H. Type IV hypersensitivity to topical estradiol in a patient tolerant to it orally. Contact Dermatitis 1996; 35:187–8.
19. Carmichael AJ, Foulds IS. Allergic contact dermatitis from oestradiol in oestrogen patches. Contact Dermatitis 1992; 26:194–5.
20. Koch P. Allergic contact dermatitis from estradiol and norethisterone acetate in transdermal hormonal patch. Contact Dermatitis 2001; 44:112–3.

21. Panhans-Gross A, Gall H, Dziuk M, Peter RU. Contact dermatitis from estradiol in transdermal therapeutic system. Contact Dermatitis 2000; 43:368–9.

22. Lamb SR, Wilkinson SM. Contact allergy to progesterone and estradiol in a patient with multiple corticosteroid allergies. Dermatitis 2004; 15:78–81.

23. Jordan WP. Clinical evaluation of contact sensitization potential of a transdermal nicotine system (Nicoderm). J Fam Pract 1992; 34:709–12.

24. Vincenzi C, Tosti A, Cirone M, et al. Allergic contact dermatitis from transdermal nicotine system. Contact Dermatitis 1993; 29:104–5.

25. Färm G. Contact allergy to nicotine from a nicotine patch. Contact Dermatitis 1993; 29:214–5.

26. Buckley DA, Wilkinson SM, Higgins EM. Contact allergy to a testosterone patch. Contact Dermatitis 1998; 39:91–2.

27. Shouls J, Shum KW, Gadour M, Gawkrodger DJ. Contact allergy to testosterone in an androgen patch: control of symptoms by pre-application of topical steroid. Contact Dermatitis 2001; 45:124–5.

28. Stoukides CA, Stegman M. Diffuse rash associated with transdermal fentanyl. Clin Pharm 1992; 11:222.

29. Mancuso G, Berdondini RM, Passarini B. Eosinophilic pustular eruption associated with transdermal fentanyl. J Eur Acad Dermatol Venereol 2001; 15:70–2.

30. Chew A-L, Maibach HI. Ten Genotypes of Irritant Contact Dermatitis. In: Chew A-L, Maibach HI, eds. Irritant Dermatitis. Berlin-Heidelberg: Springer, 2006:5–9.

31. Weltfriend S, Ramon M, Maibach HI. Irritant Dermatitis (Irritation). In: Zhai H, Maibach HI, eds. Dermatotoxicology. 6th ed. FL: CRC Press, Taylor & Francis Group, 2004:182.

32. Levin C, Maibach HI. Transdermal Drug Delivery System—an Overview. In: Zhai H, Maibach HI, eds. Dermatotoxicology. 6th ed. FL: CRC Press, Taylor & Francis Group, 2004:651.

33. The Antihypertensive Patch Italian Study (APIS) Investigators. One year efficacy and tolerability of clonidine administered by the transdermal route in patients with mild to moderate hypertension—a multicentre open label study. Clin Auton Res 1993; 3:379–83.

34. Clonidine Prescription Information. PDR 2007. 61st ed. New Jersey: Medical Economics Company, Inc, 2007:846.

35. Fillingim J, Matzek KM, Hughes EM, et al. Long-term treatment with transdermal clonidine in mild hypertension. Clin Ther 1989; 11(3):398–408.

36. Breidthart J, Schumacher H, Mehlburger L. Long-term (5 year) experience with transdermal clonidine in the treatment of mild to moderate hypertension. Clin Auton Res 1993; 3:385–90.

37. Muller P, Imhof PR, Burkhart F, et al. Human pharmacological studies of a new transdermal system containing nitroglycerin. Eur J Clin Pharmacol 1982; 22:473.

38. Ramey JT, Lockey RF. Allergic and non-allergic reactions to nitroglycerin. Allergy Asthma Proc 2006; 27(3):273–80.

39. Kounis NG, Zavras GM, Papadaki PJ, et al. Allergic reactions to local glyceryl trinitrate administration. Br J Clin Pract 1996; 50(8):437–9.

40. Vaillant L, Biette S, Machet L, et al. Skin acceptance of transcutaneous nitroglycerin patches: a prospective study of 33 patients. Contact Dermatitis 1990; 23(3):142–5.

41. Samsioe G. Hormone replacement therapy: expanding treatment options with transdermal delivery. Curr Ther Res 1999; 60(3):161–7.

42. Buvat J, Buvat-Herbaut M, Desmons F, et al. Les patches a l'estradiol. Un progress dans le traitment de la menopause. Gynecologie 1989; 40:53.

43. Erkkola R, Holma P, Jarvi T, et al. Transdermal oestrogen replacement therapy in a Finnish population. Maturitas 1991; 13:275.

44. Grall JY. Estrogenotherapie substitutive par voie transdermique: sur quels criteres choisir la posologie initiale? Tempo Med 1990; 97:1.

45. Janaud A. Estraderm TTS dans le traitment des troubles lies a la menopause: resultas d'une etude long terme chez 324 femmes. Gaz Med 1990; 97:1.

46. Kerzel C, Keller PJ. Ein transdermales therapeutisches Systemzur homonellen Therapie klimekterischer. Ausfallserschienungen. Multizentrische Studie. Geburtshilfe Frauen-heilkunde 1987; 47:565.

47. Muck AO. Transdermals Therapeutisches System zur physiologischen Otrogensustitui-tion. Therapiewoche 1990; 40:41.

48. Ibarra de Palacios P, Schmidt G, Sergejew T, et al. Comparative study to evaluate skin irritation and adhesion of Estradot® and Climara® in healthy postmenopausal women. Climacteric 2002; 5:383–9.

49. Jarupanich T, Lamlertkittikul S, Chandeying V. Efficacy, safety and acceptability of a seven-day transdermal estradiol patch for estrogen replacement therapy. J Med Assoc Thai 2003; 86:836–45.

50. Toole J, Silagy S, Maric A, et al. Evaluation of irritation and sensitization of two 50µg/day oestrogen patches. Maturitas 2002; 43:257–63.

51. Samsioe G. Transdermal hormone therapy: gels and patches. Climacteric 2004; 7:347–56.

52. Zieman M. The introduction of a transdermal hormonal contraceptive (Ortho Evra™/Evra™). Fertil Steril 2002; 77(Suppl. 2):S1–2.

53. Creasy GW, Abrams LS, Fischer AC. Transdermal contraception. Semin Reprod Med 2001; 19(4):373–80.

54. Logsdon S, Richards J, Omar HA. Long-term evaluation of the use of the transdermal contraceptive patch in adolescents. Sci World J 2004; 4:512–6.

55. Hasford J, Fagerstrom KO, Hausten K-O. A naturalistic cohort study on effectiveness, safety and usage pattern of an over-the-counter nicotine patch. Eur J Clin Pharmacol 2003; 59:443–7.

56. Campbell I. Nicotine replacement therapy in smoking cessation. Thorax 2003; 58:464–5.

57. Russell MAH, Stapleton JA, Feyerabend C, et al. Targeting heavy smokers in general practice: a randomized, controlled trial of transdermal nicotine patches. Br Med J 1993;308–12.

58. Smith EW, Smith KA, Maibach HI, et al. The local side effects of transdermally absorbed nicotine. Skin Pharmacol 1992; 5(2):69–76.

59. Mulligan SC, Masterson JG, Devane JG, et al. Clinical and pharmacokinetic properties of transdermal nicotine patch. Clin Pharmacol Ther 1990; 47:331–7.

60. Abelin T, Buehler A, Müller P, et al. Controlled trial of transdermal nicotine patch in tobacco withdrawal. Lancet 1989; 1:7–10.

61. Rose JE, Levin ED, Behm FM, et al. Transdermal nicotine facilitates smoking cessation. Clin Pharmacol Ther 1990; 47:323–30.

62. Abelin T, Ehrsam R, Bühler-Reichert A, et al. Effectiveness of transdermal nicotine system in smoking cessation studies. Methods Find Exp Clin Pharmacol 1989; 11:205–14.

63. Hurt RD, Lauger GG, Offord KP, et al. Nicotine replacement therapy with the use of a transdermal nicotine patch—a randomized double-blind placebo-controlled trial. Mayo Clin Proc 1990; 65:1529–37.

64. Kornitzer M, Bousten M, Dramaix M, et al. Combined use of nicotine patch and gum in smoking cessation: a placebo-controlled clinical trial. Prev Med 1995; 24:41–7.

65. Daughton DM, Heatly SA, Prendergrast JJ, et al. Effects of transdermal nicotine delivery as an adjunct to low-intervention smoking cessation therapy: a randomized, placebo-controlled, double-blind study. Arch Intern Med 1991; 51:749–52.

66. Eichelberg D, Stolze P, Block M, et al. Contact allergies induced by TTS treatment. Methods Find Exp Clin Pharmacol 1989; 11:223–5.

67. Chik Z, Johnston A, Chew SL, et al. Pharmacokinetics of a new testosterone transdermal delivery system, TDS®-testosterone in healthy males. Br J Clin Pharm 2005; 61(3):275–9.

68. Schulthesis D, Hiltl D-M, Meschi MR, et al. Pilot study of the transdermal application of testosterone gel for penile skin for the treatment of hypogonadotropic men with erectile dysfunction. World J Urol 2000; 18:431–5.

69. Hameed A, Brothwood T, Boulox P. Delivery of testosterone replacement therapy. Curr Opin Investig Drugs 2003; 4(10):1213–9.

70. Meikle AW. Transdermal testosterone, a viewpoint of the article: transdermal testosterone, by: McClellan KJ, Goa KL. Drugs 1998; 55(2):253–8.

71. Dobs AS, Meile W, Arver S, et al. Pharmacokinetics, efficacy, and safety of a permeation-enhanced testosterone transdermal system in comparison with bi-weekly injections of testosterone enanthate for the treatment of hypogonadal men. J Clin Endocrinol Metab 1999; 84(10):3469–78.

72. Duragesic® prescription information. PDR 2007. 61st ed. New Jersey: Medical Economics Company, Inc., 2007:3331.

73. Freynhagen R, Von Giesen HJ, Busche P, et al. Switching from reservoir to matrix systems for the transdermal delivery of fentanyl: a prospective, multicenter pilot study in outpatients with chronic pain. J Pain Symptom Manage 2005; 30(3):289–97.

74. Marier JF, Lor M, Potvin D, et al. Pharmacokinetics, tolerability, and performance of a novel matrix transdermal delivery system of fentanyl relative to the commercially available reservoir formulation in healthy subjects. J Clin Pharmacol 2006; 46:642–53.

75. Radbruch L, Elsner F. Clinical experience with transdermal fentanyl for the treatment of cancer pain in Germany. Keio J Med 2004; 53(1):23–9.

76. Jeal W, Benfield P. Transdermal fentanyl. A review of its pharmacological properties and therapeutic efficacy in pain control. Drugs 1997; 53(1):109–38.

77. Levin C, Maibach HI. Animal, human, and in vitro test methods for predicting skin irritation. In: Zhai H, Maibach HI, eds. Dermatotoxicology. 6th ed. FL: CRC Press, Taylor & Francis Group, 2004:679–93.

78. Draize JH, Woodward G, Calvery HO. Methods for the study of skin irritation and toxicity of substances applied to the skin and mucous membranes. J Pharmacol Exp Therapeutics 1944; 82:377–90.

79. Patrick E, Maibach H. Comparison of the time course, dose response and mediators of chemically induced skin irritation in three species. In: Frosch P, Dooms-Goossens A, Lachapelle J-M et al, eds. Current Topics in Contact Dermatitis. New York: Springer-Verlag, 1989.

80. Mezie M, Sager RW, Stewart WG, et al. Dermatitic effect of nonionic surfactants. I. Gross, microscopic, and metabolic changes in rabbit skin treated with nonionic surface-active agents. J Pharm Sci 1966; 55:584–90.

81. Murphy J, Watson E, Wirth PW, Skierkowski P, Folk RM, Peck G. Cutaneous irritation in the topical application of 30 antineoplastic agents to New Zealand white rabbits. Toxicology 1979; 14:117–30.

82. Patil S, Patrick E. Animal, human and in vitro test methods for predicting skin irritation. In: Marzulli FN, Maibach HI, eds. Dermatotoxicology Methods: The Laboratory Worker's Vade Mecum. Washington DC: Taylor and Francis, 1998:89–104.

83. Weil C, Scala R. Study of intra- and inter-laboratory variability in the results of rabbit eye and skin irritation tests. Toxicol Appl Pharmacol 1971; 19:276–360.

84. Edwards C. Hazardous substances. Proposed revision of test for primary skin irritants. Federal Register 1972; 37(27)(625-27):636.

85. Nixon GA, Tyson CA, Wertz WC. Interspecies comparison of skin irritancy. Toxicol Appl Pharmacol 1975; 31(3):481–90.

86. Shillaker R, Bell G, Hodgson JT, Padgham MDJ. Guinea pig maximization test for skin sensitisation: the use of fewer test animals. Arch Toxicol 1989; 63(4):283–8.

87. Patil SM, Patrick E, Maibach HI. Animal, human and in vitro test methods for predicting skin irritation. In: Marzulli FN, Maibach HI, eds. Dermatotoxicology, 5th ed. Washington DC: Taylor & Francis, 1996;412–3.

88. Levin C, Maibach HI. Animal, human, and in vitro test methods for predicting skin irritation. In: Zhai H, Maibach HI, eds. Dermatotoxicology. 6th ed. FL: CRC Press, Taylor & Francis Group, 2004:681.

89. Justice J, Travers J. The correlation between animal tests and human tests in assessing product mildness. Proc Sci Section Toilet Goods Assoc 1961; 35:12–7.

90. Frosch PJ, Schulze-Dirks A, Hoffmann M, Axthelm I, Kurte A. Efficacy of skin barrier creams. The repetitive irritation test (RIT) in the guinea pig. Contact Dermatitis 1993; 28:94–100.

91. Wahlberg J. Measurement of skin fold thickness in the guinea pig. Assessment of edema-inducing capacity of cutting fluids in responses to certain irritants. Contact Dermatitis 1993; 28:141–5.

92. Marzulli F, Maibach HI. The rabbit as a model for evaluating skin irritants: A comparison of results obtained on animals and man using repeated skin exposure. Food Cosmet Toxicol 1975; 13:533–40.

93. Anderson C, Sundberg K, Groth O. Animal model for assessment of skin irritancy. Contact Dermatitis 1986; 15:143–51.

94. Calandra J. Comments on the guinea pig immersion test. CFTA Cosmet J 1971; 3(3):47.

95. MacMillan F, Ram R. A comparison of the skin irritation produced by cosmetic ingredients and formulations in the rabbit, guinea pig and beagle dog to that observed in the human. In: Maibach HI, ed. Animal Models in Dermatology. Edinburgh: Churchill Livingstone, 1975:399–402.

96. Gupta B, Mathur A. Dermal exposure to irritants. Vet Hum Toxicol 1992; 34(5):405–7.

97. Kooyman D, Snyder F. Tests for the mildness of soaps. Arch Dermatol Syphilol 1942; 46:846–55.

98. Uttley M, Van Abbe N. Primary irritation of the skin: mouse ear test and human patch test procedures. J Soc Cosmet Chem 1973; 24:217–27.

99. Patrick E, Maibach HI. A novel predictive assay in mice. Toxicologist 1987; 7:84.

100. Humphrey D. Measurement of cutaneous microvascular exudates using Evans blue. Biotech Histochem 1993; 68(6):342–9.

101. Trush M, Enger P, Kensler TW. Myeloperoxidase as a biomarker of skin irritation and inflammation. Food Chem Toxicol 1994; 32(2):143–7.

102. Skog E. Primary irritant and allergic eczematous reactions in patients with different dermatoses. Acta Derm Venereol 1960; 40:307–12.

103. National Academy of Sciences and Committee For The Revision of NAS Publication 1138. Principles and procedures for evaluating the toxicity of household substances. Washington, DC: National Academy of Sciences, 1977. 23–59.

104. Kligman A, Woodling W. A method for the measurement and evaluation of irritants on human skin. J Invest Dermatol 1967; 49:78–94.

105. Phillips L, Steinberg M, Maibach HI, Akers WA. A comparison of rabbit and human skin responses to certain irritants. Toxicol Appl Pharmacol 1972; 21:369–82.

106. Wigger-Alberti W, Hinnen U, et al. Predictive testing of metalworking fluids: a comparison of 2 cumulative human irritation models and correlation human irritation models and correlation with epidemiological data. Contact Dermatitis 1997; 36(1):14–20.

107. Frosch PJ, Kligman AM. The soap chamber test. A new method for assessing the irritancy of soaps. J Am Acad Dermatol 1979; 1:35–41.

108. Clarys P, Manou I, et al. Influence of temperature on irritation in the hand/forearm immersion test. Contact Dermatitis 1997; 36(5):240–3.

109. Allenby C, Basketter D, et al. An arm immersion model of compromised skin. (I) Influence on irritant reactions. Contact Dermatitis 1993; 28(2):84–8.

110. Zhai H, Willard P, et al. Evaluating skin-protective materials against contact irritants and allergens. An in vivo screening human model. Contact Dermatitis 1998; 38(3):155–8.

111. Levin C, Maibach HI. Transdermal drug delivery system—an overview. In: Zhai H, Maibach HI, eds. Dermatotoxicology. 6th ed. Boca Raton, FL: CRC Press, Taylor & Francis Group, 2004:684–6.

112. Holdiness MR. A review of contact dermatitis associated with transdermal therapeutic systems. Contact Dermatitis 1989; 20:3–9.

113. Hogan DJ, Maibach HI. Adverse dermatologic reactions to transdermal drug delivery systems. J Am Acad Dermatol 1990; 22:811–4.

114. Kahawara K, Tojo K. Skin irritation in transdermal drug delivery systems: a strategy for its reduction. Pharm Res 2007; 24(2):339–408.

115. Dmochowski RR, Starkman JS, Davila GW. Transdermal drug delivery for overactive bladder. Int Braz J Urol 2006; 32:513–20.

116. Rozenfeld V, Zaslau S, New Geissel K, et al. Transdermal oxybutynin: novel drug delivery for overactive bladder. P&T Drug Forecast 2004; 29(6):367–76.
117. Physicians' Desk Reference 2007, 61st ed. New Jersey: Medical Economics Company, Inc., 2007:3394.
118. Zobrist RH, Quan D, Thomas HM, et al. Pharmacokinetics and Metabolism of trandermal oxybutynin: in vitro and in vivo performance of a novel delivery system. Pharm Res 2003; 20(1):103–9.
119. Nitti VR, Sanders S, Statskin DR, et al. Transdermal delivery of drugs for urologic applications: basic principles and applications. Urology 2006; 67:657–64.
120. Grosso A, Gates C. Drug review: transdermal oxybutynin in overactive bladder. Hospital Pharm 2004; 11:467–8.
121. Chancellor M. Transdermal oxybutynin, a viewpoint for the article: transdermal oxybutynin. Drugs Aging 2003; 20(11):865.
122. Amsterdam JD, Bodkin JA. Selegiline transdermal system in prevention of relapse of major depressive disorder: a 52-week, double-blind, placebo-substitution, parallel-group clinical trial. J Clin Pharmacol 2006; 26:579–86.
123. U. S. Food and Drug Administration. Updates: first depression patch approved. http://www.fda.gov/fdac/departs/2006/306_upd.html (last accessed October 24, 2007).
124. López FA. ADHD: new pharmacological treatments on the horizon. J Dev Behav Pediatr 2006; 5:410–6.
125. U. S. Food and Drug Administration. FDA approves methylphenidate patch to treat attention deficit hyperactivity disorder in children. http://www.fda.gov/bbs/topics/NEWS/2006/NEW01352.html (last accessed October 24, 2007).
126. Trommer H, Neubert RHH. Overcoming the stratum corneum: the modulation of skin penetration, a review. Skin Pharmacol Physiol 2006; 19:106–21.
127. Artusi M, Nicoli S, Colombo P, et al. Effect of chemical enhancers and iontophoresis on thioclochiside permeation across rabbit and human skin in vitro. J Pharm Sci 2004; 93(10):2431–8.
128. Wang C, Laroche CJ, Levin C, et al. Transdermal drug delivery system—an overview. In: Zhai H, Maibach H, eds. Dermatotoxicology. 7th ed. FL: CRC Press, Taylor & Francis Group, 2007.
129. Narashima NS, Shoba Rani R. Effect of magnetic field on the permeation of salbutamol sulfate and terbutaline sulfate. Indian Drugs 1999; 36:663–4.
130. Tinkle S, et al. Skin as route of exposure and sensitization in chronic beryllium disease. Environ Health Perspect 2003; 111:1202–8.
131. Sivamani RK, Wu GC, Stoeber B, et al. Clinical testing of microneedles for transdermal drug delivery. In: Bronaugh RL, Maibach HI, eds. Percutaneous Absortion: drugs—cosmetics—mechanisms—methodology. 4th ed. Boca Raton, FL: Taylor & Francis Group, 2005:843–9.
132. Homick JL, Reschke MF, Degioanni J, Cintron-Trevino NM, Kohl RL. Transdermal scopolamine in the prevention of motion sickness—evaluation of the time course of efficacy. Aviat Space Environ Med 1983; 54:994–1000.

Photosensitivity Induced by Exogenous Agents: Phototoxicity and Photoallergy

Haw-Yueh Thong and Howard I. Maibach
Department of Dermatology, School of Medicine, University of California San Francisco, San Francisco, California, U.S.A.

INTRODUCTION

Sunlight is the most potent environmental agent influencing life on earth. Historically, sun exposure has been believed to be healthful and beneficial. It has only recently become apparent that many of the effects of solar radiation are detrimental.

In the past decade, abnormal reactions to ultraviolet (UV) radiation, namely, photosensitivity induced by drugs, cosmetics, and many industrial and environmental chemicals have become an important health problem.

Exogenous photosensitizers can be categorized into those administered systemically and agents applied topically. Systemically administered agents are mostly medications, while topically applied ones may include sunscreen ingredients, cosmetic agents, and antibacterials (1–3). Table 1 listed medications and other agents which increase sensitivity to light reported by the Food and Drug Administration (FDA) (4).

Cutaneous photosensitivity requires the presence of a photosensitizer and exposure to its action spectrum, defined as the spectral range of electromagnetic radiation where photons are absorbed by the agent. Photosensitizers usually have a low molecular weight (200–500 Da) and are planar, di- or tricyclic, or polycyclic in configurations, often with heteroatoms in their structures enabling resonance stabilization. For most photosensitizers, the action spectrum is identical to its absorption spectrum (5,6).

Definitions of photosensitivity are numerous and frequently inconsistent. In the broadest sense, any toxicity induced by photons can be termed as photosensitivity. Photosensitivity may involve either *phototoxicity* (photoirritation) (nonimmunologic) or *photoallergy* (immunologic). The action spectrum for photoreactions to exogenous agents usually at least includes the ultraviolet-A (UVA) rays for both phototoxicity and photoallergy (7). Table 2 listed the characteristics of phototoxicity and photocontact allergy (7–9). Note that compounds which elicit a phototoxic response may also be capable of initiating a photoallergic reaction.

Phototoxicity (photoirritation or chemical photoirritation) is used to describe all nonimmunologic light-induced toxic skin reactions, and has been defined as a nonimmunologic sunlight-induced skin response (dermatitis) to a photoactive chemical, with the response being likened to an exaggerated sunburn (10). There are at least two mechanisms for phototoxicity: photodynamic, which requires oxygen, and nonphotodynamic, which does not. Reactions induced by porphyrin molecules, coal tar derivatives, and many drugs are photodynamic. The reaction induced by psoralens, for the most part, is nonphotodynamic. Acute phototoxic reactions are characterized by erythema and edema followed by hyperpigmentation. Long-term UV phototoxicity results in chronic sun damage

TABLE 1 Medications and Other Agents that Increase Sensitivity to Light

Primary classes of medications responsible for photosensitizing reactions (examples by generic name)

1. Antihistamines

Astemizole	Azatadine	Brompheniramine
Buclizine	Carbinoxamine	Chlorpheniramine
Clemastine	Cyclizine	Cyproheptadine
Dexchlorpheniramine	Dimenhydrinate	Diphenhydramine
Diphenylpyraline	Doxylamine	Hydroxyzine
Meclizine	Methapyrilene	Methdilazine
Orphenadrine	Pheniramine	Promethazine
Pyrilamine	Terfenadine	Trimeprazine
Tripelennamine	Triprolidine	

2. Coal tar and derivatives—examples by brand name

Alphosyl	Aquatar	Denorex medicated shampoo
DHS tar gel shampoo	DOAK shampoo	Estar
Ionil T. Plus	LAVATAR	Medotar
T/Derm tar emollient	Tegrin shampoo	T/Gel therapeutic shampoo
Zetar shampoo		

3. Contraceptives, oral, and estrogens (birth control pills, female sex hormones)

Estrogens

Chlorotrianisene	Diethylstilbestrol	Estradiol
Estrogens, conjugated	Estrogens, esterified	Estopipate

Progesterones

Ethinyl estradiol	Medroxyprogesterone	Megestrol
Norethindrone	Norgestrel	Quinestrol

4. Nonsteroidal anti-inflammatory drugs (antiarthritics)

Diclofenac	Diflunisal	Fenoprofen
Flurbiprofen	Ibuprofen	Ketoprofen
Meclofenamate	Naproxen	Phenylbutazone
Piroxicam	Sulindac	Suprofen
Tolmetin		

5. Phenothiazines (major tranquilizers, antiemetics)

Acetophenazine	Butaperazine	Carphenazine
Chlorpromazine	Ethopropazine	Fluphenazine
Mesoridazine	Methdilazine	Methotrimeprazine
Perphenazine	Piperacetazine	Prochlororperazine
Promazine	Promethazine	Propiomazine
Thiethylperazine	Thioridazine	Trifluoperazine
Triflupromazine	Trimeprazine	

6. Psoralens

Methozsalen	Triozsalen

7. Sulfonamides (antibiotics)

Acetazolamide	Sulfacytine	Sulfadiazine
Sulfadoxine	Sulfamethizole	Sulfamethoxazole
Sulfasalazine	Sulfapyrazone	Sulfisoxazole

8. Sulfonylureas (oral hypoglycemics)

Acetohexamide	Chlorpropamide	Glipizide
Glyburide	Tolazamide	Tolbutamide

(Continued)

TABLE 1   Medications and Other Agents that Increase Sensitivity to Light (*Continued*)

Primary classes of medications responsible for photosensitizing reactions (examples by generic name)

9. Thiazide diuretics

Bendroflumethiazide	Benzthiazide	Chlorothiazide
Chlorothalidone	Cyclothiazide	Hydrochlorothiazide
Hydroflumethiazide	Methyclothiazide	Ploythiazide
Trichlormethiazide		

10. Tetracyclines (antibiotics)

Chlortetracycline	Demeclocycline	Doxycycline
Methacycline	Minocycline	Oxytetracycline
Tetracycline		

11. Tricyclic antidepressants

Amitriptyline	Amoxapine	Desipramine
Doxepin	Imipramine	Nortriptyline
Protyiptyline	Trimipramine	

Other photosensitizing agents

Classification/use	Agents
Antifungals	Fentichlor/jadit/multifungin
Antimicrobials, antiseptics	Bithionol/chlorhexidine/hexachlorophene
Artificial sweeteners	Calcium cyclamate/cyclamates/sodium cyclohexylsulfamate
Coal tar and coal tar derivatives for psoriasis and chronic eczema and in hair shampoos	Anthracene/many phenolic agents/naphthalene/ phenanthrene/pitch/thiophene
Cosmetics and dyes	Acridine/eosin/erythrocine/fluorescein/ methylene blue/methyl violet/orange red/ paraphenylenediamine/rose bengal/toluidine blue/trypaflavin/trypan blue
Deodorant and bacteriostatic agents in soaps	Halogenated carbanilides/halogenated phenols/halogenated salicylanilides
Fluorescent brightening agent for cellulose, nylon, or wool fibers	Blankophor
Melanogenics (furocoumarins)	Methoxypsoralens/petroleum products/psoralen
Perfumes and toiletries (essential oils)	Ethereal oils/musk ambrette/oil of bergamot/oil of cedar/oil of citron/oil of lavender/oil of lemon/oil of lime/oil of rosemary/oil of sandalwood
Perfumes, flavoring, spices	*Rutaceae* (plant)/*Umbelliferae* (plant)
Tattoos	Cadmium sulfide
Sunscreens with a reported photosensitizing ingredient	
6-Acetoxy-2,4-dimethyl-*m*-dioxane (preservative in sunscreens)	
Benzophenones	
Cinnamates	
Oxybenzone	
PABA esters	
PABA-Pabagel, Pabanol, Presun, and others	
Herbal supplements	
Ginkgo biloba	
St John's wort	

Abbreviation: PABA, *para*-aminobenzoic acid.

TABLE 2 Characteristic of Phototoxicity and Photocontact Allergy

	Phototoxicity	Photocontact allergy
Clinical presentation	Sunburn reaction: erythema, edema, vesicles, and bullae; frequently resolves with hyperpigmentation	Eczematous lesions, usually pruritic
Pathophysiology	Direct tissue injury (photodynamic or nonphotodynamic)	Type IV delayed hypersensitivity response
Occurrence after first exposure	Yes	No
Onset of eruption after exposure	Minutes to hours	24–48 hr
Dose of agent needed for eruption	Large	Small
Action spectrum	Usually similar to absorption	Usually higher wavelength than absorption
Cross-reactivity with other agents	Rare	Common
Diagnosis		
Topical agent	Clinical	Photopatch tests
Systemic agent	Clinical + phototests	Clinical + phototests; possibly photopatch tests
Examples	Acridine	Halogenated phenolic compounds
	Anthracene	Coumarins
	Coal tar	Musk ambrette
	Fluoroquinolones	Fentichlor
	Phenanthrene	Dichlorophene
	Phenothiazine	Bromochloro-salicylamilide (multifungin)
	Psoralens	Chloro-2-phenylphenol
	Sulfonamides	Sunscreens
	Sulfonylureas	para-Aminobenzoic acid (PABA)
	Tetracyclines	Benzophenon-3
		Glyceryl PABA
		Digalloyl trioleate
		2-Hydroxy-4 methoxybenzophenone (mexenone)
		Phenothiazines
		Promethazine hydrochloride
		Diphenhydramine
		Others
		8-Methoxypsoralen (rare)
		Sandalwood oil
		Benzocaine
		Quindoxin
		Optical brighteners

and skin cancer formation (7). In general, phototoxicity is much more common than photoallergy.

Photoallergy is an uncommon acquired altered reactivity dependent on an immediate antibody or a type IV delayed cell-mediated reaction (7). Solar urticaria is an example of the former, whereas photoallergy to exogenous chemicals (photocontact allergy) is an example of the latter. Typically, photoallergy has a sensitization phase, occurs only in sensitized individuals, and requires only minimal concentration of the photoallergen. Photoallergy to systemic drugs does occur but is difficult to characterize. Much of our knowledge concerning photo-contact allergy was based on the halogenated salicylanilide class of chemicals that caused an outbreak in the early 1960s (11–13). Photocontact allergy, although relatively uncommon, proved to be particularly troublesome. A minority of affected patients developed a persistent photodermatitis for many years despite avoidance of further contact with the offending chemical (14,15).

EVALUATION OF PHOTOTOXICITY AND PHOTOALLERGY

Historically, the majority of systemically administered drugs have not undergone controlled testing for determining their potential for photoirritation (phototoxicity). Yet a number were later identified as phototoxic to humans.

Today's litigious social climate requires an extensive testing regimen for any new product that is placed on the market by industry. The FDA (16) required all topically applied dermatologic drugs routinely to be tested for photoirritation in both animals and humans if they absorb light in the UVA, ultraviolet-B (UVB), or visible spectrum; and short-term photoirritation testing in animals, perhaps followed by photoirritation and photoallergy studies in humans, should be considered for all drug substances and formulation components that absorb UVB, UVA, or visible radiation (290–700 nm) and (*i*) are directly applied to the skin or eyes, or significantly partition to one of these areas when administered systemically or (*ii*) are known to affect the condition of the skin or eye. Such nonclinical tests can identify some photoirritating drug products before widespread clinical exposure occurs, allowing appropriate precautions to be implemented.

Testing should be conducted under conditions of simulated sunlight to be clinically relevant. Even though a particular substance has ground state absorption in UVA or UVB after it absorbs radiation, a transient or stable photoproduct may be produced that absorbs in a different absorption range (17,18).

NONCLINICAL TESTING
Phototoxicity
Approaches to Identifying Photochemical Irritants
Photochemical irritants are usually activated by the ultraviolet radiation (UVR) portion of the sun's radiation, which involves wavelengths in the range 280 to 400 nm. UVA is responsible for almost all reactions. Therefore, information regarding the UV/visible radiation absorption spectrum for the chemical, as appropriate, is important in making a testing decision. Screening tests for evaluating phototoxic potential should begin with an examination of the test chemical under UVR. Fluorescence under UVR examination suggests that the chemical may be photoirritating and may require further investigation (19).

A spectroscopic scan will determine if a drug/chemical absorbs between 290 and 700 nm of the electromagnetic spectrum (16). Chemicals/drug products that do not absorb between 290 and 700 nm will not be photoactivated and therefore cannot be direct photochemical photosensitizers. Note that some drugs elicit a photosensitivity reaction which is unrelated to the UV absorbance of the administered drug. These secondary mechanisms include perturbation of heme synthesis and increased formation of other light-absorbing endogenous molecules resulting from administration of non-light–absorbing drugs (e.g., aminolevulinic acid). Such effects may be identified from standard toxicologic testing.

Once an absorption spectrum between 290 and 700 nm is identified, additional phototoxicity screening can be performed with in vitro tests (20). For some products, the 3T3 in vitro phototoxicity assay (21,22) could be an acceptable test for nonclinical photoirritation (16,22).

Medina et al. (23) proposed a multiple endpoint analysis (MEA) model system of reconstituted human epidermis designed to predict in vitro the phototoxicity potential of test chemicals and finished products: a set of well-known phototoxic and non-phototoxic compounds were tested using reconstituted human epidermis grown in chemically defined medium. Test chemicals were topically applied for 24 hours, in the presence or absence of UVA light, and consequently analyzed for tissue viability [lactate dehydrogenase (LDH) release], tissue histology, and the release and mRNA expression of the proinflammatory mediator interleukin-8. Using this MEA strategy, the phototoxic potential of all chemicals tested was classified correctly: strong phototoxicants were detected by LDH release and morphologic changes, whereas the weak phototoxic products (such as 6-methyl coumarin) did not induce changes in tissue viability or morphology, but increased interleukin-8 release and mRNA expression.

Taken into account the MEA approach, human epidermis reconstituted in vitro in chemically defined medium represents a very useful model for assessing skin irritation and phototoxicity.

Lee et al. (24) also examined in vitro phototoxicity test using artificial skin with melanocytes. The model showed better epidermal structures, stronger resistance to UVA exposure, and photobiologic responses closer to in vivo human skin. Among the measured cytokines, interleukin-6 could be the most reliable in vitro marker indicative of phototoxic potential.

Exploratory Studies

The mouse, rabbit, guinea pig, and other mammalian species can be used for exploratory work, with humans as the ultimate test subjects. It is advised that human tests should not be undertaken prior to familiarization with and performance of animal tests (19).

The rabbit in particular has a large area of the back, which can be divided into four test sections, enabling a reduction in the number of test animals required. Appropriate animal models (generally mice or guinea pigs, but also rabbits or swine) have been discussed by Marzulli and Maibach (25) and Lambert et al. (26).

Gerberick and Ryan (27) proposed a predictive mouse ear swelling model for investigating topical phototoxicity: using a xenon arc UV solar simulator delivering UV radiation from 290 to 400 nm (UVB + UVA) or 320 to 400 nm (UVA) depending on the filters, the phototoxic potential of nine known phototoxins and three negative test materials was successfully demonstrated. Based on the time of onset of the phototoxic response following test material application and irradiation, both immediate (20–30 minutes) and delayed-type (48–96 hours) phototoxic responses were demonstrated using this model with anthracene and 8-methoxypsoralen, respectively. The optimal time for irradiation after application of 8-methoxypsoralen to the ears was 30 to 60 minutes. The phototoxic response to 8-methoxypsoralen was dependent upon the UVA dose and, when tested at a constant UVA dose, the response was concentration dependent. To obtain an optimal phototoxic response to 7-methoxycoumarin, both UVB and UVA radiation were required.

A classic example of exploratory studies of phototoxicity was performed by Marzulli and Maibach (10,28), using a simple approach to identify bergapten (5-methoxypsoralen) as the principal phototoxic component of oil of bergamot. The basic scheme is as follows.

A source of UVR with over 90% of the UV radiation (300–400 nm) output at 365 nm was provided by a Hanovia Inspectolite (no longer available).[a] When used with no. 16125, type EH-4 bulb, red purple Corning 7–39 (5874) filter, and frosted glass cutoff at 290 nm,[b] total output at 10 cm from the source is about 3000 and 1900 J/cm^2 at 15 cm.[c,d]

The test chemical (0.05 mL) is applied to skin, and after 5 minutes it is irradiated for 25 to 40 minutes (animals[e]–humans) at a distance of 8 to 10 cm. The skin is examined for erythema and edema at 24 and 48 hours and again at seven days. Positive (using 0.01% 5-methoxypsoralen or 8-methoxypsoralen in 70% ethanol) and negative (vehicle) controls are similarly exposed for comparison. Modification may be needed depending on the nature of the chemicals being investigated, which is especially true for oral medications.

Photoallergy

Test procedures designed to identify potentially photosensitizing chemicals evolved in the wake of the photosensitivity outbreak caused by halogenated

---

[a] Hanovia Inspectolite: high-pressure glass mercury vapor lamp.

[b] The sun emits a polychromatic continuum of different wavelengths; low-pressure fluorescent sun lamps emit a continuum mainly in the UVB or UVA; high-pressure mercury arcs provide discontinuous line spectra; and high intensity solar simulators, based on xenon, xenon–mercury, or doped tungsten may mimic solar UVR, but require special filtration to shape the UVB spectrum and remove intense visible and infrared radiation (19). In performing any phototoxicity study, it is imperative that the spectral characteristics of the optical source must be known. A photodermatologist will choose a specific UV source to match best a given biologic action spectrum (if known) in order to achieve the greatest efficiency in delivering a photobiologically significant dose (29).

[c] Experimentalists currently engaged in photobiologic work need to report the source and output of radiation used in their experiments. They should employ sources with output of UVA and UVB and should specify exposure time and distance of source to the skin. The UVA should be about 10 J/cm^2 and the UVB about 0.1 J/cm^2. Irradiance from the UVR source can be measured with a UV radiometer at an appropriate distance. For correct readings, the radiometer is calibrated by the supplier, with the intended source. Irradiance is measured in mW/cm^2, dose in J/cm^2, and exposure time (t) in minutes (19,30).

[d] In the United States, General Electric Co. (Baltimore, Maryland, U.S.A.), Sylvania Corporation (Danvers, Massachusetts, U.S.A.), Solar Light Co., Inc. (Philadelphia, Pennsylvania, U.S.A.), and Elder Pharmaceuticals (Bryan, Ohio, U.S.A.) market lamps with UVA and UVB outputs. Xenon Corp. (Wilmington, Massachusetts, U.S.A.) manufactures solar simulators. Optronics (Orlando, Florida, U.S.A.), Eppley (Newport, Rhode Island, U.S.A.), and G. Gamma Scientific (San Diego, California, U.S.A.) market radiometers. United Detector Tech. (Santa Monica, California, U.S.A.) calibrates radiometers. Schoeffel Co. (Westwood, New Jersey, U.S.A.) is a source for detectors and simulators (31).

[e] Among animal models that have proved useful in predicting human phototoxicity are the mouse, rabbit, swine, guinea pig, squirrel monkey, and hamster, in that approximate order of effectiveness (10).

salicylanilides (11,13). Information was gathered primarily from studies of patients (photopatch testing) and attempts to induce photosensitization experimentally in guinea pigs (32).

The role of UV radiation in photoallergy is less clear. Absorption of UV energy by the sensitizer in the skin is required for both induction and elicitation. Schimidt and Kingston (33) noted that irradiation of the photosensitizer in vitro followed by repeated topical application of the irradiated solution is ineffective in inducing photocontact sensitization, suggesting that the formation of stable photoproducts that can act as potential contact sensitizers is an unlikely mechanism. The most plausible explanation is that absorption of photons of specific energy by the sensitizer leads to the formation of an excited molecule, which can interact with other molecules normally found in the skin to form an antigen or hapten (34).

Test procedures for identifying photocontact allergens have received less attention than methods designed to detect ordinary contact sensitizers. Efforts to induce photocontact sensitivity have thus far not been standardized. Nonclinical testing for photoallergy has been eliminated from the 2003 FDA guidance because the predictive ability of these tests was considered to be questionable (16,22).

In theory, the variables that influence ordinary contact sensitization such as the vehicle, concentration, and frequency of application (28) can similarly affect the induction of photosensitization. Furthermore, there is the added important factor of UV radiation. The wavelength dependence (action spectrum), energy requirements (dose) for both induction and elicitation, and absorption characteristics of the chemical must be determined.

Screening Tests

For screening of novel agents with unknown action spectra, however, it is necessary to use a UV source with a broad emission spectrum (34). The sources commonly used in the past were fluorescent tubes such as the FS20 sunlamp bulbs, with emission primarily in the UVB region, or blacklight fluorescent bulbs, which emit primarily in the UVA range, or a combination of both. More recently, xenon arc solar simulators have been used which offer the advantage of providing spectra similar to sunlight.

Animal Testing

Of the animals tested so far, the use of guinea pigs allows the study to act as a preliminary test for the selection of non-photoirritant concentrations for photo-allergy testing and reduction of animal numbers; and the mouse ear swelling model appears to be the most sensitive (35–37). The basic scheme of the mouse ear swelling model proposed by Gerberick and Ryan (37) is as follows.

Cyclophosphamide-pretreated BALB/c mice were induced by topical treatment of the dorsal skin surface on three consecutive days and challenged on the ears five days after the last induction. For each induction and challenge treatment, mice were consecutively irradiated with UVA ($10 \, \text{J/cm}^2$) and UVB ($45 \, \text{mJ/cm}^2$) radiation 30 minutes to 1 hour after test material application. The ear thickness changes observed in the photoallergy test mice were then compared with the changes observed in the contact allergy, vehicle/radiation, and phototoxicity control mice.

Vohr et al. (38) presented a modified local lymph node test which made it possible to quickly and reliably differentiate between irritative and allergic skin reactions with extremely simple parameters. The Integrated Model for the

Differentiation of Skin Reactions test combines measurement of cell proliferation in draining lymph nodes with measurement of primary ear swelling after topical application of the test substance on three consecutive days, and can employ UV radiation after application of the substance and, therefore, make differentiation possible between different types of skin photoreaction (photoallergy and photo-irritation) after both topical and systemic administration.

Human Testing

Kaidbey and Kligman (39) proposed *photomaximization test* which is conducted in human and is essentially a repeated insult technique that entails an exaggerated exposure to both chemical and UV and follows a design similar to that of the maximization test (40). The UV source is a 150-W xenon arc solar simulator. The emission spectrum is continuous extending from about 290 to 410 nm with a peak at about 350 nm, and closely resembles the UVB spectrum of midday sunlight at 41°N and 70° sun elevation (41).

The test procedure is as follows.

A 5% concentration of the test agent in an appropriate base (such as hydrophilic ointment USP) is delivered to the skin by plastic tuberculin syringes at a concentration of 10 μL/cm^2. The material is spread uniformly with thin glass rods and the sites covered with nonwoven cotton cloth (Webril®; BBA Nonwovens, Simpsonville, Inc., Simpsonville, South Carolina, U.S.A.) (Curity®; Tyco Healthcare Group, LP/Kendall, Mansfield, Massachusetts, U.S.A.) and sealed to the skin with clear occlusive tape (Blenderm®; 3M Co., St. Paul, Minnesota, U.S.A.). Twenty-four hours later, the patches are removed and the sites exposed to three minimal erythema doses (MEDs) from the solar simulator. The MED is individually determined beforehand by exposing the skin sites to 25% increments of radiation.[f]

After a rest period of 48 hours, a similar occlusive application is made to the same site for another 24 hours, followed again by exposure to three MEDs. This sequence is repeated for a total of six exposures over a period of three weeks.

The subjects are then challenged after a rest period of 14 days by a single exposure to a fresh skin site. An occlusive application is made with the test agent (1.0% concentration) for 24 hours, followed by exposure to 4.0 J/cm^2 UVA. The UVA is obtained from the same source by filtering the radiation through a 2-mm Schott WG345 filter (50% transmission at about 345 nm).

The sites are examined 48 and 72 hours after irradiation. Unirradiated control sites are sealed and then covered with three or four layers of opaque adhesive tape. Development of erythema and edema or a vesicular dermatitis in the irradiated but not in the unirradiated sites signifies the induction of photocontact sensitivity. Each substance is usually examined in 25 volunteers.

Modification of the photomaximization procedure has been proposed (42). With the tests the investigators (39,42) were able to photoallergic contact sensitize normal human volunteers relatively readily to certain methylated coumarin derivatives, e.g., tetrachlorosalicylanilide, 3,5-dibromosalicylanilide (3,5-DBS), chlorpromazine, and sodium omadine. A lesser number of positive induction responses were noted with tribromosalicylanilide contaminated with 47% DBS, 4,5-DBS, jadit, and bithionol. Negative results, however, were noted with *para-*

---

[f] The dose required to produce minimal but uniform erythema with a clear border 24 hours after exposure is the MED.

aminobenzoic acid and musk ambrette, which have been clinically reported to produce photoallergic contact reactions. These chemicals were thus considered as weak photosensitizers. A comprehensive review of the photosensitizing chemicals is provided by Kaidbey (34).

CLINICAL TESTING

Integral to the evaluation of photosensitivity are phototests and photopatch tests (43,44). Approximately, 7% to 20% of patients who undergo photopatch tests have clinically relevant positive photopatch test results, eventuating in the diagnosis of photoallergic contact dermatitis (45–48). Phototests are specialized tests that confirm the presence of photosensitivity, whereas the photopatch test responses can help differentiate between contact allergy, phototoxicity, and photoallergy (Table 3). A crescendo reaction pattern in the irradiated sites indicates the presence of a cell-mediated immunity process, which is highly suggestive of photocontact allergy. In general, the diagnosis of photocontact dermatitis is suspected by the clinical picture, including the character and distribution of the eruption and the histology. Confirmation and identification of the offending chemical depend on photopatch testing. The procedures and interpretation for phototests and photo-patch tests are outlined in Table 3 (45,49,50). Variations have been proposed (49).

The interpretation of photopatch test results is usually straightforward. Difficulties arise when there is marked enhancement of a positive or weakly positive reaction to a chemical in the unirradiated site by UV. Several authors had demonstrated that exceedingly small doses of UVA are sufficient to provoke a response in photosensitized individuals, especially when relatively large

TABLE 3 Outline of Phototest and Photopatch Test

	Phototest	Photopatch test
Materials	UV radiation source	UV radiation source Patch test materials
Method	MED of UVA or UVB is measured (*i*) while the subject is taking the suspected medication and (*ii*) after discontinuing the same medication	Two sets of patch test are applied for 48 hr; after removal, one set is irradiated with UVA at a dose below MED (5–10 J/cm^2 or 50% of MED, whichever is smaller), and the other set is protected from UV dose
Reading time	24 hr	48 and 96 hr
Interpretation	If MED (UVA or UVB) is much lower while the subject is taking the medication, this suggests a photosensitive (phototoxic or photoallergic) reaction to the drug	Reaction at both sites suggests contact allergy Reaction at both sites and a much stronger reaction at the irradiated site suggest both contact allergy and photoallergy Reaction at the irradiated site with a decrescendo pattern suggests phototoxicity Reaction at the irradiated site with a crescendo pattern suggests photoallergy

Abbreviations: MED, minimal erythema dose; UV, ultraviolet; UVA, ultraviolet-A; UVB, ultraviolet-B.

concentrations of the sensitizers (1.0% or 0.1%) are employed (12,51,52). In these cases, photopatch testing should be carefully repeated by quantitative methods. The procedures are as follows (34):

1. Measured amounts of the chemical in a suitable vehicle should be delivered to the skin and the unirradiated site quickly and rigorously sealed with several layers of opaque material to prevent stray radiation, since small amounts of UVA can reach the skin surface through ordinary tape and trigger a reaction in the unirradiated patch test sites in highly sensitive individuals. Epstein (53) termed the reaction a "masked" photopatch test and cautioned that it can lead to an erroneous diagnosis of contact sensitivity.
2. If a definite and clear enhancement is still observed despite the above procedures, other explanations must be invoked, such as nonspecific enhancement of contact allergy by UV, modification of local cellular immunologic responses, formation of cross-reaction photoproducts, and so on. Such possibilities have not been adequately investigated.
3. Another explanation is the existence of dual sensitivity, i.e., contact and photocontact allergy. Photopatch testing with serial dilutions of the sensitizer should then be performed. A positive photopatch test at a drug concentration that fails to elicit a response in the unirradiated test site is suggestive of dual sensitization.

CONCLUSIONS

Photosensitivity induced by exogenous agents have become increasingly prevalent over the past few decades because of increased opportunities for sun exposure and increasing numbers of photosensitizing chemicals available. Useful laboratory procedures are available for identifying chemicals that are potentially capable of producing phototoxicity or photoallergy. Although chemicals can be ranked for their photosensitizing potential under a defined set of laboratory conditions, the possible incidence of photoallergic reactions with normal usage cannot be predicted. Agents suspected of being photosensitizers on clinical grounds can be further evaluated using photopatch testing.

Compared to contact sensitization, experience with human testing on photosensitivity has been limited. Photosensitivity induced by exogenous agents is a very complex issue in dermatotoxicology. Factors that influence induction, such as concentration, vehicle, action spectrum, and UV dose, need to be further investigated. For the interested readers, detailed descriptions are found in Refs. (54,55).

REFERENCES

1. Gould JW, Mercurio MG, Elmets CA. Cutaneous photosensitivity diseases induced by exogenous agents. J Am Acad Dermatol 1995; 33(4):551–73.
2. Lankerani L, Baron ED. Photosensitivity to exogenous agents. J Cutan Med Surg 2004; 8(6):424–31.
3. Wynn RL. Drugs that cause photosensitivity. Gen Dent 2006; 54(6):384–6.
4. Levine JI. Medications that Increase Sensitivity to Light: A 1990 Listing. 12/90, U.S. Department of Health & Human Services, FDA 91-8280, 1990.
5. Moore DE. Drug-induced cutaneous photosensitivity: incidence, mechanism, prevention and management. Drug Saf 2002; 25(5):345–72.

6. Kochevar IE. Basic principles in photomedicine and photochemistry. In: Lim HW, Soter NA, eds. Clinical Photomedicine. New York: Marcel Dekker, 1993:1.

7. Epstein JH. Phototoxicity and photoallergy. Semin Cutan Med Surg 1999; 18(4):274–84.

8. Selvag E. Phototoxicity and photoallergy. Nord Med 1998; 113(10):335–7.

9. Lugovic L, Situm M, Ozanic-Bulic S, et al. Phototoxic and photoallergic skin reactions. Coll Antropol 2007; 31(Suppl. 1):63–7.

10. Marzulli FN, Maibach HI. Perfume phototoxicity. J Soc Cosmet Chem 1970; 21:695–715.

11. Calnan CD, Harman TTM, Wells GC. Photodermatitis from soaps. Br Med J 1961; 2:1266.

12. Epstein JH, Wuepper KD, Maibach HI. Photocontact dermatitis to halogenated salicylanilides and related compounds. A clinical and histological review of 26 patients. Arch Dermatol 1968; 97(3):236–44.

13. Wilkinson DS. Photodermatitis due to tetrachlorosalicylanilide. Br J Dermatol 1961; 73:213–9.

14. Wilkinson DS. Patch test reactions to certain halogenated salicylanilides. Br J Dermatol 1962; 74:302–6.

15. Jillson OF, Baughman RD. Contact photodermatitis from buthionol. Arch Dermatol 1963; 88:409–16.

16. CDER/FDA. Guidance for Industry Photosafety Testing, 2003. (http://www.fda.gov/cder/guidance/index.htm)

17. Becker L, Eberlein-Konig B, Przybilla B. Phototoxicity of nonsteroidal anti-inflammatory drugs: in vitro studies with visible light. Acta Derm Venereol 1996; 76(5):337–40.

18. Navaratnam S, Claridge J. Primary photophysical properties of ofloxacin. Photochem Photobiol 2000; 72(3):283–90.

19. Marzulli FN, Maibach HI. Photoirritation (phototoxicity) testing in humans. In: Zhai H, Maibach HI, eds. Dermatotoxicology. 6th ed., Vol. 44. Boca Raton, FL: CRC Press, 2004:871.

20. Nilsson R, Maurer T, Redmond N. Standard protocol for phototoxicity testing. Contact Dermatitis 1993; 28:285–90.

21. Spielmann H, Balls M, Dupuis J, et al. The international EU/COLIPA in vitro phototoxicity validation study: results of phase II (Blind Trial): part 1: the 3T3 NRU phototoxicity test. Toxicol In Vitro 1998; 12(3):305–27.

22. Jacobs AC, Brown PC, Chen C, et al. CDER photosafety guidance for industry. Toxicol Pathol 2004; 32(Suppl. 2):17–8.

23. Medina J, Elsaesser C, Picarles V, et al. Assessment of the phototoxic potential of compounds and finished topical products using a human reconstructed epidermis. In Vitro Mol Toxicol 2001; 14(3):157–68.

24. Lee JH, Kim JE, Kim BJ, et al. In vitro phototoxicity test using artificial skin with melanocytes. Photodermatol Photoimmunol Photomed 2007; 23:73–80.

25. Marzulli FN, Maibach HI. Photoirritation (phototoxicity, phototoxic dermatitis). In: Zhai H, Maibach HI, eds. Dermatotoxicology. 6th ed., Vol. 17. Boca Raton, FL: CRC Press, 2004:341–52.

26. Lambert LA, Wamer WG, Kornhauser A. Animal models for phototoxicity testing. In: Marzulli FN, Maibach HI, eds. Dermatotoxicology Methods. Vol. 19. New York: Taylor and Francis, 1998:229–41.

27. Gerberick GF, Ryan CA. A predictive mouse ear-swelling model for investigating topical phototoxicity. Food Chem Toxicol 1989; 27(12):813–9.

28. Marzulli FN, Maibach HI. Use of graded concentrations in studying skin sensitization in man. Food Chem Toxicol 1974; 12:219–77.

29. Sliney DH. Measuring and quantifying ultraviolet radiation exposures. In: Zhai H, Maibach HI, eds. Dermatotoxicology. 6th ed., Vol. 45. Boca Raton, FL: CRC Press, 2004:879–900.

30. Urbach F. Testing the efficacy of sunscreens: effect of choice of source and spectral power distribution of ultraviolet radiation, and choice of endpoint. Photodermatology 1989; 6:177–81.

31. Anderson TF. Artificial light sources. In: De Leo VA, ed. Dermatologic Clinics. Vol. 4. Philadelphia, PA: W.B. Saunders, 1986:203–15.

32. Herman PS, Sams WM, Jr. Soap Photodermatitis: Photosensitivity to Halogenated Salicylanilides. Springfield, IL: Thomas, 1972.
33. Schmidt RJ, Kingston T. Testing with musk ambrette and congeners in a case of photosensitivity dermatitis and actinic reticuloid syndrome (PD/AR). Photodermatology 1984; 1:195–8.
34. Kaidbey KH. The evaluation of photoallergic contact sensitizers in humans. In: Marzulli FN, Maibach HI, eds. Dermatotoxicology. 4th ed., Vol. 22. Washington, DC: Hemisphere, 1991:595.
35. Maguire HC, Kaidbey KH. Experimental photoallergic contact dermatitis: a mouse model. J Invest Dermatol 1982; 79:147–52.
36. Miyachi Y, Takigawa M. Mechanisms of contact photosensitivity in mice. III. Predictive testing of chemicals with photoallergenic potential in mice. Arch Dermatol 1983; 119:736–9.
37. Gerberick GF, Ryan CA. A predictive mouse ear-swelling model for investigating topical photoallergy. Food Chem Toxicol 1990; 28(5):361–8.
38. Vohr HW, Blumel J, Blotz J, et al. An intra-laboratory validation of the integrated model for the differentiation of skin reactions (IMDS): discrimination between (photo)allergic and (photo)irritant skin reactions in mice. Arch Toxicol 2000; 73(10–11):501–9.
39. Kaidbey KH, Kligman AM. Photomaximization test for identifying photoallergic contact sensitizers. Contact Dermatitis 1980; 6:161–9.
40. Kligman AM. The identification of contact allergens by human assay. III. The maximization test. A procedure for screening and rating contact sensitizers. J Invest Dermatol 1966; 48:393–409.
41. Berger DS. Specification and design of solar ultraviolet simulators. J Invest Dermatol 1969; 53:192–9.
42. Kaidbey KH. The evaluation of photoallergic contact sensitizers in humans. In: Marzulli FN, Maibach HI, eds. Dermatotoxicology. 2nd ed. Washington, DC: Hemisphere, 1983:405–14.
43. Rosen C. Photo-induced drug eruptions. Semin Dermatol 1989; 8:149–57.
44. Bilsland D, Diffey BL, Farr PM, et al. Diagnostic phototesting in the United Kingdom. British Photodermatology Group. Br J Dermatol 1992; 127(3):297–9.
45. Neumann NJ, Holzle E, Plewig G, et al. Photopatch testing: the 12-year experience of the German, Austrian, and Swiss photopatch test group. J Am Acad Dermatol 2000; 42(2 Pt 1):183–92.
46. Fotiades J, Soter NA, Lim HW. Results of evaluation of 203 patients for photosensitivity in a 7.3-year period. J Am Acad Dermatol 1995; 33(4):597–602.
47. Deleo VA, Suarez SM, Maso MJ. Photoallergic contact dermatitis: results of photopatch testing in New York, 1985 to 1990. Arch Dermatol 1992; 128:1513.
48. Bryden AM, Moseley H, Ibbotson SH, et al. Photopatch testing of 1155 patients: results of the U.K. multicentre photopatch study group. Br J Dermatol 2006; 155(4):737–47.
49. Meola T. Evaluation of the photosensitive patient. In: Lim HW, Soter NA, eds. Clinical Photomedicine. New York: Marcel Dekker, 1993:153.
50. Amin S, Lauerma A, Maibach HI. Diagnostic tests in dermatology: patch and photopatch testing and contact urticaria. In: Zhai H, Maibach HI, eds. Dermatotoxicology. 6th ed. Boca Raton, FL: CRC Press, 2004:1007.
51. Osmundsen PE. Contact photodermatitis due to tribromosalicylanilide. Br J Dermatol 1968; 80:228–34.
52. Willis I, Kligman AM. Photocontact allergic reactions. Elicitation by low doses of long ultraviolet rays. Arch Dermatol 1969; 100:535–9.
53. Epstein S. "Masked" photopatch test. J Invest Dermatol 1963; 41:369–70.
54. Lim HW, Hoenigsmann H, Hawk JLM. Photodermatology. New York: Informa Healthcare, 2007.
55. Zhai H, Wilhelm K-P, Maibach HI, eds. Dermatotoxicology. 7th ed. New York: Informa Healthcare, 2007.

23 Systemic Toxicity Caused by Absorption of Drugs and Chemicals Through Skin

Haw-Yueh Thong, Susi Freeman, and Howard I. Maibach
Department of Dermatology, School of Medicine, University of California San Francisco, San Francisco, California, U.S.A.

INTRODUCTION

The skin forms an effective two-way barrier that controls the loss of chemicals from the body as well as the absorption of many foreign chemicals into the body. However, many chemicals do enter via the skin and some, when specifically applied to the skin, have been found to be sufficiently well absorbed to produce systemic toxicity.

FACTORS AFFECTING ABSORPTION

Many drugs for topical use on the skin and mucous membranes are capable of producing systemic side effects whose occurrence and severity depend largely on factors that affect the absorption of topically applied drugs. The skin barrier plays a critical role in determining drug absorption. Any factors which may affect the barrier function have the potential to affect absorption (1). The factors affecting percutaneous absorption can be summarized in Table 1.

The Integrity of the Barrier

Apart from follicular orifices and sweat gland ducts which may provide additional pathways for absorption, the stratum corneum layer of the epidermis is the skin's main barrier to transepidermal absorption. This barrier function can be ascribed to the macroscopical structure of the stratum corneum, which consists of alternating lipoidal and hydrophilic regions. Anything that alters the structure or function of the stratum corneum will affect epidermal absorption. The integrity of this barrier, with resultant increase in percutaneous absorption, is reduced by any inflammatory process of the skin, such as any form of dermatitis or psoriasis. Similarly, removal of the stratum corneum by stripping or damage by alkalis, acids, etc. will increase percutaneous absorption. Stratum corneum can also act as a reservoir for drugs.

The Physicochemical Properties of the Substance

The physicochemical characteristics of the drug, such as partition coefficient and molecular weight, play an important role in determining the facility of percutaneous absorption. Absorption decreases with increasing molecular size. It is affected by the relative water/lipid solubility of the drug and the relative solubility of the drug in its vehicle compared with its solubility in the stratum corneum.

TABLE 1   Factors Affecting Percutaneous Absorption

The integrity of the skin barrier
The physicochemical properties of the substances
The vehicle containing the drug
The site of application
Occlusion
Age
Temperature
Metabolism

The Vehicle Containing the Drug

Another factor to consider in transdermal drug delivery is the vehicle in which the drug is formulated as it acts on the release of drug from the formulation. The greater the affinity of a vehicle for the drug it contains, the less the percutaneous absorption of the drug.

Moreover, vehicles may also interact with human stratum corneum, thereby affecting its barrier function, causing increased drug absorption. Surfactants and penetration enhancers are well-known examples.

Physical properties of vehicles, especially the degree of occlusion they produce, affect percutaneous absorption, as discussed under section Occlusion below (e.g., greases).

Structural or chemical damage to the barrier layer can also be caused by the vehicle used; vehicles such as dimethyl sulfoxide (DMSO) cause greatly increased percutaneous absorption.

In general, a higher concentration of the drug in its vehicle enhances penetration.

Site of Application

Drug absorption is affected by regional anatomic variations and special cuticular structures such as nails and follicles (2). Regional differences in permeability of skin largely depend on the thickness of the intact stratum corneum. According to the findings of a study by Feldmann and Maibach (3) the highest total absorption of hydrocortisone is that from the scrotum, followed (in decreasing order) by absorption from the forehead, scalp, back, forearms, palms, and plantar surfaces.

Occlusion

Skin occlusion produces profound changes, including hydration status, barrier permeability, epidermal lipids, DNA synthesis, microbial flora, and numerous molecular and cellular processes (4). The penetration of topical drugs may be increased by the use of an occlusive covering, by a factor of 10 or more. This is because of increased H_2O retention in the stratum corneum, increased blood flow, increased temperature, and increased surface area after prolonged occlusion (skin wrinkling).

Age

Human skin changes dramatically with increasing age. Morphological and physiological changes in aged skin may affect the percutaneous absorption of compounds and thus their potential for localized, as well as systemic, efficacy (5).

However, the greatest toxicological response to topical administration has been seen in the infant. The preterm infant does not have intact barrier function and hence is more susceptible to systemic toxicity from topically applied drugs (6,7).

A normal full-term infant probably has a near fully developed stratum corneum with complete barrier function (8), topical application of the same amount of a compound to both adult and newborn results in a 2.7 times greater systemic availability in the newborn. This is because the ratio of surface area to body weight in the newborn is three times that in the adult. Therefore, given an equal area of application of a drug to skin of the newborn and adults, the proportion absorbed per kilogram of body weight is much more in the infant.

Temperature
Increased skin temperature usually enhances penetration by increasing hydration and blood flow (9).

Metabolism
Like the liver, the skin is capable of metabolizing drugs and foreign substances. It contains many of the enzyme systems of the liver, and its metabolizing potential has been estimated to be about 2% that of the liver (10).

Enzymes of the cytochrome P450 (P450 or CYP) super family are the most versatile and important class of drug-metabolizing enzymes that are induced in human skin in response to xenobiotic exposure. At the same time, CYP have numerous important roles in endogenous and exogenous substrate metabolism in the skin such as, fatty acids, eicosonoids, sterols, steroids, vitamin A, vitamin D, and the metabolism of therapeutic drugs thus capable of modulating drug bioavailability (11,12).

SYSTEMIC SIDE EFFECTS CAUSED BY TOPICALLY APPLIED DRUGS AND COSMETICS

Topically applied drugs and cosmetics can cause allergic or irritant contact dermatitis. However, this type of side effect, usually limited to the skin, is outside the scope of the present article. The reader is referred to the textbooks of Frosch et al. (13) and Fisher (14) for references to contact dermatitis. Systemic side effects from topically applied chemicals can sometimes result from either a toxic (irritant) reaction or a hypersensitivity reaction. The latter can be an anaphylactic type of reaction, which is the extreme manifestation of the contact urticaria syndrome (15). Many topical drugs and cosmetics have reportedly caused anaphylactic reactions.

While anaphylactic reactions to topical medicaments from immunologic contact urticaria are uncommon, their potentially serious nature warrants attention.

However, reports of toxic (as distinct from allergic) reactions to applied drugs and cosmetics are more numerous and include many medicaments that have been safely used for many years but that can be toxic under special circumstances.

TOPICALLY APPLIED DRUGS AND COSMETICS CAUSING SYSTEMIC SIDE EFFECTS

Table 2 is a list of topical drugs/cosmetics causing systemic side effects, followed by a detailed discussion of each chemical.

TABLE 2 Topical Drugs/Cosmetics Causing Systemic Side Effects

Antibiotics
  Chloramphenicol
  Clindamycin
  Gentamycin
  Neomycin
Antihistamines
  Diphenhydramine hydrochloride
  Diphenylpyraline hydrochloride
  Promethazine
Antimicrobials
  Boric acid
  Castellani's paint
  Hexachlorophene
  Homosulfanilamide
  Iodine, povidone-iodine
  Phenol
  Resorcinol
  Silver sulfadiazine
  Trichlorocarbanilide
Arsenic
Carmustine
Camphor
Cosmetic agents
DEET
DMSO
DNCB
Ethyl alcohol
Fumaric acid monoethyl ester
Local anesthetics
  Benzocaine
  Lidocaine
Mercurials
Monobenzone
2-Naphthol
Insecticides
  Lindane
  Malathion
Podophyllum resin
Salicylic acid
Selenium sulfide
Silver nitrate
Steroids
  Corticosteroids
  Sex hormones
Tars
  Coal tar
  Dithranol
5-FU
Minoxidil
Tacalcitol
Monochloroacetic acid

See text for detail.
Abbreviations: DEET, diethyltoluamide; DMSO, dimethyl sulfoxide; DNCB,
dinitrochlorobenzene; 5-FU, 5-Fluorouracil.

Antibiotics
Chloramphenicol
Oral administration of chloramphenicol may lead to aplastic anemia (16). A case of marrow aplasia with a fatal outcome after topical application of chloramphenicol in eye ointment was described by Abrams et al. (17). There have been three earlier reports of bone marrow aplasia after the use of chloramphenicol-containing eye drops. However, Walker et al. (18) reviewed seven cases of idiosyncratic hemato-poietic reactions associated with topical chloramphenicol reported in the literature and found that there was refutable evidence for the existence of such a response, and supported the view that topical chloramphenicol was not a risk factor for inducing dose-related bone marrow toxicity.

Clindamycin
Topical clindamycin is widely used in the treatment of acne vulgaris. It is estimated that 4% to 5% clindamycin hydrochloride is absorbed systemically (19). The degree of absorption largely depends on the vehicles, ranging from 0.13% (acetone) to 13.92% (DMSO) (20). Several cases of topical clindamycin-associated diarrhea have been reported (21–23).

Pseudomembranous colitis is a well-recognized side effect of systemic administration of clindamycin. Cases of pseudomembranous colitis have been reported after topical administration (24,25). The authors concluded that all patients receiving topical clindamycin should be warned to discontinue therapy and consult their physician if intestinal symptoms occur.

Gentamycin
Ototoxicity is a well-known hazard of systemic gentamycin administration. However, topical application to large thermal injuries of the skin has similarly caused ototoxic effects, ranging from mild to severe hearing loss, with an associated decrease of vestibular function (26). In the two patients described, serum levels of gentamycin measured were 1.0 to 3.0 µg/mL and 3.3 to 4.3 µg/mL, respectively. Drake (27) described a woman who developed tinnitus each time she treated her paronychia with gentamycin sulfate cream 0.1%. Use of gentamycin ear drops may also be associated with ototoxic reactions (28–30).

Neomycin
Just as ototoxicity is a well-known hazard of parenteral neomycin administration, so has deafness been reported after almost any form of local treatment, including treatment of skin infections and burns (31–34), application as an aerosol for inhalation, instillation into cavities (35), irrigation of large wounds (36), and use of neomycin-containing eardrops (30,37). Kellerhals (38) reported 13 cases of inner ear damage in which the use of eardrops containing neomycin and polymyxin was incriminated. All cases had perforated tympanic membranes, and the paper concludes that these drops (and also those containing chloromycetin, colistin, and polymyxin), should not be used in such cases for periods longer than 10 days.

Antihistamines
Diphenhydramine Hydrochloride
Diphenhydramine hydrochloride is an antihistamine with anticholinergic proper-ties that is frequently used both orally and topically for the temporary relief of

pruritus. Toxic encephalopathy caused by topically applied diphenhydramine has been reported (39). Significant systemic absorption may occur following vigorous administration of topical diphenhydramine in patients with varicella–zoster lesions (40–42). The patients often presented with mental confusion associated with hallucinations. Concomitant use of oral diphenhydramine may increase the risk of toxicity. A complete resolution of mental status abnormalities could occur within 24 hours after discontinuation of all diphenhydramine-containing products.

Diphenylpyraline Hydrochloride
Diphenylpyraline hydrochloride has been used topically in Germany for the treatment of eczematous and other itching dermatoses. Symptomatic psychosis has been observed in 12 patients, 9 of whom were children. The amounts of the active drug applied ranged from 225 to 1350 mg. The first symptoms of intoxication were psychomotor restlessness in all cases, usually within 24 hours. Other symptoms included disorientation, and optic and acoustic hallucinations. All symptoms disappeared four days after discontinuation of the topical medication (43).

Promethazine
Topical promethazine intoxication has been reported (44). Bloch and Beysovec (45) reported a 16-months-old male weighing 11.5 kg who was treated with 2% promethazine cream for generalized eczema. After approximately 15 to 20 g of the cream had been applied, the child fell asleep. He woke a few hours later with abnormal behavior, loss of balance, inability to focus, irritability, drowsiness, and failure to recognize his mother. One day later all symptoms had spontaneously disappeared. A diagnosis of promethazine toxicity through percutaneous absorption was made. Known symptoms of promethazine toxicity include disorientation, hallucinations, hyperactivity, convulsions, and coma.

Shawn and McGuigan (46) also reported two cases in which dermal absorption of promethazine hydrochloride resulted in a toxic neurological syndrome which included central nervous system (CNS) depression, acute excitomotor manifestations, ataxia and visual hallucinations, and peripheral anticholinergic effects.

Antimicrobials
Boric Acids
The toxicity of this mildly bacteriostatic substance is dealt with elsewhere (47). Poisoning and fatal cases have been reported in adults and infants (48–51). Undoubtedly, the use of borates should be abandoned because of their limited therapeutic value and high toxicity. In recent times, few cases of borate intoxication have been published, probably due to its disappearing use.

Castellani's Solution
Castellani's solution (or paint) is an old medicament mainly used for the local treatment of fungal skin infections. It contains boric acid, 800 mg; magenta, 400 mL; phenol, 4 g; resorcinol, 8 g; acetone, 4 mL; alcohol, 8.5 mL; and water, 100 mL.

Lundell and Nordman (52) reported a case in which two applications of Castellani's solution severely poisoned a six-week-old boy who became cyanotic with 41% methemoglobin. The authors stated that this case demonstrated that the application of Castellani's to napkin eruptions and other areas where absorption was rapid may cause serious complications.

Another case report (53) stated that hours after the application of Castellani's paint to the entire body surface except the face of a six-week-old infant for severe seborrheic eczema, the child became drowsy and had shallow breathing. The authors stated that phenol was detected in the urine of 4 out of 16 children treated with Castellani's paint.

Hexachlorophene

Since 1961, hexachlorophene (54) has been extensively used in hospital nurseries, mainly for reducing the incidence of staphylococcal infections among the newborn. In addition, it has been an ingredient of many medical preparations, cosmetics, and other consumer goods.

Hexachlorophene readily penetrates damaged skin, and its absorption through intact skin has also been demonstrated (55–57).

In 1972 in France, as a result of the accidental addition of 6.3% hexachlorophene to batches of baby talcum powder, 204 baby fell ill and 36 died from respiratory arrest (58,59). This report was followed by animal experiments with hexachlorophene confirming that the drug is neurotoxic. Exposures of 160 to 250 mg/kg have resulted in death (54).

Consequently in 1972, the U.S. Food and Drug Administration (FDA) banned the use of hexachlorophene to prescription use only, or as a surgical scrub and hand wash for health care personnel. Hexachlorophene was excluded from cosmetics except as a preservative in levels not exceeding 0.1%.

Because of the high absorption through damaged skin and its proven neurotoxicity, hexachlorophene is contraindicated for the treatment of burns or application to otherwise damaged skin. Premature infants are also at risk. The safety of hexachlorophene for routine bathing of babies is still controversial. Plueckhahn et al. (60) and Hopkins (61) have reviewed the benefits and risks of hexachlorophene.

4-Homosulfanilamide (Sulfamylon Acetate)

4-Homosulfanilamide is a topical sulfanomide that was used for the treatment of large burns. It has now been largely replaced by silver sulfadiazine. Sulfamylon is a carbonic anhydrase inhibitor and caused hyperchloremic metabolic acidosis in patients with extensive burns treated with its topical application, caused by percutaneous absorptions of the drug (62,63). Reversible pulmonary complications (64) and methemoglobinuria (65) have also been reported.

Iodine and Povidone Iodine

Povidone iodine (Betadine) is a water-soluble complex that retains that broad-range microbiocidal activity of iodine without the undesirable effects of iodine tincture (66). However, toxicity still occurs from povidone iodine percutaneously absorbed, mainly when it is used on large areas of burnt skin. Hunt et al. (67) reviewed 17 patients with burns ranging from 4% to 85% TBSA treated with povidone-iodine ointment to both partial- and full-thickness burns. Peak serum iodine levels in patients treated within 24 hours of injury ranged from 595 to 4900 µg/dL. The amount of iodine absorbed was directly related to the size of the burn. Serum iodine levels continued to rise until the drug was discontinued and remained elevated for as long as seven days after discontinuance. Iodine excretion was directly related to renal function. The highest serum and lowest urinary iodine levels were present in patients who developed renal failure and thus the drug is contraindicated in any patient with impaired renal function. Thyroid function was not affected.

Irrigation of povidone iodine considered as a safe and effective procedure, is frequently used for deep infections. Labbe et al. (68) reported a case of intoxication by iodine in a 68-year-old man after subcutaneous irrigations of Betadine at a concentration of 20% for a subcutaneous infection of the thigh. Abnormalities of cardiac conduction, lactic acidosis, acute renal failure, hypocalcemia and thyroid dysfunction were the manifestations of the intoxication confirmed by a very high level of total blood iodine and urine iodine.

Povidone-iodine toxicity is comprehensively dealt with elsewhere (69).

Phenol (Carbolic Acid)

Phenol is no longer widely used as a skin antiseptic, but in dilutions of 0.5% to 2.0% it is sometimes prescribed as an antipruritic in topical medicaments and is used for phenol face peels and as a nail cauterizer.

As much as 25% of phenol is absorbed from 2 mL of a solution of 2.5 g phenol/L water applied to the skin of the forearm and left on for 60 minutes (70). The toxic dose for adults has been estimated to be 8 to 15 g.

Phenol-induced ochronosis has been reported (71) in patients who for many years treated leg ulcers with wet dressing containing phenol.

There have been several case reports of fatal reactions to percutaneously absorbed phenol. One was caused by accidental spillage of phenol (72), one due to treatment of burns with a phenol-containing preparation (73), and another due to the application of phenol to wounds (74). A one-day-old child died after application of 2% phenol to the umbilicus (75).

Several cases of sudden death or intra- or postoperative complications have been reported after phenol chemical peels (76–79). Systemic manifestations of phenol toxicity may develop after 5 to 30 minutes post dermal application, and may produce nausea, vomiting, lethargy or coma, hypotension, tachycardia or bradycardia, dysrhythmias, seizures, acidosis, hemolysis, methemoglobinemia, and shock (79). Major cardiac arrhythmias were noted in 10 out of 43 patients during phenol face peels (80). However, this item is rather controversial, and some authors feel that when the procedure is done over more than one hour, and when the dose applied is carefully monitored, phenol face peels are not risky (81,82). Poisoning due to phenol ingestion is dealt with elsewhere (83).

Resorcinol

Resorcinol is used for its keratolytic properties in the treatment of acne vulgaris. It is also a constituent of the antifungal Castellani's solution. Formerly, leg ulcers were treated with external applications of resorcinol-containing applications.

Resorcinol can penetrate human skin. It has an antithyroid activity similar to that of methyl thiouracil, although it is chemically unrelated to any of the known groups of antithyroid drugs. Clinical case reports from patients undergoing resorcinol therapy for dermatological indications reveal thyroid side effects when copious amounts of resorcinol-containing ointments are applied to integrity-compromised skin for months to years. Effect levels were greater than 34 mg/kg/day (84). Several cases of myxedema caused by percutaneous absorption of resorcinol, especially from ulcerated surfaces, have also been described (85,86).

Methemoglobinemia in children, caused by absorption of resorcinol applied to wounds, has been reported (87,88). Cunningham (89) reported a case in which an ointment containing 12.5% resorcinol applied to the napkin area of an infant produced cyanosis, hemolytic anemia, and hemoglobinemia. In the literature, the author found seven cases of acute poisoning in babies as a consequence of topical resorcinol application; in some instances to limited areas, five fatalities were recorded.

A case of severe poisoning of a six-week-old infant due to two applications of Castellani's paint has been described (52).

Although the use of resorcinol in young children and for leg ulcers should be avoided, topical resorcinol, when used for acne vulgaris, appears to be safe (90).

Silver Sulfadiazine

Sulfadiazine silver cream is widely used for the topical treatment of burns. Intended primarily for the control of pseudomonas infections, this bactericidal agent acts on the cell membranes and cell walls of a variety of gram-positive and gram-negative bacteria, as well as on yeasts. Its relative freedom from appreciable side effects has contributed to its popularity.

Absorption of sulfonamide from burns to 17% to 46% body area treated with sulfadiazine silver showed 20% to 25% of the daily topical dose could be accounted for as conjugated sulfonamide. Unconjugated drug represented from 35% to 95% of the total output. Total plasma, sulfonamide concentration did not exceed 10 µg/mL (91).

Prolonged topical application of silver sulfadiazine cream can induce argyria and adverse effects of sulphonamides (92,93). Silver is rapidly absorbed through the burn wound. It provokes hepatic, renal and neurologic tissue toxicity. Renal and hepatic function tests are not correlated with serum silver levels. Monitoring concentration of silver in blood and/or urine is necessary, especially in patients treated with silver sulfadiazine cream for cutaneous burns.

Nephrotic syndrome following topical therapy has been reported (94). Chaby et al. (95) also reported a case of a woman with acute renal failure following repeated applications of topical silver sulfadiazine on pyoderma gangrenosum wounds. Silver concentration in blood was 1818 nmol/L (N < 92 nmol/L) and 1381 nmol/L (N < 9 nmol/L) in urine. Sulfadiazine concentration in blood was undetectable. All the signs regressed after withdrawal of silver sulfadiazine and after several sessions of hemodialysis.

Several authors have reported leukopenia during treatment with silver sulfadiazine (96–100). Current evidence suggests a causal relationship of silver sulfadiazine with leukopenia, although the mechanism of this reaction is unknown. Examination of bone marrow aspirates show hyperplasia with no evidence of maturation arrest. The drug presumably affects the white blood cells peripherally (98). The sulfadiazine-induced leukopenia is at its nadir within two to four days of starting therapy. The leukocyte count returns to normal levels within two to three days and recovery is not affected by continuation of therapy. The erythrocyte count is not affected. Other proposed mechanisms of leukopenia include an allergic reaction of bone marrow toxicity (99,101).

Triclocarban (Trichlorocarbanilide)

Triclocarban is a bacteriostatic agent used as an antimicrobial in toilet soap since 1956. The percutaneous absorption has been studied by Scharpf et al. (102), who showed that after a simple shower employing a whole-body lather with approximately 6 g of soap containing 2% trichlorocarbanilide (TCC), about 0.23% of the applied dose of TCC was recovered in feces after six days, and 0.16% of the dose in the urine after two days. At all sampling times, blood levels of radioactivity were below the detection limit of 10 ppb. There have been several reports (103) of methemoglobinemia presumably induced by topical TCC in neonates.

Arsenic

The toxicity, mutagenesis, and carcinogenesis of ingested or inhaled arsenic are dealt with elsewhere (104–106). Fowler's solution, long used orally in the treatment of psoriasis, contained arsenic. Arsenical keratoses and malignancies are well recognized long-term reactions to this.

Carmustine

Topical carmustine (BCNU) has been used for the treatment of mycosis fungoides, lymphomatoid papulosis, and parapsoriasis en plaques. Percutaneous absorption of BCNU has been demonstrated in man. Zackheim et al. (107) treated 91 patients with mycosis fungoides and related disorders with topical BCNU. Mild to moderate reversible bone marrow depression occurred in three patients. Their data suggest that hematological toxicity arises primarily from the shorter intensive schedules; the prolonged use of up to 100 mg/wk appears to be safe. Although an occasional mild elevation in the blood urea nitrogen (BUN) or serum glutamic oxaloacetic transaminases/Aspartate aminotransferase (SGOT/AST) was noted in patients treated with courses exceeding 600 mg, no such changes were seen with lower doses. In the study of Zackheim et al. (107), there were no apparent long-term harmful effects on the hematopoietic system or internal organs.

Camphor

Camphor is a pleasant-smelling cyclic ketone of the hydroaromatic terpene group. When rubbed on the skin, camphor is a rubefacient but, if not vigorously applied, produces a feeling of coolness. It is an ingredient of a large number of over-the-counter remedies (with a camphor content of 1/20%), taken especially for symptomatic relief of "chest congestion" and muscle aches, but its effectiveness is rather dubious.

Camphor is readily absorbed from all sites of administration, including topical application to the skin.

The compound is classified as a Class IV chemical, that is, a very toxic substance. Hundreds of cases of intoxications have been reported, usually after accidental ingestion in children (47,107–111).

Cosmetic Agents

The use of henna dye is traditional in Islamic communities. The dye is used on nails, skin, and hair by married ladies, and traditionally it is also used by the major participants in marriage ceremonies, when the bridegroom and best man also apply henna to their hands.

Henna consists of the dried leaves of *Lawsonia alba* (family Lythraceae), a scrub cultivated in North Africa, India, and Sri Lanka. The coloring matter, lawsone, is a hydroxynaphthoquinone and is associated with fats, resin, and henna tannin in the leaf. Dyeing hair or skin with powdered henna is a somewhat lengthy procedure, and to speed up this process, Sudanese ladies mix a "black powder" with henna; this accelerates the fixing process of the dye merely to a matter of minutes. This black powder is *p*-phenylenediamine. The combination of henna and "black powder" is particularly toxic, and over 20 cases of such toxicity, some fatal, have been noted in Khartoum alone in a two-year period. Initial symptoms are those of angioedema with massive edema of the face, lips, glottis, pharynx, neck, and bronchi. These occur within hours of the application of the dye mix to the skin. The symptoms may then progress on the second day to anuria and acute renal failure, with death occurring on the third day. Dialysis has helped some patients, but others have died from renal tubular necrosis (112). Whether this toxicity is due to *p*-phenylenediamine per se (probably grossly impure) or whether its toxicity is potentiated in its combination with henna powder is unknown. Systemic administration of the "black powder" leads to similar symptoms, and several deaths due to ingestion with suicidal intent have been reported (113,114).

Diethyltoluamide
This has been used as an insect repellent since 1957. Although diethyltoluamide has an overall low incidence of toxic effects, prolonged use in children has been discouraged because of reports of toxic encephalopathy (115,116). In one case, the bedding, nightclothes, and skin of a 3.5-year-old girl were sprayed with a total amount of 180 mL of 15% diethyltoluamide for two weeks; shaking and crying spells, slurred speech, and confusion developed. Improvement occurred after vigorous medical treatment including anticonvulsants. In another report, one of two children displaying signs of severe toxic encephalopathy died after prolonged hospitalization. At autopsy, edema of the brain and congestion of the meninges was found.

Dimethyl Sulfoxide
The toxicology of topical DMSO has been investigated by Kligman (117). In this study, 9 mL of 90% DMSO was applied twice daily to the entire trunk of 20 healthy volunteers for three weeks. The following laboratory tests were done: complete blood count, urinalysis, blood sedimentation rate, SGOT/AST, BUN, and fasting blood sugar determination. At the end of the study, all laboratory values remained normal. Except for the appearance of cutaneous signs as erythema, scaling, contact urticaria, stinging, and burning sensations, the drug was tolerated well by all but two individuals, who developed systemic symptoms. In one, a toxic reaction developed on day 12 characterized by a diffuse erythematous and scaling rash accompanied by severe abdominal cramps; the other had a similar rash and complained of nausea, chills, and chest pains. These signs, however, abated in spite of continuous administration of the drug.

To investigate possible side effects of chronic exposure to DMSO, another 20 volunteers were painted with 9 mL of 90% DMSO applied to the entire trunk, once daily for a period of 26 week. Neither clinical nor laboratory investigations showed adverse effects of the drug. However, most subjects did experience the well-known DMSO-induced disagreeable oyster-like breath odor, to which they eventually became insensitive. One fatality due to a hypersensitivity reaction has been reported (118).

Dinitrochlorobenzene
Dinitrochlorobenzene (DNCB), a potent contact allergen, has been used with some success for the treatment of recalcitrant alopecia areata; today, however, its use has

been discouraged because suspicion has been aroused that DNCB may be mutagenic. Another drawback for its use is its ability to potentiate epicutaneous sensitization to nonrelated allergens (119). DNCB is absorbed in substantial amounts through the skin, and about 50% of the applied dose is ultimately recoverable in the urine (120).

A possible systemic reaction to DNCB has been reported (121): a 25-year-old man was treated with 0.1% DNCB in an absorbent ointment base for alopecia areata after prior sensitization. After two months of daily applications, the patient experienced generalized urticaria, pruritus, and dyspepsia; discontinuance of the drug led to cessation of all symptoms, which recurred after reintroduction of DNCB therapy.

Ethyl Alcohol

Twenty-eight children with alcohol intoxication from percutaneous absorption were described by Gimenez et al. (122) from Buenos Aires, Argentina. Apparently, in that area, it is (or was) a popular procedure to apply alcohol-soaked cloths to the abdomens of babies as a home remedy for the treatment of disturbances of the gastrointestinal tract such as cramps, pain, vomiting, and diarrhea, or because of crying, excitability, and irritability. The children were of both sexes and ranged in age from 33 months to 1 year (mean: 12 months, 27 days). Alcohol-soaked cloths had been applied on the babies' abdomens under rubber panties, and the number of applications varied from one to three; it was estimated that each application contained approximately 40 cm^3 ethanol. Medical consultation took place from 1 to 23 hours after application. Alcohol breath and abdominal erythema were valuable clues to the diagnosis.

All 28 children showed some degree of CNS depression, 24 showed miosis, 15 hypoglycemia, 5 convulsions, 5 respiratory depression, and 2 died. Eleven cases showed blood alcohol from 0.6 to 1.49 g%. Of the two who died, one was autopsied: the findings were consistent with ethyl alcohol intoxication.

More recently, a case of acute ethanol intoxication in a preterm infant of 1800 g due to local application of alcohol-soaked compresses on the legs as a treatment for puncture hematomas was reported (123).

Topically applied ethanol in tar gel (124) and beer-containing shampoo (125) have caused Antabuse effects in patients on disulfiram for alcoholism, through percutaneous absorption.

Fumaric Acid Monoethyl Ester

The effect of systemically and/or topically administered fumaric acid monoethyl ester (ethyl fumarate) on psoriasis was studied by Dubiel and Happle (126) in six patients. Two patients who had been treated with locally applied ointments, consisting of 3% or 5% ethyl fumarate in petrolatum, developed symptoms of renal intoxication.

Local Anesthetics

Benzocaine

Methemoglobinemia has been reported following the topical application of benzocaine to both skin and mucous membranes (127–130). However, this is an uncommon occurrence (131); most cases occurred in infants (132).

Lidocaine

Lidocaine hydrochloride is widely used for both topical and local injection anesthesia. When the drug is applied to mucous membranes, blood levels simulate those resulting from intravenous injection (133). Serum lidocaine concentrations higher than 6 µg/mL are associated with toxicity (134), whose signs are CNS stimulation followed by depression and later inhibition of cardiovascular function. Cases of central nervous toxicity, especially seizures, following topical application of local anesthetics have been reported (135–137). Systemic toxicity from viscous lidocaine applied to the oral cavity in two children has been described (138,139). In one, the mother had been applying lidocaine hydrochloride 2% solution to the infant's gums with her finger five to six times daily for a week; the child experienced two generalized seizures within an hour. Urine examined by thin-layer chromatography revealed a large amount of lidocaine, and a blood level of 10 µg/mL was determined (139). The other child had a seizure after having received 227.8 mg/kg oral viscous lidocaine for stomatitis herpetica over a 24-hour period. In this case, however, ingestion and resorption from the gastrointestitnal tract may have contributed to the clinical picture. It has been suggested that for pediatric patients viscous lidocaine should be applied with an oral swab to individual lesions, thus limiting buccal absorption by decreasing the surface area exposed to lidocaine (138).

Lidocaine–prilocaine cream (EMLA) is a widely used local anesthetic with few side effects when used properly. Intoxication with a lidocaine–prilocaine preparation may have serious consequences, such as changes in intracardiac conduction, excitation or depression of the CNS (140,141) and methemoglobinemia (142–144).

Mercurials

The toxicology of mercury is comprehensively dealt with elsewhere (145). With a few exceptions, the use of mercury in medicine is considered to be outdated. However, attention should be paid to the possibility of mercurial poisoning even nowadays, as mercury may still be present in many drugs, and in many countries even in over-the-counter remedies and cosmetic creams, often without mention on the label.

Although there are considerable differences between various mercurials regarding the rate of absorption through the skin, all mercurial preparations are a potential hazard and may cause intoxication. Metallic mercury is readily absorbed through intact skin; absorption of ammoniated mercury chloride in psoriatic patients was demonstrated by Bork et al. (146).

Young (147) examined 70 psoriatic patients treated with an ointment containing ammoniated mercury before, during, and after treatment. Symptoms and signs of mercurial poisoning could be detected in 33 of them.

Nephrotic syndrome has been reported in a 24-year-old man using an ammoniated mercury-containing ointment for psoriasis (148,149). Nephrotic syndrome due to topical mercury has also been reported (150,151). Minimal change disease, facial mercury pigmentation, raised levels of mercury in the blood and urine, and possible neuropsychiatric toxicity secondary to mercury exposure in cosmetic creams has been reported (152–156).

There have been two case reports (157,158) of children who died following the treatment of an omphalocele with merbromin (an organic mercurial antiseptic).

In view of the risks of both systemic side effects and contact allergic reactions to mercurials, there hardly seems to be any justification for continuing the use of these drugs in dermatological therapy.

Monobenzone

Monobenzone (monobenzyl ether of hydroquinone) is used topically by patients with extensive vitiligo to depigment their remaining normally pigmented skin. A patient who had been applying the drug for one year had an anterior linear deposition of pigment on both corneas. In 11 additional patients with vitiligo who were using monobenzone, acquired conjunctival melanosis occurred in two patients and pingueculae in three (159).

2-Naphthol (β-Naphthol)

2-Naphthol is used in peeling pastes for the treatment of acne, and between 5% and 10% of a cutaneous dose has been recovered from the urine (160,161).

The extensive application of 2-naphthol ointments has been responsible for systemic side effects, including vomiting and death (162,163). Hemels (161) concludes that 2-naphthol-containing pastes should be applied only for short periods of time and to a limited area not exceeding 150 cm^2.

Insecticides

Lindane

Lindane is the δ isomer of benzene hexachloride. It is widely used in the treatment of scabies and pediculosis, usually in a 1% lotion applied to the entire body and left on for 24 hours (in the case of scabies). The percutaneous absorption of the drug has been studied (164–166). The general toxicology is dealt with elsewhere (167).

Intoxication from excessive topical therapeutic application of Lindane has been documented (168–172).

The issue of possible toxic reactions to a single therapeutic application of Lindane, notably CNS toxicity, has not yet been settled (168,172–174).

Most authors seem to agree that the benefits to be derived from the use of Lindane as a scabicide and pediculicide outweigh the risks involved (175–178). The risk of toxicity appears minimal when Lindane is used properly according to directions.

Solomon et al. (175) in their review on Lindane toxicity give the following observations and recommendations:

1. Lindane should not be applied after a hot bath.
2. The regimen of application for 24 hour may be unnecessarily long; 8 to 12 hours may be sufficient (177).
3. A concentration weaker than 1.0% may suffice, particularly for badly excoriated patients.
4. Lindane 1% should be used with extreme caution if at all in pregnant women, very small infants, and people with massively excoriated skin. Rassmussen (177) does not agree on this point.
5. Lindane treatment should not be repeated within eight days, and then only if necessary.

Malathion
The detailed toxicity of malathion is dealt with elsewhere (167,179). Malathion is used in the treatment of lice, a single application of 0.5% in a solution being customary. Used in this way, it is generally safe.

Ramu et al. (180) reported on four children with an intoxication following hair washing with a solution containing 5% malathion in xylene for the purpose of louse control. Malathion is also a weak but definite skin sensitizer (181).

Podophyllum/Podophyllin
The toxicity of podophyllum was reviewed in 1982 (182). Of greatest concern are the number of case reports revealing that following podophyllin painting of large condylomas, after subdermal injection into plantar warts, or following accidental ingestion, podophyllin may cause fatal or near fatal intoxication due to CNS influence, coma, respiratory depression, etc, and cardiovascular crisis (183–185). There is no known antidote. Irreversible peripheral neuropathy is a sequel in survivors. Warnings against use of volumes exceeding 0.4 to 0.9 mL have been issued (183).

Podophyllum 20% in tincture of benzoin is still indicated for isolated venereal warts (186). Its use is contraindicated in pregnancy. Following application it should be washed off after a specific period of time.

Salicylic Acid
The general toxicology of salicylates is dealt with elsewhere (187), including its absorption through the skin (188). Salicylic acid is widely used in dermatology as a topical application for its keratolytic properties. Cases of salicylate poisoning after topical use of salicylic acid have been reported several times. Taylor and Halprin (189) used 6% salicylic acid in a gel base under plastic suit occlusion in adults with extensive psoriasis. During their five-day study, serum salicylates never exceeded 5 mg/100 mL and no patient developed toxicity. However, toxicity was noted by von Weis and Lever (190); they found serum salicylate levels ranging from 46 to 64 mg/100 mL salicylic acid therapy for extensive lesions may be especially dangerous for children. An unpublished review (191) revealed 13 deaths associated with the widespread use of salicylic acid preparations, and all but three occurred in children. This compound should not be used on large areas (more than 25%) of the skin of a child.

In 1952, Young collected eight fatal cases of salicylate poisoning with symptoms of vomiting, tinnitus, stupor, Cheyne–Stokes respiration, and nuchal rigidity.

von Weiss and Lever (190) reported three adults with extensive psoriasis who were treated with an ointment containing 3% or 6% salicylic acid six times daily. Between the second and fourth days, symptoms of salicylism developed in all three patients.

The levels of salicylic acid in the serum ranged from 46 to 64 mg/100 mL. Within one day after discontinuation of the ointment, the symptoms had largely disappeared. The serum salicylic acid in the serum decreased to zero within a few days.

The same authors also recorded 13 deaths resulting from intoxication with salicylic acid following the application of salicylic ointment to the skin, reported in literature up to 1964, and several nonfatal intoxications. The 13 deaths included three patients with psoriasis, five cases of scabies, three of dermatitis, one of lupus vulgaris, and one of congenital ichthyosiform erythroderma. Ten of the fatal cases occurred in children, three of them being under three years of age.

The most dramatic account in the literature is that of two plantation workers in Bougainville, in the Solomon Islands, who were painted twice a day with an alcoholic solution of 20% salicylic acid to tinea imbricate involving about 50% of the body. The victims were comatose within six hours and dead within 28 hours (192).

Wechelsberg (193) reported a three-months-old baby with scaly erythroderma treated in a hospital with 1% salicylic acid in soft paraffin. After 10 days, the child began to vomit and lose weight. Later hyperpnea developed and an increasing somnolence. When the treatment was stopped, the child recovered rapidly.

A case of salicylic acid intoxication leading to coma in an adult patient with psoriasis who had been treated with 20% salicylic acid in petrolatum was also described (194).

Methyl salicylate is widely available as a component in many over-the-counter brands of creams, ointments, lotions, liniments and medicated oils intended for topical application to relieve musculoskeletal aches and pains. Methyl salicylate continues to be a relatively common source of pediatric exposures. Persistent reports of life-threatening and fatal toxicity were found (195). In addition, excessive usage of these preparations in patients receiving warfarin may result in adverse interactions and bleedings (196,197). Methyl salicylate in topical analgesic preparations may cause irritant or allergic contact dermatitis and anaphylactic reactions (196). Caution is advised in special circumstances, such as during childhood, pregnancy, lactation and concomitant therapy with other drugs.

Selenium Sulfide

Ransone et al. (198) reported a case of systemic selenium toxicity in a woman who had been shampooing her hair two or three times weekly for eight months with selenium sulfide suspension.

Silver Nitrate

Ternberg and Luce (199) observed fatal methemoglobinemia in a three-year-old girl suffering from burns involving 82% of the body surface, who was treated with silver nitrate solution.

Another complication of the use of silver nitrate in the treatment of large burns is electrolyte disturbance, especially in children. Due to the hypotonicity of the silver nitrate dressings, hyponatremia, hypokalemia, and hyperchloremia may develop (200,201). Also, loss of other water-soluble minerals and vitamins may occur. Postmortem examinations of patients treated with silver nitrate have revealed that silver has been deposited in internal organs, showing that absorption of silver from topical preparation does occur (202). It should be mentioned that the excessive use of silver-containing drugs has led to local and systemic argyria (203) and to renal damage involving the glomeruli and proteinuria (204).

Steroids

Corticosteroids

It has been amply documented that topically applied glucocorticoids are absorbed through the skin (205). Systemic absorption in quantities sufficient to replace endogenous production is not uncommon. However, iatrogenic Cushing's syndrome resulting from the use of topical steroids is rare (206) except for topical steroid abuse (207). Pascher (208) summarized the relevant data of 12 cases.

Systemic side effects of topical corticosteroids occur more frequently in children than adults (209) and occur in patients with liver disease because of retarded degradation of the drug (210). The two main causes of systemic side effects are hypercorticism leading to an iatrogenic Cushing's syndrome and suppression of the hypothalamic–pituitary–adrenal axis (211).

It is not easy to provide data on "safe" uses of topical corticosteroids, but as for the potent corticosteroid clobetasol 17-propionate 0.05% the dose is recommended to be limited to 45 g/wk (212).

Sex Hormones
Estrogens
Topical application of estrogen-containing preparations may lead to resorption of these hormones and systemic estrogenic effects.

Beas et al. (213) reported on seven children with pseudoprecocious puberty due to an ointment containing estrogens. The common fact found in every patient was the use of the same ointment for treatment or prevention of ammoniacal dermatitis for a period of 2 to 18 months with 2 to 10 applications daily. Endocrinological and radiological studies had excluded other possible causes of sexual precocity. The most important clinical signs were intense pigmentation of mammillary areola, linea alba of the abdomen and the genitals, mammary enlargement, and the presence of pubic hair. Three female patients also had vaginal discharge and bleeding. Estrogenic contamination of the ointment was suspected and confirmed by a biological test of the vaginal opening of castrated female guinea pigs. After discontinuation of the incriminated topical drug, all symptomatology progressively disappeared in every patient.

Pseudoprecocious puberty has also been observed in young girls after contact with hair lotions and other substances containing estrogens (214–216). Such contact has led to gynecomastia in young boys (217,218). Gynecomastia in a 70-year-old man from exposure to 0.01% dienestrol cream used by his wife for atrophic vaginitis and as a lubricant before intercourse has been reported (219).

Estrogen cream for the treatment of baldness has also caused gynecomastia, which was persistent in the reported case (220). In adult males, both oral and topical administration of estrogens may result first in pigmentation of the areola and then in gynecomastia (221,222).

Tars
Coal Tar
A case of methemoglobinemia in an infant following the five-day application of an ointment containing 2.5% crude coal tar and 5% benzocaine to about half the body surface has been reported (223).

Dithranol
Dithranol has been used since 1916 for the treatment of psoriasis. Although it causes irritant dermatitis and discoloration of the skin, its use is generally considered to be devoid of systemic side effects (224,225).

5-Fluorouracil

5-Fluorouracil (5-FU) remains one of the most frequently used chemotherapy drugs for the treatment of several different malignancies, including carcinomas of the breast, colon, and skin. The mechanism of 5-FU antitumor action (and most host toxicities) depends on anabolism of the drug to cytotoxic nucleotides, which in turn can act at multiple sites including inhibition of thymidylate synthase or incorporation into RNA and DNA.

An administered dose of 80% to 90% of 5-FU is degraded by dihydropyrimidine dehydrogenase (DPD; EC 1.3.1.2), the initial rate-limiting enzyme in pyrimidine catabolism. Cancer patients with decreased DPD activity are at increased risk for severe toxicity including diarrhea, stomatitis, mucositis, myelosuppression, neurotoxicity, and in some cases, death. The cause of this potentially life-threatening toxicity appears to be decreased catabolism, resulting in markedly prolonged exposure to 5-FU. Johnson et al. (226) reported the first known cancer patient who developed life-threatening complications after treatment with topical 5-FU and was shown, subsequently, to have profound DPD deficiency. The authors concluded that the presence of this metabolic defect combined with topical 5-FU (a drug demonstrating a narrow therapeutic index) results in the unusual presentation of life-threatening toxicity after treatment with a topical drug.

Minoxidil

Minoxidil is a $K(+)$ channel opener able to cause relaxation of vascular smooth muscles and modify cell growth and/or cell migration. Since 1987 when it became commercially available, topical minoxidil has been used widely in the treatment of hair loss and seemed to be well tolerated and sufficiently safe. Nevertheless, there are some reports referring that scalp application may cause hypotension, tachycardia, and even myocardial infarction (227–229). This strongly suggests that minoxidil, even topically applied, may be systemically absorbed and reach pharmacologically active blood concentrations. Smorlesi et al. (230) reported a case of fetal malformation caused by topically applied minoxidil in a pregnant woman. Georgala et al. (231) reported three young patients with alopecia areata treated with minoxidil solution 2% and all of them experienced cardiovascular side effects. It is thus suggested that minoxidil, when topically applied in children, may be systemically absorbed to some extent and cause several side effects.

Tacalcitol

Recently, various analogs of 1,25-$(OH)_2D_3$ with potent differentiation stimulating activity on keratinocytes but insufficient calcium-mobilizing activity have been developed (tacalcitol, calcipotriol and 22-oxacalcitriol). However, since the agents can be easily absorbed through the skin lesions, severe hypercalcemia may develop when these ointments were abundantly applied to patients with psoriasis (232,233). Knackstedt et al. (234) reported a case of acute necrotic pancreatitis induced by severe hypercalcemia due to tacalcitol ointment. Monitoring of calcium level may be important to prevent such complication.

Monochloroacetic Acid

Monochloroacetic acid ($ClCH_2COOH$, MCA) is widely used in industrial fields. MCA is generally used as an 80% solution, as flakes or as the sodium salt. MCA is highly corrosive to tissues and is 25 to 40 times more toxic than acetic, dichloroacetic, or trichloroacetic acids (235). There have been many fatal occupational and domestic accidents that have involved skin exposure to MCA (236–238). Toshina et al. (239) reported a worker with 10% total body surface area exposure to 80% MCA solution, who despite immediate water washing, developed third grade chemical burn, then became unconscious after 90 minutes and died six hours later. It was thus suggested that MCA would be absorbed by the momentary cutaneous contact. The authors suggested that important serum biochemical abnormalities should be closely monitored in the early stage, since coma and mortality could frequently be followed several hours later.

COMMENT

This chapter summarized literature citations and the basic aspects of percutaneous penetration. The purpose is to alert the reader to the potential for systemic toxicity from topical exposure. Demonstrating causality (rather than association) requires careful documentation. Combining knowledge of the inherent molecular and animal toxicology, cutaneous penetration, and metabolism with the adverse human reaction literature permits a more precise determination of causality. With each of the examples presented here, the original citations combined with the further documentation noted here should permit more discriminate causality judgments.

Documenting causality between a chemical and putative adverse effect often is incomplete—both in a given case and in the pharmacoepidemiology. Naranjo (Table 3) provided a robust algorithm to semiquantitatively

TABLE 3   Naranjo Adverse Drug Reaction Probability Scale

Question	Yes	No	Don't know	Score[a]
Are there previous *conclusive* reports on this reaction?	+1	0	0	
Did the adverse event appear after the suspected drug was administered?	+2	−1	0	
Did the adverse reaction improve when the drug was discontinued or a *specific* antagonist was administered?	+1	0	0	
Did the adverse reaction reappear when the drug was readministered?	+2	−1	0	
Are there alternative causes (other than the drug) that could on their own have caused the reaction?	−1	+2	0	
Did the reaction reappear when a placebo was given?	−1	+1	0	
Was the drug detected in the blood (or other fluids) in concentrations known to be toxic?	+1	0	0	
Was the reaction more severe when the dose was increased or less severe when the dose was decreased?	+1	0	0	
Did the patient have a similar reaction to the same or similar drug in *any* previous exposure?	+1	0	0	
Was the adverse event confirmed by any objective evidence?	+1	0	0	

[a] Probability of the adverse reaction or drug interaction was drug-related: score >9, highly probable; 5 to 8, probable; 1 to 4, possible; and ≤0, doubtful.
Source: From Ref. 240.

establish—or deny—such a relationship (240). When Naranjo's system is more widely utilized, we will have better assurance of causality.

REFERENCES

1. Wiechers JW. The barrier function of the skin in relation to percutaneous absorption of drugs. Pharm Weekbl Sci 1989; 11(6):185–98.
2. Stoughton RB. Percutaneous absorption of drugs. Ann Rev Pharmacol Toxicol 1989; 29:55–69.
3. Feldmann RJ, Maibach HI. Regional variation in percutaneous penetration of ^{14}C cortesol in man. J Invest Dermatol 1967; 48:181.
4. Zhai H, Maibach HI. Effects of skin occlusion on percutaneous absorption: an overview. Skin Pharmacol Appl Skin Physiol 2001; 14(1):1–10.
5. Roskos KV, Maibach HI. Percutaneous absorption and age. Implications for therapy. Drugs Aging 1992; 2(5):432–49.
6. Nachman RL, Esterly NB. Increased skin permeability in pre-term infancts. J Pediatr 1971; 89:628–32.
7. Greaves SJ, Ferry DG, Mcqueen EG, et al. Serial hexachlorophene blood levels in the premature infant. NZ Med J 1975; 81:334–6.
8. Rasmussen JE. Percutaneous absoption in children. In: Dobson RL, ed. Year Book of Dermatology. Chicago: Year Book Medical, 1979:15–38.
9. Danon A, Ben-Shimon S, Ben-Zvi Z. Effect of exercise and heat exposure on percutaneous absorption of methyl salicylate. Eur J Clin Pharmacol 1986; 31(1):49–52.
10. Pannatier A, Jenner B, Testa B, et al. The skin as a drug-metabolizing organ. Drug Metab Rev 1978; 8:319–43.
11. Baron JM, Merk HF. Drug metabolism in the skin. Curr Opin Allergy Clin Immunol 2001; 1(4):287–91.
12. Ahmad N, Mukhtar H. Cytochrome p450: a target for drug development for skin diseases. J Invest Dermatol 2004; 123(3):417–25.
13. Frosch PJ, Menne T, Lepoittevin J-P. Allergic contact dermatitis in humans—experimental and quantitative aspects. In: Lepoittevin J-P, ed. Contact Dermatitis. 4th ed. Berlin/Heidelberg, Germany: Springer, 2006:189–98.
14. Fisher AA. Contact Dermatitis. 3rd ed. Philadelphia, PA: Lea and Febiger, 1986.
15. Amin S, Lahti A, Maibach HI. Contact urticaria and the contact urticaria syndrome (immediate contact reactions). In: Zhai H, Maibach HI, eds. Dermatotoxicology. 6th ed. Boca Raton, FL: CRC Press, 2004:817–48 (chap. 42).
16. Wilson AJ, Mielke CH. Haematological consequences of poisoning. In: Haddad LM, Winchester JF, eds. Poisoning and Drug Overdose. Philadelphia, PA: W.B. Saunders, 1983:893 (chap. 96).
17. Abrams SM, Degnan TH, Vinciguerra V. Marrow aplasia following topical application of chloramphenicol eye ointment. Arch Intern Med 1980; 140:576.
18. Walker S, Diaper CJ, Bowman R, Sweeney G, Seal DV, Kirkness CM. Lack of evidence for systemic toxicity following topical chloramphenicol use. Eye 1998; 12(5):875–9.
19. Barza M, Goldstein JA, Kane A, Feingold DS, Pochi PE. Systemic absorption of clindamycin hydrochloride after topical application. J Am Acad Dermatol 1982; 7:208.
20. Franz TJ. On the bioavailability of topical formulations of clindamycin hydrochloride. J Am Acad Dermatol 1983; 9:66.
21. Stoughton TB. Topical antibiotics for acne vulgaris: current usage. Arch Dermatol 1975; 106:740.
22. Voron DA. Systemic absorption of topical clindamycin. Arch Dermatol 1978; 114:708.
23. Becker LE, Bergstresser PR, Whiting DA. Topical clindamycin therapy for acne vulgaris: a cooperative clinical study. Arch Dermatol 1981; 117:482.
24. Milstone EB, Mcdonald AJ, Scholhamer CF. Pseudomembranous colitis after topical application of clindamycin. Arch Dermatol 1986; 117:154.
25. Akhavan A, Bershad S. Topical acne drugs: review of clinical properties, systemic exposure, and safety. Am J Clin Dermatol 2003; 4(7):473–92.

26. Dayal VS, Smith EL, McCain WG. Cochlear and vestibular gentamycin toxicity: a clinical study of systemic and topical usage. Arch Otolaryngol 1974; 100:338.
27. Drake TE. Reaction to gentamycin sulfate cream. Arch Dermatol 1984; 110:638.
28. Mittelman H. Ototoxicity of "ototopical" antibiotics: past, present, and future. Trans Am Acad Opththal Otolaryngol 1972; 76:1432.
29. Conlon BJ, Smith DW. Topical aminoglycoside ototoxicity: attempting to protect the cochlea. Acta Otolaryngol 2000; 120(5):596–9.
30. Matz G, Rybak L, Roland PS, et al. Ototoxicity of ototopical antibiotic drops in humans. Otolaryngol Head Neck Surg 2004; 130(Suppl. 3):S79–82.
31. Macdonald RH, Beck M. Neomycin: a review with particular reference to dermatological usage. Clin Exp Dermatol 1983; 8(3):249–58.
32. Friedmann I. Aerosols containing neomycin. Lancet 1977; 1:1662.
33. Anonymous. Warning on aerosols containing neomycin. Lancet 1977; 1:1115.
34. Bamford MFM, Jones LF. Deafness and biochemical imbalance after burns treatment with topical antibiotics in young children. Arch Dis Child 1978; 53:326.
35. Masur H, Whelton PK, Whelton A. Neomycin toxicity revisited. Arch Surg 1976; 3:822.
36. Kelly DR, Nilo EN, Berggren RB. Deafness after topical neomycin wound irrigation. N Engl J Med 1969; 280:1338.
37. Goffinet M. A propos de la toxicite cliniquement presumable de certainties gouttes otiques. Acta Otorhinolaryngol Belg 1977; 31:585.
38. Kellerhals B. Horschaden durch ototxische Ohrtropcen. Ergebnisse einer Umfrage. HNO (Berl) 1978; 26:49.
39. Filloux F. Toxic encephalopathy caused by topically applied diphenhydramine. J Pediatr 1986; 108(6):1018–20.
40. Chan CY, Wallander KA. Diphenhydramine toxicity in three children with varicella-zoster infection. DICP 1991; 25(2):130–2.
41. Bernhardt DT. Topical diphenhydramine toxicity. Wis Med J 1991; 90(8):469–71.
42. Reilly JF, Jr., Weisse ME. Topically induced diphenhydramine toxicity. J Emerg Med 1990; 8(1):59–61.
43. Cammann R, Hennecke H, Beier R. Symptomatische Psychosen nach Kolton-Gelee-Applikation. Psychiatr Neurol Med Psychol 1971; 23:426.
44. Vidal Pan C, Gonzalez Quintela A, Galdos Anuncibay P, Mateo Vic J. Topical promethazine intoxication. DICP 1989; 23(1):89.
45. Bloch R, Beysovec L. Promethazine toxicity through percutaneous absorption. Contin Pract 1982; 9:28.
46. Shawn DH, Mcguigan MA. Poisoning from dermal absorption of promethazine. Can Med Assoc J 1984; 130(11):1460–1.
47. Sue Y-J, Pinkert H. Baby powder, borates, and camphor. In: Haddad LM, Shannon MW, Winchester JF, eds. Clinical Management of Poisoning and Drug Overdose. 3rd ed. Philadelphia, PA: W.B. Saunders, 1998:1161–4.
48. Maxson WT. Case report of boric acid poisoning from topical application. J Ky State Med Assoc 1954; 52(6):423–4.
49. Searle A. Boric acid poisoning. Clin Proc Child Hosp Dist Columbia 1956; 12(1):13–6.
50. Jordan JW, Crissey JT. Boric acid poisoning; a report of fatal adult case from cutaneous use; a critical evaluation of the use of this drug in dermatologic practice. AMA Arch Derm 1957; 75(5):720–8.
51. Kaufmann HJ, Held U, Salzberg R. Fatal transcutaneous resorption of boric acid in an infant. Dtsch Med Wochenschr 1962; 87:2374–8.
52. Lundell E, Nordman R. A case of infantile poisoning by topical application of Castellani's solution. Ann Clin Res 1973; 5:404.
53. Rogers SCF, Burrows D, Neill D. Percutaneous absorption of phenol and methylalcohol in magenty paint B.P.C. Br J Dermatol 1978; 98:559.
54. Langford CP, Bartlett R, Haddad LM. Phenol and related agents. In: Haddad LM, Shannon MW, Winchester JF, eds. Clinical Management of Poisoning and Drug Overdose. 3rd ed. Philadelphia, PA: W.B. Saunders, 1998:958.
55. Tyrala EE, Hillman LS, Hillman RE, Dodson WE. Clinical pharmacology of hexachlorophene in newborn infants. J Pediatr 1977; 91:481.

56. Curley A, Hawk RE, Kimbrough RD, Nathenson G, Finberg L. Dermal absorption of hexachlorophene infancts. Lancet 1971; 2:296.

57. Alder VD, Burman D, Coroner-Beryl D, Gillespie WA. Absorption of hexachlorophene from infant's skin. Lancet 1972; 2:384.

58. Pine WI. Hexachlorophene: why FDA concluded that hexachlorophene was too potent and too dangerous to be used as it once was? FDA Consumer 1972; 6:24.

59. Editorial. Hexachlorophene today. Lancet 1982; 1:500.

60. Plueckhahn VC, Ballard BA, Banis JM, Collins RB, Flett PT. Hexachlorophene preparations in infant antiseptic skin care: benefit, risk and the future. Med J Aust 1978; 2:555.

61. Hopkins J. Hexachlorophene: more bad news than good. Food Cosmet Toxicol 1979; 17:410.

62. Otten H, Plempel M. Antibiotika und Chemotherapeutika in Einzeldarstellungen. Chemotherapeutika mit braitem Wirkungsbereich. Sulgonamide. In: Otten H, Plempel M, Siegenthaler G, eds. Antibiotika-Fibel. Stuttgart: Thieme Verlag, 1975:110–45.

63. Liebman PR, Kennelly MM, Hirsch EF. Hypercarbia and acidosis associated with carbonic anhydrase inhibition: a hazard of topical mafenide acetate use in renal failure. Burns 1982; 8:395.

64. Albert TA, Lewis NS, Warpeha RL. Late pulmonary complications with use of mafenide acetate. J Burn Care Rehab 1982; 3:375.

65. Ohlgisser M, Adler MN, Ben-Dov B, Taitelman U, Birkhan HJ, Bursztein S. Methemoglobinaemia induced by mafenide acetate in children. A report of two cases. Br J Anaesth 1978; 50:299.

66. Connell JF, Jr., Rousselot LM. Povidone-iodine, extensive surgical evaluation of a new antiseptic. Am J Surg 1964; 108:849.

67. Hunt JL, Sato R, Heck EL, Baxter CR. A critical evaluation of povidone-iodine absorption in thermally injured patients. J Trauma 1980; 20(2):127–9.

68. Labbe G, Mahul P, Morel J, Jospe R, Dumont A, Auboyer C. Iodine intoxication after subcutaneous irrigations of povidone iodine. Ann Fr Anesth Reanim 2003; 22(1):58–60.

69. Shannon MW. Bromine and iodine compounds. In: Haddad LM, Shannon MW, Winchester JF, eds. Clinical Management of Poisoning and Drug Overdose. 3rd ed. Philadelphia, PA: W.B. Saunders, 1998:809–10.

70. Baranowski-Dutkiewicz B. Skin absorption of phenol from aqueous solutions in men. Int Arch Environ Health 1981; 49:99.

71. Cullison D, Abele DC, O'Quinn JL. Localized exogenous ochronosis. Report of a case and review of the literature. J Am Acad Dermatol 1983; 8:882.

72. Johnstone RT. Occupational Medicine and Industrial Hygiene. St. Louis: C.V. Mosby, 1948:216.

73. Cronin TD, Brauer RO. Death due to phenol contained in Foille. J Am Med Assoc 1949; 139:777.

74. Deichmann WB. Local and systemic effects following skin contact with phenol—a review of the literature. J Ind Hyg 1949; 31:146.

75. Von Hinkel GK, Kitzel HW. Phenolvergiftungen bei Neugeborenen durch kutane Resorption. Dtsch Gesundheitwes 1968; 23:240.

76. Del Pizzo A, Tanski EL. Chemical face peeling—malignant therapy for benign disease? Plast Reconstr Surg 1980; 66:121 (editorial).

77. Unlu RE, Alagoz MS, Uysal AC, et al. Phenol intoxication in a child. J Craniofac Surg 2004; 15(6):1010–3.

78. Botta SA, Straith RE, Goodwin HH. Cardiac arrhythmias in phenol face peeling: a suggested protocol for prevention. Aesthetic Plast Surg 1988; 12(2):115–7.

79. Todorovic V. Acute phenol poisoning. Med Pregl 2003; 56(Suppl. 1):37–41.

80. Truppman ES, Ellerby JD. Major electocardiographic changes during chemical face peeling. Plast Reconstr Surg 1979; 63:44.

81. Tromovitch TA. Safety of chemical face peels. J Am Acad Dermatol 1982; 7:137 (letter).

82. Baker TJ. The voice of polite dissent. Plast Reconstr Surg 1979; 63:262.

83. Langford CP, Bartlett R, Haddad LM. Phenol and related agents. In: Haddad LM, Shannon MW, Winchester JF, eds. Clinical Management of Poisoning and Drug Overdose. 3rd ed. Philadelphia, PA: W.B. Saunders, 1998:958–9.
84. Lynch BS, Delzell ES, Bechtel DH. Toxicology review and risk assessment of resorcinol: thyroid effects. Regul Toxicol Pharmacol 2002; 36(2):198–210.
85. Berthezene F, Fournier M, Bernier E, Mornex R. L'Hypothyroidie induite par la resorcine. Lyon Med 1973; 230:319.
86. Thomas AE, Gisburn MA. Exogenous ochronosis and myxoedema from resorcinol. Br J Dermatol 1961; 73:378.
87. Flandin C, Rabeau H, Ukrainczyk M. Intolerance a la resorcine. Test Cutane Soc Dermatol Syph 1953; 12:1804.
88. Murray MC. An analysis of sixty cases of drug poisoning. Arch Pediatr 1926; 43:193.
89. Cunningham AA. Resorcin poisoning. Arch Dis Child 1956; 31:173.
90. Yeung D, Kanto S, Nacht S, Gans EH. Percutaneous absorption, blood levels and urinary excretion of resorcinol applied topically in humans. Int J Dermatol 1983; 22:321.
91. Hoffmann S. Silver sulfadiazine: an antibacterial agent for topical use in burns. A review of the literature. Scand J Plast Reconstr Surg 1984; 18(1):119–26.
92. Wang XW, Wang NZ, Zhang OZ, Zapata-Sirvent RL, Davies JW. Tissue deposition of silver following topical use of silver sulphadiazine in extensive burns. Burns Incl Therm Inj 1985; 11(3):197–201.
93. Maitre S, Jaber K, Perrot JL, Guy C, Cambazard F. Increased serum and urinary levels of silver during treatment with topical silver sulfadiazine. Ann Dermatol Venereol 2002; 129(2):217–9.
94. Owens CJ, Yarbrough DR, Brackett NR. Nephrotic syndrome following topically applied sulfadiazine therapy. Arch Intern Med 1972; 134:332.
95. Chaby G, Viseux V, Poulain JF, De Cagny B, Denoeux JP, Lok C. Topical silver sulfadiazine-induced acute renal failure. Ann Dermatol Venereol 2005; 132(11 Pt 1):891–3.
96. Chan CK, Jarrett F, Moylan JA. Acute leukopenia as an allergic reaction to silver sulfadiazine in burn patients. J Trauma 1976; 16:395.
97. Jarrett F, Ellerbe S, Demling R. Acute leukopenia during topical burn therapy with silver sulfadiazine. Am J Surg 1978; 135:818.
98. Fraser GL, Beaulieu JT. Leukopenia secondary to sulfadiazine silver. J Am Med Assoc 1978; 21:1928.
99. Viala J, Simon L, Le Pommelet C, Philippon L, Devictor D, Huault G. Agranulocytosis after application of silver sulfadiazine in a 2-month old infant. Arch Pediatr 1997; 4(11):1103–6.
100. Wilson P, George R, Raine P. Topical silver sulphadiazine and profound neutropenia in a burned child. Burns Incl Therm Inj 1986; 12(4):295–6.
101. Gamelli RL, Paxton TP, O'Reilly M. Bone marrow toxicity by silver sulfadiazine. Surg Gynecol Obstet 1993; 177(2):115–20.
102. Scharpf LG, Hill ID, Maibach HI. Percutaneous penetration and disposition of tricarban in man. Arch Environ Health 1975; 30:7.
103. Ponte C, Richard J, Bonte C, Lequien P, Lacombe A. Methemoglobinemies chez le nouveau-nie. Discussion du role etiologique du trichlorcarbanilide. Ann Pediatr 1974; 21:359.
104. Hall AH. Arsenic and arsine. In: Haddad LM, Shannon MW, Winchester JF, eds. Clinical Management of Poisoning and Drug Overdose. 3rd ed. Philadelphia, PA: W.B. Saunders, 1998:784.
105. Tchounwou PB, Centeno JA, Patlolla AK. Arsenic toxicity, mutagenesis, and carcinogenesis—a health risk assessment and management approach. Mol Cell Biochem 2004; 255(1–2):47–55.
106. Thomas DJ, Styblo M, Lin S. The cellular metabolism and systemic toxicity of arsenic. Toxicol Appl Pharmacol 2001; 176(2):127–44.
107. Zackheim HS, Feldman RJ, Lindsay E, Maibach HI. Percutaneous absorption of 1,3-bis(2-chloro-ethyl)-1-nitrosurea (cbcnu, carmustine) in mycosis fungoides. Br J Dermatol 1977; 97:65.

108. Skolglund RR, Ware LL, Jr., Schanberger JE. Prolonged seizures due to contact and inhalation exposure to camphor. Clin Pediatr 1977; 16:901.
109. Gossweiler B. kampfervergiftungen heute. Schweiz Rundsch Med Prax 1982; 71:1475.
110. Committee on Drugs. Camphor—who needs it? Pediatrics 1978; 62:404.
111. Siegel E, Wason S. Camphor toxicity. Pediatr Clin North Am 1986; 33(2):375–9.
112. D'acry PF. Fatalities with the use of a henna dye. Pharm Int 1982; 3:217.
113. El-Ansary EH, Ahmed MEK, Clague HW. Systemic toxicity of para-phenylenediamine. Lancet 1983; 1:1341.
114. Cronin E. Immediate-type hypersensitivity to henna. Contact Dermatitis 1980; 5:198.
115. Grybowsky J, Weinstein D, Ordway N. Toxic encephalopathy apparently related to the use of an insect repellent. N Engl J Med 1961; 264:289.
116. Zadicoff C. Toxic encephalopathy associated with use of insect repellant. J Pediatr 1979; 95:140.
117. Kligman AM. Dimethyl sulfoxide—part 2. J Am Med Assoc 1965; 193:151.
118. Bennett CC. Dimethyl sulfoxide. J Am Med Assoc 1980; 244:2768.
119. Degroot AC, Nater JP, Bleumink K, De Long MCJM. Does DNCB therapy potentiate epicutaneous sensitization to non-related contact allergens? Clin Exp Dermatol 1981; 6:139.
120. Feldmann RJ, Maibach HI. Absorption of some organic compounds through the skin in man. J Invest Dermatol 1970; 54:399.
121. Mcdaniel DH, Blatchley DM, Welton WA. Adverse systemic reaction to dinitrochlorobenzene. Arch Dermatol 1982; 118:371 (letter).
122. Gimenez ER, Vallejo NE, Roy E, et al. Percutaneous alcohol intoxication. Clin Toxicol 1968; 1:39.
123. Castot A, Garnier R, Lanfranchi E, et al. Effects systematiques indesirables des medicaments appliqués sur la peau chez l'enfant. Therapie 1980; 35:423.
124. Ellis CN, Mitchell AJ, Beardsley GR, Jr. Tar gel interaction with disulfiram. Arch Dermatol 1979; 115:1367.
125. Stoll D, King LE, Jr. Disulfiram—alcohol skin reaction to beer-containing shampoo. J Am Med Assoc 1980; 244:2045 (letter).
126. Dubiel W, Happle R. Behandlungsversuch mit Fumarsaure mono-athylester bei Psoriasis vulgaris. Z Haut Geschlechtskr 1972; 47:545.
127. Haggerty RJ. Blue baby due to methemoglobinemia. N Engl J Med 1962; 267:13303.
128. Meynadier J, Peyron JL. Resorption transcutanee des medicaments. Rev Pract (Paris) 1982; 32:41.
129. Steinberg JB, Zepernick RGL. Methemoglobinemia during anesthesia. J Pediatr 1962; 61:885.
130. Olson ML, McEvoy GK. Methemoglobinemia induced by local anesthetics. Am J Hosp Pharm 1981; 38:89.
131. American Medical Association. Drug Evaluations. 3rd ed. Littleton, Mass: Publishing Sciences Group, 1977:269.
132. Liebelt EL, Shannon MW. Small doses, big problems: a selected review of highly toxic common medications. Pediatr Emerg Care 1993; 9(5):292–7.
133. Adriani J, Zepernick R. Clinical effectiveness of drugs used for topical anesthesia. J Am Med Assoc 1964; 118:711.
134. Seldon R, Sasahara AA. Central nervous system toxicity induced by lidocaine. J Am Med Assoc 1987; 202:908.
135. Wehner D, Hamilton GC. Seizures following topical application of local anesthetics to burn patients. Ann Emerg Med 1984; 13(6):456–8.
136. Serizawa M, Aihara M, Takei Y, Sata Y, Nakazawa S. Lidocaine induced seizure following topical application of local anesthetics: case report. No To Hattatsu 1999; 31(3):280–1.
137. Brosh-Nissimov T, Ingbir M, Weintal I, Fried M, Porat R. Central nervous system toxicity following topical skin application of lidocaine. Eur J Clin Pharmacol 2004; 60(9):683–4.
138. Giard MJ, Uden DL, Whitelock DJ. Seizures induced by oral viscous lidocaine. Clin Pharm 1983; 2:110.

139. Mofenson HC, Caraccio TR, Miller H, Greensher J. Lidocaine toxicity from topical mucosal application. Clin Pediatr 1983; 22:190.
140. Rincon E, Baker RL, Iglesias AJ, Duarte AM. CNS toxicity after topical application of EMLA cream on a toddler with molluscum contagiosum. Pediatr Emerg Care 2000; 16(4):252–4.
141. Wieringa JW, Ketel AG, Van Houten MA. Coma in a child after treatment with the 'magic salve' lidocaine–prilocaine cream. Ned Tijdschr Geneeskd 2006; 150(33):1805–7.
142. Touma S, Jackson JB. Lidocaine and prilocaine toxicity in a patient receiving treatment for mollusca contagiosa. J Am Acad Dermatol 2001; 44(Suppl. 2):399–400.
143. Sinisterra S, Miravet E, Alfonso I, Soliz A, Papazian O. Methemoglobinemia in an infant receiving nitric oxide after the use of eutectic mixture of local anesthetic. J Pediatr 2002; 141(2):285–6.
144. Couper RT. Methaemoglobinaemia secondary to topical lignocaine/prilocaine in a circumcised neonate. J Paediatr Child Health 2000; 36(4):406–7.
145. Bates BA. Mercury. In: Haddad LM, Shannon MW, Winchester JF, eds. Clinical Management of Poisoning and Drug Overdose. 3rd ed. Philadelphia, PA: W.B. Saunders, 1998:750.
146. Bork K, Morsches B, Holzmann H. Zum Problem der QuecksilberResorption aus weisser Prazipatatsalbe. Arch Dermatol Forsch 1973; 248:37.
147. Young E. Ammoniated mercury poisoning. Br J Dermatol 1960; 72:449.
148. Silverberg DS, Mccall JT, Hung JC. Nephrotic syndrome with use of ammoniated mercury. Arch Intern Med 1967; 120:581.
149. Turk JL, Baker H. Nephrotic syndrome due to ammoniated mercury. Br J Dermatol 1968; 80:623.
150. Lyons TJ, Christer CN, Larsen FS. Ammoniated mercury ointment and the nephritic syndrome. Minn Med 1975; 58:383.
151. Soo YO, Chow KM, Lam CW, et al. A whitened face woman with nephrotic syndrome. Am J Kidney Dis 2003; 41(1):250–3.
152. Tang HL, Chu KH, Mak YF, et al. Minimal change disease following exposure to mercury-containing skin lightening cream. Hong Kong Med J 2006; 12(4):316–8.
153. Dyall-Smith DJ, Scurry JP. Mercury pigmentation and high mercury levels from the use of a cosmetic cream. Med J Aust 1990; 153(7):409–10 (see also 414–415).
154. Mcrill C, Boyer LV, Flood TJ, Ortega L. Mercury toxicity due to use of a cosmetic cream. J Occup Environ Med 2000; 42(1):4–7.
155. Weldon MM, Smolinski MS, Maroufi A, et al. Mercury poisoning associated with a Mexican beauty cream. West J Med 2000; 173(1):15–8 (discussion 19).
156. Tlacuilo-Parra A, Guevara-Gutierrez E, Luna-Encinas JA. Percutaneous mercury poisoning with a beauty cream in Mexico. J Am Acad Dermatol 2001; 45(6):966–7.
157. Stanley-Brown EG, Frank JE. Mercury poisoning from application to omphalocele. J Am Med Assoc 1971; 216:2144 (letter to the editor).
158. Clark JA, Kasselberg AG, Glick AD, O'neill JA, Jr. Mercury poisoning from merbromin (MercurochromeR) therapy of omphalocele. Clin Pediatr 1982; 21:445.
159. Hedges TR, III, Kenyon KR, Hanninen LA, Mosher DB. Corneal and conjunctival effects of monobenzone in patients with vitiligo. Arch Ophthalmol 1983; 101:64.
160. Harkness RA, Beveridge GW. Isolation of b-naphthol from urine after its application to skin. Nature (Lond) 1966; 211:413.
161. Hemels HGWM. Percutaneous absorption and distribution of 2-naphthol in man. Br J Dermatol 1972; 87:614.
162. Osol A, Farrar GE, Jr. The Dispensatory of the United States of America. 24th ed. Philadelphia, PA: Lippincott, 1947.
163. Windholz M, Budavari S, Stroumtsos LY, Fertig MN, eds. The Merck Index: An Encyclopedia of Chemicals and Drugs. 9th ed. Rahway, NJ: Merck, 1976:291.
164. Feldmann RJ, Maibach HI. Percutaneous penetration of some pesticides and herbicides in man. Toxicol Appl Pharmacol 1974; 28:126.
165. Ginsburg CM, Lowry W, Reisch JS. Absorption of lindane (gamma benzene hexachloride) in infants and children. J Pediatr 1977; 91:998.

166. Hosler J, Tschanz C, Higuite C. Topical application of Lindane cream (Kwell) and antipyrine metabolism. J Invest Dermatol 1980; 74:51.

167. Carlton FB, Simpson WM, Jr., Haddad LM. The organophosphates and other insecticides. In: Haddad LM, Shannon MW, Winchester JF, eds. Clinical Management of Poisoning and Drug Overdose. 3rd ed. Philadelphia, PA: W.B. Saunders, 1998:836–45.

168. Lee B, Groth P. Scabies: transcutaneous poisoning during treatment. Pediatrics 1977; 59:643.

169. Telch J, Jarvis DA. Acute intoxication with lindane (gamma benzene hexachloride). Can Med Assoc J 1982; 126:662.

170. Davies JE, Dedhia HV, Morgade C, et al. Lindane poisonings. Arch Dermatol 1983; 119:142.

171. Bhalla M, Thami GP. Reversible neurotoxicity after an overdose of topical lindane in an infant. Pediatr Dermatol 2004; 21(5):597–9.

172. Pramanik AK, Hansen RC. Transcutaneous gamma benzene hexachloride absorption and toxicity in infants and children. Arch Dermatol 1979; 115(10):1224–5.

173. FDA. Gamma benzene hexachloride (Kwell) and other products alert. FDA Drug Bull 1976; 6:28.

174. Matsuoka LY. Convulsions following application of gamma benzene hexachloride. J Am Acad Dermatol 1981; 5:98.

175. Solomon LM, Fahrner L, West DP. Gamma benzene hexachloride toxicity. A review. Arch Dermatol 1977; 113:353.

176. Shacter B. Treatment of scabies and pediculosis with lindane preparations: an evaluation. J Am Acad Dermatol 1981; 5:517.

177. Rasmussen JE. The problem of lindane. J Am Acad Dermatol 1981; 5:507.

178. Kramer MS, Hutchinson TA, Rudnick SA, et al. Operational criteria for adverse drug reactions in evaluating suspected toxicity of a popular scabicide. Clin Pharmacol Ther 1980; 27:149.

179. Jamal GA, Hansen S, Pilkington A, et al. A clinical neurological, neurophysiological, and neuropsychological study of sheep farmers and dippers exposed to organophosphate pesticides. Occup Environ Med 2002; 59(7):434–41.

180. Ramu A, Slonim EA, Egal F. Hyperglycemia in acute malathion poisoning. Israel J Med Sci 1973; 9:631.

181. Milby TH, Epstein WL. Allergic sensitivity to malathion. Arch Environ Health 1964; 9:434.

182. Cassidy DE, Drewry J, Fanning JP. Podophyllum toxicity: a report of a fatal case and a review of the literature. J Toxicol Clin Toxicol 1982; 19:35.

183. Von Krogh G, Longstaff E. Podophyllin office therapy against condyloma should be abandoned. Sex Transm Infect 2001; 77(6):409–12.

184. Slater GE, Rumack BH, Peterson RG. Podophyllin poisoning. Systemic toxicity following cutaneous application. Obstet Gynecol 1978; 52(1):94–6.

185. Tomczak RL, Hake DH. Near fatal systemic toxicity from local injection of podophyllin for pedal verrucae treatment. J Foot Surg 1992; 31(1):36–42.

186. Chamberlain MJ, Reynolds AL, Yeoman WV. Toxic effect of podophyllum application in pregnancy. Br J Med 1972; 3:291.

187. Krenzelok EP, Kerr F, Proudfoot AT. Salicylate toxicity. In: Haddad LM, Shannon MW, Winchester JF, eds. Clinical Management of Poisoning and Drug Overdose. 3rd ed. Philadelphia, PA: W.B. Saunders, 1998:675.

188. Birmingham BK, Greene DS, Rhodes CT. Systemic absorption of topical salicylic acid. Int J Dermatol 1979; 18(3):228–31.

189. Taylor JR, Halprin K. Percutaneous absorption of salicylic acid. Arch Dermatol 1975; 106:740.

190. Von Weiss JF, Lever WF. Percutaneous salicylic acid intoxication in psoriasis. Arch Dermatol 1964; 90:614.

191. U.S. Department of Health, Education and Welfare, Food and Drug Administration, OTC Antimicrobial II Advisory Panel. Cited by Rasmussen, J.E. percutaneous absorption in children. In: Dobson RL, ed. Year Book of Dermatology. Chicago: Year Book Medical, 1979:28.

192. Lindsey CP. Two cases of fatal salicylate poisoning after topical application of an antifungal solution. Med J Aust 1968; 1:353.
193. Wechselsberg K. Salizylsaure-Vergiftung durch perkutane Resorption 1%-iger Salizyl-vaseline. Anasth Prax 1969; 4:103.
194. Treguer GL, Le Bihan G, Coloignier M, Le Roux P, Bernard JP. Intoxication salicylee par application locale de vaseline salicylee a 20% chez un psoriasique. Nouv presse Med 1980; 9:192.
195. Davis JE. Are one or two dangerous? Methyl salicylate exposure in toddlers J Emerg Med 2007; 32(1):63–9.
196. Chan TY. Potential dangers from topical preparations containing methyl salicylate. Hum Exp Toxicol 1996; 15(9):747–50.
197. Joss JD, LeBlond RF. Potentiation of warfarin anticoagulation associated with topical methyl salicylate. Ann Pharmacother 2000; 34(6):729–33.
198. Ransone JW, Scott NM, Knoblock EC. Selenium sulfide intoxication. N Engl J Med 1973; 9:631.
199. Ternberg JL, Luce E. Methemoglobinemia: a complication of the silver nitrate treatment of burns. Surgery 1968; 63:328.
200. Editorial. Burns and silver nitrate. J Am Med Assoc 1965; 193:230.
201. Connely DM. Silver nitrate—Ideal burn wound therapy? NY State J Med 1920; 70:1642.
202. Bader KF. Organ deposition of silver following silver nitrate therapy of burns. Plast Reconstr Surg 1966; 37:550.
203. Marshall JP, Schneider RP. Systemic argyria secondary to topical silver nitrate. Arch Dermatol 1977; 113:1072.
204. Zech P, Colon S, Labeeuw R, Blanc-Brunat N, Richard P, Porol M. Syndrome nephrotique avec depot d'argent dans les membranes glomerulaires au cours d'une argyrie. Nouv presse Med 1973; 2:161.
205. Feldmann RJ, Maibach HI. Penetration of ^{14}C hydrocortisone through normal skin. Arch Dermatol 1965; 91:661.
206. Hengge UR, Ruzicka T, Schwartz RA, Cork MJ. Adverse effects of topical glucocortico-steroids. J Am Acad Dermatol 2006; 54(1):1–15.
207. Nnoruka E, Okoye O. Topical steroid abuse: its use as a depigmenting agent. J Natl Med Assoc 2006; 98(6):934–9.
208. Pascher F. Systemic reactions to topically applied drugs. Int J Dermatol 1978; 17:768.
209. Feiwell M, James VHT, Barnett ES. Effect of potential topical steroids on plasma-cortisol levels of infants and children with eczema. Lancet 1969; 1:485.
210. Burton TT, Cunliffe WJ, Holti G, Wright W. Complications of topical corticosteroid therapy in patients with liver disease. Br J Dermatol 1974; 9(Suppl. 10):22.
211. May P, Stern EJ, Ryter RJ, Hirsch FS, Michel B, Levy RP. Cushing syndrome from percutaneous absorption of triamcinolone cream. Arch Intern Med 1976; 136:612.
212. Van Der Harst LCA, Smeenk G, Burger PM, Van Der Rhee JH, Polano MK. Waardebe-paling en risicoschatting van de uitwendige behandeling met clobetasol-17-propionaat (Dermovate). Ned Tijdschr Geneeskd 1978; 122:219.
213. Beas F, Vargas L, Spada RP, Merchak N. Pseudoprecocious puberty in infants caused by a dermal ointment containing estrogens. J Pediatr 1969; 75:127.
214. Bertaggia A. A case of precocious puberty in a girl following the use of an estrogen preparation on the skin. Pediatria (Napoli) 1968; 76:579.
215. Landolt R, Murset G. Vorzeitige Pubertatsmerkmale als Folge unbeabsichtigter Ostrogenverabreichung. Schweiz Med Wochenschr 1968; 98:638.
216. Ramos AS, Bower BF. Pseudosexual precocity due to cosmetics ingestion. J Am Med Assoc 1969; 207:369.
217. Stoppelman MRH, Van Valkenburg RA. Pigmentaties en gynecomastie ten gevolge van het gebruik van stilboestrol bevattend haarewater bij kinderen. Ned Tijdschr Geneeskd 1955; 99:3925.
218. Edidin EV, Levitsky LL. Prepubertal gynecomastia associated with estrogen-containing hair cream. Am J Dis Child 1982; 136:587.
219. Diraimondo CV, Roach AC, Meador CK. Gynecomastia from exposure to vaginal estrogen cream. N Engl J Med 1980; 302:1089 (letter).

220. Gabrilove JL, Luria M. Persistent gynecomastia resulting from scalp injunction of estradiol: a model for persistent gynecomastia. Arch Dermatol 1978; 114:1672.
221. Bazex A, Salvader R, Dupre A, Christol B. Gynecomastie et hyperpigmentation areolaire après oestrogenotherapie locale antiseborrheque. Bull Soc Fr Dermatol Syphiligr 1967; 74:466.
222. Goebel M. Mamillenhypertorphie mit Pigmentierung nach lokaler Oestrogentherapie im Kindesalter. Hautarzt 1969; 20:521.
223. Goluboff N, MacFadyen DJ. Methemoglobinemia in an infant. J Pediatr 1955; 47:222.
224. Gay MW, Moore WJ, Morgan JM, Montes LF. Anthralin toxicity. Arch Dermatol 1972; 105:213.
225. Farber EM, Harris DR. Hospital treatment of psoriasis. Arch Dermatol 1970; 101:381.
226. Johnson MR, Hageboutros A, Wang K, High L, Smith JB, Diasio RB. Life-threatening toxicity in a dihydropyrimidine dehydrogenase-deficient patient after treatment with topical 5-fluorouracil. Clin Cancer Res 1999; 5(8):2006–11.
227. Ranchoff RE, Bergfeld WF. Topical minoxidil reduces blood pressure. J Am Acad Dermatol 1985; 12:586–7.
228. Leenen FH, Smith DL, Unger WP. Topical minoxidil: cardiac effects in bald man. Br J Clin Pharmacol 1988; 26:481–5.
229. Satoh H, Morikaw S, Fujiwara C, Terada H, Uehara A, Ohno R. A case of acute myocardial infarction associated with topical use of minoxidil (RiUP) for treatment of baldness. Jpn Heart J 2000; 41:519–23.
230. Smorlesi C, Caldarella A, Caramelli L, Di Lollo S, Moroni F. Topically applied minoxidil may cause fetal malformation: a case report. Birth Defects Res A Clin Mol Teratol 2003; 67(12):997–1001.
231. Georgala S, Befon A, Maniatopoulou E, Georgala C. Topical use of minoxidil in children and systemic side effects. Dermatology 2007; 214(1):101–2.
232. Sato K. Drug-induced hypercalcemia. Clin Calcium 2006; 6(1):67–72.
233. Kawaguchi M, Mitsuhashi Y, Kondo S. Iatrogenic hypercalcemia due to vitamin D3 ointment (1,24(OH)$_2$D$_3$) combined with thiazide diuretics in a case of psoriasis. J Dermatol 2003; 30(11):801–4.
234. Knackstedt C, Winograd R, Koch A, Abuzahra F, Trautwein C, Wasmuth HE. Acute necrotic pancreatitis induced by severe hypercalcaemia due to tacalcitol ointment. Br J Dermatol 2007; 56(3):576–7.
235. Rogers DR. Accidental fatal monochloroacetic acid poisoning. Am J Forensic Med Pathol 1995; 16:115–6.
236. Kulling P, Anderson H, Bostrom K, et al. Fatal systemic poisoning after skin exposure to monochloroacetic acid. Clin Toxicol 1992; 30:643–52.
237. Kato J, Dote T, Shimizu H, Shimbo Y, Fujihara M, Kono K. Lethal acute lung injury and hypoglycemia after subcutaneous administration of monochloroacetic acid. Toxicol Ind Health 2006; 22(5):203–9.
238. Pirson J, Toussaint P, Segers N. An unusual cause of burn injury: skin exposure to monochloroacetic acid. J Burn Care Rehabil 2003; 24(6):407–9 (discussion 402).
239. Toshina Y, Dote T, Usuda K, et al. Hepatic injury and glucogenesis after subcutaneous injection of monochloroacetic acid in rats. Environ Health Prev Med 2004; 9:58–62.
240. Naranjo CA, Busto U, Sellers EM, et al. A method for estimating the probability of adverse drug reactions. Clin Pharmacol Ther 1981; 30(2):239–45.

Solvent and Vehicle Effects on the Skin

Michael S. Roberts and Audrey Gierden
Department of Medicine, Princess Alexandra Hospital, University of Queensland, Woolloongabba, Queensland, Australia

Jim E. Riviere and Nancy A. Monteiro-Riviere
Center for Chemical Toxicology Research and Pharmacokinetics, College of Veterinary Medicine, North Carolina State University, Raleigh, North Carolina, U.S.A.

INTRODUCTION

The effects of solvents and vehicles on the skin are important since skin is the largest organ of the human body and provides protection against the external environment. In addition, the skin enables us to maintain a state of homeostasis. However, skin and its barrier properties may be altered when exposed to various chemical agents. Exposure to solvents and vehicles can occur after occupational or accidental spillage, topical application of cosmetics, sunscreens, insect repellents, as well as following the topical application of drugs for therapeutic purposes.

This chapter provides an update on our earlier work (1). As discussed earlier in this book, the outermost layer of the skin, the stratum corneum (SC), is the main skin barrier and is composed of keratinized dead epidermal cells that are thin, less than 1 μm, and 30 to 40 μm in diameter. Figure 1 shows a transmission electron microscopy (TEM) image of the SC (1). The lipid bilayers between the cells can be easily visualized by after fixing in Trump's fixative and postfixing in phosphate-buffered ruthenium tetroxide prior to being processed for TEM. Desmosomes are evident in lipid bilayers, especially in areas associated with friction in the environment. Disintegration of the desmosomes, most evident in the outermost SC, is frequently associated with the creation of lacunae (1). Desmosomes usually span the entire width of the intercellular space but, with jet fuel JP-8+100 treatment, desmosomes are degraded and separated from the central core leaving a space (lacunae) between the desmosomes (2), similar to what was found for hydrocarbon solvents in our earlier work (1). The lacunae are probably also due to the extracted lipid lamellae (1). The main lipids in the SC are ceramides, cholesterol, and free fatty acids (3).

MECHANISMS BY WHICH SOLVENTS AFFECT SKIN PERMEABILITY

Figure 2 shows that solvents can cause a range of structural alterations when applied on the skin. In general, either the lipid bilayer or the SC proteins are affected. Solvents can selectively extract skin lipids from intercellular lamellae, corneocytes, or even the follicles, as illustrated in Figure 3A for cyclohexane. *n*-Octanol, laurocapram, isopropyl myristate, and oleic acid are able to extract ceramides; this would generate a dilatation between adherent cornified cells thus enhancing the intercellular penetration pathway. Figure 3B shows such an effect occurring after extraction by a cyclohexane:ethanol (4:1) solvent. Polar enhancers such as *N*-methyl-2-pyrrolidone (NMP) and dimethylsulfoxide (DMSO) partly

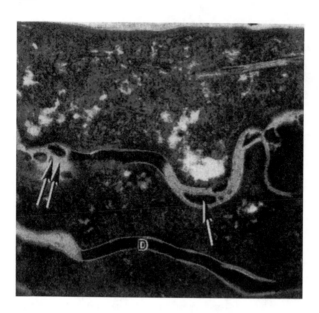

FIGURE 1 A cross section of human stratum corneum showing corneocytes packed with keratin and intercellular lipid regions containing lipid bilayers and desmosomes (D), as well as degenerating desmosomes (*arrow*) that lead to the formation of lacunae (*double arrow*) ruthenium tetroxide postfixation (×48,750). *Source*: From Ref. 1.

extract sphingolipids (4). Some water-soluble solvents affect the intercellular lipid layers at or near the polar head group, disturbing the hydration spheres. Others act mainly between the hydrophobic tails of the lipids, causing their organization to be disturbed and increasing their fluidity (5). Some solvents also interact with the proteins, leading to a conversion of keratin from α-helix to β-sheet, often accompanied by the uncoiling of the filaments. Hygroscopic enhancers affect the integrity of desmosomes and other proteic junctions that maintain the SC cohesion, leading to fissuring and splitting of the corneocytes or squamous cells. In summary, it is most likely that solvent will interact with the SC components with multiple mechanisms.

The penetration of a solvent through the skin and its effects also depend on its characteristics such as its molecular weight (MW), lipophilicity, concentration, and viscosity.

Methyl groups are often associated with the greatest enhanced permeability of solvents. For example, solvents resulting in the highest permeability enhancements include: DMSO, NMP, dimethylformamide, and dimethylacetamide. Each has one or more methyl groups directly linked to heteroatom (S or N) (6). The extent of solvent effects depends on the duration and area of solvent contact, the body site, and whether the site is occluded.

MECHANISM OF INDIVIDUAL SOLVENTS/PERMEATION ENHANCERS/VEHICLES
Water

The effects of water on the skin are discussed by Roberts and Bouwstra in Chapter 7 of the companion volume (7). In brief, the effects of water occur mainly within the corneocytes due, in part, to its interaction with complex mixture of water soluble and compounds with a high affinity for water (called natural moisturizing factor) therein. While the lipid lamellae are relatively unaffected by skin hydration level, lacunae from desmosome degradation are filled with water in over-hydrated situations (8).

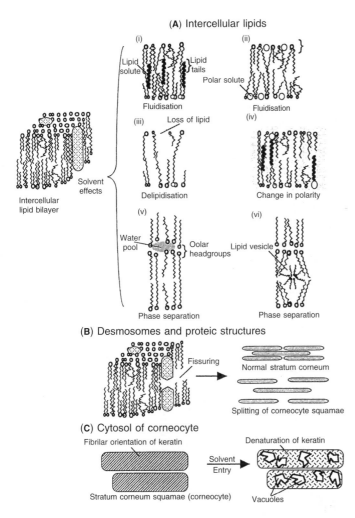

FIGURE 2 Sites of Solvent action in the stratum corneum. (**A**) In the intercellular lipid layer, the processes involving the intercellular lipids include: (i) interaction of lipid solutes (lipophilic enhancers) with intercellular or corneocyte envelope lipids, resulting in increasing the fluidity of the lipid tails; and/or (ii) interaction of polar solutes (polar enhancers) with the polar head groups of the intercellular or corneocyte envelope lipids, increasing their fluidity; (iii) solvent extraction of lipid components; and/or (iv) solvents changing the polarity of the intercellular and/or corneocyte envelope lipids; (v) formation of water pools in the polar head group region; and (vi) forming of lipid vesicles in the lipid tail region. (**B**) Damage to the desmosomes and protein-like bridges may lead to a fissuring of the intercellular lipid layer and splitting of the corneocyte squamae. (**C**) Entry into the corneocyte may be associated with disruption of keratin and vacuolization. *Source*: Adapted from Ref. 1.

Alcohols and Glycols

The alcohols and glycols are semipolar solvents which can have a range of effects on the skin. Ethanol can extract lipids from the SC and may displace bound water molecules at the lipid head group–membrane interface region thus promoting interdigitation of the hydrocarbon chains (4). It can also improve solute partitioning

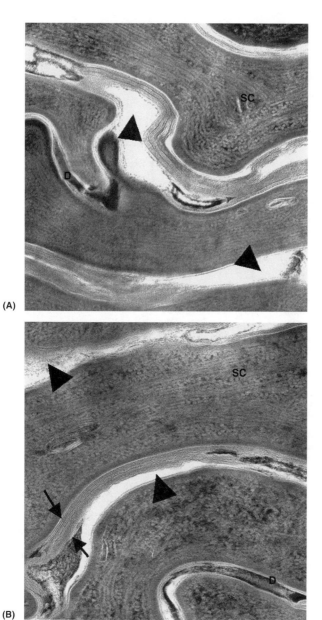

FIGURE 3 Transmission electron micrographs of SC showing: (**A**) areas (*arrowhead*) devoid of intercellular lipid between the SC layers due to extraction with cyclohexane; and (**B**) the intercellular space with compact lipid lamellae (*arrows*) and desmosome attachment (D). Large spaces (*arrowhead*) representative of devoid lipid lamellae caused by cyclohexane and ethanol (4:1) extraction (×140,300). *Abbreviations*: D, desmosomes; SC, stratum corneum. *Source*: From Ref. 14.

in the SC through its action in changing its solubility properties of the SC (9). In general, the enhancing abilities of alcohols depend on the number of carbon atoms in the chain (10). Propylene glycol competes with water for the Hbond binding sites thus solvating keratin and it intercalates itself in the polar head groups of the lipid bilayers (10). Glycerol is a humectant and, accordingly, glycerol-containing moist-urizers produce long-lasting moisturization by binding and holding water. Glycerol can prevent humidity-induced crystal phase transitions in SC lipids. In addition, it can facilitate desquamation by promoting the proteolytic degradation of the corneodesmosomes and induce the maturation of corneocytes.

Acetone
Acetone disrupts the organization of the lipid bilayer by selectively removing lipids from intercellular lipid domains (11). Acetone mainly removes nonpolar lipids such as sterol esters, free fatty acids, triglycerides, and alkenes and to a lesser extent polar sphingolipids and free sterols (12). The alterations in the intracellular domain caused by acetone are not uniform. Figure 4 shows that both acetone and ethanol leads to lipid extraction from the SC.

Dimethylsulfoxide
DMSO is a powerful aprotic solvent that creates solvent-filled spaces when applied onto skin and, in concentrations above 60%, disturbs the lipid bilayer organization (10). DMSO also denatures protein and, when applied on human skin, leads to the intercellular keratin conformation changing from α-helix to β-sheet. DMSO further interacts with the intercellular lipids in the SC, distorting the packing geometry—probably by interaction with the head groups of bilayer lipids. After treatment with DMSO, highly enlarged intercellular space and expanded lacunae can be observed, with the desmosomes also appearing to be swollen (1).

Pyrrolidones
NMP and 2-pyrrolidone (2P) are the most widely used enhancers of this group. Pyrrolidones can enhance penetration of both lipophilic and hydrophilic drugs (10). As pyrrolidones can cause adverse reactions, their clinical usefulness is limited (10).

Urea and Derivatives
Urea is a natural moisturizing agent, which is present in the skin and, when applied in formulations, can swell the desmosomes in the SC layers and promote desquamation (10).

Terpenes
Terpenes are highly lipophilic, aliphatic compounds found in essential oils that are on the FDA's generally regarded as safe (GRAS) list. They disrupt the SC lipid organization (10).

Fatty Acids
The penetration-enhancing effect of fatty acids also depends on their nature, unsaturated fatty acids being more efficient enhancers than saturated ones and additional double bonds increasing enhancing efficiency further by causing kinks in

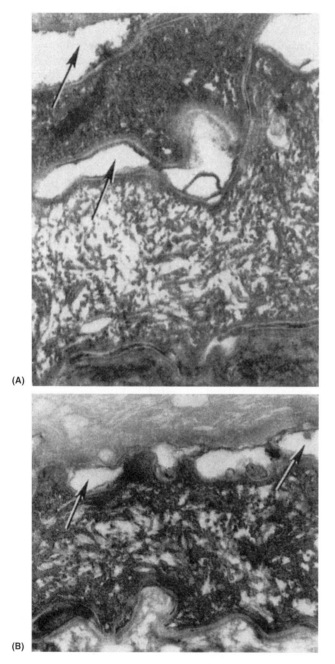

FIGURE 4 (**A**) Transmission electron micrograph of human stratum corneum after exposure to acetone showing lipid extraction in the upper layers of stratum corneum (*arrows*) but with the intercellular lamellar being largely intact in the lower layers (×32,000). (**B**) Transmission electron micrograph of human stratum corneum after exposure to ethanol showing a similar lipid extraction effect (*arrows*) as seen for acetone (×32,000).

the intercellular lipid tail structure (10). For saturated fatty acids, a 10- or 12-carbon alkyl chain linked to a polar group is an optimal enhancer whereas, for unsaturated alkyl chains, an 18-carbon chain length is preferred. A bent *cis* configuration also has a higher likelihood of disturb the bilayer lipids organization (10). A synergistic mechanism has been observed between oleic acid and benzyl alcohol, the polar penetration route was increased probably by interaction with polar and nonpolar SC lipids (10).

Hydrocarbons

Hydrocarbons are usually classified as being either low or high in MW. High-MW hydrocarbons (e.g., petroleum jelly) are occlusive. Naturally anhydrous, petroleum jelly moisturizers can reduce water loss by more than 98%, when compared with many other oils which lead to 20% to 30% reduction. Petroleum jelly also can diffuse into the intercellular lipid domain (13).

Exposure to hydrocarbons can markedly disrupt the SC (1). As discussed earlier, Figure 3A shows that focal areas of lipid lamellae detachment occurs after exposure to cyclohexane whereas Figure 3B shows that focal areas lacking lipid are evident within the intercellular spaces of the SC following the application of a mixture of cyclohexane and ethanol in a 4:1 ratio. Focal areas lacking the normal compact lipid lamellae within the intercellular lipid bilayers of the SC were noted. Many other methods were used to extract lipids from the abdominal, inguinal, and back regions of the pig. In general, the mean total lipid concentration depended on the extraction solvents and body region, and was reproducible across different sites. This study had demonstrated that extraction of lipids increased the transepidermal water loss similar to repeated tape stripping. In addition, it suggested strategies that could alter the lipid composition that could increase the absorption of topical compounds for enhanced drug delivery (14).

JP-8 jet fuel is mostly composed of aliphatic and aromatic hydrocarbons. Topical application of hydrocarbons were applied to in vivo pigs after one day and after repeated exposures for four days and then removed on the fifth day. Figure 5B,C shows both light and electron micrographs of skin from the back of the pig after repetitive treatments with different jet fuels, Jet A, JP-8, and JP-8 + 100. After four days of repeated application a disorganized stratum granulosum (SG)–SC interface with loosely packed filaments, numerous lacunae, and remnants of keratohyalin granules can be observed, relative to control (Fig. 5A). Repetitive treatments with jet fuels by electron microscopy showed focal areas of vacuoles devoid of lipid within the intercellular space of the SG layers. All jet fuels, especially JP-8 + 100, showed cleft formations within the intercellular lipid lamellar bilayers (Fig. 5C) (2).

Ultrastructural studies of ruthenium tetroxide staining of the lipid bilayers between the SC layers after one day of exposure to aliphatic and aromatic hydrocarbons revealed large lacunae resulting from lipid extraction in the SC intercellular lipid layers after exposure to fabric soaked in JP-8 (Fig. 6B), fabric soaked in *o*-xylene (Fig. 6C), and fabric soaked in tetradecane (Fig. 6D), relative to control (Fig. 6A) (15).

Ultrastructural observations after treatment of skin with both aromatic and aliphatic hydrocarbons for four days and evaluated on the fifth day caused similar damages to the SC lipid bilayers, but the intensity of damaged was enhanced with prolonged exposure to the aromatic and aliphatic hydrocarbons (Fig. 7B,C,D) compared to control (Fig. 7A) (15).

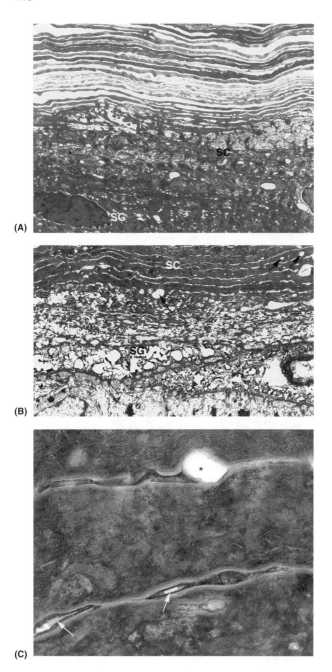

FIGURE 5 Effect of jet fuels on pig skin histology. (**A**) Normal skin, showing SC and SG with normal electron-dense keratohyalin granules and tightly packed filaments ($\times$9600) and (**B**) repeated application over four days showing the loosely packed filaments in the SG ($\times$7500). (**C**) Transmission electron microscopy of the SC layers following repeated application over four days ($\times$117,000). White arrows and astrick depict vacuoles devoid of lipid. White arrow depicts desmosome separation from the central core. *Abbreviations*: D, desmosomes; SC, stratum corneum; SG, stratum granulosum. *Source*: From Ref. 2.

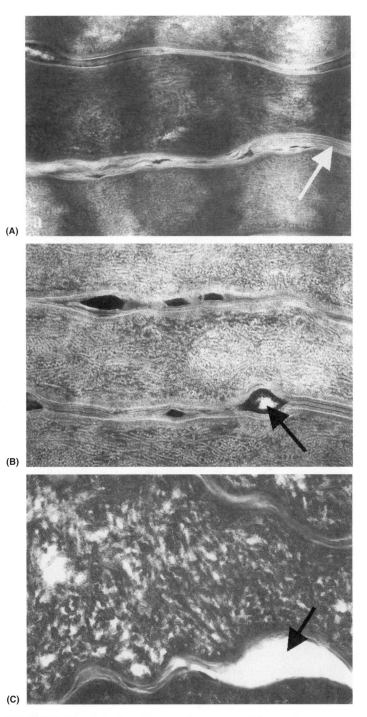

FIGURE 6 Transmission electron micrographs of the stratum corneum cell layers following one-day exposure to (**A**) control fabric, (**B**) fabric soaked in JP-8, (**C**) fabric soaked in *o*-xylene. *Source*: From Ref. 15. (*Continued*)

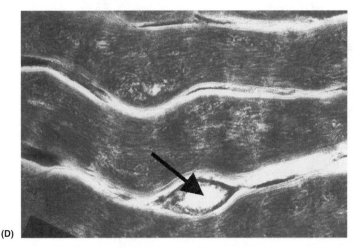

(D)

FIGURE 6 (*Continued*) (**D**) fabric soaked in tetradecane. Note the intact lipid bilayers (*white arrow*) and expanded intercellular spaces (*black arrows*) where the intercellular lipid lamellae appeared extracted (×70,000, ruthenium tetroxide staining). *Source*: From Ref. 15.

Cutting Fluids

Cutting fluids are either oil–water mixtures or strictly synthetic aqueous formulations, they are used in the metal machine industry when cutting metal in order to lubricate and reduce heat generation. Aqueous cutting fluids usually include a surfactant (e.g., linear alkylbenzene sulfonate), a biocide (e.g., triazine, TRI), a fatty acid performance lubricant (e.g., sulfurized ricinoleic acid), and a corrosive inhibitor (e.g., triethanolamine, TEA). In order to simulate both types of cutting fluids, the compounds were formulated in either mineral oil or polyethylene glycol 200 to mimic this exposure. They are usually alkaline and soap like, thereby can denature keratin and extract lipids and water from the skin (16). Figure 8A and B depicts dermal inflammation, intracellular epidermal edema, and epidermal infiltrates observed after treatment with lubrication oils. Dermal edema and dermal inflammation were pronounced with TEA and TRI.

QUANTITATING SOLVENT INTERACTIONS WITH THE SKIN

Quantitative structure permeability relationships are often used to describe chemical absorption across membranes including the skin (17–19). The form of these equations, based on linear solvation or free energy relationships (LSER, LFER), involves defining a multiple regression equation linking the parameter of interest, say membrane permeability (K_p) to a number of molecular descriptors ($A,B,C...$) (e.g., hydrogen bonding, molecular size, solubility, polarizability, etc.) via strength coefficients ($a,b,c...$) that relate the parameter of interest to the solute molecular properties. The general form of such equations is thus

$$K_p = \text{Intercept} + aA + bB + cC...$$

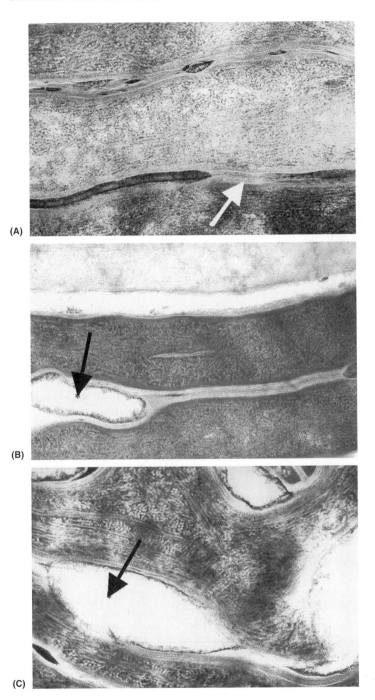

FIGURE 7 Transmission electron micrographs after ruthenium tetroxide staining of the lipid bilayers between the stratum corneum cell layers following four-day of exposures to (**A**) control fabric, (**B**) fabric soaked in JP-8, (**C**) fabric soaked in *o*-xylene. *Source*: From Ref. 15. (*Continued*)

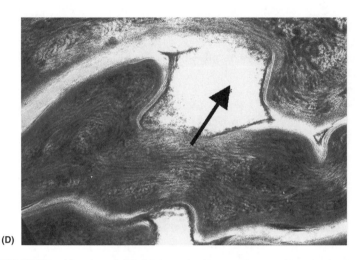

(D)

FIGURE 7 (*Continued*) (**D**) fabric soaked in tetradecane. Note the intact lipid bilayers (*white arrow*) in control, and expanded intercellular spaces (*black arrow*) in treated samples where the intercellular lipid lamellae were extracted (×70,000). *Source*: From Ref. 15.

The data used to define such relationships are obtained from chemical exposure in water. These types of relationships have found wide applicability in many fields. However, under normal exposure conditions say for skin, as discussed earlier exposure to chemicals most often occurs in solvents or other complex mixtures which may modulate the intermolecular interactions seen between solute–solvent–membrane (skin) that define the LSER equation. This has prohibited use of equations defined in aqueous systems to be used to predict chemical absorption from other solvents or vehicles. In many cases, solvent effects on penetrant penetration can be correlated to specific physical–chemical properties of the solvent (19).

An approach to compensate for these solvent–solute–membrane interactions is to add another term to the basic LSER model that takes into account the physical–chemical nature of these interactions (20,22). This could be incorporated as a mixture factor (MF) as

$$K_p = \text{Intercept} + m\text{MF} + aA + bB + cC...$$

where the MF is a physical–chemical property of the vehicle (e.g., hydrogen bonding, Henry's constant, ovality) calculated based on the weight percentages of the vehicle components. The parameter selected is that which significantly improves the predictability (R^2, Q^2) of the base equation over that without a MF, determined by correlating the vehicle component weighted MF to the residual plot of the original equation (Fig. 9). This approach has worked for different forms of LFER across two skin model systems (diffusion cells, isolated perfused skin flap). In addition to this approach illustrating the impact the vehicle effect has on chemical dermal absorption, it also provides a method to quantitate this effect using available chemical properties of specific solute and solvent combinations.

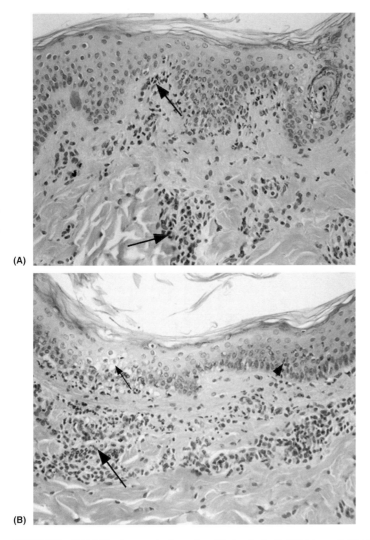

FIGURE 8 (A) Light micrograph of porcine skin treated with 5% linear alkyl benzene sulfonate, 5% triethanolamine, and 2% triazine for eight hours depicting dermal inflammation (*arrows*). (B) depicts intracellular epidermal edema (*small arrow*), epidermal infiltrates (*arrow head*), and dermal inflammation (*large arrow*). (Hematoxylin and eosin, ×175.)

CONCLUSION

Most solvents affect the SC, but to what extent depend on their ability to enter the skin and interact with lipid and protein components in both the intercellular and the cellular regions. But the nature of the interactions between the solvents and the epidermal components are numerous. In addition, solvents can be chemically transformed by enzymes present in the skin, resulting in either detoxification or in generation of toxic derivatives of what was previously an inert compound (23).

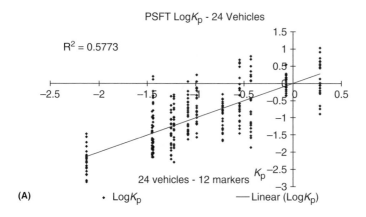

(A)

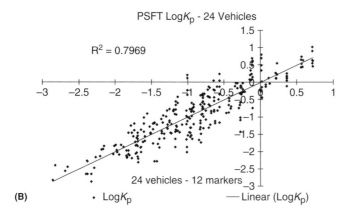

(B)

FIGURE 9 Illustration of the effect of a mixture factor on improving quantitative structure permeability relationship prediction of chemical dermal absorption of 12 compounds in 24 vehicles in porcine skin flow-through diffusion cells. (**A**) No mixture factor and (**B**) mixture factor equal to 1/(vapor pressure) of weighted vehicle components. *Abbreviation*: PSFT, porcine skin flow-through.

ACKNOWLEDGMENTS

MR thanks the National Health and Medical Research Council of Australia (NHMRC) for their support. JR and NAMR acknowledge support from the U.S. Air Force Office of Scientific Research (AFOSR) and the National Institutes of Occupational Safety and Health (NIOSH).

REFERENCES

1. Menon GK, Lee SH, Roberts MS. Ultrastructural effects of some solvents and vehicles on the stratum corneum and other skin components: evidence for an extended mosaic-partitioning model of the skin barrier. In: Roberts MS, Walters KA, eds. Dermal Absorption and Toxicity Assessment. Vol. 91. New York: Blackwell Publishing, 1998:727–51.

2. Monteiro-Riviere NA, Inman AO, Riviere JE. Skin toxicity of jet fuels: ultrastructural studies and the effects of substance P. Toxicol Appl Pharmacol 2004; 195:339–47.
3. Bouwstra JA, Honeywell-Nguyen PL, Gooris GS, Ponec M. Structure of the skin barrier and its modulation by vesicular formulations. Prog Lipid Res 2003; 42:1–36.
4. Ogiso T, Paku T, Iwaki M, Tanino T. Percutaneous penetration of fluorescein isothiocyanate-dextrans and the mechanism for enhancement effect of enhancers on the intercellular penetration. Biol Pharm Bull 1995; 18:1566–71.
5. Suhonen TM, Bouwstra JA, Urtti A. Chemical enhancement of percutaneous absorption in relation to stratum corneum structural alterations. J Control Release 1999; 59:149–61.
6. Estrada E, Uriarte E, Gutierrez Y, Gonzalez H. Quantitative structure–toxicity relationships using TOPS-MODE. 3. Structural factors influencing the permeability of commercial solvents through living human skin. SAR QSAR Environ Res 2003; 14:145–63.
7. Roberts MS, Bouwstra JA. Skin hydration—a key determinant in topical absorption. In: Walters KA, Roberts MS, eds. Chapter 7 in Dermatological and Cosmeceutical Development. Marcel Dekker.
8. Bouwstra JA, de Graaff A, Gooris GS, Nijsse J, Wiechers JW, van Aelst AC. Water distribution and related morphology in human stratum corneum at different hydration levels. J Invest Dermatol 2003; 120:750–8.
9. Williams AC, Barry BW. Penetration enhancers. Adv Drug Deliv Rev 2004; 56:603–18.
10. Trommer H, Neubert RHH. Overcoming the stratum corneum: the modulation of skin penetration—a review. Skin Pharmacol Physiol 2006; 19:106–21.
11. Tsai JC, Sheu HM, Hung PL, Cheng CL. Effect of barrier disruption by acetone treatment on the permeability of compounds with various lipophilicities: implications for the permeability of compromised skin. J Pharm Sci 2001; 90:1242–54.
12. Sznitowska M, Janicki S, Williams AC. Intracellular or intercellular localization of the polar pathway of penetration across stratum corneum. J Pharm Sci 1998; 87:1109–14.
13. Ghadially R, Halkiersorenson L, Elias PM. Effects of petrolatum on stratum corneum structure and function. J Am Acad Dermatol 1992; 26:387–96.
14. Monteiro-Riviere NA, Inman AO, Mak V, Wertz P, Riviere JE. Effect of selective lipid extraction from different body regions on epidermal barrier function. Pharm Res 2001; 18:992–8.
15. Muhammad F, Monteiro-Riviere NA, Riviere JE. Comparative in vivo toxicity of topical JP-8 jet fuel and its individual hydrocarbon components: identification of tridecane and tetradecane as key constituents responsible for dermal irritation. Toxicol Pathol 2005; 33:258–66.
16. Monteiro-Riviere NA, Inman AO, Barlow BM, Baynes RE. Dermatotoxicity of cutting fluid mixtures: in vitro and in vivo studies. Cutan Ocul Toxicol 2006; 25:235–47.
17. Abraham MH, Chadha HS, Martins F, Mitchell RC, Bradbury MW, Gratton JA. A review of the correlation and prediction of transport properties by an LFER method: physiochemical properties, brain penetration and skin permeability. Pesticide Sci 1999; 55:78–88.
18. Moss GP, Dearden JC, Patel H, Cronin MTD. Quantitative structure-permeability relationships (QSPRs) for percutaneous absorption. Toxicol In Vitro 2002; 16:299–317.
19. Potts RO, Guy RH. Predicting skin permeability. Pharm Res 1992; 9:663–9.
20. van der Merwe D, Riviere JE. Cluster analysis of the dermal penetration and stratum corneum/solvent partitioning of ten chemicals in twenty-four chemical mixtures in porcine skin. Skin Pharmacol Physiol 2006; 19:198–206.
21. Riviere JE, Brooks JD. Predicting skin permeability from complex chemical mixtures. Toxicol Appl Pharmacol 2005; 208:99–110.
22. Riviere JE, Brooks JD. Prediction of dermal absorption from complex chemical mixtures: incorporation of vehicle effects and interactions into a QSPR framework. SAR QSAR Environ Res 2007; 18:31–44.
23. Rowse DH, Emmett EA. Solvents and the skin. Clin Occup Environ Med 2004; 4:657–730.

25 United States Environmental Protection Agency Perspectives on Skin Absorption and Exposure

Michael Dellarco
U.S. Environmental Protection Agency, National Center for Environmental Assessment, Washington, D.C., U.S.A.

DERMAL EXPOSURE

The U.S. Environmental Protection Agency (EPA) defines exposure as the contact of a contaminant with the outer boundary of the body (skin and openings such as mouth and nostrils) (1). Humans are exposed dermally to environmental contaminants in water, soil, and air, or as pure chemicals or chemical mixtures in consumer products or in occupational settings. Because the Agency utilizes exposure information to estimate local and systemic risks associated with chemical contact, the focus of dermal exposure includes absorption of a chemical through the skin and its distribution to one or more target organs where it may exert a toxic action (Fig. 1). The anatomical site of contact is directly related to the activity being performed at the time of exposure. Depending on the media and anatomical site where contact occurs, the same contaminants can be absorbed very differently. Several factors can influence the extent of dermal exposure. These include:

- Reduction or increases in the chemical contact with skin due to normal clothing;
- Protective clothing and gloves worn by workers and the amount of protection they offer;
- Individual differences in dermal exposure due to differing degrees of speed, care, and dexterity in performing work;
- Variance in the amount of material available for dermal absorption due to actions such as wiping the affected area with the hand; and
- The physical state of the chemical contaminant: solid, liquid, or vapor.

Several individual factors may influence dermal penetration such as variance of skin penetrability in different parts of the body and variability of skin penetrability due to the age and skin condition of an individual. In some cases skin temperature, which can affect the blood flow rate, hydration of the skin, and the effects of soaps and surfactants can influence dermal penetration of chemical compounds (2–4). The amount of chemical that absorbs into skin may be altered significantly by epidermal metabolism. Studies have shown that the activity of hydrolytic, oxidative, reductive, and conjugative enzymes in the epidermis can be 80–90% of those in the liver and many of these enzymes are inducible (5). However, these factors generally are not considered in dermal absorption models for environmental exposures. Desquamation, the epidermal turnover rate due to the flaking off of outer surface flakes and the generation of new cells at the base of the epidermis can affect dermal absorption for

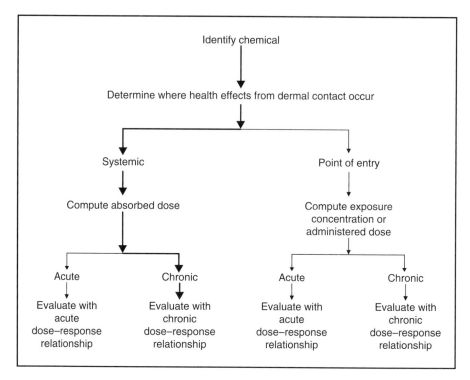

FIGURE 1 Dermal risk assessment process. Bolded arrows show relationship to U.S. Environmental Protection Agency risk assessments.

some chemcials. Reddy et al. (6) developed theoretical calculations that indicate that for highly lipophilic (log $K_{o/w}$ > about 4) or high molecular weight chemicals (> about 350 Da), the epidermal turnover can significantly reduce absorption into the systemic circulation. Washing may not always remove chemical from skin, particularly for lipophilic chemicals. In a study conducted by Fenske et al. (7), results indicated incomplete removal of the pesticide Captan from hands of human volunteers after handwashing. The volunteers washed their hands twice after exposure to Captan and analysis of the contaminant remaining on the skin was analyzed immediately after washing or at one hour after washing. Volunteers whose hands were washed immediately after exposure had a Captan removal efficiency of 77.8% and those that washed one hour later showed a removal efficiency of 68.4%. Zendzian (8) has demonstrated that washing the chemical application site in rats with a solvent at the end of the exposure period can actually increase dermal absorption of the chemical. Similarly, Kligner et al. (3) showed that dermal absorption could be enhanced for certain industrial chemicals when workers washed with soap and water.

The amount of chemical coverage on the skin surface can influence the amount of dermal absorption. The transfer efficiency from a contaminated surface to the skin or liquid solution may be highly variable due to the nature and extent of the contact or the deposition of chemical residue due to solubility or evaporation of the liquid (9,10). Chemical coverage of the skin in a solid, such as in sediment, soil, or in a powder, may be incomplete or exceed the exposed skin surface area by piling up on itself (11). Reddy and Bunge (12) have calculated dermal penetration from skin that is partly and completely covered with a chemical. Results of their calculations indicate that increasing the area fraction covered increased dermal absorption proportionally if the chemical was distributed in a few large piles, but did not produce a proportional increase in the amount absorbed if the chemical was distributed on the surface in many small piles. These calculations were consistent with some experimental observations. Reddy and Bunge (12) examined the effect of applied dose on dermal absorption of pesticides measured in rats in vivo. Results for four liquids showed that dermal absorption increased as the applied dose increased for pesticides in a liquid form. In contrast, dermal absorption of eight pesticides that were solids at skin temperature did not increase proportionally with applied dose, and in some cases was independent of applied dose.

Passive diffusion is considered to be the main processes of dermal penetration of chemicals through the stratum corneum (1,13). After a chemical passes through the stratum corneum it can transfer through the viable epidermis into the dermal blood supply and be transported to the systemic circulation (5). Quantitating dermal absorption is a key step in constructing dermal exposure assessments. Both in vivo and in vitro methods can be used to estimate dermal absorption.

In vivo techniques can be used to measure dermal penetration either directly or indirectly (14–17). Direct methods measure the chemical in the blood or excreta, on tape strips that remove stratum corneum or by a biological or pharmacological response. Indirect methods estimate dermal absorption by measuring the disappearance of the chemical from the surface of the skin. These kinds of studies in humans provide the most relevant dermal penetration data but they often are limited due to costs and ethical considerations associated with testing toxic compounds in humans. Laboratory animal experiments can be conducted which permits analysis of absorbed material at the site of application and in body tissues and excreta to provide more complete information (18–21). However, anatomical and physiological differences between animals and humans may make interpretation of results difficult. Dermal penetration in most laboratory animals has been shown to overestimate human dermal absorption in both in vivo and in vitro techniques. Depending on the approach and experimental conditions, results can vary in a wide and unpredictable manner (4,22,23). Nonetheless the EPA's Office of Pesticides Program uses an in vivo protocol in the rat to evaluate pesticide registrations where dermal absorption is a concern when there are no studies in humans (19). The protocol requires a minimum of three doses at log intervals at concentrations spanning application of the pesticide. Doses are applied as mass per unit area (mg/cm^2) application site. A minimum of 24 rats are used at each dose, and exposed in groups of 4 for 0.5, 1.0, 2.0, 4.0, 10.0, and 24.0 hours to a radiolabeled form of the test chemical. Animals are sacrificed at each time interval and examined for the chemical at the application site and in various tissues and organs. Analysis of the application enclosure, skin wash, excreta, and cage wash provides an opportunity to obtain a material balance for the chemical. With these data it is possible to estimate the dose, skin penetration, distribution, and fate of the chemical in the rat. Other parts of the EPA do not use this protocol. They rely on published studies from the literature or in vitro dermal absorption methods to estimate dermal exposure when studies are unavailable.

In Vitro Methods

In vitro dermal absorption methods provide skin permeation rate measurements where fraction absorbed or permeability constants can be determined (1,16,21,24). These methods are appealing because of their efficiency and economy and because they eliminate ethical concerns for studies with toxic or corrosive chemicals in animals or humans. Viable or non-viable skin is used. Samples are generally obtained from the abdomen from elective surgical procedures or from cadavers. In both cases diffusion across the stratum corneum is considered to be the rate-limiting step for dermal absorption. Absorption through the stratum corneum is believed to depend on chemical specific factors such as molecular weight, solubility, and polarity. Though good correlations have been reported between in vivo and in vitro methods for some chemicals (25,26) appropriate care must be taken to simulate in vivo conditions. Results can vary due to factors such as skin species used, type of skin preparation used, choice of receptor fluid, humidity, and temperature (24,27). Moreover, some lipophilic compounds can absorb into skin but may not partition readily into the receptor fluid. Material in skin must be included with that found in the receptor fluid for determination of total percutaneous absorption and estimates of dermal exposure (24). Use of surfactants or other receptor fluids can impair metabolic activity in skin or affect the penetration of some chemicals through the skin (1,24).

Two different types of in vitro procedures can be used to study dermal exposure: the infinite dose and finite dose procedure (1,24,28,29). An infinite dose is achieved when the maximum rate of absorption of a chemical concentration is attained and maintained. In this case the vehicle volume is sufficiently large such that it is not depleted during the course of the exposure event. This represents a steady state situation and permits estimation of permeability coefficients that can be used in environmental exposure and risk assessments. It is applicable to several dermal exposure events such as bathing or swimming in chemically contaminated water. A finite dose occurs when the maximum absorption rate for a given chemical is not achieved or is achieved but not maintained. In this case the chemical concentration in the vehicle changes over time due to absorption into the skin and evaporation from the site of application. This applies to a wide range of dermal exposure events where the amount of time for chemical to penetrate through the skin is less than the amount of time of chemical contact with the skin.

ESTIMATING DERMAL EXPOSURE

Quantitative exposure assessments for contaminants in water and air are based on the use of a permeability constant (K_p), which measures the rate of penetration into the skin. K_p is usually measured in the laboratory from in vitro studies at steady state. For exposure to soil, percutaneous absorption is usually expressed as the fraction of the applied dose absorbed from both in vivo and in vitro studies. Many of the permeability coefficients are based on predictive methods that commonly use octanol–water partition coefficients ($K_{o/w}$) and molecular weight due to a lack of experimentally derived permeability coefficients for many chemicals (1,16,22). Most experimentally derived permeability coefficients are determined using the pure chemical deposited onto skin in a volatile solvent (e.g., acetone or ethanol) or the chemical in an aqueous solution. A number of factors may influence dermal absorption estimation such as physical and chemical characteristics of the contaminant (including factors such as corrosivity, solubility, and vapor pressure), matrix composition, physiological characteristics of the skin (including anatomical site or species), amount of surface area contact, and rate and mechanism of absorption.

Permeability of Chemicals in Water

While there is a large number of permeability coefficient measurements for chemicals in water, most are for small organic chemicals and pharmaceuticals. Correspondingly fewer chemicals of importance in environmental or occupational exposures have been measured. This is particularly true for highly lipophilic chemicals (log $K_{o/w} > 4$); many of interest to the EPA. The large number of chemicals in commerce and the time and expense to conduct permeability coefficient tests has prompted investigation of equations to predict chemical permeability (30,31). Vecchia and Bunge (31) compared 22 different equations to estimate permeability coefficients with experimental values collected by Flynn (30). Their results indicated that most of the equations adequately predicted K_p for chemicals of low molecular weight (50–150 Da) but that high molecular weight chemicals (450–550 Da) were best predicted by equations developed specifically for them.

In those instances where measured permeability coefficients are not available, the EPA advocates the use of equations to predict chemical permeability. Initially, the approach described by Flynn (30) and the equation of Potts and Guy (32) were used to generate an algorithm for organic compounds in aqueous solutions.

$$\text{Log } K_p = 2.72 + 0.71 \log K_{o/w} - 0.0061 \text{ MW}$$

where K_p, dermal permeability coefficient for a compound in water (cm/hr); $K_{o/w}$, octanol/water partition coefficient (dimensionless); MW, molecular weight.

Recently, this approach has been refined to provide more precision and accuracy (24). First, the original Flynn database was modified by removing the in vivo studies (ethyl benzene, styrene, and toluene) to develop K_p correlations based only on in vitro measurements using human skin. This produced a modified Potts and Guy equation for Log K_p:

$$\text{Log } K_p = -2.80 + 0.66 \log K_{o/w} - 0.0056 \text{ MW}$$

where K_p, dermal permeability coefficient for a compound in water (cm/hr); $K_{o/w}$, octanol/water partition coefficient (dimensionless); MW, molecular weight.

Second, statistical analyses of the regression equation using Mandel's approach (33) were conducted to develop acceptable boundaries for predicted K_p in an acceptable size range such that:

$$-0.06831 \leq 0.5103 \times 10^{-4} \text{ MW} + 0.05616 \log K_{o/w} \leq 0.5577$$

$$-0.3010 \leq -0.5103 \times 10^{-4} \text{ MW} + 0.05616 \log K_{o/w} \leq 0.1758$$

This approach does not work well for compounds with a very small or very large $K_{o/w}$. This is due to the limited permeability of these compounds through skin in aqueous solutions. For these compounds the EPA advocates use of a modified Potts and Guy equation.

Beyond aqueous solutions, studies have shown that strong surfactants (e.g., sodium lauryl sulfate) can increase dermal penetration of chemicals in aqueous solutions by as much as 3 or 4 times the normal penetration rate (8). Surfactants can also alter the lipid composition on the skin altering penetration and cause skin irritation, which can further affect dermal penetration (16). Despite its importance to environmental and occupational exposures, little has been reported about dermal absorption from non-aqueous liquid vehicles, though the EPA recently published a protocol for industrial chemicals using this approach with isopropyl myristate (24).

Permeability of Chemicals in Soil

In soil, the amount of chemical that can be absorbed by the skin is largely determined by the interactions that occur between the soil matrix and the chemical. These interactions depend on the physical and chemical properties of the chemical compound and the soil and can be highly variable (34). These effects can be reversible or irreversible. Reversible processes, such as adsorption and desorption, can control the rate of chemical transfer from soil. Irreversible processes, such as sequestration, can permanently bind the chemical to soil particles to reduce the amount of chemical that can be absorbed into skin. Adsorption and desorption, sequestration of contaminants in soils and sediments, and soil–water interactions have been well reported in the literature, but few of these studies address dermal absorption of chemically contaminated soil. Those that do show interactions with the organic material control contaminant adsorption and desorption except for soils with low organic content or high clay content.

Interactions between the contaminant and the soil have been shown to affect the rate of chemical transfer from the soil to skin. Partitioning of non-polar organic chemicals into the organic fraction of the soil matrix occurs due to the high affinity of the organic fraction for non-polar organic chemicals (34). Soil organic material has a solubility limit. If the amount of chemical in the soil exceeds the solubility limit, then a neat chemical will remain (11,35,36).

Information about soil or sediment adherence, contact rates, and frequencies for typical exposures are limited. Studies have been conducted to demonstrate soil and sediment loadings on skin for various activities. These studies have focused on soil or sediment adherence to various body parts, especially the hands (37,38). However more studies are warranted with different types of soils, a wider variety of time activity patterns and climatic conditions to obtain a more complete picture about the factors that affect soil or sediment loading on skin for exposure assessment.

Dermal Contact and Transfer from Treated Surfaces

Historically, hand press or hand wipe methods have been used to estimate the amount of contaminant transferred to the skin following dermal contact with a surface.

Studies have been conducted to estimate the transfer efficiency of pesticides applied to various kinds of floors such as hardwood, vinyl, and carpets. Surfaces have been treated with pesticides such as chlorpyrifos, diazinon, heptachlor, isophenfos, malathion, cis and trans permethrin, and piperonyl butoxide and examined for residue transfer to skin after surface contact (39–41). Similar studies have been conducted for polychlorinated biphenyls (PCBs) on concrete Slayton et al. (42).

However, these methods do not adequately account for the activity being performed at the time of exposure or the frequency of exposure based on activity patterns. Approaches have been developed, such as the microactivity and macroactivity approach, that are currently being used to quantify activity patterns and exposure frequencies in children (43). In addition, methodologies for analyzing hand-to-mouth transfer of contaminants and the dermal spatial distribution of contaminants following contact and transfer also have been developed.

DERMAL EXPOSURE ESTIMATES

The exposure assessment evaluates the type and magnitude of exposures to chemicals of potential concern at a site. The exposure assessment considers the source from which a chemical is released to the environment, the pathways by which chemicals are transported through the environmental medium, and the routes by which individuals are exposed. Parameters necessary to quantitatively evaluate dermal exposures, such as permeability coefficients, soil absorption factors, body surface area exposed, and soil adherence factors, are developed in the exposure assessment. In this chapter, the dermal assessment is evaluated for two exposure media: water and soil. The EPA's *Policy for Risk Characterization* (44) states that each EPA risk assessment should present information on a range of exposures (e.g., provide a description of risks to individuals in average and high end portions of the exposure distribution). Generally, within the Superfund program, to estimate exposure to an average individual (i.e., a central tendency), the 95% upper confidence limit on the arithmetic mean is chosen for the exposure point concentration, and central estimates (i.e., arithmetic average, 50th percentile, median) are chosen for all other exposure parameters. This guidance document provides recommended central tendency values for dermal exposure parameters, using updated information from the Exposure Factors Handbook (45). In comparison with the average exposure, dermal exposure is defined as the amount of material in contact with the skin and available for absorption. The skin loading rate, expressed as mg/cm^2-hour, normally varies across anatomical regions of the body and is estimated by subdividing the exposed dermal regions sampling purposes. Therefore, the total dermal exposure, expressed as mg/hr, is calculated as follows:

$$\text{Dermal Exposure} = \sum (\text{SLR}_1 \times \text{SA}_1) + \cdots + (\text{SLR}_n \times \text{SA}_n)$$

where SLR, skin loading rate for each anatomical region (mg/cm^2-hour); SA, exposed skin area for each anatomical region (cm^2).

Dermal Exposure to Chemical Contaminants in Water and Soil

The approach for estimating the dermal absorption of compounds in water is based on the use of a permeability coefficient, whereas the procedure for estimating the dermal absorption of soil-bound compounds is based on the use of an absorption fraction.

For dermal exposure to chemicals in water and air, the average daily dose absorbed (DAD, in mg/kg-day) is given by the following equation:

$$\text{DAD} = \frac{\text{DA}_{\text{event}} \times \text{EV} \times \text{ED} \times \text{EF} \times \text{A}}{\text{BW} \times \text{AT}} \tag{1}$$

where DAD, dermally absorbed dose (mg/kg-day); DA_{event}, absorbed dose per event (mg/cm^2-event); A, skin surface area available for contact (cm^2); EV, event frequency (events/day); EF, exposure frequency (days/yr); ED, exposure duration (years); BW, body weight (kg); AT, averaging time (days); for noncarcinogenic effects AT = ED, and for carcinogenic effects AT = 70 years, or 25,550 days.

For dermal exposure to soil, the average daily dose exposed is given by a similar equation:

$$DAD = \frac{DA_{event} \times EF \times ED \times A}{BW \times AT} \tag{2}$$

where DAD, dermally absorbed dose (mg/kg-day); DA_{event}, absorbed dose per event (mg/cm^2-event); A, skin surface area available for contact (cm^2); EF, exposure frequency (events/yr); ED, exposure duration (years); BW, body weight (kg); AT, averaging time (days); for noncarcinogenic effects AT = ED, and for carcinogenic effects AT = 70 years, or 25,550 days.

DA_{event} is a function of the permeability coefficient K_p for water and air exposure; for soil exposure, DA_{event} is a function of the absorption fraction.

REFERENCES

1. Environmental Protection Agency. Dermal exposure assessment: principles and applications. January, 1992. EPA/600/8-91/011B.
2. Gordon SM, Wallace LA, Callahan PJ, Kenny DV, Brinkman MC. Effect of water temperature on dermal exposure to chloroform. Environ Health Perspect 1998; 106:337–45.
3. Klingner T, Boeniger MF. In-use testing and interpretation of chemical resistant glove performance. Appl Occup Environ Hyg 2002; 17:368–78.
4. Zendzian RP. Pesticide residues in the washed skin and its potential contribution to dermal toxicity. J Appl Toxicol 2003; 23:121–36.
5. Roberts MS. Targeted drug delivery to the skin and deeper tissues: role of physiology, solute structure and disease. Clin Exp Pharmacol Physiol 1997; 24(11):874–9.
6. Reddy MB, Guy RH, Bunge AL. Does epidermal turnover reduce percutaneous penetration? Pharm Res 2000; 17:1–6.
7. Fenske RA, Schulter C, Lu C, Allen EH. Incomplete removal of the pesticide captan from skin by standard handwash exposure assessment procedures. Bull Environ Contam Toxicol 1998; 61(2):194–201.
8. Zendzian RP. Pesticide residue in the washed skin and its potential contribution to dermal toxicity. J Appl Toxicol 2003; 23:121–36.
9. Geer LA, Cardello N, Dellarco MJ, et al. Comparative analysis of passive dosimetry and biomonitoring for assessing chlorpyrifos exposure in pesticide workers. Ann Occup Hyg 2004; 48:683–95.
10. Stinchcomb AL, Pirot F, Touraille GD, Bunge AL, Guy RH. Chemical uptake into human stratum corneum in vivo from volatile and non-volatile solvents. Pharm Res 1999; 16:1288–93.
11. Bunge AL, Parks JM. Soil contamination: theoretical descriptions. In: Roberts MS, Walters KA, eds. Dermal Absorption and Toxicity Assessment. New york: Marcel Dekker, 1998:669–96.
12. Reddy MB, Bunge AL. Dermal absorption from pesticide residues. Data analysis. In: De Raat WK, Kruse J, Verhaar H, eds. Practical Applicability of Toxicokinetic and Biologically Based Modeling in the Risk Assessment of Chemicals. Dordrecht. The Netherlands: Kluwer Academic Press, 2000.
13. Moody RP, Chu I. Dermal exposure to environmental contaminants in the Great Lakes. Environ Health Perspect 1995; 103(Suppl. 9):103–14.
14. Higo N, Naik A, Bommannan DB, et al. Validation of reflectance infrared spectroscopy as a quantitative method to measure percutaneous absorption in vivo. Pharm Res 1993; 10:1500–6.
15. Pirot F, Kalia Y N, Stinchcomb AL, et al. Characterization of the permeability barrier of human skin in vivo. Proc Natl Acad Sci 1997; 94:1562–7.

16. Bunge AL, McDougal J. Dermal uptake. In: Olin SS, ed. Exposure to Contaminants in Drinking Water. Estimating Uptake Through the Skin and by Inhalation. Boca Raton, Florida: CRC Press, 1999.
17. Wester RC, Maibach HI. In vivo methods for percuaneous absorption measurements. In: Bronaugh RL, Maibach HI, eds. Percutaneous Absorption. 2nd ed. New York: Marcel Dekker, 1999.
18. Environmental Protection Agency. Subchapter E, Pesticide Programs. Data requirements for registration. 1993. 40 CFR 158.
19. Zendzian, RP. Pesticide Assessment Guidelines. Subdivision F: Hazard Evaluation, Humans and Domestic Animals. 1994. Series 85-3.
20. European Commission (EC). Commission Directive 94/79/EC amending Council Directive 91/414/EEC concerning the placing of plant protection products on the market. Official Journal of the European Communities, Vol. L354, 21 December, 1994.
21. Organisation for Economic Co-Operation and Development (OECD). OECD guidance document for the conduct of skin absorption studies. Draft 2000a. December 2000.
22. Vecchia BE. Estimating Dermal Absorption: Data Analysis, Parameter Estimation, and Sensitivity to Parameter Uncertainties. Golden, Colorado: Colorado School of Mines, 1997.
23. Ross HJ, Dong MH, Krieger RI. Conservatism in pesticide exposure assessment. Reg Toxicol Pharmacol 2000; 31:53–8.
24. Environmental Protection Agency. Federal Register: Rules and Regulations. 2004b, 2004; 69(80):22402–41.
25. Feldmann RJ, Maibach HI. Percutaneous penetration of some pesticides and herbicides in man. Toxicol Appl Pharmacol 1974; 28:126–32.
26. Franz TJ. Percutaneous absorption: on the relevance of in vitro data. J Invest Dermatol 1975; 64(3):190–5.
27. Zendzian R, Dellarco M. Validating in vitro dermal absorption studies: an introductory case study. In: Salem H, Katz SA, eds. Alternative Toxicological Methods. Boca Raton: CRC Press, 2000.
28. Organisation for Economic Co-Operation and Development (OECD). OECD guideline for the testing of chemicals. Draft. 2000b. New guidelines 428. Skin absorption: in vitro method. December, 2000.
29. Sartorelli P, Andersen HR, Angerer J, et al. Percutaneous penetration studies for risk assessment. Environ Toxicol Pharmacol 2000; 8:133–52.
30. Flynn GL. Physicochemical determinants of skin absorption. In: Gerrity TR, Henry CJ, eds. Principles of Route-to-Route Extrapolation for Risk Assessment. New York: Elsevier, 1990:93–127.
31. Vecchia BE, Bunge AL. Estimating skin permeability of organic chemicals from aqueous solutions. In: Hadgraft J, Guy RH, eds. Transdermal Drug Delivery Systems. 2nd ed. New York: Marcel Dekker, 2000.
32. Potts RO, Guy RH. Predicting skin permeability. Pharm Res 1992; 9:663–9.
33. Mandel J. The regression analysis of collinear data. J Res Nat Bur Stand 1985; 90:465–78.
34. National Environmental Policy Institute (NEPI). Assessing the bioavailability of organic compounds in soil for use in human health risk assessments. Bioavailability Project Policy, Organics Task Force. NEPI, Washington, DC. Fall, 2000.
35. Macalady, DL, Bunge, AL. Partial pressure data as an insight into mechanisms of dermal absorption of soil contaminants. Conference on Hazardous Waste Research, Denver, CO, 23–25, May. 2000.
36. McCarley KD, Bunge AL. Physiologically relevant two-compartment pharmacokinetic models for skin. J Pharm Sci 2000; 89:1212–35.
37. Kissel JC, Richter KY, Fenske RA. Field measurements of dermal soil loadings attributable to various activities: implications for exposure assessment. Risk Anal 1996; 16(1):115–25.
38. Kissel JC, Richter KY, Fenske RA. Factors affecting soil adherence to skin in hand-press trials. Bull Environ Contam Toxicol 1996; 56:722–8.
39. Bernard C, Willaims R, Krieger R. Exploring the determinants of human exposure to insecticide residue deposited on carpeted surfaces. International Society of Exposure Analysis (ISEA) Annual Meeting, Monterey CA, 2000.

40. Clothier JM. Dermal Transfer efficiency of pesticides from new, vinyl sheet flooring to dry and wetted palms. Human Exposure & Atmospheric Sciences Division, National Exposure Research Laboratory (NERL), Environmental Protection Agency (EPA), Research Triangle Park, North Carolina. EPA/600/R-00/029. February, 2000.

41. Rohrer C, Hiebe T, Melny L, Berry M. Pesticide transfer efficiency from household surfaces to food. International Society of Exposure Analysis (ISEA) Annual Meeting, Monterey CA, 2000.

42. Slayton TM, Valberg PA, Wait AD. Estimating dermal transfer from PCB-contaminated porous surfaces. Chemosphere 1998; 36:3003–14.

43. Zartarian VG, Ozkaynak H, Burke JM, et al. A modeling framework for estimating children's residential exposure and dose to chlorpyrifos via dermal residue contact and nondietary Ingestion. Environ Health Perspect 2000; 108:505–14.

44. Environmental Protection Agency. Risk Characterization Program. Memorandum from Carol Browner. March 21, 1995.

45. Environmental Protection Agency. Exposure Factors Handbook (CD-ROM). February, 1999. EPA/600/C-99/001.

26 Dermal Absorption of Chemicals: Some Australian Regulatory Considerations

Utz Mueller
Food Standards Australia New Zealand, Canberra BC, Australia

Andrew Bartholomaeus
Drug Safety and Evaluation Branch, Therapeutic Goods Administration, Woden, Australia

Mark Jenner
Scitox Assessment Services, Kambah, Australia

INTRODUCTION

A wide range of chemicals in formulated products are used in, and around, the average residential dwelling and occupational workplace. Intentional or inadvertent exposure to these chemicals may occur via the dermal, inhalation, and oral routes. However, the main route of exposure for the majority of products is the dermal route. A key step in the regulation of chemicals that are used in these settings is to ascertain their safety. This is usually done with a risk assessment. An important element of a risk assessment is to provide a quantitative estimate of the extent of both dermal exposure and the resultant internal (or systemic) dose. This chapter focuses on the estimation of internal dose once dermal exposure has been determined. Practical aspects of the process of extrapolation from animal data in the estimation of human risk are also discussed using data for two insect repellents, picaridin, and dimethyl phthalate (DMP), as examples.

GENERAL CONSIDERATIONS
What is "The Dose"

A key concept in risk assessment of dermal exposures is that of internal (or systemic) dose versus exposure (or applied) dose. Estimates of exposure must be expressed in a manner that can be compared with dose–response data. Systemic exposure to a chemical may be considered as the outcome of a two-step process, governed by the duration and extent of exposure (i.e., the amount deposited and surface area of contamination) and the chemical's ability to penetrate the skin and reach the systemic circulation. As discussed later in this chapter, under some circumstances, the *internal dose* is not necessarily directly proportional, or even related, to the *applied dose* (exposure) to the skin. Further, there are many ways in which the internal dose can be described. One of the most common approaches is to estimate the achieved internal dose in terms of an equivalent oral dose, which allows direct comparison with the results of oral toxicity studies. From toxicokinetic data, the amount absorbed into the systemic circulation following oral dosing can be calculated. So, for example, if an orally administered compound is 80% absorbed from the gut, the effective internal dose following an oral dose of 100 mg/kg body weight (bw) is 80 mg/kg bw. If following a dermal dose of 100 mg/kg bw only 20% is absorbed the internal dose is 20 mg/kg bw, i.e., the internal dose is one-quarter that achieved from an oral dose of the same compound or equal to that following an oral dose of 25 mg/kg bw. So, if we wish to estimate the likely toxicological effects of such a dermal exposure utilizing studies employing oral dosing, we would look at the effects observed at a dose equal to, or as close as possible to 25 mg/kg bw PO, as this gives the same internal dose. The difficulty with this approach is that toxicokinetic data are generally very limited for workplace, agricultural, and domestic chemicals. In general kinetic data are available only for the rat. Although most dermal absorption studies are also conducted in the rat, the key toxicological findings may have been identified in the dog or the rabbit. For most nonpharmaceutical compounds, no information is available on the internal dose or the metabolite profile in these species. Consequently, there is no information to support the generally held assumption that the internal dose in these species will be comparable at comparable milligram per kilogram body weight doses. In fact, it is well known that internal dose scales more accurately between species in relation to dose per square meter of surface area rather than dose per unit of body weight.

ESTIMATING DERMAL ABSORPTION
Study Guidelines
The Organisation for Economic Cooperation and Development (OECD) Test Guidelines (427 and 428) for performing in vivo and in vitro dermal absorption studies are designed to simulate occupational or residential exposure scenarios insofar as they use a finite dose and limit exposure to no more than 10% of the total body surface area (1,2). Under conditions of finite dose, the maximum absorption rate though skin may never be reached, or if it does it will not be maintained for very long. During dermal absorption studies, the concentration of the pesticide in the donor fluid or on the skin will change due to evaporation and/or uptake of chemical into the skin, as may occur when the in vitro test cell or in vivo application site is not occluded. A finite dose study enables the estimation of maximal absorption rate (dermal flux) as well as total absorption (overall internal exposure). Most occupational and domestic exposure to chemicals can be considered as being incidental and undesirable. In most cases, this exposure is episodic and occurs over discrete intervals separated by relatively prolonged exposure-free periods. Moreover, such exposure is unlikely to contaminate much more than 10% of the total body surface area, especially if dermal personal protective clothing such as overalls or gloves are worn during use.

The Elements of Quantitative Risk Assessment
Conventional toxicological databases submitted to regulatory agencies usually consist of toxicity tests conducted using experimental animals. The designs for their conduct have become standardized to a large extent and international guidelines have been developed to achieve consistency in experimental techniques. In general, groups of test animals are exposed to a number of dose levels (usually three) of the substance and a further (control) group is left unexposed. The treatment levels are selected so that the highest dose will cause some obvious toxic effects, while the lowest dose should not result in toxicity. During the course of the study, a range of observations is made and the findings in each treated group are compared with the control group.

Ideally, physiologically-based pharmacokinetics models should be used to extrapolate animal data to humans, but such models require extensive additional data that are not usually considered to be cost-effective for pesticides, industrial chemicals, or cosmetics.

Approaches to systemic dose assessment following dermal exposure vary significantly between regulatory bodies, with varying degrees of sophistication employed in each. The principal sources of this variation derive from whether a no observed (adverse) effect level [NO(A)EL] for risk assessment is based on repeat-dose dermal toxicity studies in experimental animals (as in the U.S.A.) or on route-to-route (i.e., oral-to-dermal) extrapolation that incorporates a correction for the relatively lesser extent of dermal absorption in humans, as is the preferred option in the European Union (EU). Each approach has its strengths and weaknesses but, provided the assessment paradigms yield conservative (i.e., worst-case) estimates of systemic exposure, safety standards based on them will usually provide acceptable protection of those potentially exposed. This chapter will discuss some of the pitfalls with each approach using examples taken from the open literature.

Use of Repeat-Dose Dermal Toxicity Studies to Characterize the Toxicological Hazard

The systemic dose resulting from dermal application is usually not proportional to the dermal dose applied (except for the most readily absorbed compounds or for very low dose rates). As higher doses are applied, the dermal flux rate plateaus and essentially reaches a limiting value. Systemic exposure is however proportional to the surface area of application. Consequently, studies performed with substantial doses of a compound (i.e., hundreds of mg/kg bw) applied to a small proportion of the animal's surface area (typically 10 cm^2 or around 2–3% of the rat body surface area assuming a body weight of 200–250 g) are not useful for hazard identification or characterization, as even a broad range of dermal doses may result in essentially similar levels of systemic exposure. We describe an example of where dermal toxicity studies for the well-known insect repellent "picaridin" are inadequate to define the toxicological hazard. These toxicity studies are reported in peer-reviewed journals.

Picaridin Case Study

Picaridin [IUPAC: (RS)-sec-butyl (RS)-2-(2-hydroxyethyl)piperidine-1-carboxylate] is a repellent for biting insects such as mosquitoes and is a mixture of two diastereoisomers in an approximately 1:1 ratio, each being a racemate (3).

In 1999, Wahle et al. (4,5) and Astroff et al. (6) published a series of studies that reported the effects of lifelong dermal dosing with picaridin in rats and mice and on multigeneration reproduction in rats. Each study involved the daily application of undiluted picaridin to a shaved 10 cm^2 dermal area in rats or 5 cm^2 in mice for five days per week. The animals wore Elizabethan collars to prevent oral ingestion and the application sites were not occluded. The increase in applied "doses" namely 50, 100, or 200 mg/kg bw per day in all studies was achieved simply by increasing the volume of undiluted picaridin applied to the same surface area. Although acanthosis and hyperkeratosis developed at application sites, no systemic toxicity was observed at up to and including the highest dose, and so the NO(A)EL was 200 mg/kg bw per day.

In addition to dissipating from the application sites by dermal absorption, the vapor pressure of picaridin is sufficiently high (5.9×10^{-2} Pa at 25°C) for the chemical to have been lost from the uncovered test sites by evaporation. This loss was not quantified. Evaporative losses are unlikely to have been consistent across the treatment groups because of the differing application volumes of undiluted picaridin, and are a possible source of dosing error.

No experimentally determined dermal flux rate for picaridin is available in the open literature. However, sufficient physicochemical information for picaridin is available to permit an estimate. Magnusson et al. (7) have correlated known maximal in vitro flux rates (J_{max}) with readily available physicochemical properties such as molecular weight (MW, g/mol), melting point (MP, K), octanol–water partition coefficient (K), water solubility (S, mol/L), and number of atoms available for H-bonding (HB). They classified skin penetrants as "good" ($J_{max} > 10^{-5.52}$ mole/cm^2/hr), "bad" ($J_{max} < 10^{-8.84}$ mole/cm/hr), or "intermediate" on mean ± 1 SD. Good penetrants had MW ≤ 152, log $S > -2.3$, HB ≤ 5, log $K < 2.6$, MP ≤ 432. Bad penetrants had MW > 213, log $S < -1.6$, HB ≥ 4, log $K > 1.2$, MP ≥ 223. Considering picaridin has an MW of 229, a log octanol–water partition coefficient (log K) of 2.21, and a log aqueous solubility (log S) of -1.42, it could be classified as a "bad" penetrant. As a bad penetrant, the maximal flux rate will be in the order of $10^{-8.84}$ mole/cm^2/hr or 0.3 µg/cm^2/hr. If we assume that picaridin has a maximal dermal flux rate of 0.3 µg/cm^2/hr (at 1 mg/cm^2, the lowest tested application dose in rats), then the application to 10 cm^2 of rat skin or a 5 cm^2 of mouse skin for six hours a day would yield systemic doses in the order of 18 and 9 µg, respectively, regardless of whether the applied dose was increased from 50 to 200 mg/kg bw per day. These studies may therefore not have yielded data appropriate for establishing dose–response relationships.

The fixed dosing area used in the rat and mouse chronic dosing studies also provides an additional confounder, in that the ratio of dosed surface area (5 or 10 cm^2) to body weight will reduce over the dosing duration of 18 months in mice and 24 months in rats. For example, in rats that are fed ad libitum, their body weight will approximately double from 250 g at the start of dosing to around 500 g at killing (8). So, while the amount of picaridin applied to the skin is adjusted for the change in body weight, the effective "systemic" exposure will decline as the body weight increases.

More seriously, although no systemic toxicological effects were observed at doses up to 200 mg/kg bw per day, we cannot necessarily conclude that a NO(A)EL of 200 mg/kg bw per day was an appropriate value to use for human risk assessment. This is because, had the same nominal doses of picaridin been applied to a greater surface area, systemic exposures would have risen proportionally. For example, the use of 30 cm^2 test sites would have yielded a maximum systemic exposure of around 54 µg per rat. Thus, for insect repellents that may be applied to 30% or more of a user's skin (> 6000 cm^2 assuming an adult human total surface area of 2 m^2) at surface loadings that exceed the threshold level required to saturate the absorption process, repeat-dose dermal studies in animals using currently accepted test methods can easily lead to misleading estimates of both the true systemic dose and the NO(A)EL. It is important to recognize the limitations in "tailoring" an adequate margin of safety simply using a higher application dose without the concomitant increase in systemic dose.

Other important factors that need to be considered are that in humans the extent of absorption from various anatomical areas is not uniform. For example, the extent of absorption from the volar forearm is 5 to 10 times less than that from the face and neck [based on hydrocortisone kinetics; (9)], thus absorption from the face and neck will contribute much more to the systemic exposure than material applied to the forearms. Furthermore, consumers are not being exposed to the pure active constituent, but to formulated products containing 10% to 20% (w/w) picaridin, in the presence of other chemicals. Owing to its low aqueous solubility (8.6 mg/mL), picaridin products are likely to include nonaqueous solvents such as ethanol to ensure adequate dissolution. As discussed later in this chapter, use of solvents, which may enhance the dermal absorption, is likely to further increase the systemic exposure. Under these circumstances, the combined effect of large treatment areas and dermal absorption enhancers could erode the margin of safety significantly below the value estimated.

Oral-to-Dermal Route of Exposure Extrapolation
The picaridin case study demonstrates the difficulties and limitations inherent in the use of dermal toxicity studies in the characterization of the potential hazards of a substance for risk assessment purposes. If toxicity studies for dermally applied substances are not conducted by the dermal route, then an extrapolation from the effects observed following, usually, oral administration to that expected following dermal exposure is necessary.

Route-to-route extrapolation is defined as the prediction of an equivalent dose and dosing regimen which produce the same toxicological response as that obtained for a given dose and dosing regimen by another route while taking into account differences in metabolism and differences in kinetics (AUC, C_{max}, half-life).

INTERPRETATION OF IN VITRO AND IN VIVO DERMAL ABSORPTION DATA

A 2004 review of in vitro dermal absorption studies by the OECD, in conjunction with the consideration of draft Test Guidelines for in vitro and in vivo determination of percutaneous absorption (1,2), concluded that dermal absorption in rats may either under- or overpredict that in humans depending on the class of chemical involved. The use of viable human skin in appropriately designed in vitro studies was considered likely to be a better predictor than in vivo studies in rats. Thus, the general order of relevance for dermal absorption data would be: human in vivo studies, human cadaver skin in vitro studies, rat in vivo studies, and rat skin in vitro studies. For many chemicals, studies in pigs, or using pig skin in vitro, may be superior to rat studies due to the closer similarity between pig and human skin, but these are not commonly available.

A hybrid approach, recommended by the European Centre for Ecotoxicology and Toxicology of Chemicals (9) and adopted by the EU and Australian regulatory authorities, uses the ratio of the dermal absorption values obtained from excised human and rat skin in vitro to "adjust" the value obtained from a rat in vivo study (i.e., the absorption value in live rats is multiplied by the ratio of that in human excised skin to that in rat excised skin in vitro). This approach has some merit as it recognizes the greater relevance of the physiological sink conditions in the live

TABLE 1   Absorption Rates of Phthalate Esters Across Rat and Human Skin

Compound	Absorption rate (μg/cm^2/hr)			Rat in vivo: rat in vitro	Human in vitro: rat in vitro
	Rat in vivo[a]	Rat in vitro[b]	Human in vitro[b]		
DMP	20–25	41.6	3.95	~0.60	0.1
DEP	36.7	41.4	1.27	0.89	0.03
DBP	33–40	9.33	0.07	~4.29	0.008
DEHP	3.30	2.24	1.06	~1.47	0.5

[a] Five to eight milligrams of radiolabeled compound in ethanol was applied to a 1.3 cm^2 area under a nonocclusive dressing and urine and feces were collected over 24-hour intervals for seven days. Absorption rates derived from the limited information provided, based on total recovery minus recovery from cover and skin at application site.
[b] The exposure period necessary to obtain a steady state for rat skin was under eight hours for all phthalates except DEHP (53 hours). For human skin, exposures of 30 hours were needed for most phthalates and 72 hours for DEHP.
Abbreviations: DBP, dibutyl phthalate; DEHP, di-2-ethyl hexyl phthalate; DEP, diethyl phthalate; DMP, dimethyl phthalate.
Source: From Refs. 10, 11.

rat but compensates for the generally greater permeability of rat skin relative to human skin.

The forgoing points may be illustrated using phthalate esters as an example. As shown in Table 1, absorption rates of phthalate esters across rat skin in vivo are generally comparable to those obtained with excised rat skin in vitro with the exception of dibutyl phthalate (DBP), where the in vivo rate exceeds the in vitro rate by fourfold. However, values from both sources overestimate absorption rates measured across human skin in vitro, but without a consistent relationship: absorption rates across human and rat skin in vitro differ by 2-, 11-, 33-, and 133-fold for di-2-ethyl hexyl phthalate (DEHP), DMP, diethyl phthalate (DEP), and DBP, respectively. The absorption rate of DBP across human skin in vitro (2.5–3.95 μg/cm^2/hr) is similar to the value of 3.0 μg/cm^2/hr obtained by Reifenrath et al. (12) across pig skin in vitro.

PERCENT ABSORPTION VS. DERMAL FLUX RATES

In occupational risk assessments, especially those involving pesticides, a conventional approach to estimating human systemic exposure is to perform an in vivo dermal absorption study in rats using radiolabeled material, and then calculate the percentage of applied material absorbed. This percentage is then used in conjunction with estimates of the amount (mass) of the chemical likely to become deposited on the skin during preparation and application, derived from measurements in exposed workers or by use of the U.K. Pesticide Operators Exposure Model or U.S. Environmental Protection Agency Pesticide Handler's Exposure database.

Using percent absorption as the basis for calculating systemic dose has the advantage of being quick and simple but has a number of serious flaws. Generally, relatively large doses of a compound are applied to a small proportion of the animal's surface area giving rise to high surface loadings (up to 1–5 mg/cm^2) that approach or exceed those necessary to result in the maximal dermal flux rate for the applied material. Under these conditions, the amount absorbed per unit time and area remains constant or near constant as the amount applied increases. Consequently, the "percent absorbed" value becomes a

TABLE 2 Absorption Rate of Dimethyl Phthalate (DMP) in Various Vehicles Through Human and Rat Skin In Vitro

Species/volume applied	DMP applied (mg)	Maximum absorption rates (μg/cm^2/hr)		
		Propylene glycol	Octanol	Ethyl decanoate
Human skin				
200 μL	2	2.5	1.4	2.5
10 μL	0.1	0.81	0.98	0.65
1.25 μL	0.0125	0.17	0.24	0.25
Rat skin				
200 μL	2	4	31	51
5 μL	0.05	5.9	7.7	13
DMP solubility (mg/mL)		541	>600	>600

Source: From Ref. 13.

function of the amount applied rather than the propensity of the material to cross the dermal barrier.

Table 2 demonstrates this principle for DMP in various vehicles, using human and rat skin in vitro. As the amount of DMP in propylene glycol applied to a 2.5 cm^2 area of human skin is increased from 12.5 to 100 and then to 2000 μg, the flux rate increases by 5-fold and then by 3-fold despite the amount applied having increased by 8-fold and 20-fold, respectively. Similar results are observed for DMP in the other vehicles. Thus, even at surface loadings of less than 1 mg/cm^2, DMP has reached a near maximal dermal penetration rate.

Using the data with human skin as an example, we will compare the flux rate and percentage absorption approaches with systemic dose calculation, based on the scenarios of exposure with a concentrate or a dilute preparation over a six-hour period. At an application rate of 2 mg per 2.5 cm^2, or 800 μg/cm^2, the amount absorbed over 6 hours becomes 6 hours$\times$2.5 μg/cm^2/hr, or 15 μg/cm^2, which is 1.9% of that which was applied. If the skin exposure was at the lowest level tested (12.5 μg per 2.5 cm^2 or 5 μg/cm^2), the dermal flux would be 0.17 μg/cm^2/hr, yielding a total absorption of 1.02 μg/cm^2 over six hours, or 20.4% of the material in contact with the skin.

Thus, as observed in the EU Guidance Document on Dermal Absorption (14), "...There is an inverse relation between concentration (area dose) and percentage absorption. At low concentrations the absorbed test substance expressed as a percent of applied dose per time interval is in general higher than the percentage absorption at high concentration." As demonstrated here, the difference can involve an order of magnitude.

It follows that the test concentration applied in dermal absorption studies should approximate those used in the intended industrial/agricultural application, which will to some extent compensate for the inherent error in a "percentage absorption" value. It is also advisable to perform exposure estimates for pesticide mixer/loaders (who handle concentrates) separately from those of workers applying diluted spray mixtures, wherever the experimental data permit. However, in most scenarios that do not involve dilute preparations, the primary determinant of systemic exposure following dermal contact with a chemical will be the surface area exposed and duration of exposure, rather than the amount of material deposited.

Confounding Factors

The ideal data for chemical risk assessment following dermal absorption is derived in studies using human skin in vitro or in vivo from the exact formulation of material for which the risk assessment is being conducted. In practice, this is rarely possible and a risk assessment must be performed from studies on the principal (or active) ingredient of toxicological interest in a formulation and at a concentration different to that under consideration. Dermal penetration studies will usually have been conducted in vivo in rats and possibly also in vitro with human and rat skin. Risk assessors seldom have access to a complete and high-quality database, and in some cases the temptation may be to use dermal absorption estimates derived from studies not specifically designed for this purpose, such as median lethal dose studies. Estimation of dermal absorption from a comparison of dermal and oral median lethal dose studies is particularly unsound. Dermal median lethal dose studies usually involve application of high doses to relatively small surface areas. The actual systemic dose will be related more to the surface area of application and duration of contact than to the amount of test material applied. Furthermore, toxicity is frequently determined by peak concentrations in plasma. In acute oral dosing studies, the rate of absorption from the gastrointestinal tract, especially following gavage administration, is frequently quite rapid and results in higher chemical levels in plasma than does absorption from the skin, which is usually slower and more even. Based on these considerations, it is clear that the results of median lethal dose studies are inappropriate for the estimation of the extent of dermal absorption.

Effects of Vehicle on Dermal Absorption

As the rate at which a compound penetrates the skin depends on the nature of the vehicle in which it is applied, dermal penetration studies are ideally conducted using the final product formulation. Unfortunately, in the real world, such studies are not always available. Risk assessors need to be aware however that vehicle effects may range from negligible to substantial. The vehicle in which a chemical is applied to the skin may affect dermal permeability in a number of ways. Rat skin in vitro, and probably also in vivo is susceptible to excessive hydration effects, decreasing the barrier properties of the skin and increasing permeation [(10) and references therein]. The relative solubility, and degree of saturation, of the chemical under investigation in the receptor fluid, compared with the application vehicle, may also affect rate of penetration as this determines the thermodynamic activity [(13) and references therein]. Clearly, vehicles that defat, such as organic solvents, or physically damage the skin, such as phenols, cresols, or strong emulsifying agents like dodecylbenzene sulfonates, will reduce or destroy the barrier properties of the skin.

Looking again at DMP, Hilton et al. (13) examined the effect of a range of vehicles on the rate of absorption across excised rat or human skin (Table 2). Epidermal membranes were prepared from Sprague–Dawley rats and human abdominal epidermal membranes. After confirming the permeability/integrity of the membranes by measuring the penetration of tritiated water, they were cut into disks and placed onto the receptor chamber of a glass diffusion cell with an exposed surface 2.54 cm^2. The diffusion cell receptor chambers were filled with a known volume of 50% v/v aqueous ethanol and 0.2, 0.01, or 0.00125 mL of the dosing solution (10 mg/mL of ^{14}C-DMP in one of propylene glycol, octanol, and ethyl decanoate) was applied to the skin surface. At regular intervals, up to 54 hours after exposure, the receptor fluid was analyzed for DMP content. The steady-state rate of absorption was calculated from the linear portion of a plot of cumulative amount of DMP penetrated versus time. As shown in Table 2, at high application rates of 0.8 mg/cm^2 of DMP, human skin was comparable or markedly less permeable to DMP than rat skin. The degree of variability (1- to 20-fold) was dependent on the solvent used. The degree of penetration through rat skin was highly dependent on solvent with a greater than 10-fold difference in steady-state flux rate between ethyl decanoate and propylene glycol as solvents, but a much lesser effect was seen across human skin with less than a 2-fold difference between octanol and the other two solvents. At lower application volumes little difference in the penetration of DMP across human skin was noted between the three solvents. Similarly with rat skin the variation in penetration rate with solvent was much less at low application rates.

This study highlights a potential confounding factor in the extrapolation of rat dermal penetration studies for DMP to man, rat skin being far more sensitive to solvent effects than human skin. That this difference is exacerbated at high application rates is also directly relevant to the interpretation of dermal toxicity studies in the rat and extrapolation of the results of these studies to humans. The absence of data in the same series of studies for the penetration of undiluted DMP is an unfortunate omission in the current context. The previous study evaluated above, indicates that the steady-state absorption rate of neat DMP is similar to that of low concentrations of DMP in octanol or ethyl decanoate obtained in this study.

Conversely, Reifenrath et al. (12) found no meaningful difference between the penetration rates for DMP in the presence or absence of diethyl-*m*-toluamide (DEET), both applied at 320 µg/cm^2, when tested in vitro on viable human and pig skin. They also found that four other vehicles had negligible effect on the penetration rate of DEET, although a skin-forming polymer markedly reduced penetration. The formulations investigated are shown in Table 3.

Evaporation was a significant source of test compound loss (Table 4). The evaporation rate for a 320 µg/cm^2 application of DEET to human or pig skin in vitro was approximately 10 and 8 µg/cm^2/hr during the first 15 minutes for pig and human skin, respectively, decreasing to approximately 2 µg/cm^2/hr at 60 minutes

TABLE 3 Formulations Tested

	A	B	C	D	D'	E
Diethyl-*m*-toluamide	195 mg	195 mg	195 mg	144 mg	144 mg	256 mg
Silicone polymer (Dow corning)	66.8	—	—	—	—	—
Acrylate polymer (Carboset 515)	—	66.8	—	—	—	—
High molecular weight fatty acid (1010 Dimer acid)	—	—	66.8	—	—	—
Skin forming polymer	—	—	—	332	166	—
Isopropanol	—	—	—	5 mL	5 mL	—
Dimethyl phthalate	—	—	—	—	—	256
Ethanol	5 mL	5 mL	5 mL	—	—	5 mL

10 µL of formulation to 1.2 cm^2 of skin.
Source: From Ref. 12.

TABLE 4 Disposition of Applied Radioactivity (% of Applied Dose) after 50 Hours—Pig Skin

N	Formulation	Evaporation	Penetration	Recovery
5–6	A	40	23	89
	B	39	22	92
	C	33	23	92
	Control[a]	38	22	85
3	D	34	4	87
	Control	66	19	93
7–8	D′	49	15	95
	Control	60	26	96
9	D[b]	51	3	94
	Control	73	13	93
6–9	Pure DMP	50	18	
	Pure DEET diethyl-*m*-toluamide	40	21	
	E	DEET/DMP 38/46	DEET/DMP 20/21	

[a] Neat DEET.
[b] Determined over 25 hours of exposure.
Abbreviations: DEET, diethyl-*m*-toluamide; DMP, dimethyl phthalate.
Source: From Ref. 12.

for both. Peak penetration rates in pig skin were similar for both DEET and DMP at 2.5 and 3 $\mu g/cm^2/hr$, respectively, and the peaks occurred at similar times (10–12 and 8–10 hours, respectively). The combined formulation (E) displayed a plateau for absorption from about 5 hours for DMP and from 10 hours for DEET, but the overall extent of absorption was similar.

DEET and DMP are absorbed across pig skin to a similar extent. The combination of the two repellents in the one formulation does not substantially alter the amount of applied DMP or DEET absorbed but does result in a prolonged, more even penetration curve than that is seen with either compound alone. The peak penetration rate of 3 $\mu g/cm^2/hr$ for DMP across pig skin in vitro is similar to the steady-state rate observed for human skin in vitro of 2.5 to 4 $\mu g/cm^2/hr$ discussed elsewhere in this chapter.

CONCLUSIONS
Dermal Absorption Studies
Given that nonaqueous solvents can enhance dermal penetration of chemicals, especially across rat skin, dermal absorption studies should be performed with the intended market product or similar formulation. It is highly desirable for risk assessments to include at least in vitro studies with human skin, as this is likely to prevent overestimates of systemic exposure based solely on data from rats. In vivo human studies should be mandatory for chemicals that are intended to be applied dermally.

Since dermal flux rate and percentage absorption are dependent on surface loading, studies should include measurements of absorption from both concentrated and diluted preparations (e.g., spray mixture), according to the intended use pattern. The range of surface loadings should be sufficient to demonstrate the highest attainable steady-state flux rate, and define the threshold surface loading at which maximum flux occurs.

OECD TG 427 is more suited to simulating incidental, episodic, finite exposures involving a small proportion of the body surface area (e.g., pesticide application) than to infinite exposures on large areas (e.g., use of insect repellents).

Risk assessors should be aware that estimates of percentage absorption using in vivo and in vitro data are largely an artifact of experimental design, especially at surface loadings that approach or exceed the threshold for saturation of dermal flux. In many studies, the apparent percentage absorption is inversely proportional to surface loading and does not accurately measure the inherent ability of the test chemical to penetrate the skin. Percentage absorption values are closest to physiological reality at low dermal surface loadings, as would occur on exposure to dilute preparations such as agricultural spray mixtures. They are most inaccurate when modeling systemic exposure to pure test chemicals or concentrated formulations. Percentage absorption values should only be used for estimating systemic exposure if they have been derived from studies in which the concentration of the applied test chemical and the dermal surface loading are similar to those associated with in-use exposure.

Interpretation of in vitro and in vivo dermal absorption studies is not straightforward and requires detailed knowledge of the experimental protocol and findings. When preparing evaluation reports, risk assessors should completely describe the composition of the test material and the conditions under which it is applied, including the area of the application site. In addition to the apparent percentage absorption, the dermal flux rate and/or rates of excretion of the chemical and its metabolites at steady state should be stated. In the absence of this information, the accuracy of systemic exposure and risk assessments can become seriously compromised.

Use of Median Lethal Dose Studies

Inferences on dermal absorption based on comparing the results of acute oral and dermal median lethal dose studies are highly error prone and likely to underestimate its true extent.

Dermal Toxicity Studies

Despite their apparent advantages in eliminating the need for route-to-route extrapolation, dermal toxicity studies may actually be inferior to oral studies for dermal risk assessment purposes. Especially in the absence of adequate data on dermal absorption and toxicokinetics by oral and dermal administration, it is difficult to design a dermal toxicity study so as to achieve a range of predictable internal (systemic) doses suitable for characterizing dose–response relationships.

Dermal dose delivery is subject to artifacts that do not affect oral dosing, such as evaporation, mechanical removal from the application site, and changes in the ratio of the dosed surface area to body weight, as may occur as animals grow during long-term studies.

The internal (systemic) dose can seldom be defined in terms of external milligram dose per kilogram body weight, or even the surface loading. It is likely to be related more closely to the application area and duration of contact.

Standard protocols for dermal toxicity studies involve applying large amounts of the test chemical to no greater than 10% of the body surface area, which is the technically feasible upper limit in laboratory rodents. When the rate of absorption is saturated, systemic exposure is limited by the area of skin to which the chemical has been applied. Consequently, systemic dose may not increase proportionally to external dose, leading to overestimates of the systemic NO(A)EL.

The limitations of dermal toxicity studies are most severe when modeling exposure to concentrated formulations applied over large areas of the body, as occurs with the use of insect repellents and some personal care products. Ideally, risk assessment of a chemical intended for personal application should include:

- A dermal absorption study in human volunteers, which includes pharmacokinetic measurement of systemic exposure to the test chemical, and
- A complete toxicological database of studies performed in experimental animals via the oral route, also including pharmacokinetic measurement of systemic exposure that enables complete definition of dose–exposure and dose–response relationships.

REFERENCES

1. OECD guideline for the testing of chemicals—guideline 427: skin absorption: in vivo method. Paris: Organisation for Economic Co-operation and Development, 2004:1–8 (adopted April).
2. OECD guideline for the testing of chemicals—guideline 428: skin absorption: in vitro method. Paris: Organisation for Economic Co-operation and Development, 2004:1–8 (adopted April).
3. WHO Specifications and evaluations for public health pesticides. Icaridin (1-piperidinecarboxylic acid 2-(2-hydroxyethyl)-1-methylpropylester), 2004. (http://www.who.int/whopes/quality/en/Icaridin_spec_eval_Oct_2004.pdf)
4. Wahle BS, Sangha GK, Elcock LE, et al. Carcinogenicity testing in the CD-1 mouse of a prospective insect repellent (KBR 3023) using the dermal route of exposure. Toxicology 1999; 142(1):29–39.
5. Wahle BS, Sangha GK, Lake SG, et al. Chronic toxicity and carcinogenicity testing in the Sprague–Dawley rat of a prospective insect repellent (KBR 3023) using the dermal route of exposure. Toxicology 1999; 142(1):41–56.
6. Astroff AB, Freshwater KJ, Young AD, et al. The conduct of a two-generation reproductive toxicity study via dermal exposure in the Sprague–Dawley rat-a case study with KBR 3023 (a prospective insect repellent). Reprod Toxicol 1999; 13(3):223–32.
7. Magnusson BM, Pugh WJ, Roberts MS. Simple rules defining the potential of compounds for transdermal delivery or toxicity. Pharm Res 2004; 21(6):1047–54.
8. Chevalier S, Ferland G, Tuchweber B. Effect of age and diet on retinol absorption. FASEB J 1996; 10(9):1085–90.
9. ECETOC (European Centre for Ecotoxicology and Toxicology of Chemicals). Percutaneous Absorption: Monograph No. 20. Brussels/Belgium: ECETOC, 1993.
10. Scott RC, Dugard PH, Ramsey JD, et al. In vitro absorption of some o-phthalate diesters through human and rat skin. Environ Health Perspect 1987; 74:223–7.
11. Elsisi AE, Carter DE, Sipes GI. Dermal absorption of phthalate diesters in rats. Fundam Appl Toxicol 1989; 12(1):70–7.
12. Reifenrath WG, Hawkins GS, Kurtz MS. Evaporation and skin penetration characteristics of mosquito repellent formulations. J Am Mosq Control Assoc 1989; 5(1):45–51.
13. Hilton J, Woollen BH, Scott RC, et al. Vehicle effects on in vitro percutaneous absorption through rat and human skin. Pharm Res 1994; 11(10):1396–400.
14. European Commission. Guidance Document on Dermal Absorption. Sanco/222/2000 rev 7, 19 March 2004. (http://ec.europa.eu/food/plant/protection/evaluation/guidance/wrkdoc20_rev_en.pdf)

27 International Perspectives in Dermal Absorption

Janet Kielhorn and Stephanie Melching-Kollmuß

Fraunhofer Institute of Toxicology and Experimental Medicine, Hannover, Germany

INTRODUCTION

This chapter is based on the preparatory work and on the final version of an International Programme on Chemical Safety (IPCS) Environment Health Criteria (EHC) document on Dermal Absorption (1) and the views of experts (IPCS Task Group Members: R. Bronaugh, A. L. Bunge, J. Heylings, S. Kezic, J. Krüse, U. Mueller, M. Roberts, J. J. M. van de Sandt, K. A. Walters, F. M. Williams) invited to the Task Group Meeting from 28 June to 1 July, 2005 in Hannover, Germany, to discuss the document. This chapter highlights some of the aspects discussed, which are presented in more detail in the IPCS EHC document.

The purpose of the IPCS EHC document was to present an overview of dermal (percutaneous) absorption and its measurement, in particular with regard to the risk assessment of chemicals. A further aim was to present and discuss current topics of interest in the field of percutaneous penetration. In the last few years, partly due to regulatory pressures, there have been several initiatives to accelerate progress in the fields of international harmonization of methodology and protocols, culminating in the publication of the Organisation for Economic Co-operation and Development (OECD) test guidelines for skin absorption studies in 2004 (2–4) and the European Evaluations and Predictions of Dermal Absorption of Toxic Chemicals (EDETOX) project (5). Further, available data on permeation have been collected into databases, and progress has been made in developing quantitative structure–activity relationships (QSARs) linking physicochemical properties to permeation data so that in the future it may be possible to predict the data for a large number of chemicals rather than undertake expensive testing of chemicals. In addition, projects have been initiated to investigate risk assessment processes. In spite of these successes in interdisciplinary international harmonization, there are still a number of controversial topics in the assessment of dermal absorption that are under discussion. A way forward in the form of recommendations by the Task Group experts is proposed.

The IPCS EHC document concentrates on dermal absorption from occupational, environmental, or consumer exposure, which may involve exposure to liquids, solids, or vapors. The exposure to liquids is usually intermittent; volatile substances may evaporate from the skin surface. Occupational exposure may be single or repeated, thus requiring risk assessment and control.

The steps between the presence of a chemical in the environment and systemic exposure may be divided into two phases (6). The first phase is the dermal exposure to the chemical (amount, area, and duration). This is affected by a number of factors, such as the properties of the chemical, the work process, the individual's behavior and work practices, type of clothing, type of protective equipment, etc. The IPCS EHC deals only with the second phase, that from exposure of the skin to systemic exposure—dermal absorption.

Although interest in dermal absorption for risk assessment purposes is comparatively recent, research into the factors involved in the passage of compounds through the skin has been conducted for other purposes for several decades. Some scenarios where dermal absorption considerations are important include:

■ The development of transdermal drug delivery systems;
■ Dermatological formulations for localized transport;
■ Safety assessment of cosmetics; and
■ Risk assessment of occupational, environmental, or consumer exposure.

Although these applications involve dermal absorption, they all have different aims and approaches. For some drugs, it may be important that the substance passes through the skin and into the bloodstream. For cosmetics and sunscreen lotions, it may not be necessary or desirable for the product to penetrate the skin; instead, the product may simply remain in the upper skin layers.

In occupational and consumer scenarios, the skin absorption of chemicals such as pesticides needs to be minimized. Risk assessment is usually performed to determine the extent to which exposure to a particular substance is acceptable and therefore the extent to which the substance is safe to use. For many chemicals, there is no information on dermal absorption.

This chapter does not cover all the contents of the IPCS EHC. Thus skin structure, transport mechanisms including theoretical aspects, and details of in vitro or in vivo measurements are not discussed here (see Ref. 1 for more details). This chapter reflects some of the discussion of controversial topics and the conclusions and recommendations of the Task Group.

CONTROVERSIAL TOPICS IN THE ASSESSMENT OF DERMAL ABSORPTION
QSARs/QSPERs

There has been much interest in the potential to predict dermal absorption thereby avoiding costly in vitro and in vivo testing. This is partly due to ethical issues with respect to human and laboratory animal experiments and partly due to economic and time considerations as a result of increasing legislation in the risk assessment of industrial chemicals e.g., the proposed new European chemicals strategy: Registration, Evaluation, and Authorization of Chemicals, which requires generation of toxicity data for thousands of chemicals.

QSARs are generally used to relate properties of chemicals to biological effects or transport properties and are an observation of the association between an outcome and the properties likely to affect that outcome. Descriptors of hydrophobicity, molecular size, and possibly hydrogen bonding (which may describe non-covalent interactions with skin proteins) are of importance for the development of QSARs (7). QSARs, when applied to predicting the permeability coefficients needed to estimate dermal absorption, are sometimes known as quantitative structure–permeability relationships (QSPRs or QSPeRs). For recent overviews of QSPeRs for permeation into human skin from water, see this volume and (7–12).

The OECD guidelines are not strict protocols. However, the acceptance and use of these guidelines should lead to a more reliable database. It is debated whether reliable QSPeRs be constructed from such an improved database, or whether stricter protocols are necessary [e.g., that suggested by a CEFIC Working Group (13)]. However, some are of the opinion that the present data are sufficient to derive reliable QSPeRs (13). The acceptance of QSARs/QSPeRs themselves is still a matter of controversy. On the one hand, dermal absorption data are lacking for thousands of chemicals; on the other hand, variability of data is controversial. Further guidance is needed on the use of QSPeR data in risk assessment. At present, most QSPeRs give estimates of permeability coefficient (K_p) values, or relative absorption over 24 hours, which need to be "translated" into a parameter that can be applied in risk assessment.

Relevance of Percutaneous Measurements to Data Required by Risk Assessors: Finite and Infinite Exposures

Ideally, estimates of dermal absorption required by risk assessors should be as close as possible to real exposure conditions. To achieve this, experiments should be conducted under finite-dose conditions, using vehicles, concentrations of chemicals, and periods of exposure that reflect in-use conditions (14,15). In practice, many in vitro dermal absorption studies are carried out under infinite exposure conditions. At present, there are attempts to use modeling to link permeability coefficients measured under infinite (steady-state conditions) to conditions more typical of occupational exposure (nonsteady-state conditions) (13,16).

Use of In Vitro Studies in Risk Assessment

There is still a debate regarding how in vitro data could or should be used in risk assessment (17). An evaluation of available data on in vitro dermal absorption was performed under the auspices of the OECD (18). As the available studies comparing the in vitro and in vivo test results contained many variables (different species, thickness and types of skin, exposure duration, vehicles, etc.), an evaluation/consensus was difficult. However, a number of studies, mostly more recent, have been conducted which show that an in vitro approach can predict absorption in vivo, for example, rodent studies using fluazifop butyl (19,20), testosterone (21), triclosan (22), phenoxyethanol (23,24), butoxyethanol, and ethoxyethanol (25,26). In humans, studies with glycol ethers using human skin in vitro (27) gave a reasonably good prediction of in vivo penetration in man (28). Further studies have examined a number of in vitro parameters using both rodent and human skin in comparison to in vivo studies, e.g., with caffeine (29), propoxur (30), *ortho*-phenylphenol (31). This data together with that derived from pesticides (32) and from 12 chemicals (33) show that there is an agreement between absorption data obtained from in vitro and in vivo rodent models at similar exposure levels and that it is now accepted that in vitro human absorption data can be extrapolated to estimate human in vivo absorption in risk assessments.

Studies on inter- and intra-laboratory variation reinforce the need to conduct carefully controlled in vitro and in vivo dermal absorption studies (34,35). Some of these topics (e.g., skin thickness, vehicle effects, receptor fluids, tape stripping) have also been addressed in a recent European project (5). The acceptance of in vitro measurements in lieu of in vivo studies by regulatory authorities necessitates controlled study conditions using accepted protocols.

Consequences of Reservoir Effect for Risk Assessment

Another controversial issue is the presence of test substance in the various skin layers—i.e., absorbed into the skin but not passed into the receptor fluid. In particular, very lipophilic compounds are difficult to investigate in vitro due to their low solubility in most receptor fluids. If the amount retained in the skin is also considered to be absorbed, a more acceptable but conservative estimate can be made. Water-soluble substances can be tested more accurately in vitro because they more readily diffuse into the receptor fluid. If skin levels are included in the overall absorption value, data from in vitro methods seem to adequately reflect those from in vivo experiments and support their use as a replacement of in vivo testing (36).

Different approaches are taken by various bodies. European Centre for Ecotoxicology and Toxicology of Chemicals (37) base their measurements of percutaneous absorption on receptor fluid values only. In the cosmetic guidelines issued by the European Cosmetic Toiletry and Perfumery Association (38) and the Scientific Committee on Cosmetic Products and Non-Food Products Intended for Consumers (39), the material remaining in the epidermis and dermis in addition to that in the receptor fluid is considered as being systemically available, but not the test substance remaining in the stratum corneum at the end of the study. In OECD Test Guideline 428 (4), skin absorption may sometimes be expressed using receptor fluid data alone. However, when the test substance remains in the skin at the end of the study (e.g., lipophilic test substances), it may need to be included in the total amount absorbed. The OECD guidance document (2) notes that skin fractionation (e.g., by tape stripping) may be performed to further define the localization of the test substances within the skin as required by the objectives of the study. Alternatively, distribution within the skin can be determined by taking vertical sections and using autoradiography or other analytical techniques to visualize the test substance. A recent publication has discussed this topic and concludes that when the movement of chemicals from a skin reservoir to the receptor fluid is shown to occur, it is appropriate to add skin levels to receptor fluid values to obtain a more realistic estimate of dermal absorption (40).

Single- vs. Multiple-Exposure Regimes

It is suggested that experiments using multiple-dosing regimes would be more comparable with occupational exposure scenarios. However, most data from dermal absorption studies are from single-exposure regimes. Data on the effects of repeated exposure are scarce and conflicting. Some data show that repeated exposures may alter dermal absorption (e.g., Ref. 41,42), but others show no differences. For example, the effects of single and multiple dosing (for 14–21 days) on the dermal absorption of six test compounds (methylprednisolone aceponate, azone, malathion, estradiol, hydrocortisone, and testosterone) have been compared. No significant changes in absorption were observed following multiple dosing (43–46). In a repeated-dose experiment with caffeine, the amount recovered from each skin compartment mirrored the number of doses applied (47).

Barrier Integrity Test in Skin Penetration Studies

OECD Test Guideline 428 (4) recommends the use of a barrier integrity test when performing skin penetration studies for regulatory submission. It has been recommended that before and, in some cases, after the experiment, the barrier integrity of the skin should be checked by physical methods, such as transepidermal water loss or transcutaneous electrical resistance, or using the tritium method, where the permeation of tritiated water through the skin is determined and compared with standard values (2,4,48). However, there is much debate at the moment as to whether barrier integrity tests actually correlate to epidermal properties (49). If skin samples exhibit a permeability coefficient (K_p) for tritiated water above 2.5×10^{-3} cm/hr, they are rejected as being "damaged." In a recent study (50) on K_p values from 1110 human skin samples, 230 (21%) were rejected because they did not fulfill the barrier integrity criteria. However, it is likely that many of these rejected samples were atypical rather than damaged, resulting in an underestimation of absorption in such an individual. Further, this is an unnecessary wastage of valuable human skin samples, leading to a truncation of the actual population frequency distribution of K_p at high K_p.

Regulatory Risk Assessment

Assessment of dermal absorption is becoming an increasingly important aspect of the overall risk assessment of chemicals. Inhalation exposures to chemicals have decreased as a result of improved control technologies and reduction of occupational exposure limits (OELs), thereby increasing the contribution of dermal exposure. In certain scenarios, dermal exposure may be greater than respiratory exposure, and in rare cases e.g., with glycol ethers, intoxications due to skin exposure have been documented.

Most of the above controversial topics are related to the risk assessment of dermal absorption depending on the data available. In only a few cases are reliable data from human volunteer studies available. How can risk to dermal exposure of chemicals be assessed in lieu of this? As mentioned above it is now generally accepted by experts in the field that a well-conducted in vitro study using human skin can be used to estimate in vivo exposure. However, there are only limited data from well-conducted studies e.g., only about 50% of the data collected for the EDETOX database of in vitro and in vivo studies satisfied the criteria for study design (5,17,51).

Further, some regulatory bodies do not accept in vitro data and prefer to extrapolate from data gathered from other routes of exposure or to use a default assumption of 100% absorption, even for chemicals that do not penetrate the skin well. Others use a default assumption of 10% for those chemicals with a molecular weight > 500 and log $K_{o/w}$ less than -1 or higher than 4. The expectations from predictive modeling to generate absorption data are now being reduced as it is realized that reliable QSPeRs (see above) have to be based on reliable data, and further that for risk assessment, K_p from a finite dose is needed rather than a QSPeR model based on an infinite aqueous dose that may overpredict absorption by several fold.

Dermal Absorption in Susceptible Populations

Risk assessment of dermal exposure is mostly related to healthy, adult individuals. However, skin contact with chemicals occurs in everyday life, and all of the population are potentially exposed.

In the last few years, the awareness that children are a potentially susceptible population for exposure to toxic environmental agents has increased (52). Although full-term neonates have a well-developed stratum corneum, the stratum corneum of premature infants is less effective (53,54). Furthermore, risks from dermal exposure to environmental chemicals may differ between children and adults for a variety of reasons, including differing behavioral patterns, anatomical and physiological differences, and developmental differences of vital organs such as the brain, which may result in different end organ effects (55).

Enhanced dermal absorption has also been reported in skin affected by disease. Certain genetic defects in lipid metabolism or in the protein components of the stratum corneum produce scaly or ichthyotic skin with abnormal barrier lipid structure and function (56). The inflammatory skin diseases psoriasis and atopic dermatitis also show decreased barrier function. Impaired barrier functions of clinically normal skin in atopic dermatitis may predispose inflammatory processes evoked by irritants and allergens. This is a point of concern, since the prevalence of atopic dermatitis in industrialized countries is dramatically increasing.

The skin barrier can be compromised in a variety of ways: physical damage (e.g., burned, shaved), chemical damage (e.g., detergents, solvents), occluded skin (e.g., wearing of gloves), increased hydration (e.g., excessive hand washing), and even psychological stress (54,57). The compromised skin barrier makes the skin more permeable and facilitates dermal uptake. It is more susceptible to irritants, sensitizers, and disease. A compromised skin barrier is not a rarity and therefore, when evaluating the health risk associated with skin exposure, susceptible subgroups in the population should be considered.

Skin Notation

The skin notation was introduced almost 50 years ago as a qualitative indicator of hazard related to dermal absorption at work. It is designated if skin exposure to a defined area, duration, etc. increases the systemic dose by a given percentage, compared with inhalation exposure at the OEL; and/or realistic dermal exposure at the workplace has been shown to cause adverse effects (6). However, in different countries there are different understandings and definitions. A major complication is that the skin notation is often used as an instrument for risk management (58). Workplace exposure needs to be assessed in quantitative terms, and a qualitative hazard indicator, such as the skin notation, is not very useful for risk assessment or management. It has been suggested that skin notation should relate to the potential for toxicity following relevant dermal exposure (58,59).

In many countries, compounds considered as a skin hazard are identified by skin notation on the list of OELs. In general, the notation has the purpose of drawing attention to the fact that cutaneous exposure to these compounds can significantly contribute to total systemic exposure. Irritating and corrosive compounds do not have a skin notation.

A review of the use of the skin notation used by many international health and safety authorities identified inconsistencies (60). For example, the U.K. Health and Safety Executive currently assigns a skin notation to over 120 chemicals, while the American Conference of Governmental Industrial Hygienists (ACGIH) applies the skin notation to over 160 substances. The ACGIH notations have been criticized in the past for inconsistencies in documentation. Varying criteria for assignment are due to a lack of information on dermal absorption rates of chemicals (61). The German criteria for designation of a skin notation (discussed in Ref. 62) are that the maximal allowable concentration for the substance is not sufficient to protect dermally exposed persons from adverse effects on their health. The German definition has therefore introduced adverse health effects as part of the criterion, but does not include quantitative terms (58).

The National Institute for Occupational Safety and Health in the United States is currently revising its criteria for skin notation. There is an obvious need for harmonization of the skin notation both within the EU and within the United States and a strong argument for a quantitative component.

Dermal Absorption of Nanoparticles

This is a very recent controversial topic although nanoparticles in themselves have been present in the environment for a long time. However, the manufacture of nanoparticles for a particular purpose/application is comparatively new and is a booming industry. Nanoscale materials have at least one dimension less than 100 nm, a scale 1000 times smaller than most microscale materials. This significant reduction in size has resulted in topical products containing nanoscale materials and has generated concern about the potential nanoparticle skin exposure. Cosmetic products containing non-ghosting sunscreens and nanoliposome-based skin care products, certain window sprays, paints, varnishes, and coatings are examples of nanoscale products (63). It is, however, unclear exactly how well nanoparticles will penetrate the skin and what the toxicological impact will be (64,65). When nanoparticles are administered in the dermis, they localize to regional lymph nodes, potentially via skin macrophages and Langerhans cells, raising potential concern for immunomodulation if nanoparticles penetrate the skin (65). Potential sources of toxicity may be skin or organ cytotoxicity, long-term toxicity subsequent to accumulation in skin and other organs, metabolism to toxic particles, and toxicity of photoactivated nanoparticles (64).

In cosmetic products, solid lipid nanoparticles have been used since the early 1990s as an alternative system to emulsions, liposomes, and polymeric nanoparticles (66). Emphasis has been placed on measuring the skin absorption of drugs incorporated in the solid lipid nanoparticles rather the penetration of solid lipid nanoparticles per se (67,68). Solid lipid nanoparticles can lead to macrophage cytotoxicity at high concentrations but, in general, appear to be safe, toxicologically acceptable carrier systems (69).

Nanoscale material science is an emerging field in which the benefits and adverse consequences of exposure and dermal absorption are not yet understood. Objective research will be critical over the next 5 to 10 years to promote responsible development that maximizes positive biological interaction and minimal adverse health effects.

CONCLUSIONS AND RECOMMENDATIONS OF THE IPCS TASK GROUP

In addition to reviewing the EHC document, the members of the IPCS Task Group were asked to give their expert opinion as to conclusions that could be made on the basis of the document and any recommendations for regulators or for further research. The Task Group formulated the following text (1):

1. Human skin in vitro and in vivo should be universally recognized as the gold standard in dermal absorption risk assessment.
2. In vitro and in vivo human experimental studies using standardized, well-controlled methods are needed to appropriately assess human dermal

absorption of chemicals, including formulated products that come into contact with the skin.

3. Further efforts are needed to improve and harmonize methodology in order to minimize variability in in vitro dermal absorption measurements. Interlaboratory comparative studies should include appropriate internal and external quality controls, i.e.,:
   a. Use of a validated analytical technique;
   b. Use of a standard membrane and test solution as an additional control;
   c. Cross-check using pure reference chemicals;
   d. Confirmation of barrier integrity;
   e. Consistent and appropriate skin preparation; and
   f. Other recommendations of the OECD test guidelines (2,4).

4. There should be more research aimed at addressing the lack of repeated-dose dermal absorption experiments that simulate relevant exposure conditions.

5. In risk assessment, maximum flux, either measured or estimated from molecular weight, should be used in preference to K_p or percentages of the chemical absorbed. Adjustment should be made to account for non-saturating exposure.

6. Collection of more data on highly lipophilic chemicals under in-use conditions is needed to facilitate understanding of the effect of various vehicles, receptor fluids, and mixtures on results obtained in dermal absorption studies.

7. There is a need for more in vivo and in vitro data on the dermal absorption of chemicals in damaged skin (e.g., mechanical damage, ultraviolet damage, skin irritants, sensitizers, and solvents) and in diseased skin to assist the risk assessment process.

8. Greater efforts should be made to correlate in vitro and in vivo data and to develop reliable prediction models.

9. The regression of the absorption time course will always give a more accurate estimate of dermal absorption parameters than the usual techniques and may be more valuable in finite-dose estimation, in comparing different dose exposure scenarios, and in extrapolating to different occupational exposure situations.

10. Further efforts to evaluate QSARs for risk assessment purposes, and to prepare guidance on their use, are encouraged. However, the inherent limitations of QSARs to mimic a highly complex biological process must be recognized, and approaches being developed in the pharmaceuticals area to model drug–skin component interactions hold promise for the future.

11. Databases containing measured and well-defined skin absorption data are a key first step in the development of QSARs and for research to improve understanding of the dermal absorption process for chemicals. Such databases have been developed by industry, researchers, and government institutions and should be supported, maintained, and updated. Means of sharing data should be explored, recognizing that in some instances the data are proprietary.

12. Noting that different sectors (pesticides, industrial chemicals, cosmetics, pharmaceuticals, etc.) have long established but different usages for some key terms (e.g., permeation, penetration, absorption, resorption, systemic absorption), it is important that terms are clearly defined in scientific articles to aid interpretation. Similarly, care needs to be taken in making comparisons between studies.

13. It needs to be recognized that emerging technologies such as nanoparticles may have unanticipated toxicological consequences following contact with the skin.

14. Development and standardization of noninvasive and semi-invasive human in vivo methods, such as stratum corneum stripping, Fourier transform infrared, Raman, multiphoton, and confocal spectroscopy, and microdialysis, should be encouraged.

REFERENCES

1. IPCS. Dermal Absorption, International Programme on Chemical Safety. Environmental Health Criteria 235. Geneva: World Health Organization, 2006. (http://www.who.int/ipcs/publications/ehc/en/index.html)
2. OECD. Guidance document for the conduct of skin absorption studies (ENV/JM/MONO(2004)2). OECD Environmental Health and Safety Publications Series on Testing and Assessment No. 28, Environment Directorate, Organisation for Economic Co-operation and Development, Paris, 2004:1–31. (http://appli1.oecd.org/olis/2004doc.nsf/linkto/env-jm-mono(2004)2)
3. OECD guideline for the testing of chemicals. Skin absorption: in vivo method. 427. Adopted: April 2004. Organisation for Economic Co-operation and Development, Paris, 2004:1–8.
4. OECD guideline for the testing of chemicals. Skin absorption: in vitro method. 428. Adopted: April 2004. Organisation for Economic Co-operation and Development, Paris, 2004:1–8.
5. EDETOX. Evaluations and Predictions of Dermal Absorption of Toxic Chemicals website. European Union Framework V: Quality of Life, Environment and Health Key Action Funding. (Accessed September 6, 2007 at http://www.ncl.ac.uk/edetox)
6. Johanson G. Dermal absorption and principles for skin notation. In: Occupational exposure limits—approaches and criteria. Proceedings from a NIVA course held in Uppsala, Sweden, September 24–28, 2001 (Stockholm: National Institute for Working Life [Arbete och hälsa 17], 2003:79–86).
7. Moss GP, Dearden JC, Patel H, et al. Quantitative structure–permeability relationships (QSPRs) for percutaneous absorption. Toxicol In Vitro 2002; 16:299–317.
8. Vecchia BE, Bunge AL. Skin absorption databases and predictive equations. In: Guy R, Hadgraft J, eds. Transdermal Drug Delivery. 2nd ed. New York: Marcel Dekkar, 2003:57–141.
9. Vecchia BE, Bunge AL. Evaluating the transdermal permeability of chemicals. In: Guy R, Hadgraft J, eds. Transdermal Drug Delivery. 2nd ed. New York: Marcel Dekker, 2003:25–55.
10. Walker JD, Rodford R, Patlewicz G. Quantitative structure–activity relationships for predicting percutaneous absorption rates. Environ Toxicol Chem 2003; 22(8):1870–84.
11. Fitzpatrick D, Corish J, Hayes B. Modelling skin permeability for risk assessment—the future. Chemosphere 2004; 55:1309–14.
12. Geinoz S, Guy RH, Testa B, et al. Quantitative structure–permeation relationships (QSPeRs) to predict skin permeation: a critical evaluation. Pharm Res 2004; 21(1):83–91.
13. Jones AD, Dick IP, Cherrie JW, et al. Research Report, TM/04/07. CEFIC workshop on methods to determine dermal permeation for human risk assessment. European Chemical Industry Council, December 2004:1–86. (http://www.iom-world.org/pubs/IOM_TM0407.pdf)
14. Benford DJ, Cocker J, Sartorelli P, et al. Dermal route in systemic exposure. Scand J Work Environ Health 1999; 25:511–20.
15. EC. Guidance Document on Dermal Absorption. European Commission, Sanco/222/2000 rev. 7, 2004:1–15. (http://www.eu.int/comm/food/plant/protection/evaluation/guidance/wrkdoc20_rev_en.pdf)
16. Krüse J, Kezic S. Interpretation and extrapolation of dermal permeation data using a mechanistically based mathematical model. In: Brain KR, Walters KA, eds. Perspectives in Percutaneous Penetration. Vol. 9a. Cardiff: STS Publishing, 2004:96.
17. Williams F. In vitro studies—how good are they at replacing in vivo studies for measurement of skin absorption? Environ Toxicol Pharmacol 2006; 21(2):199–203.

18. OECD. Test guidelines programme (ENV/JM/TG(2000)5). Percutaneous absorption testing: is there a way to consensus? Organisation for Economic Co-operation and Development, Paris, 2000:1–42.
19. Clark NW, Scott RC, Blain PG, et al. Fate of fluazifop butyl in rat and human skin in vitro. Arch Toxicol 1993; 67(1):44–8.
20. Ramsey J D, Woollen BH, Auton T R, et al. The predictive accuracy of in vitro measurements for the dermal absorption of a lipophilic penetrant (fluazifop-butyl) through rat and human skin. Fundam Appl Toxicol 1994; 23:230–6.
21. Lee F W, Earl L, Williams F M. Interindividual variability in the percutaneous penetration of testosterone through human skin in vitro. Toxicology 2001; 168:63.
22. Moss T, Howes D, Williams F M. Percutaneous penetration and dermal metabolism of triclosan (2,4,4′-trichloro-2′-hydroxydiphenyl ether). Food Chem Toxicol 2000; 38(4): 361–70.
23. Roper C S, Howes D, Blain PG, et al. Percutaneous penetration of 2-phenoxy ethanol through rat and human skin. Food Chem Toxicol 1997; 35:1009–16.
24. Roper C S, Howes D, Blain PG, et al. A comparison of the absorption of a series of ethoxylates through rat skin in vitro. Toxicology 1998; 12:57–65.
25. Lockley DJ, Howes D, Williams F M. Percutaneous penetration and metabolism of 2-ethoxyethanol. Toxicol Appl Pharmacol 2002; 180(2):74–82.
26. Lockley DJ, Howes D, Williams F M. Cutaneous metabolism of glycol ethers. Arch Toxicol 2004; 17:1–16.
27. Wilkinson SC, Williams F M. Effects of experimental conditions on absorption of glycol ethers through human skin in vitro. Int Arch Occup Environ Health 2002; 75(8):519–27.
28. Jakasa I, Mohammadi N, Krüse J, et al. Percutaneous absorption of neat and aqueous solutions of 2-butoxyethanol in volunteers. Int Arch Occup Environ Health 2004; 77:79–84.
29. Meuling WJ, van de Sandt J JM, Roza L. Percutaneous penetration of [^{14}C]-caffeine in human volunteers: a mass balance approach. In: Brain KR, Walters KA, eds. Perspectives in Percutaneous Penetration. Vol. 8a. Cardiff: STS Publishing, 2002:105.
30. van de Sandt J JM, Meuling WJ A, Elliott GR, et al. Comparative in vitro–in vivo percutaneous absorption of the pesticide propoxur. Toxicol Sci 2000; 58:15–22.
31. Cnubben NH, Elliott GR, Hakkert B C, et al. Comparative in vitro–in vivo percutaneous penetration of the fungicide ortho-phenylphenol. Regul Toxicol Pharmacol 2002; 35:198–208.
32. O'Connor J, Cage S. In vitro skin absorption—can it be used in isolation for risk assessment purposes?. In: Brain KR, Walters KA, eds. Perspectives in Percutaneous Penetration. Vol. 9a. Cardiff: STS Publishing, 2004:92.
33. van Ravenzwaay B, Leibold E. A comparison between in vitro rat and human and in vivo rat skin absorption studies. Hum Exp Toxicol 2004; 23(9):421–30.
34. van de Sandt JJM, van Burgsteden JA, Carmichael PL, et al. In vitro predictions of skin absorption of caffeine, testosterone, and benzoic acid: a multi-centre comparison study. Regul Toxicol Pharmacol 2004; 39:271–81.
35. Chilcott RP, Barai N, Beezer AE, et al. Inter- and intralaboratory variation of in vitro diffusion cell measurements: an international multicenter study using quasi-standardized methods and materials. J Pharm Sci 2005; 94(3):632–8.
36. EC. Technical guidance document (TGD) in support of Commission Directive 93/67/ EEC on risk assessment for new notified substances. European Commission, Part 1, 2003:1–303. (http://ecb.jrc.it/technical-guidance-document/)
37. ECETOC. Percutaneous absorption. Monograph No. 20. Brussels, Belgium, European Centre for Ecotoxicology and Toxicology of Chemicals, 1993:1–80.
38. Diembeck W, Beck H, Benech-Kieffer F, et al. Test guidelines for in vitro assessment of dermal absorption and percutaneous penetration of cosmetic ingredients. European Cosmetic, Toiletry and Perfumery Association. Food Chem Toxicol 1999; 37(2–3): 191–205.
39. SCCNFP. Basic Criteria for the In Vitro Assessment of Dermal Absorption of Cosmetic Ingredients. Updated October 2003, Scientific Committee on Cosmetic Products and Non-Food Products Intended for Consumers, (SCCNFP/0750/03), 2003:1–9.

40. Yourick JJ, Koenig ML, Yourick DL, et al. Fate of chemicals in skin after dermal application: does the in vitro skin reservoir affect the estimate of systemic absorption? Toxicol Appl Pharmacol 2004; 195(3):309–20.
41. Roberts MS, Horlock E. Effect of repeated application of salicylic acid to the skin on its percutaneous absorption. J Pharm Sci 1978; 67:1685–7.
42. Wester RC, Maibach HI. Percutaneous absorption: short-term exposure, lag time, multiple exposures, model variations, and absorption from clothing. In: Marzulli FN, Maibach HI, eds. Dermatotoxicology. 5th ed. Washington, DC: Hemisphere Publishing Corp., 1996:35–48.
43. Wester RC, Maibach HI, Bucks DA, et al. Malathion percutaneous absorption after repeated administration to man. Toxicol Appl Pharmacol 1983; 68(1):116–9.
44. Wester RC, Melendres J, Sedik L, et al. Percutaneous absorption of azone following single and multiple doses to human volunteers. J Pharm Sci 1994; 83:124–5.
45. Bucks DAW, Maibach HI, Guy RH. Percutaneous absorption of steroids: effect of repeated application. J Pharm Sci 1985; 74:1337–9.
46. Tauber U, Matthes H. Percutaneous absorption of methylprednisolone aceponate after single and multiple dermal application as ointment in male volunteers. Arzneimittel-forschung 1992; 42(9):1122–4.
47. Pendlington RU, Sanders DJ, Bourner CB, et al. Development of a repeat dose in vitro skin penetration model. In: Brain KR, Walters KA, eds. Perspectives in Percutaneous Penetration. Vol. 9a. Cardiff: STS Publishing, 2004:79.
48. USEPA. In vitro dermal absorption rate testing of certain chemicals of interest to the Occupational Safety and Health Administration; Final rule. Fed Regist 2004; 69(80): 22402–41.
49. Gordon Research Conference. Gordon Research Conference on Barrier Function of Mammalian Skin. Mount Molyoke College, South Hadley, Massachusetts, August 7–12, 2005. (http://www.grc.uri.edu/programs/2005/barrier.htm)
50. Roper CS, Crow LF, Madden S. Should we use a barrier integrity test for skin barrier function of human skin in skin penetration studies?. In: Brain KR, Walters KA, eds. Perspectives in Percutaneous Penetration. Vol. 9a. Cardiff: STS Publishing, 2004:69.
51. Soyei S, Williams F. A database of percutaneous absorption, distribution and physico-chemical parameters. In: Brain KR, Walters KA, eds. Perspectives in Percutaneous Penetration. Vol. 9a. Cardiff: STS Publishing, 2004:84.
52. Daston G, Faustman E, Ginsberg G, et al. A framework for assessing risks to children from exposure to environmental agents. Environ Health Perspect 2004; 112(2):238–56.
53. Barker N, Hadgraft J, Rutter N. Skin permeability in the newborn. J Invest Dermatol 1987; 88(4):409–11.
54. USEPA. Dermal exposure assessment: principles and applications. Interim Report, EPA/600/8-91/011B. Washington, DC, United States Environmental Protection Agency, Office of Health and Environmental Assessment, 1992:1–389. (http://www.epa.gov/nceawww1/pdfs/derexp.pdf)
55. Mancini AJ. Pediatric dermatology. Pediatr Ann 2005; 34(3):161–2.
56. Madison KC. Barrier function of the skin: "La raison d'etre" of the epidermis. J Invest Dermatol 2003; 121(2):231–41.
57. Choi EH, Brown BE, Crumrine D, et al. Mechanisms by which psychologic stress alters cutaneous permeability barrier homeostasis and stratum corneum integrity. J Invest Dermatol 2005; 124(3):587–95.
58. Nielsen JB, Grandjean P. Criteria for skin notation in different countries. Am J Ind Med 2004; 45(3):275–80.
59. Sartorelli P. Dermal exposure assessment in occupational medicine. Occup Med 2002; 52(3):151–6.
60. Fiserova-Bergerova V, Pierce J, Droz P. Dermal absorption potential of industrial chemicals: criteria for skin notation. Am J Ind Med 1990; 17:617–35.
61. Semple S. Dermal exposure to chemicals in the workplace: just how important is skin absorption? Occup Environ Med 2004; 61(4):376–82.
62. Drexler H. Assignment of skin notation for MAK values and its legal consequences in Germany. Int Arch Occup Environ Health 1998; 71:503–5.

63. Scientific Committee on Emerging and Newly Identified Health Risks (SCENIHR 002/ 005). Opinion on the appropriateness of existing methodologies to assess the potential risks associated with engineered and adventitious products of nanotechnologies, 2005. (http://europa.eu.int/comm/health/ph_risk/committees/04_scenihr/docs/scenihr_o _003.pdf)
64. Tsuji JS, Maynard AD, Howard PC, et al. Research strategies for safety evaluation of nanomaterials. Part IV: risk assessment of nanoparticles. Toxicol Sci 2006; 89(1):42–50.
65. Kim S, Lim YT, Soltesz EG, et al. Near-infrared fluorescent type II quantum dots for sentinel lymph node mapping. Nat Biotechnol 2004; 22(1):93–7.
66. Muller RH, Radtke M, Wissing SA. Solid lipid nanoparticles (SLN) and nanostructured lipid carriers (NLC) in cosmetic and dermatological preparations. Adv Drug Deliv Rev 2002; 54(Suppl. 1):131–55.
67. Santos Maia C, Mehnert W, Schaller M, et al. Drug targeting by solid lipid nanoparticles for dermal use. J Drug Target 2002; 10(6):489–95.
68. Borgia SL, Regehly M, Sivaramakrishnan R, et al. Lipid nanoparticles for skin penetration enhancement—correlation to drug localization within the particle matrix as determined by fluorescence and parelectric spectroscopy. J Control Release 2005; 110(1):151–63.
69. Scholer N, Zimmermann E, Katzfey U, et al. Effect of solid lipid nanoparticles (SLN) on cytokine production and the viability of murine peritoneal macrophages. J Micro-encapsul 2000; 17(5):639–50.

Structure–Activity Relationships and Prediction of Photoallergic and Phototoxic Potential

Martin D. Barratt
Marlin Consultancy, Carlton, Bedford, U.K.

INTRODUCTION

The physical, chemical, and toxicological properties of a chemical are all derived from and related to the unique molecular structure of that chemical; it follows therefore that the various properties of the chemical are also interrelated. This principle forms the basis for the prediction of toxicity from chemical structure. If a mechanistic hypothesis can be proposed which links structural features of a group of related chemicals with a particular toxicological end point, in this case photoallergy, then a structure–activity relationship can be established.

Photoallergy is an acquired altered reactivity of the skin to light in the presence of a photoreactive chemical or photosensitizer (1). Photosensitizers are chemicals that react chemically with the skin on the absorption of light of the wavelengths present in sunlight. The majority of photosensitizers are phototoxic, rather than photoallergic. Phototoxic chemicals, or phototoxins, will elicit a response upon the first exposure if there is sufficient light energy of the appropriate wavelength and a sufficient amount of phototoxin present. Phototoxic responses in the skin can be likened to primary irritation responses.

For photoallergy, the response is mediated via the formation of conjugates between the photosensitizer and cells or proteins in the skin (2). By analogy with allergic contact dermatitis, photoallergic responses require more than one and often many exposures to the photoallergen in the presence of light before photoallergy is induced.

In order to behave as a photoallergen, a chemical must therefore possess certain properties: it must be able to absorb wavelengths of light present in sunlight and upon absorption of that light, it must be able to generate a chemical species capable of binding to proteins in the skin either directly or after subsequent chemical transformation or metabolism. The protein–photoallergen conjugate then acts as an antigen leading to induction and/or elicitation of an allergic response in an identical manner to that observed in contact allergy. At a sufficiently high dose, most photoallergens also exhibit phototoxicity.

Relationships between the structure and properties of chemicals can be programmed into knowledge-based systems. DEREK for Windows (DEREK is an acronym for Deductive Estimation of Risk from Existing Knowledge) (3,4) is one such system for the qualitative prediction of chemical toxicity that is now in widespread use in the chemical and pharmaceutical industries.

This chapter describes rules (structural alerts) for the identification of several classes of potential photoallergens and phototoxins from their chemical structures.

Each rule is underpinned by its putative chemical mechanism, together with examples of known photoallergens or phototoxins considered to be acting by that mechanism.

STRUCTURAL ALERTS FOR PHOTOALLERGENS AND PHOTOTOXINS

Rules for the identification of potential toxicity are called structural alerts; structural alerts are substructures of chemicals that have been found to correlate with specific toxicological end points. Structural alerts, derived for a number of classes of photoallergens and phototoxins, are shown below. The names of known photoallergens and phototoxins supporting each class of structural alerts are listed in Table 1, together with their Chemical Abstracts Service (CAS) numbers and references to supporting literature. A more detailed description of the derivation of structural alerts for photoallergens and phototoxins is to be found elsewhere (5).

TABLE 1   Photoallergens and Phototoxins (with Chemical Abstracts Service Numbers) Classified by Reaction Type

Halogenated phenolic compounds
   3,3′,4′,5-Tetrachlorosalicylanilide [1154-59-2]
   3,4′,5-Tribromosalicylanilide [87-10-5]
   Buclosamide [575-74-6]
   Bithionol [97-18-7]
   Fentichlor [97-24-5]
   Multifungin [3679-64-9]
   Lomefloxacin [98079-51-7]
   Ciprofloxacin [85721-33-1]
   Fleroxacin [79660-72-3]
Halogenated aromatic compounds with other heteroatoms
   Chlorpromazine [50-53-3]
   Carprofen [53716-49-7]
   Dicloran (2,6-dichloro-4-nitroaniline) [99-30-9]
   Diclofenac [15307-86-5]
   Aceclofenac [89796-99-6]
Sulfonamides
   Sulfanilamide [63-74-1]
   Sulfamethoxazole [723-46-6]
   Tolbutamide [64-77-7]
   Glibenclamide [10238-21-8]
Aromatic dinitro and trinitro compounds
   Musk ambrette [83-66-9]
   Moskene [116-66-5]
   Musk xylene [81-15-2]
Diaryl ketones
   Ketoprofen [22071-15-4]
   Tiaprofenic acid [33005-95-7]
   Fenofibrate [49562-28-9]
   Suprofen [40828-46-4]
Imino-*N*-oxides
   Chlorodiazepoxide [58-25-3]
   Olaquindox [23696-28-8]
   Sodium omadine [3811-73-2]

(Continued)

TABLE 1 Photoallergens and Phototoxins (with Chemical Abstracts Service Numbers) Classified by Reaction Type (*Continued*)

Tetracyclines
    Demeclocycline [127-33-3]
    Doxycycline [564-25-0]
    Minocycline [10118-90-8]
    Tetracycline [60-54-8]
Coumarins and furocoumarins
    6-Methylcoumarin [92-48-8]
    7-Methylcoumarin [2445-83-2]
    7-Methoxycoumarin [531-59-9]
    7-Ethoxy-4-methylcoumarin [87-05-8]
    Psoralen [66-97-7]
    5-Methoxypsoralen [484-20-8]
    8-Methoxypsoralen [298-81-7]

Halogenated Aromatic Photoallergens

Halogenated Phenolic Compounds

The following structural alerts for halogenated phenolic compounds have been identified (5):

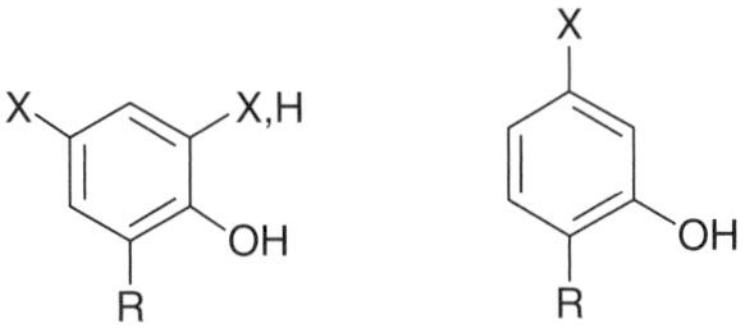

where $X = Cl$, Br, I and $R = S$ or amido.

Halogenated phenolic compounds of this type have been shown to bind covalently to proteins on irradiation with ultraviolet (UV) light (6,7). The mechanism of protein conjugate formation is thought to proceed via generation of a reactive aryl carbon free radical from loss of a halogen, on irradiation with UV light; free radicals have been detected and characterized using electron spin resonance spectroscopy on UV irradiation of several of these chemicals (8,9). Loss of halogen appears to take place more readily when the halogen is separated from the hydroxyl group by two or three aromatic carbon atoms.

A related structural alert is for halogenated fluoroquinolone derivatives; structures of fluoroquinolones are usually represented as the keto form, however, the photoreactivity is more easily explained using the aromatic enol form. The structural alert contains a halogen atom linked via four aromatic carbons to a phenolic OH with the difference that the hydroxyl and halogen are on different rings. There is also a heteroatom at aromatic carbon-5.

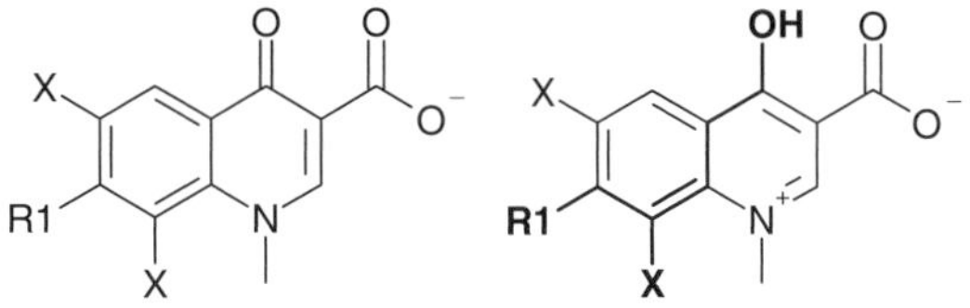

One or two X = F, Cl, Br, or I

R1 = N, O, or S

The photoallergen amiodarone (10) is a benzophenone derivative (see below); however, its photoallergic potential is more easily explained by the above rule.

Amiodarone

Halogenated Aromatic Compounds with Other Heteroatoms

Structural alerts for halogenated aromatic compounds containing heteroatoms other than oxygen (phenols) have been proposed. The first of these is:

where X=Cl, Br, or I, and R=NH or S; Car=aromatic carbon.

This structural alert is analogous to one of the alerts for halogenated phenols in that the phenolic oxygen is replaced by nitrogen or sulfur.

A second alert for the prospective identification of dihalogenated analog is as follows:

where R_1=an aromatic ring and/or R_2=NO$_2$.

General Discussion

Halogenated aromatic compounds probably form the largest group of potentially photoallergic and phototoxic chemicals. A great many of them are photoallergens. Whether they are photoallergens or phototoxins, in many cases, will depend on the dose. Highly photoreactive chemicals such as 3,3′,4′,5-tetrachlorosalicylanilide (11) and the Bayer pharmaceutical BAYy3118 (12) are phototoxic at high doses, and also photoallergenic at lower doses.

Halogenated aromatic chemicals are likely to be photoallergens or photo-toxins if they absorb UV–visible light of a wavelength with energy sufficient to break a carbon–halogen bond; these properties may comprise a more general rule for halogenated aromatic photoallergens.

Sulfonamides

The mechanism of photochemical action of a number of sulfanilamide derivatives has been investigated extensively by Chignell and coworkers (13–15). In the case of sulfanilamide itself, either direct or indirect evidence was obtained for photoinduced homolytic bond cleavage at four different points in the chemical structure (see below).

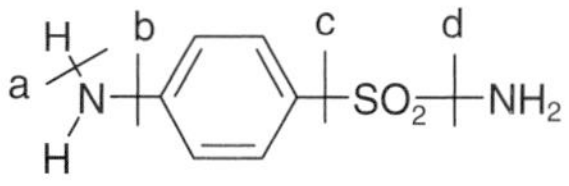

sulfanilamide

For derivatives of sulfonamide, the major point of cleavage appears to be bond "d." The presence of an aromatic substituent on the nitrogen of the sulfonamide, however, appears to inhibit cleavage at this point.

The structural alert for the prospective identification of sulfonamide photo-allergens is as follows:

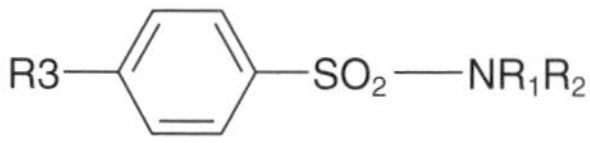

or

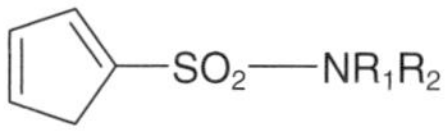

The rule is intended not to fire if R_1 or R_2 is an aromatic group, but allowed if R_3 is a primary, secondary, or tertiary amino group.

Aromatic Dinitro and Trinitro Compounds

The nitro musks are aromatic nitro compounds used in the perfume industry; several of these chemicals have been shown to possess photoallergic potential, the most potent example being musk ambrette (16) which is now prohibited by the International Fragrance Association and the U.S. Food and Drug Administration on account of its carcinogenicity (17).

Structural alerts, for dinitro and trinitro compounds, have been drawn up to identify potential photoallergens of these classes.

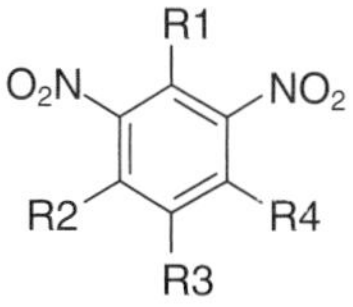

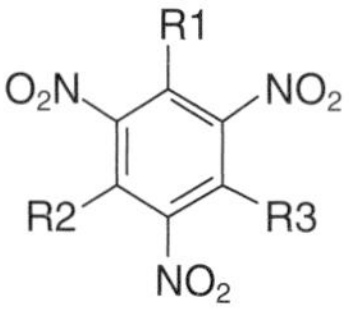

For the dinitro compounds R_1 can be hydrogen or a primary substituent (not secondary or tertiary) up to four carbon atoms long, R_2, $R_4 = H$, methyl, or methoxy and $R_3 = $ hydrogen or any sp^2 or sp^3 carbon. For the trinitro compounds, R_1 can be hydrogen or a primary substituent up to four carbon atoms long, R_2, $R_3 = H$, methyl, or methoxy. These requirements are based on the hypothesis that to be photoaller-gens, the chemicals must be capable, on photolysis, of forming nitro radical anions that are coplanar with the aromatic ring (18); conjugation with the aromatic ring confers an increased reactivity on the nitro radical anions which then go on to be metabolized into reactive intermediates (19).

Diaryl Ketones

A number of drugs containing the diaryl ketone chromophore have been found to behave as photoallergens (20–23). Chemicals containing the diaryl ketone chromophore are also generally phototoxic via a variety of free radical reactions, depending on the nature of the substituents present on the ring systems.

The mechanism of action for the photoallergic potential of diaryl ketones is understood to involve excitation to the triplet state, followed by hydrogen abstraction from the α-carbon of a peptide bond and recombination of the free radicals so formed (24), i.e.,

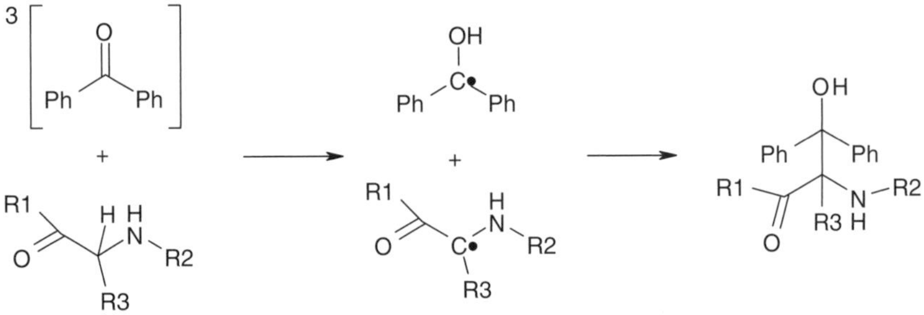

The photoallergens identified so far are either benzophenones or benzoylthiophenes. The presence of an *ortho* substituent with a labile hydrogen on either ring, e.g., hydroxyl, amino, or thiol, results in deactivation of the phototoxic and photoallergic effects via an internal hydrogen transfer mechanism, resulting in quenching of the triplet state

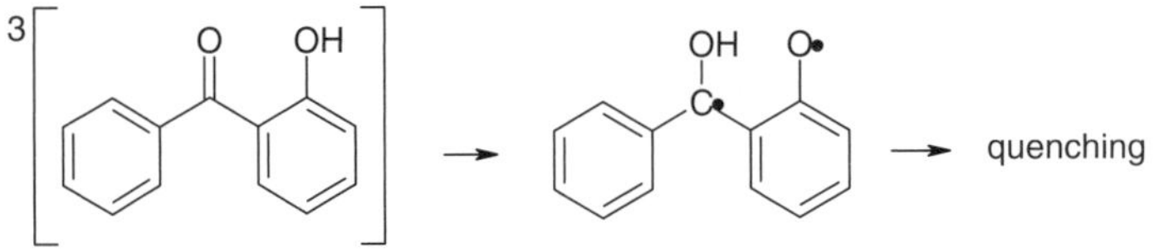

The structural alerts for diaryl ketones are

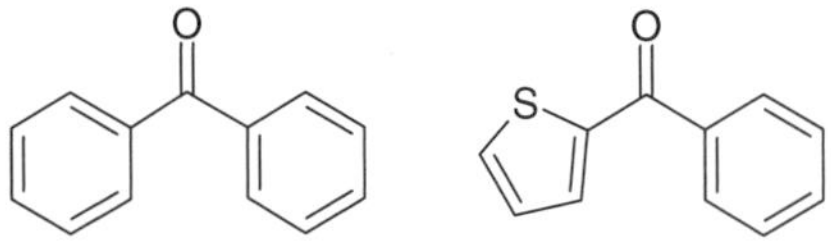

The presence of OH, NH_2, NHR, or SH on either ring in a position *ortho* to the ketone group will prevent the rule from firing.

Imino-*N*-Oxides

Several imino-N-oxides have been shown to be photoallergens, e.g., chlorodiazepoxide (25), olaquindox (26), and sodium omadine (27). Structural alerts for these chemicals are shown below:

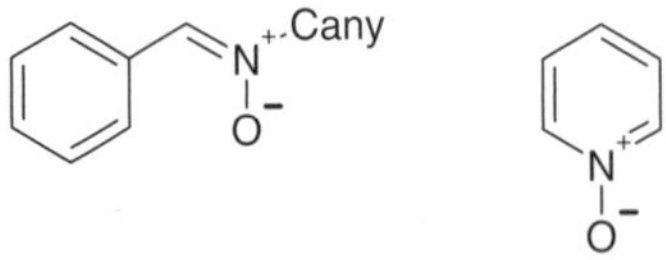

Cany = any carbon atom.

The mechanism of action of imino-*N*-oxides is believed to be via isomerization to highly reactive oxaziridines on irradiation with UV light (28) followed by covalent binding to skin proteins

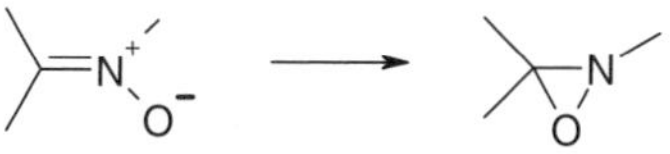

Several chemicals containing the above structural alerts have been found to bind covalently to proteins on irradiation with UV light (6,28–30), indicating their potential to be photoallergens.

Tetracyclines

Most of the evidence from studies of photosensitization by tetracyclines supports the view that the primary event is a phototoxic effect arising from the generation of singlet oxygen, rather than a photoallergic effect from the photochemical binding of a tetracycline ligand to skin protein (31,32). The role of singlet oxygen in the process is demonstrated by the fact that phototoxicity is increased in the presence of deuterium oxide and decreased in the presence of sodium azide (33). It has also been shown that tetracyclines can also be converted to a number of phototoxic photoproducts on irradiation with UV light (33,34).

A structural alert for the prospective identification of tetracycline phototoxicity is as follows:

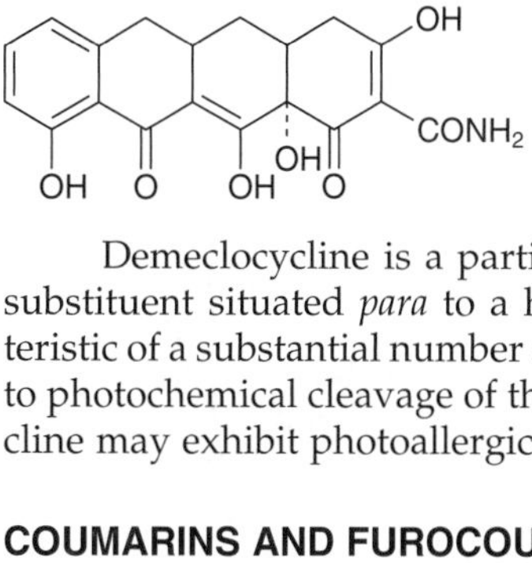

Demeclocycline is a particularly potent tetracycline that contains a 7-chloro substituent situated *para* to a hydroxyl group. This chemical grouping is characteristic of a substantial number of haloaromatic photoallergens which are active due to photochemical cleavage of the carbon–halogen bond, indicating that demeclocycline may exhibit photoallergic as well as phototoxic potential.

COUMARINS AND FUROCOUMARINS

A number of coumarins and furocoumarins are reported to be photoallergens (35) and have also been shown to photobind to proteins (6,36,37), including 8-methoxypsoralen, better known as a chemical that binds photochemically to DNA.

A proposed mechanism for the photochemical reaction of these chemicals, e.g., 6-methylcoumarin, with proteins is that the chemicals undergo photodimerization on irradiation with UV light and it is the photodimer that then reacts covalently with skin proteins.

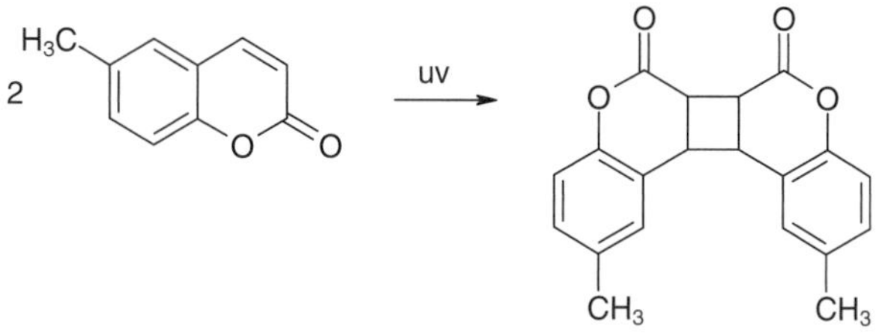

The rationale behind this hypothesis is that the resonance stabilization of 6-methyl coumarin renders it insufficiently reactive to form conjugates with proteins in the absence of irradiation. In the absence of the resonance stabilization, the photodimer is now able to bind covalently to protein via an acylation mechanism. Further support to this hypothesis is given by the fact that unlike 6-methylcoumarin, dihydrocoumarin is reported to be a contact allergen (38).

6-Methylcoumarin, 7-methyl coumarin, 7-methoxycoumarin, and 7-ethoxy-4-methylcoumarin are all reported to be photoallergens, but coumarin itself is not a photoallergen. Of the furocoumarins, psoralen, 5-methoxypsoralen, and 8-methoxypsoralen are all reported to be photoirritant (phototoxic), but 5,8-dimethoxypsoralen is inactive (38). On the basis of the above data, the structural alert for these chemicals is

where R_2 or R_3 must be sp^2 or sp^3 carbon or O-sp^2 or O-sp^3 carbon and O-alkyl substituents on both R_1 and R_4 will prevent the rule from firing.

HOW IMPORTANT ARE PARTITION PARAMETERS?

The toxicity of a chemical depends on two factors. First it must be transported from its site of administration to its site of action; then it must bind to or react with a receptor or target; i.e., biological activity is a function of partition and reactivity (39).

In the foregoing sections, some criteria for predicting from its chemical structure, whether or not a chemical may possess the requisite photochemical reactivity to be a photoallergen or phototoxin have been explored. In order to be photoallergens or phototoxins, all of the chemicals used to support the proposed structural alerts must be capable of partitioning to their sites of activity simply from the fact that they are all active chemicals. Other chemicals, however, may possess the appropriate photochemical reactivity to be photoallergens or photo-toxins, but as a result of their polarity and/or size, may not penetrate the skin sufficiently to be active in vivo. This point is exemplified by Rose Bengal, a potent photosensitizer, which has been shown to cause only negligible phototoxicity when applied topically to normal skin (40). Rose Bengal is a polar molecule with a high molecular weight, both properties that preclude it from penetrating readily through the skin.

For chemicals where the route of administration is via the gut, similar criteria will apply.

A STRATEGY FOR THE IDENTIFICATION OF PHOTOALLERGENS AND PHOTOTOXINS

Using the structural alerts, the structure of the chemical is examined to see if it has the reactivity potential to be a photoallergen or phototoxin. This process can be carried out either by inspection or by using a computerized expert system such as

DEREK for Windows (3,4). If no structural alert is found, either the chemical does not possess the requisite reactivity, or its reactivity is outside the scope of the current structural alerts. In many cases, absence of photochemical reactivity may be confirmed by inspection of the chemical structure. For chemicals that do not possess the appropriate photochemical reactivity, no further evaluation is required. For chemicals that are found to possess the appropriate photochemical reactivity, the second step is to assess their skin permeability/partition parameters. This involves the use of physicochemical parameters such as log octanol/water partition coefficient (log P) and the molecular weight or molecular volume of the chemical, from which an assessment of skin permeability can be made (41,42).

One major advantage of a strategy such as the one outlined above is that it allows the evaluation of the photoallergic or phototoxic potential of a new chemical even before it has been synthesized. Such an approach is extremely valuable for reducing the use of animals either in screening out potentially toxic chemicals or in providing data for making positive classifications of toxicity.

REFERENCES

1. Epstein JH. Photoallergy—a review. Arch Dermatol 1972; 106:741–8.
2. Kochevar IE. Photoallergic responses to chemicals. Photochem Photobiol 1979; 30:437–42.
3. Sanderson DM, Earnshaw CG. Computer prediction of possible toxic action from chemical structure; The DEREK system. Hum Exp Toxicol 1991; 10:261–73.
4. Ridings JE, Barratt MD, Cary R, et al. Computer prediction of possible toxic action from chemical structure: an update on the DEREK system. Toxicology 1996; 106:267–79.
5. Barratt MD. Structure–activity relationships and prediction of the phototoxicity and phototoxic potential of new drugs. Altern Lab Anim 2004; 32:511–24.
6. Barratt MD, Brown KR. Photochemical binding of photoallergens to human serum albumin: a simple in vitro method for screening potential photoallergens. Toxicol Lett 1985; 24:1–6.
7. Pendlington RU, Barratt MD. Molecular basis of photocontact allergy. Int J Cosmet Sci 1990; 12:91–103.
8. Delahanty JN, Evans JC, Rowlands CC, et al. An electron spin resonance study of the free radicals formed on ultraviolet irradiation of the photoallergens fentichlor and bithionol. J Chem Soc Faraday Trans I 1987; 83:135–9.
9. Chignell CF. Free radicals in drug-induced photosensitivity reactions: spin trapping study of photoallergenic halogenated salicylanilides. In: Hayaishi O, Niki E, Kondo M, et al. eds. Medical, Biochemical and Chemical Aspects of Free Radicals. Amsterdam: Elsevier Science Publishers, 1989:209–12.
10. Son EA, Yugai SG. Case of photodermatosis due to long term treatment with amiodarone. Klin Med 1992; 70:46.
11. Wilkinson DS. Photodermatitis due to tetrachlorosalicylanilide. Br J Dermat 1961; 73:213–9.
12. Reavy HJ, Traynor NJ, Gibbs NK. Photogenotoxicity of skin phototumorigenic fluoroquinolone antibiotics detected using the comet assay. Photochem Photobiol 1997; 66:368–73.
13. Chignell CF, Kalyanaraman B, Mason RP, et al. Spectroscopic studies of cutaneous photosensitizing agents—I. Spin trapping of photolysis products from sulfanilamide, 4-aminobenzoic acid and related compounds. Photochem Photobiol 1980; 32:563–71.
14. Chignell CF, Kalyanaraman B, Sik RH, et al. Spectroscopic studies of cutaneous photosensitizing agents—II. Spin trapping of photolysis products from sulfanilamide and 4-aminobenzoic acid using 5,5-dimethyl-1-pyrroline-1-oxide. Photochem Photobiol 1981; 34:147–56.

15. Motten AG, Chignell CF. Spectroscopic studies of cutaneous photosensitizing agents—III. Spin trapping of photolysis products from sulfanilamide analogs. Photochem Photobiol 1983; 37:17–26.
16. Ford RA. Photoallergenicity testing of fragrance material. A review on photoallergy by musk ambrette in male human patients. Nippon Koshohin Kagakkaishi 1984; 8:301–4.
17. Wisneski HS, Havery DC. Nitro musks in fragrance products: update of FDA findings. Cosmet Toiletries 1996; 111:73–6.
18. Motten AG, Chignell CF, Mason RP. Spectroscopic studies of cutaneous photosensitizing agents—VI. Identification of the free radicals generated during the photolysis of musk ambrette, musk xylene and musk ketone. Photochem Photobiol 1983; 38:671–8.
19. Beijersbergen van Henegouwen GMJ. Medicinal photochemistry; phototoxic and photo-therapeutic aspects of drugs. In: Testa B, Meyer UA, eds. Advances in Drug Research. Vol. 29. London: Academic Press, 1997:79–170.
20. Mozzanica N, Pigatto PD. Contact and photocontact allergy to ketoprofen, clinical and experimental study. Contact Dermatitis 1990; 23:336–40.
21. Ophaswongse H, Maibach HI. Topical nonsteroidal anti-inflammatory drugs: allergic and photoallergic contact dermatitis and phototoxicity. Contact Dermatitis 1993; 29:57–64.
22. Jeanmougin M, Manciet JR, Deprost Y, et al. Photoallergy induced by fenofibrate. Ann Dermatol Venereol 1993; 120:549–54.
23. Kurumaji Y, Ohshiro Y, Miyamoto C, et al. Allergic photocontact dermatitis due to suprofen, photo-patch testing and cross-reaction study. Contact Dermatitis 1991; 25:218–23.
24. Bosca F, Miranda MA. Photosensitizing drugs containing the benzophenone chromophore. J Photochem Photobiol B 1998; 43:1–26.
25. Garcia-Bravo B, Rodriguez-Pichardo A, Camacho F. Contact dermatitis from diazepoxides. Contact Dermatitis 1994; 30:40.
26. Francalanci S, Gola M, Giorgini S. Occupational photocontact dermatitis from olaquindox. Contact Dermatitis 1986; 15:112–4.
27. Maguire HC, Jr., Kaidbey K. Experimental photoallergic contact dermatitis: a mouse model. J Invest Dermatol 1982; 79:147–52.
28. Bakri A, Beijersbergen van Henegouwen GMJ, de Vries H. Photobinding of some 7-chloro-1,4-benzodiazepines to human plasma protein in vitro and photopharmacology of diazepam in the rat. Pharm Weekbl Sci 1988; 10:122–9.
29. De Vries H, Bojarski J, Donker AA, et al. Photochemical reactions of quindoxin, carbadox and cyadox with protein, indicating photoallergic properties. Toxicology 1990; 63:85–95.
30. Pöhlmann H, Theil FP, Franke P, et al. In vitro- und in vivo-Untersuchungen zur fotochemische Reaktivität von Methaqualon-1-oxid. Pharmazie 1986; 41:856–8.
31. Hasan T, Kochevar IE, McAuliffe DJ, et al. Mechanism of tetracycline phototoxicity. J Invest Dermatol 1984; 83:179–83.
32. Lasarow RM, Isseroff RR, Gomez EC. Quantitative in vitro assessment of phototoxicity by a fibroblast-neutral red assay. J Invest Dermatol 1992; 98:725–9.
33. Shea CR, Olack GA, Morrison H, et al. Phototoxicity of lumidocycline. J Invest Dermatol 1993; 101:329–33.
34. Drexel RE, Olack GA, Jones C, et al. Lumitetracycline: a novel new tetracycline photoproduct. J Org Chem 1990; 55:2471–8.
35. Kaidbey KH, Kligman AM. Photomaximisation test for identifying contact sensitisers. Contact Dermatitis 1980; 6:161–9.
36. Schoonderwoerd SA, Beijersbergen van Henegouwen GMJ, Persons CC, et al. Photobinding of 8-methoxypsoralen, 4,6,4'-trimethylangelicin and chlorpromazine to Wistar rat epidermal biomacromolecules in vivo. J Photochem Photobiol 1991; 10:257–68.
37. Schmitt IM, Chimenti S, Gasparro FP. Psoralen-protein photochemistry—a forgotten field. J Photochem Photobiol 1995; 27:101–7.
38. Opdyke DL. Die Struktur-Aktivität-Beziehungen einiger substituiter Cumarine in bezug auf Hautreaktionen. Dragoco Report (German Fragrance Edition) 1981; 28:71–6.

39. Dearden JC. Physico-chemical descriptors. In: Karcher W, Devillers J, eds. Practical Applications of Quantitative Structure–Activity Relationships (QSAR) in Environmental Chemistry and Toxicology. Dordrecht, The Netherlands: Kluwer Academic Publishers, 1990:25–59.
40. Wachter E, Dees C, Harkins J, et al. Topical Rose Bengal: preclinical evaluation of pharmacokinetics and safety. Lasers Surg Med 2003; 32:101–10.
41. Potts RO, Guy R. Predicting skin permeability. Pharm Res 1992; 9:663–9.
42. Barratt MD. Quantitative structure–activity relationships for skin permeability. Toxicol in Vitro 1995; 9:27–37.

29 Potential Regulatory Use of (Q)SARs to Develop Dermal Irritation and Corrosion Assessment Strategies

Ingrid Gerner
Weidenauer Weg, Berlin, Germany

Etje Hulzebos, Emiel Rorije, and Betty Hakkert
National Institute for Public Health and the Environment, Expertise Centre for Substances, Bilthoven, The Netherlands

John D. Walker
TSCA Interagency Testing Committee, Office of Pollution Prevention and Toxics, U.S. Environmental Protection Agency, Washington, D.C., U.S.A.

Matthias Herzler
Federal Institute for Risk Assessment, Safety of Substances and Preparations, Thielallee, Berlin, Germany

Horst Spielmann
Federal Institute for Risk Assessment, Centre for Alternative Methods to Animal Experiments—ZEBET, Diedersdorfer Weg, Berlin, Germany

INTRODUCTION

Legislation on the control of chemicals requires assessment of their inherent properties in order to predict risks for human health and the environment. In the European Union (EU), chemicals legislation is based on the "Dangerous Substances Directive" of 1967 (Directive 67/548/EEC) and its subsequent amendments (1). While legislative requirements for hazard assessment are clear, efforts to harmonize ideas between industry and the member states with respect to risk assessment have been slow for some end points. Therefore, in the EU, these initiatives are described in the *White Paper on a Strategy for a Future Chemicals Policy* as a framework for the Registration, Evaluation, and Authorization of Chemicals (REACH) (2). This new EU policy underlines the needs for the development of valid in vitro and (quantitative) structure–activity relationship [(Q)SAR] models for toxicological assessment of all untested chemicals that are already on the market. This policy makes use of all available information on a chemical prior to any considerations on further testing, especially prior to any in vivo testing. The REACH text has now been outlined (3).

Dermal contact constitutes one of the most common routes of human exposure to chemical substances used, e.g., at home, at the work place, or in any other circumstances, where chemicals may be released intentionally or accidentally. Therefore, potential risks after dermal contact with a chemical substance need to be assessed. For hazard assessment, internationally agreed protocols for toxicity testing are provided as standardized toxicological test guidelines published by the Organization for Economic Co-operation and Development (OECD). Results of such toxicity testing are translated by applying valid toxicological models into classification and labeling of the detected hazards according to internationally harmonized systems, such as the EU system (4) or the Globally Harmonized System (GHS) of the United Nations (5).

REGULATORY ASSESSMENT OF ACUTE DERMAL TOXICITY

With respect to acute dermal contact, hazardous properties to be classified and labeled are those causing (*i*) mortality within two weeks after single contact (due to the toxic chemical being able to penetrate the skin in lethal doses), (*ii*) acute irritation or corrosion after single contact with skin, and (*iii*) skin sensitization after multiple skin contacts.

For new industrial chemicals, it has been suggested that testing for acute dermal toxicity for regulatory purposes is only appropriate for substances that have demonstrated toxic potential after oral administration (6). Among 1226 substances tested for acute dermal toxicity, according to current EU legislation for new chemicals (1), only 52 (4.2%) have been classified important for acute dermal toxicity. All of these new chemicals were previously classified for acute oral toxicity and/or for severe skin corrosion. Hence, acute systemic toxicity after dermal contact with a new industrial chemical is a rare effect. It is proposed to test only those chemicals for further acute dermal toxicity that show some acute oral toxicity and skin irritation. Assessment of hazardous properties with respect to acute dermal contact with a new industrial chemical for regulatory purposes is therefore normally restricted to assessment of skin sensitization potential and assessment of skin irritation or corrosion potential, also taking into account possible photometabolism of chemicals on and within skin tissue.

ASSESSMENT OF SKIN IRRITATION AND CORROSION POTENTIAL

In the EU, evaluation of skin irritation/corrosion potential is mandatory as part of the basic set of toxicological tests in all major chemical assessment programs, e.g., for cosmetics, industrial chemicals, and pesticides or biocides. Classification and labeling of properties of a chemical leading to skin irritation or corrosion is based on specific limit values for results observed in a standardized Draize skin irritation test using rabbits [one of the official test methods described in Annex V to Directive 67/548/EEC as well as in the OECD Test Guidelines (7), and in the Health Effects Test Guidelines of the U.S. Environmental Protection Agency (8)]. Therefore, all alternatives to this animal test should provide results that can be translated into information with respect to classification limits defined for results of a standardized Draize skin irritation test (7). REACH guidance on the assessment of the skin irritation end point assessment is currently being developed to interpret alternative methods in this way (3).

Dermal corrosion is defined as the production of irreversible damage to skin, namely visible necrosis through the epidermis and into the dermis, following the application of a test substance for up to four hours. Corrosive reactions are typified by ulcers, bleeding, bloody scabs and, by the end of observation of

14 days, by discoloration due to blanching of the skin, complete areas of alopecia, and scars. Dermal irritation is defined by Draize results demonstrating the production of reversible damage of the skin following the application of a test substance for up to four hours (1,5,9). Substances may be classified as skin irritants because they cause:

- Moderate but persistent erythema and scaling, without any signs of edema, or
- Severe edema over a period of one week, which is not accompanied by relevant erythema.

These definitions as well as toxicological experience demonstrate one of the principal difficulties for comparisons between results of the Draize rabbit test and results of alternative techniques: two substances may receive the same classification and labeling based on different effects, in different skin tissues, caused by different mechanisms. Therefore, the Draize test with rabbits can only be replaced by alternative methods if these methods are combined within testing and assessment strategies that take into account relevant mechanisms of skin irritation or corrosion. Within these strategies, classification and labeling for skin irritation/corrosion can be derived by evaluating:

- Specific physicochemical properties and peculiarities of the chemical structure using (Q)SARs and
- Biological reactivity using results of specific in vitro test methods.

Development of toxicological models such as (Q)SARs, in vitro test methods, and their combination is based on biological/biochemical mechanisms for triggering corrosion or skin irritation by a chemical substance (10). Several mechanisms and a cascade of reactions can lead to erythema, edema, crust formation, and necrosis to skin. As a result of an extensive evaluation of data submitted within the EU notification procedure for new chemicals, systems to support alternative testing methods and strategies for local irritation and corrosion were developed using the data submitted to regulators (11,12). Development of these systems and strategies has to take into account that there is either no general "irritation/corrosion potential" with respect to dermal contact with a chemical, or skin corrosive lesions are produced by mechanisms different from those that cause skin irritation (13,14). Furthermore, it is crucial to assure that alternative methods model exclusively irritation to *skin* tissues and not irritation to other living tissues such as, e.g., that of the eye. When evaluating the new chemicals database of the BfR (13), it was found that the results of a Draize test on rabbit skin in many cases differ from the results of a Draize test on rabbit eyes with the same substance. Several chemicals that did not cause skin irritation caused irritation or even corrosion of eye tissues, and vice versa (14).

- Among 1855 chemicals tested for skin irritation/corrosion potential, 1004 (54.1%) did not induce any signs of irritation in the skin of rabbits, while 132 chemicals (7.1%) had to be labeled "R38, irritating to skin," and 106 chemicals (5.7%) caused skin corrosion; the remaining 613 substances (33.0%) showed skin irritation properties below the limit for classification. Using the European Chemicals Bureau (ECB) chemical database of new chemicals, Hoffmann and colleagues from the Joint Research Centre (JRC) of the European Commission have recently published very similar percentages for skin lesion potential of industrial chemicals (15).

■ Among the 1004 chemicals that did not induce any signs of skin irritation, 87 substances (8.7%) had to be labeled "R36, irritating to eyes," and 110 (11.0%) caused serious damage to eyes.

■ Among 132 chemicals labeled R38 due to their skin irritation potentials, 20 (15.2%) caused only slight conjunctival irritation, which was reversible within three days!

The regulatory acceptance of alternative assessment tools and their combination within testing and assessment strategies will depend on their ability to translate into internationally accepted classification and labeling systems. Therefore, demonstration of links between the alternatives [such as (Q)SARs, in vitro, or ex vivo methods] and the mechanisms known to induce lesions of the skin would increase regulatory acceptance of these techniques. Furthermore, a proper description of (Q)SARs and in vitro methods is required to evaluate what they are really predicting.

(Q)SARs should be reported according to the OECD principles on (Q)SARs (16–19). The information required is the definition of the end point, the algorithm, the applicability domain (AD), the evaluation process and—this is very important—the mechanism that the (Q)SAR is predicting. This means that (Q)SARs need to give information comparable to OECD guidelines on testing. A guidance document on these OECD principles has been drafted and is available on the ECB website (20). This text is currently being reviewed by the OECD and the final version will be released by the end of 2006 or early in 2007.

The general (Q)SAR model description is needed, but is not sufficient to evaluate the prediction of the skin irritation potential of a specific chemical. Therefore, the assessment has to include how the chemical can be assessed by the specific model, e.g., whether the substance is in or outside the AD, as well as the performance of the model for that specific type of chemicals. The reliability of the model prediction should be assessed. This evaluation of the prediction results and scoring of their reliability is similar to evaluation of the results of a chemical being tested.

The last information level is to put the outcome of the first steps and their reliability into the overall assessment depending on the requirements of a specific framework. This framework can be hazard assessment, EU classification and labeling purposes, and/or risk assessment but also e.g., priority setting or the waiving of testing requirements as laid down in e.g., Annex XI to the REACH text (3). These information levels indicate the information required by regulators in order to be able to use (Q)SAR and/or in vitro model outcome for regulatory purposes.

MECHANISMS LEADING TO IRRITATION OR CORROSION OF SKIN

For organic chemicals, the mechanisms that lead to skin irritation can normally be described as a two-stage process in which a chemical at first has to penetrate the stratum corneum and then trigger a biological response in the deeper epidermal or dermal layers (21,22). Harold (23) and Lansdown and Grasso (24) have described this process for surface-active agents. Surface-active agents increase skin permeability by reacting with proteins (e.g., by denaturing keratin) and subsequently cause skin irritation. Berner et al. (25) illustrated this for chemicals having a pKa <4 or ≥8. Nangia et al. (26) showed that pKa based skin irritancy is induced with minimal stratum corneum damage.

For strong inorganic acids and bases, no stratum corneum penetration is needed because they erode the stratum corneum. According to the Technical Guidance Document supporting Commission Directive 93/67/EEC on risk assessment for new notified and existing substances (27), the percutaneous absorption of acrylates, quaternary ammonium ions, heterocyclic ammonium ions, and sulfonium salts is slow, since these chemicals are binding to macromolecules in skin. As a result of binding, corrosion can occur as the stratum corneum is eroded.

At this time, the following mechanisms are proposed (10) for inducing skin irritation or skin corrosion by affecting the structure and function of the stratum corneum (28):

1. Skin irritation:
    a. Reaction with skin proteins and interference with lipids in the stratum corneum (29) by surface-active agents and
    b. Dissolution of skin fat and disintegration of skin by low molecular weight organic chemicals (30).
2. Skin corrosion:
    a. Erosion of the stratum corneum by most inorganic acids and bases and by strong organic acids with pH <2.0 and bases with pH >11.5 (31) and
    b. Binding to skin components in the stratum corneum by cationic surfactants (32); and percutaneous absorption of acrylates, quaternary ammonium ions, heterocyclic ammonium ions, and sulfonium salts (27).
3. Skin irritation and corrosion:
    a. Penetration of the stratum corneum by anionic or non-surfactant organic chemicals with sufficient hydrophobic and hydrophilic properties and
    b. Elicitation of a cytotoxic response in the epidermis or dermis, where the severity of the cytotoxic response may determine whether irritation or corrosion occurs (33).

SKIN IRRITATION/CORROSION ASSESSMENT USING STEPWISE STRATEGIES (SICRET)

Combinations of physicochemical property limits demonstrating the absence of any relevant skin lesion potential (34) and structural alerts for skin irritation/corrosion potential (35) can help to develop procedures that could be used by both regulatory authorities and industry to decide on provisional classification, thereby simplifying the identification of a relevant testing strategy and reducing (or abolishing) the need for animal testing. A decision tree model for assessment of corrosion and skin irritation avoiding any animal test was recently developed and published by regulators [Fig. 1, adopted from a publication of Walker et al. (36)].

Figure 1 describes the Skin Irritation Corrosion Rules Estimation Tool (SICRET) that was developed to allow others to estimate whether their chemicals are likely to cause skin irritation or skin corrosion. SICRET uses physicochemical property limits to identify chemicals *with no* skin corrosion or skin irritation potential. If a chemical's physicochemical properties do not meet the prescribed limits to identify chemicals *with no* skin corrosion or skin irritation potential, then the chemical's structural alerts are used to identify chemicals *with* skin corrosion or

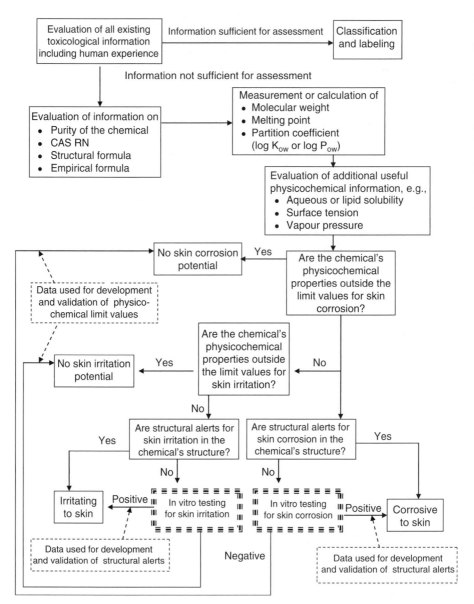

FIGURE 1 The skin irritation corrosion rules estimation tool. *Abbreviation*: CAS RN, Chemical Abstracts Service registry numbers. *Source*: Adopted from Ref. 36.

skin irritation potential. If a chemical does not contain structural alerts that indicate it has skin corrosion or skin irritation potential, then in vitro skin corrosion or skin irritation testing is conducted. If the in vitro skin corrosion or skin irritation testing is positive, then the data are included in feedback loops for development of new structural alerts to identify chemicals *with* skin corrosion or skin irritation potential.

If in vitro testing for skin corrosion or skin irritation is negative then the data are included in feedback loops for development of new physicochemical property limits to identify chemicals *with no* skin corrosion or skin irritation potential. The use of in vitro tests was proposed as a safety net to identify new structural alerts for chemicals *with* skin corrosion or skin irritation potential or new physicochemical property limits to identify chemicals *with no* skin corrosion or skin irritation potential. In summary, SICRET is a "battery approach" that uses (Q)SARs and in vitro tests to classify chemicals that cause skin irritation or skin corrosion without further animal testing.

Development and validation of in vitro and ex vivo methods has led to OECD Test Guidelines for assessment of corrosivity with alternative methods to testing with animals (37,38). Development and official validation of in vitro and ex vivo methods for assessment of skin irritation potential is a current project of the European Centre for the Validation of Alternative Methods at the European JRC in Ispra, Italy (39–41). Development and evaluation of (Q)SARs to be used within SICRET was reported in detail recently (14,34,35) and is summarized in the following chapter.

REGULATORY NEEDS FOR THE EVALUATION OF (Q)SARS

As mentioned above, regulators have already published a hazard assessment tool— SICRET (36)—with identification of physicochemical property limits for chemicals that do not cause skin irritation or corrosion (34), characterization of structural alerts for chemicals that cause skin irritation or corrosion (35), and integration of these limits and alerts into a testing and assessment strategy which also uses results of in vitro testing. This tool is in accordance with recently published guidance for developing and using (Q)SARs (20,42–46). In the following chapter, a detailed report on the development of (Q)SARs to be used within the SICRET assessment strategy will be given. Within REACH, industry has the responsibility to make chemical safety assessments and hence, industry and regulators need guidance on how to interpret (Q)SAR models, the predictions, and the overall assessment including all information available. An outline is proposed below for how (Q)SARs and other not (yet) accepted test methods can be used in the regulatory assessment of chemicals.

First, the model/methodology needs to be described in sufficient detail [see section (Q)SAR Model Evaluation]. Next, the actual (Q)SAR prediction for a specific chemical must be given and characterized with regard to its reliability [see section Evaluation of (Q)SAR Predictions]. The (Q)SAR information needs to be indented with other available information on that particular chemical to identify results relevant for, e.g., hazard evaluation, classification and labeling, priority setting and/or risk assessment in a so-called Weight of Evidence (WoE) approach before in vivo testing is carried out (see section Regulatory Decision using a WoE Approach). The SICRET tool described above can be seen as a good example for such a WoE approach which combines (Q)SARs and in vitro tests. The WoE concept has also been officially laid down in the Annex XI of the REACH text (3) as a means to conclude on the presence or absence of specific adverse health effects. The different types of information available for those toxicological/regulatory end points relevant under REACH are currently evaluated and strategies for their combined use are being developed in the REACH Implementation Projects [the so-called RIPs, e.g., RIP 3.3-2, information is available via the website of the ECB, (47)].

(Q)SAR Model Evaluation

The first information level contains the information similar to the OECD Test Guidelines, and can be structured according to the OECD principles on validation. The assessment of the model according to the OECD principles for the validation of QSARs returns: (*i*) a definition of end points, (*ii*) details of the algorithm used and how transparent this algorithm is, (*iii*) the AD of the model, e.g., the physicochemical and structural characteristics/limitations of the training set, (*iv*) the predictive performance and, if possible, (*v*) the underlying mechanism of action. These results will be reported in a standardized QSAR Model Reporting Format (QModelRF). These QModelRFs have a similar function as testing guidelines for chemicals, which also describe in general terms a test method for a certain toxicological end point, e.g., the OECD Test Guideline 404 for skin irritation.

Application of the OECD Principles to the Use of Physical–Chemical Limits (First Step in SICRET)

The defined end point for this type of rule consists of the absence of a need for EU classification for skin irritation/corrosion hazard under the EU and basically also the GHS, classification and labeling framework. In this case, the "algorithms" are given in the form of individual rules, each of them associated with its own AD and individual sensitivity, specificity, and predictivity. The underlying mechanism is that skin absorption is usually needed for skin lesions and that the physical chemical cutoff values indicates limited dermal absorption. These principles are described in detail in the following chapter.

Application of OECD Principles to the Use of Structural Alerts (in SICRET)

The defined end point for structural alerts is specific reactivity, which is related to the need for skin lesion classification and labeling. These algorithms consist of alerts including the description of the neighboring fragments, each of them having its own sensitivity, specificity, and predictivity. The mechanism explanation is given by the assumption that chemicals containing the alert are seen as susceptible to reaction with proteins, as, e.g., nucleophilic groups in proteins will attack electrophilic centers in chemicals.

The ECB is establishing an inventory of (Q)SAR models to make this type of information available, while OECD is developing a (Q)SAR toolbox that should help regulators using (Q)SAR (see the OECD and ECB websites for the latest developments).

Evaluation of (Q)SAR Predictions

The next information level contains the evaluation of the prediction of the model for a specific chemical. Only if the chemical is within the application domain of a specific algorithm or rule is a scientifically sound prediction possible. In order to characterize the reliability of the outcome of the prediction, a more detailed analysis of the AD with regard to its representative coverage of the relevant part of (physico)chemical space, to the even/uneven distribution of the training set of chemicals over the AD, and to the position of the chemical within it, is needed, as well as a description of the statistical figures of merit (sensitivity, specificity, and predictivity etc.) in internal/external validation exercises. Finally, mechanistic reasoning can help to increase or decrease the reliability of the prediction. The reporting of this information level step is similar to the information that is given for a chemical in a test report based on an OECD Test Guideline.

Regulatory Decision Using a WoE Approach

In the last information level, that is the WoE, all the information will be gathered and (Q)SAR predictions are one part of this information. In the OECD 404 testing strategy, this is already indicated, and the SICRET tool is an example of this approach (36). Even if not all information is available, according to current guidelines, the overall assessment can be used to assess the (absence of) skin lesion potential.

Prerequisites of such a WoE approach are indicated in REACH. Annex XI of the REACH (3) requires gathering all information such as in vitro, in silico [(Q)SARs], and other information, which may be less robust, but should all be evaluated to come to a conclusion on the hazard, before animal testing is warranted.

The great advantage of the three information levels approach as reported here is that information on (Q)SAR models is made transparent in a standardized way. It is expected that it will be the responsibility of the model developer to provide the necessary information on the model (model information level). The reliability of the prediction will be given by the model and/or will need to be interpreted by the user of the prediction (prediction information level). The quality of the model and its prediction can be objectively and scientifically evaluated (WoE information level). Out of the WoE approach a regulatory decision will be extracted, either that sufficient evidence is available to conclude on the absence or presence of an effect, necessity of classification and labeling etc. and whether or not further in vitro or in vivo testing is required for that specific decision.

ACKNOWLEDGMENTS

The authors wish to acknowledge Dutch Organization for Health Research and Development—ZonM, ECB and the Dutch Ministry of Housing and Spatial Planning for their financial contribution to the evaluation of (Q)SARs research. The authors are indebted Maaike van Zijverden (RIVM) for critical comments on the manuscript.

REFERENCES

1. European Commission. Commission Directive 2004/73/EC of 29 April 2004 adapting to technical progress for the twenty-ninth time Council Directive 67/548/EEC on the approximation of the laws, regulations and administrative provisions relating to the classification, packaging and labelling of dangerous substances. Off J Eur Union 2004; L152:1–311.
2. European Commission. White Paper on a Strategy for a Future Chemicals Policy. Brussels: Commission of the European Communities, 2003. (Accessed May 2006 at http://europa.eu.int/comm/environment/chemicals/whitepaper.htm)
3. ECB. REACH Text on Annex XI. (Accessed September 2006 at http://ecb.jrc.it/DOCUMENTS/REACH/REACH_PROPOSAL/COUNCIL_COMMON_POSITION_-JUNE_2006/st07524.en06.pdf)

4. European Commission. Annex VI of the Directive 67/548/EEC. General classification and labelling requirements for dangerous substances and preparations. Off J Eur Communities 2001; L225:263–314.

5. United Nations. Globally Harmonized System of classification and labelling of chemicals. UN ST/SG/AC.10/30, United Nations Publications sales no. E.03.II.E.25. United Nations, New York/Geneva, 2003.

6. Indans I, Fry T, Parson P, et al. Classification and labelling of new industrial chemicals for acute toxicity, skin and eye irritation. Hum Exp Toxicol 1998; 17:529.

7. OECD. Guideline for Testing of Chemicals No.404: Acute Dermal Irritation/Corrosion. Paris: OECD, 2002:1–13.

8. EPA (U.S. Environmental Protection Agency. Office of Pollution Prevention and Toxics). Health Effects Test Guidelines. Acute Dermal Irritation. Washington DC: EPA, 1998.

9. OECD. Harmonised system for the classification of chemicals which cause skin irritation/corrosion. In: OECD, Harmonised integrated classification system for human health and environmental hazards of chemical substances and mixtures. ENV/JM/MONO(2001)6. Paris: Organisation for economic cooperation and development, 2001:25–30.

10. Walker JD, Gerner I, Hulzebos E, et al. (Q)SARs for predicting skin irritation and corrosion: mechanisms, transparency and applicability of predictions. QSAR Comb Sci 2004; 23:721–5.

11. Zinke S, Gerner I, Graetschel G, et al. Local irritation/corrosion testing strategies: development of a decision support system for the introduction of alternative methods. Altern lab anim 2000; 28:29–40.

12. Zinke S, Gerner I. Local irritation/corrosion testing strategies: extending a decision support system by applying self-learning classifiers. Altern lab anim 2000; 28:651–63.

13. Gerner I, Graetschel G, Kahl J, et al. Development of a decision support system for the introduction of alternative methods into local irritation/corrosion testing strategies: development of a relational data base. Altern lab anim 2000; 28:11–28.

14. Gerner I, Zinke S, Graetschel G, et al. Development of a decision support system for the introduction of alternative methods into local irritancy/corrosivity testing strategies. Creation of fundamental rules for a decision support system. Altern lab anim 2000; 28:665–98.

15. Hoffmann S, Cole T, Hartung T. Skin irritation: prevalence, variability, and regulatory classification of existing in vivo data from industrial chemicals. Regul Toxicol Pharmacol 2005; 41:159–66.

16. Eriksson L, Jaworska JS, Worth AP, et al. Methods for reliability, uncertainty assessment, and applicability evaluations of classification and regression based QSARs. Environ Health Perspect 2003; 22:361–1375.

17. OECD. The Report from the Expert Group on (Quantitative) Structure Activity Relationships [(Q)SARs] on the Principles for the Validation of (Q)SARs. OECD Series on Testing and Assessment No. 49. ENV/JM/MONO(2004)24. Paris, France: OECD, 2004:206. (Accessed June 2006 at http://www.oecd.org/document/23/0,2340,en_2649_34365_33957015_1_1_1_1,00.html)

18. Walker JD, Jaworska JS, Comber MHI, et al. Guidelines for developing and using quantitative structure activity relationships. Environ Toxicol Chem 2003; 22:1653–65.

19. Walker JD, Carlsen L, Jaworska JS. Improving opportunities for regulatory acceptance of QSARs: the importance of model domain, uncertainty, validity and predictability. QSAR Comb Sci 2003; 22:346–50.

20. Worth AP, Bassan A, Gallegos A, et al. The Characterisation of (Quantitative) Structure–Activity Relationships: Preliminary Guidance. ECB Report, 2005. (Accessed August 2006 at http://ecb.jrc.it/QSAR/home.php?CONTENU=/QSAR/qsar_tools/sommaire.php)

21. Barratt MD. Quantitative structure–activity relationships for skin permeability. Toxicol In Vitro 1995; 9:27–37.

22. Schaefer H, Redelmeier TE. Principles of Percutaneous Absorption. Basel: Karger AG, 1996:21–42.

23. Harold SP. Denaturation of epidermal keratin by surface active agents. J Invest Dermatol 1959; 32:581–8.
24. Lansdown ABG, Grasso P. Physico-chemical factors influencing epidermal damage by surface active agents. Br J Dermatol 1972; 86:361–73.
25. Berner B, Wilson DR, Steffens RJ, et al. The relationship between pKa and skin irritation for a series of basic penetrants in man. Fundam Appl Toxicol 1990; 15:760–6.
26. Nangia A, Anderson PH, Berner B, et al. High dissociation constants (pKa) of basic permeants are associated with in vivo skin irritation in man. Contact Dermatitis 1996; 34:237–42.
27. European Commission. Technical guidance document on risk assessment in support of Commission Directive 93/67/EEC on risk assessment for new notified substances and Commission Regulation (EC) No 1488/94 on risk assessment for existing substances and Directive 98/8/EC of the European Parliament and of the Council concerning the placing of biocidal products on the market, 2003:214.
28. Elias PM. Structure and function of the stratum corneum permeability barrier. Drug Dev Res 1988; 13:97–105.
29. Imokawa G, Akasaki S, Minematsu Y, et al. Importance of intercellular lipids in water-retention properties of the stratum corneum: induction and recovery study of surfactant dry skin. Arch Derm Res 1989; 281:45–51.
30. Boman A. The evaluation and classification of substances with a defatting action on the skin. Ad-hoc working group on defatting substances, Stockholm, 1996, ECB/22/96-ECB/Add. 10.
31. Young JR, How MJ, Walker AP, et al. Classification as corrosive or irritant to skin of preparations containing acidic or alkaline substance without testing on animals. Toxicol In Vitro 1988; 2:19–26.
32. Schaefer H, Redelmeier TE. Principles of Percutaneous Absorption. Basel: Karger AG, 1996:165–89.
33. Barratt MD. Quantitative structure activity relationships for skin corrosivity of organic acids, bases and phenols. Toxicol Lett 1995; 75:169–76.
34. Gerner I, Walker JD, Hulzebos ET, et al. Use of physicochemical property limits to develop rules for identifying chemical substances with no skin irritation or corrosion potential. QSAR Comb Sci 2004; 23:726–33.
35. Hulzebos ET, Walker JD, Gerner I, et al. Use of structural alerts to develop rules for identifying chemical substances with skin irritation or skin corrosion potential. QSAR Comb Sci 2005; 24:332–42.
36. Walker JD, Gerner I, Hulzebos ET, et al. The skin irritation corrosion rules estimation tool (SICRET). QSAR Comb Sci 2005; 24:378–84.
37. OECD. OECD Guideline for Testing of Chemicals No. 430: In Vitro Skin Corrosion: Transcutaneous Electrical Resistance Test (TER). Paris: OECD, 2004:1–12.
38. OECD. OECD Guideline for Testing of Chemicals No. 431: In Vitro Skin Corrosion: Human Skin Model Test. Paris: OECD, 2004:1–8.
39. Botham PA. The validation of in vitro methods for skin irritation. Toxicol Lett 2004; 149:287–390.
40. Kandarova H, Liebsch M, Gerner I, et al. The EpiDerm test protocol for the upcoming ECVAM validation study on in vitro skin irritation tests—An assessment of the performance of the optimised test. Altern lab anim 2005; 33:351–67.
41. Zuang V, Balls M, Botham PA, et al. Follow-up to the ECVAM prevalidation study on in vitro tests for acute skin irritation. European centre for the validation of alternative methods skin irritation task force report 2. Altern Lab Anim 2002; 30:109–29.
42. Walker JD, Carlsen L, Hulzebos E, et al. Global government applications of analogues, SARs and QSARs to predict aquatic toxicity, chemical or physical properties, environmental fate parameters and health effects of organic chemicals. SAR QSAR Environ Res 2002; 13:607–19.
43. CEFIC (European Chemical Industry Council). Report from the workshop on regulatory acceptance of QSARs for human health and environmental endpoints, Setubal, Portugal, March 4–6, 2002:58. Report available from rbu@cefic.be

44. OECD. Organisation for Economic Co-Operation and Development Ad-Hoc Expert Group on (Q)SARS: Summary Conclusion of the 1st Meeting and Draft Work Plan. Paris: OECD, 2003.

45. Jaworska JS, Comber M, Auer C, et al. Summary of a workshop on regulatory acceptance of (Q)SARs for human and environmental endpoints. Environ Health Perspect 2003; 111:1358–60.

46. Cronin MTD, Jaworska JS, Walker JD, et al. Use of QSARs in international decision-making frameworks to predict health effects of chemical substances. Environ Health Perspect 2003; 111:1391–401.

47. http://ecb.jrc.it (Accessed June 2006).

Development of (Q)SARs for Dermal Irritation and Corrosion Assessment Using European Union New Chemicals Notification Data

Ingrid Gerner
Weidenauer Weg, Berlin, Germany

Etje Hulzebos and Emiel Rorije
National Institute for Public Health and the Environment, Expertise Centre for Substances, Bilthoven, The Netherlands

Matthias Herzler
Federal Institute for Risk Assessment, Safety of Substances and Preparations, Thielallee, Berlin, Germany

Manfred Liebsch
Federal Institute for Risk Assessment, Centre for Alternative Methods to Animal Experiments—ZEBET, Diedersdorfer Weg, Berlin, Germany

John D. Walker
TSCA Interagency Testing Committee, Office of Pollution Prevention and Toxics, U.S. Environmental Protection Agency, Washington, D.C., U.S.A.

Horst Spielmann
Federal Institute for Risk Assessment, Centre for Alternative Methods to Animal Experiments—ZEBET, Diedersdorfer Weg, Berlin, Germany

INTRODUCTION

The application of (quantitative) structure–activity relationship (Q)SARs in a regulatory context reflects a need to reduce animal testing, and was a policy aim in the European Commission's *White Paper on a Strategy for a Future Chemicals Policy* as a framework for the Registration, Evaluation and Authorization of Chemicals (REACH) (1). This policy makes use of all available relevant information on a chemical prior to any considerations on further testing, especially prior to any in vivo testing, e.g., by using (Q)SARs. In subsequent years, a number of papers have been published on commercially and publicly available (Q)SARs. In the meantime, criteria for the interpretation and evaluation of (Q)SARs, and corresponding guidance, were established (2).

In the present paper, the development of (Q)SARs for the prediction of skin irritation is reported, which is mostly based on data submitted to regulators, and comprises two main parts: one consists of exclusion rules to predict the absence of skin irritation or corrosion potential. The second provides structural alerts indicating the presence of skin irritation or corrosion potential. These (Q)SAR models are part of an integrated testing strategy (ITS), called the Skin Irritation Corrosion Rules Estimation Tool (SICRET) (3) which is comparable to the testing and assessment strategy attached to Organization for Economic Co-operation and Development (OECD) test guideline 404 (4): Like the OECD strategy, SICRET requires the assessment of all available information before any testing is started. However, if this information is not sufficient, SICRET adds to the OECD testing strategy on how (Q)SARs (which are already mentioned in OECD 404) can be used for predicting the absence or the presence of skin irritation/corrosion potential and what type of further testing is needed to make a decision on classification and labeling (see the description of SICRET and Fig. 1 in Chapter 29). Within REACH, it is permitted to go one step further: to use a weight of evidence (WoE) approach for a decision. Development and evaluation of (Q)SARs to be used within SICRET was reported in detail recently (5–9) and is summarized below.

EVALUATION OF INFORMATION SUBMITTED TO EU REGULATORS
Development of a Relational Database
A computerized database was developed in the German *Federal Institute for Risk Assessment* (BfR, former *Federal Institute for Health Protection of Consumers and Veterinary Medicine*, BgVV) with data submitted according to the new chemicals legislation in the European Union (EU) (10), using data produced according to standardized test protocols. At present, this database (11) contains the available physicochemical data and all available information on skin irritation/corrosion potential for 1855 substances (purity $\geq 95\%$).

The BfR database was created in order to develop (Q)SARs for assessing the toxic potential of chemicals. Therefore, not all the chemicals notified in the EU are considered within this database. All inorganic substances and all organic chelate complexes containing atoms of transition metals as central atoms have been discarded (because the toxicology of inorganic substances and of transition metals is different from the toxicology of "normal" organic chemicals). Thus, the database was limited to pure organic substances (purity $\geq 95\%$, with only toxicologically irrelevant impurities) that contain no heteroatoms other than oxygen, nitrogen, sulphur, phosphorus, silicon, or the halogens fluorine, chlorine, bromine, and iodine.

Within the BfR database, the chemical structure of a substance is characterized by:

■ The empirical formula,
■ The molecular weight (MW) (if applicable, subdivided into MW of the anion and MW of the cation), and
■ Specific substructures (characterizing chemical reactivity) within the structural formula.

The thermodynamic properties of a substance are characterized by:

■ The vapor pressure (Pa) at 20°C,
■ The melting point (°C) at atmospheric pressure (101.3 kPa), and
■ The boiling point (°C) at atmospheric pressure (101.3 kPa).

The toxicokinetic substance properties are characterized by:

■ The lipid solubility (g/kg) at body temperature (37°C),
■ The aqueous solubility (g/L) at room temperature (20°C), and
■ The *n*-octanol/water partition coefficient log K_{ow} at room temperature (20°C).

Physical interactions and chemical reactions with water (as an important biological medium) are characterized by:

■ The surface tension (mN/m) of an approximately saturated aqueous solution of the substance at room temperature (20°C),
■ The pH value of this aqueous solution at 20°C, and
■ The likelihood of hydrolysis of the substance in contact with water (information based on observations during solubility testing).

The skin irritation properties of a chemical observed in a Draize test on rabbit skin are characterized in this database by the following EU risk phrases denoting skin irritation or corrosion:

■ R34 = Causes burns (skin corrosion caused by a four-hour skin contact)
■ R35 = Causes severe burns (skin corrosion caused by a three-minute skin contact)
■ R38 = Irritating to skin (skin irritation caused by a four-hour skin contact), and
■ A detailed evaluation of all described effects on skin (erythema and edema scores relative to EU classification thresholds, their strength and duration, and their contribution to the overall toxicological assessment).

In order to evaluate the possibilities for the development of specific (Q)SAR models for prediction of the skin irritation and skin corrosion potential of chemicals that meet the requirements for regulatory hazard assessment, and for decisions on hazard classification and labeling with EU risk phrases (12), the BfR database was evaluated and the results of this evaluation were published in 2000, when the database contained information on approximately 1300 chemicals (7); evaluation was repeated in 2004 when the database contained data on 1833 substances (5,6).

For development of (Q)SAR models from the database, empirically derived "main groups" of chemicals have been established which can be compiled automatically by a computer. These main groups are defined according to the type of heteroatoms contained within the specific molecule. This approach proved useful to establish specific groups of chemicals (7), and the 1855 chemicals which are at the moment in the BfR database have been allocated to these groups (Table 1). A detailed description of the main groups and their specific properties has been published (7). Due to the uneven distribution of the chemicals over the 16 groups, it was decided to create only two different types of (Q)SAR models and prediction rules: rules covering all chemicals (neglecting allocation to specific main groups) and separate rules for each of the five main groups containing more than 100 individual substances (CN, C, CNHal, CNS, and CHal).

Derivation of Physicochemical Limit Values for Triggering Skin Lesions

Local effects on skin caused by acute contact with a chemical depend on the physicochemical properties that govern the toxicokinetic fate of a substance. A detailed summary of presently available information on the relationship between structure and barrier function of skin and the potential of chemicals to interfere has been published by Roberts and Walters (13). Some of the physicochemical data submitted to regulators (e.g., the information stored in the BfR database) are related to (toxico) kinetic substance properties, i.e., the probable behavior of chemicals within the water–oil emulsion on the skin surface, within the different skin tissues and when penetrating the skin, and therefore also to skin irritation potential.

TABLE 1   Relationship between Main Chemical Groups and Potential to Elicit Skin Lesions

Main group	Formula	Total	Not labeled	Labeled for skin lesions R34/R35	Labeled for skin lesions R38
CN	$C_xH_yO_zN_a$	652	605 (92.8%)	28 (4.3%)	19 (2.9%)
C	$C_xH_yO_z$	345	279 (80.9%)	13 (3.8%)	53 (15.4%)
CNHal	$C_xH_yO_zN_aHal_b$	250	231 (92.4%)	13 (5.2%)	6 (2.4%)
CNS	$C_xH_yO_zN_aS_c$	228	212 (93.0%)	5 (2.2%)	11 (4.8%)
CHal	$C_xH_yO_zHal_b$	153	106 (69.3%)	21 (13.7%)	26 (17.0%)
Si	Si-containing comp.	55	36	8	11
CNSHal	$C_xH_yO_zN_aS_cHal_b$	61	52	5	4
CS	$C_xH_yO_zS_c$	38	33	5	—
CP	$C_xH_yO_zP_d$	32	26	5	1
CSHal	$C_xH_yO_zS_cHal_b$	14	12	2	—
CNP	$C_xH_yO_zN_aP_d$	14	14	—	—
CPHal	$C_xH_yO_zP_dHal_b$	5	4	1	—
CNSP	$C_xH_yO_zN_aS_cP_d$	3	3	—	—
CNPHal	$C_xH_yO_zN_aP_dHal_b$	3	2	—	1
CNSHalP	$C_xH_yO_zN_aS_cHal_bP_d$	1	1	—	—
CSHalP	$C_xH_yO_zS_cHal_bP_d$	1	1	—	—
Total		1855	1617 (87.2%)	106 (5.7%)	132 (7.1%)

Abbreviation: Hal, halogens (fluorine, chlorine, bromine, and iodine).

Here we present our results obtained using those data related to toxicokinetic fate and to reactivity with water for the development of empirical rules, which predict the absence of skin irritation and corrosion potential. These rules can be used in combination with other information indicating the absence of hazardous properties, e.g., lack of specific chemical reactivity.

The goal of presenting the following tables (Tables 2–7) in addition to the validated prediction rules (Table 8) is to illustrate those rules, the frequency of chemicals that have the potential to cause skin lesions, and the probability of the prediction. In combination with other information such as chemical reactivity and defatting properties, these tables can be used in a WoE assessment to evaluate chemicals with specific physicochemical properties to assess if skin lesions may be expected.

Kinetic Properties
Relationship between MW and Skin Irritation/Corrosion
MW can be interpreted as a rough measure of molecular size, and it is the basis of one of the important rules for predicting the absence of skin lesions. We found that:

TABLE 2   Relationship between the Molecular Weight and the Skin Irritant/Corrosive Properties of a Chemical (Data on Molecular Weight are Available for all Chemicals of the Database)

Molecular weight (g/mol)	Number of substances in this group	Total number of substances causing skin lesions	Risk phrases R34/R35	Risk phrases R38
≤200	402	118 (29.4%)	59 (14.7%)	59 (14.7%)
201–250	312	62 (20.0%)	22 (7.1%)	40 (12.8%)
251–370	520	36 (6.9%)	16 (3.1%)	20 (3.8%)
≥371	621	22 (3.5%)	9 (1.5%)	13 (2.1%)
Total	1855	238 (12.8%)	106 (5.7%)	132 (7.1%)

TABLE 3 Relationship between the *n*-Octanol/Water Partition Coefficient (log K_{ow}) at Room Temperature (20°C) and Skin Irritant/Corrosive Properties of a Chemical

Log K_{ow} at 20°C	Number of substances in this group	Number of substances causing skin lesions	Risk phrases	
			R34/R35	R38
≤ −1.0	219	14 (6.4%)	8 (3.7%)	6 (2.7%)
> −1.0 to 1.0	246	33 (13.4%)	18 (7.3%)	15 (6.1%)
> 1.0–2.0	272	31 (11.4%)	13 (4.8%)	18 (6.6%)
> 2.0–3.0	234	35 (15.0%)	16 (6.8%)	19 (8.1%)
> 3.0–4.0	190	30 (15.8%)	8 (4.2%)	22 (11.6%)
> 4.0–6.0	222	38 (17.1%)	7 (3.2%)	31 (14.0%)
> 6.0	170	7 (4.1%)	3 (1.8%)	4 (2.4%)
Total	1553	188 (12.1%)	73 (4.7%)	115 (7.4%)

For the rest of the substances, no data on log K_{ow} were available.

TABLE 4 Relationship between the Lipid Solubility at Body Temperature and Skin Irritant/Corrosive Properties of a Chemical

Lipid solubility at 37°C (g/kg)	Number of substances in this group	Number of substances causing skin lesions	Risk phrase	
			R34/R35	R38
≤0.1	113	2 (1.8%)	1 (0.9%)	1 (0.9%)
>0.1–1.0	45	5 (11.1%)	4 (8.9%)	1 (2.2%)
>1.0–10.0	112	6 (5.4%)	4 (3.6%)	2 (1.8%)
>10.0–100.0	98	8 (8.2%)	3 (3.1%)	5 (5.1%)
>100.0	183	61 (33.3%)	25 (13.7%)	36 (19.7%)
Total	551	82 (14.9%)	37 (6.7%)	45 (8.2%)

For the rest of the substances, no data on lipid solubility were available.

TABLE 5 Relationship between the Aqueous Solubility at Room Temperature and Skin Irritant/Corrosive Properties of a Chemical

Aqueous solubility at 20°C (g/L)	Number of substances in this group	Number of substances causing skin lesions	Risk phrase	
			R34/R35	R38
≤0.1	835	78 (9.3%)	18 (2.2%)	60 (7.2%)
>0.1–1.0	202	22 (11.0%)	7 (3.5%)	15 (7.4%)
>1.0–10.0	203	27 (13.3%)	11 (5.4%)	16 (7.9%)
>10.0–100.0	166	17 (10.2%)	10 (6.0%)	7 (4.2%)
>100.0	225	37 (16.4%)	24 (10.7%)	13 (5.8%)
Total	1631	181 (11.1%)	70 (4.3%)	111 (6.8%)

For the rest of the substances, no data on aqueous solubility were available.

- No chemical with MW >1200 g/mol is classified as corrosive or irritant to skin, and
- Only six of the chemicals with MW >600 g/mol are classified for skin lesions (three substances R34, three substances R38). Five of them are salts with strong anions and strong cations (which erode the skin), the last substance is a silanol (which is very reactive with water).

Table 2 shows that the incidence of skin irritation/corrosion potential is relatively high if MW <250 g/mol, but for chemicals with MW >370 g/mol the

TABLE 6 Relationship between the Melting Point and Skin Irritant/Corrosive Properties of a Chemical

Melting point at 101.3 kPa (°C)	Number of substances in this group	Number of substances causing skin lesions	Risk phrase	
			R34/R35	R38
<1	267	107 (40.1%)	36 (13.5%)	71 (26.6%)
≥1–40	97	34 (35.0%)	20 (20.1%)	14 (14.4%)
41–120	448	14 (3.1%)	7 (1.6%)	7 (1.6%)
>120	762	28 (3.7%)	15 (2.0%)	13 (1.7%)
Total	1574	183 (11.6%)	78 (5.0%)	105 (6.7%)

For the rest of the substances, no data on melting point were available.

TABLE 7 Relationship between the Decrease of Surface Tension of Pure Water (Approximately 75 mN/m) Caused by Dissolution of a Chemical, and Local Irritant/Corrosive Potential

Surface tension of an aqueous solution (mN/m)	Number of substances in this group	Number of substances causing skin lesions	Risk phrases	
			R34/R35	R38
<15–40	26	10 (38.5%)	6 (23.1%)	4 (15.4%)
>40–50	65	15 (23.1%)	7 (10.8%)	8 (12.3%)
>50–65	320	48 (15.0%)	23 (7.2%)	25 (7.8%)
>65	618	61 (9.9%)	27 (4.4%)	34 (5.5%)
Total	1029	134 (13.0%)	63 (6.1%)	71 (6.9%)

For the rest of the substances, no data on surface tension were available.

TABLE 8 Validated PhysicoChemical Exclusion Rules for Skin Irritation/Corrosion

Class[b]	Rule	Excludes	Cutoff value 100%(±1%)
Lipid solubility (LS)			
All	LS <0.01 g/kg	R34/R35	0.010 g/kg
	Log LS <−2		−2(±0.38)
CN	LS <0.4 g/kg	R34/R35	Limited data basis for this rule[a]
CNHal	LS <400 g/kg	R34/R35	Limited data basis for this rule[a]
CNHal	LS <4 g/kg	R34/R35 or R38	Limited data basis for this rule[a]
Octanol–water partition coefficient (log K_{ow})			
All	Log K_{ow} < −3.1	R34/R35 or R38	−3.1(±0.18)
All	Log K_{ow} > 9.0	R34/R35	8.7(±1.79)
CHal	Log K_{ow} > 4.5	R34/R35	3.7(±0.07)
CN	Log K_{ow} > 4.5	R34/R35	4.2(±0.02)
CN	Log K_{ow} > 5.5	R34/R35 or R38	5.4(±0.27)
CNHal	Log K_{ow} > 3.8	R34/R35 or R38	3.7(±0.07)
CNS	Log K_{ow} < −2.0	R34/R35 (or R38)	−1.3(±0.17)
CNS	Log K_{ow} < 0.5	R38	Rule invalidated, see Ref. (13)
Melting point (MP)			
All	MP >200°C	R34/R35 or R38	430(±50) °C
C	MP >55°C	R34/R35 or R38	285(±14) °C

(Continued)

TABLE 8 Validated PhysicoChemical Exclusion Rules for Skin Irritation/Corrosion (*Continued*)

Class[b]	Rule	Excludes	Cutoff value 100%($\pm$1%)
Melting point (MP)			
CN	MP $>$180°C	R38 (and R34/35)	240($\pm$27) °C
CNS	MP $>$50°C	R34/R35	360($\pm$12) °C
CNS	MP $>$120°C	R34/R35 or R38	430($\pm$9) °C
CHal	MP $>$65°C	R34/R35	61($\pm$2) °C
Molecular weight (MW)			
C	MW $>$350 g/mol	R34/R35	272($\pm$2) g/mol
CHal	MW $>$280 g/mol	R34/R35	276($\pm$6) g/mol
CHal	MW $>$380 g/mol	R34/R35 or R38	368($\pm$9) g/mol
CN	MW $>$290 g/mol	R34/R35	281($\pm$3) g/mol
CN	MW $>$540 g/mol	R34/R35 or R38	539($\pm$13) g/mol
CNHal	MW $>$370 g/mol	R34/R35	370($\pm$7) g/mol
CNHal	MW $>$380 g/mol	R34/R35 or R38	375($\pm$1) g/mol
CNS	MW $>$620 g/mol	R34/R35	601($\pm$9) g/mol
Aqueous solubility (AS)			
C	AS $<$0.1 mg/L	R34/R35	0.207 mg/L
	Log AS <-4 g/L		-3.684 (0.005) g/L
CN and CNHal	AS $<$100 mg/L	R34/R35	100 mg/L
	Log AS <-1 g/L		-1.00 (0.01) g/L
CN and CNHal	AS $<$0.1 mg/L	R34/R35 or R38	0.200 mg/L
	Log AS <-4 g/L		-3.70 (0.3) g/L
Vapor pressure (VP)			
C	VP $<$0.0001 Pa	R38	0.0001 Pa[a])
	Log VP <-4		-4
CN	VP $<$0.001 Pa	R34/R35	0.0016 Pa[a])
	Log VP <-3		-2.80
Surface tension (ST)			
C	ST $>$62 mN/m	R34/R35	68.4 (mN/m[a])
CNS	ST $>$62 mN/m	R34/R35	58.0 (mN/m[a])

[a] No 100% values and/or $\pm$1% margins were calculated because of the low predictive value (in the external validation) and/or limited data basis for these rules.
[b] For definitions of structural classes, see Table 9.
Source: From Ref. 8.

probability of skin lesions to be labeled with EU risk phrases is clearly less than "normal" (Table 2). When interpreting these results, it may be argued that generally for chemicals with higher MW, skin absorption tends to be limited. However, very reactive chemicals that are able to erode the stratum corneum (extreme pH, strongly corrosive anions or cations, actively hydrolyzing chemicals) are not sufficiently covered by this rule.

Relationship between the *n*-Octanol/Water Partition Coefficient (log K_{ow}) and Skin Irritation/Corrosion

The logarithm of the octanol/water partition coefficient (log K_{ow}) for the partition of a chemical between a hydrophobic (*n*-octanol) and a hydrophilic solvent phase (water) is correlated with aqueous solubility (14). SAR considerations relating to local lesions can be based on this partition coefficient (15,16).

Seven categories for log K_{ow} values at room temperature (20°C) between <-1 and $>+6$ were defined (7), and the prevalence of specific local effects within these categories was calculated. Table 3 shows that generation of local effects in the skin of rabbits is more frequent if partition properties can be characterized by log K_{ow} values > -1 and $< +6$. The relation of log K_{ow} and absence of skin lesions can be interpreted knowing that most chemicals (except the very reactive ones) need to penetrate the skin in order to cause skin lesions. High and low log K_{ow} values indicate that penetration through an aqueous phase or through a lipid phase within skin tissue, respectively, will be limited (17) and therefore skin lesions are only seldom expected outside these boundaries.

Relationship between Lipid Solubility and Skin Irritation/Corrosion

Values for lipid solubility were assigned to five categories, assuming a "limit solubility at body temperature (37°C)" of 0.1 g chemical/kg standard lipid, to distinguish between "slightly soluble" and "insoluble," and a limit of 100 g/kg for characterizing "sufficient lipid solubility" (Table 4) (see Ref. 7). Table 4 shows that a higher than average percentage of the substances belonging to the latter category caused skin irritation/corrosion. However, data on lipid solubility are not mandatory according to EU regulations for new chemicals and hence, data for only 551 chemicals were available. Rorije and Hulzebos (8) showed that in a representative test dataset of 201 new chemicals, lipid solubility data were only available for very few substances and therefore external validation of the physicochemical exclusion rules could not be performed for this parameter. The rules in Table 4 are applicable for other new chemicals, but the false negative rate for an external set cannot be given.

Relationship between Aqueous Solubility and Skin Irritation/Corrosion

Prevalidation of the BfR database (7) had demonstrated that there may be an "aqueous solubility limit at room temperature (20°C)," of approximately 0.1 g/L, to differentiate between substances that are "slightly soluble" and substances that are "insoluble" in water for the purpose of a (Q)SAR rule of the type "IF aqueous solubility is <xg/L, THEN this substance probably does not cause relevant skin lesions." The aqueous solubility values above this limit were divided into three categories (Table 5). Chemicals that are corrosive normally seem to be highly soluble indicating that these chemicals may damage the skin (to be labeled R34 or R35). Chemicals characterized by a moderate skin irritation potential (labeled R38) are distributed evenly among the established classes.

Relationship between Melting Point and Skin Irritation/Corrosion

Vapor pressure and melting point are also potentially important physicochemical parameters for the prediction of possible local lesions after contact with a chemical. Therefore, data on melting points and on vapor pressure were evaluated. These evaluations demonstrated that data on vapor pressure, as submitted within the notification procedure of the EU, are often not precise and difficult to assess. Many of those data are calculated when they are below a certain value, instead of measured, e.g., those $<1 \times 10^{-5}$ Pa. Also volatile impurities can cause high vapor pressure values, which are not necessarily related to the chemical itself. Because of these problems, such data were not evaluated in detail (7). Instead, only measured data on melting points were evaluated. The melting point also characterizes an important thermodynamic property of a substance, such as the vapor pressure, but it can be assessed with more precision on the basis of the EU notification data.

Table 6 shows the relationship between melting point and skin irritation/ corrosion potential of the substances in the BfR database. Four categories of substances were defined: liquids (chemicals melting below 1°C); liquids that may change into waxes at room temperature or solids that may partially melt on contact with skin (1°C–40°C); solids with a melting point below 120°C; and solids melting above 120°C. The results of this evaluation demonstrate that:

■ Skin irritation or corrosion is caused mostly by liquids or waxes melting below 40°C, and

■ Only 42 out of the 1210 solids melting above 40°C (3.5%) are labeled for skin irritation/corrosion.

From a mechanistic point of view, the high frequency of skin lesions caused by liquids or waxes may be due to a higher absorption rate by the skin due to the duration and intensity of contact with such substances compared to contact with solids.

Reactive Properties
Relationship between Surface Activity and Skin Irritation/Corrosion
A chemical is characterized as surface active if the surface tension of pure water (approximately 75 mN/m) is reduced to values ≤50 mN/m on diluting the chemical with water. The relationship between the decrease of surface tension caused by a chemical and its local irritation/corrosion potential was evaluated. For this purpose, the submitted surface tension values were divided into values characterizing powerful surface activity (15–40 mN/m), values indicative of some surface activity (41–50 mN/m), minor surface-active properties (51–65 mN/m), and absence of any surface activity (66–80 mN/m). Table 7 demonstrates that high surface activity (low values of surface tension) is linked to severe damage to skin, whereas moderate reversible skin irritation also correlates with surface activity of a chemical in general, but less explicitly. This relation between surface activity and skin lesions shows that surface-active chemicals potentially cause skin lesions, which is also known for cationic and, to a lesser extent, anionic surface-active agents (17,18). Therefore, surface activity may not only enhance penetration but also cause important changes within skin tissues [e.g., by disturbing the intercellular lipid lamellae of the stratum corneum (13)].

Physicochemical Limits Identifying Absence of Potential to Injure Skin
The physicochemical exclusion rules that can be developed on the basis of the data listed in Tables 2–7 are of the general form:

IF *the value of a physicochemical parameter A is higher (or less) than the respective limit value*

THEN *the toxic effect B is not probable.*

This kind of exclusion rule was first developed at a time when the BfR database of new EU chemicals contained information on approximately 1300 chemicals (7), and was amended in 2004 using the then enlarged database of the BfR (5). In 2005, the limit values defined by these rules were evaluated at the National Institute of Public Health and Environment (RIVM) in Bilthoven, Netherlands (8), and externally validated by RIVM using data that were not used for their development at the BfR. Prediction rules using the evaluated and some subsequently amended limit values (8) are presented in Table 8.

In Table 8, physicochemical rules that can be used to exclude the potential of a substance to exert skin lesions leading to (EU) classification as irritating to the skin (labeled with R38) or as corrosive (labeled with R34 or R35) are listed. For comparison purposes, the cutoff values (where 100% of the training set data are correctly classified) are given in column "100%," together with the indication of the 1% margins ($\pm 1\%$) that would determine the cutoff value (where only 99% of the training set substances is correctly classified). A large margin indicates that very few irritant/corrosive substances have physicochemical properties close to the cutoff value, whereas a small margin indicates that a (relatively) large number of irritant/corrosive substances possess physicochemical properties close to the cutoff value. This information should aid the interpretation of "border-line" cases, and/or the determination of a safety margin for the cutoff values.

If the molecule is too large or too insoluble to penetrate the skin, then it is not able to do so even if other limit values are not met. For an in-depth discussion of the distribution of the training set compounds over the parameter domain and the distribution of substances around the cutoff values see the report of Rorije and Hulzebos (8). In this report, it is also shown that highly reactive chemicals should indeed be included in the first step of skin irritation evaluation before using the prediction rules, characterized above, which are based on the assumption that skin penetration is a limiting factor for skin irritation/corrosion.

Development and evaluation of these physicochemical limit values meet criteria which are defined in detail within international hazard classification systems such as the current classification criteria of the EU (12) or the hazard classification criteria published first by the OECD (19) and later by the United Nations (20). Hence, they can support regulatory classification of health hazards. We differentiate these limit values dependent on the chemical class ("main groups" containing more than 100 individual chemicals in the BfR database as discussed above and listed in Table 9). These rules are straightforward, easy to interpret, easily accessible, and based on (measured) physicochemical data that is available for every substance that has to be notified in the EU or will be within the REACH framework.

The validation of the exclusion rules (8) may serve as a model for future validation exercises with models built from confidential data. The collection of data and the model development were performed in one EU member state (BfR, Germany), the process was organized by a supranational European body [EU Joint Research Centre/European Chemicals Bureau (ECB)], and the validation itself was contracted to independent experts from a second EU member state (RIVM, the Netherlands). This external validation of the set of rules using 201 new substances not present in the training set showed ca. 99% correct predictions of noncorrosivity and ca. 97% correct predictions of nonirritancy. The relevance of the rules to the new chemicals database and their potential to reduce animal testing was demonstrated by the fact that testing for irritation/corrosion was not needed for more than 40% of the

TABLE 9   Definition of Structural Classes ("main groups") for Which Separate Skin Irritation Exclusion Rules have been Defined

Class	Structure contains only	Formula
C	Carbon (C), hydrogen (H), and oxygen (O) atoms	$C_xH_yO_z$
CN	C, H, O, and nitrogen (N) atoms	$C_xH_yO_zN_a$
CNHal	C, H, O, N, and halogen (Hal) atoms	$C_xH_yO_zN_aHal_b$
CNS	C, H, O, N, and sulphur (S) atoms	$C_xH_yO_zN_aS_c$
CHal	C, H, O, and halogen (Hal) atoms	$C_xH_yO_zHal_b$

test set chemicals. Even when considering that the latter represented only a small section of the "new chemicals universe," it appears appropriate to state that the exclusion rules could allow for waiving of skin irritation tests for a considerable share of the EU new substance notifications. In addition, the validation showed that the exclusion rule base fulfils all major regulatory information requirements, as almost all OECD principles on (Q)SARs were met satisfactorily (8).

Rules, that each apply only to a minor number of chemicals that need to be classified, should not be used as stand-alone methods for excluding skin lesion potential, but can be used in combination with other parameters.

EVALUATION OF STRUCTURAL ALERTS FOR PREDICTING SKIN LESION POTENTIAL

The molecular structure of a chemical is normally characterized by its empirical and structural formulae and by its UV, IR and NMR spectra (this information has to be submitted, e.g., within the EU notification procedure for new chemicals). The probable chemical reactivity of a substance can be deduced from its 2D structural formula, which contains information on the nature and the number of all the atoms in the molecule, and on the nature of the chemical bonds between these atoms. Therefore, this formula gives detailed information on the geometry and the topography of a molecule.

Structural alerts have been defined empirically by experts as chemical substructures that may be responsible for the specific adverse health effects caused by a particular chemical (21). These alerts define in detail e.g., substructures and their environment within a molecule, which could putatively lead to the biochemical reactions that could induce corrosion or skin irritation. Structural alerts are also derived from a knowledge of organic chemistry reaction mechanisms, which has been elaborated for the skin sensitization endpoint [for a review see Aptula and Roberts (22)] much more than for skin lesions, although attempts have also been made by Barratt and coworkers (18).

The use of structural alerts for classification and labeling purposes has only found limited application. For example, the possibility to use SARs is indicated in the EU Technical Guidance Document's section on skin lesions, but no defined structural alerts are mentioned (17). The only SARs that are given in the classification and labeling guide are those for organic (hydro)peroxides, where it is stated that any compound containing one of those alerts should be classified as a skin irritant (or skin corrosive, respectively) without testing, unless evidence to the contrary is (already) available. Neither a detailed description nor an applicability domain is given for this structural alert. Moreover, examples are missing, e.g., analogues. It remains unclear why peroxides and hydroperoxides have been specifically selected. From the literature, a large number of structural alerts, other than the (hydro)peroxide alerts, are known. Several of these alerts are based on organic chemistry rules or rules of thumb, evaluated over time. Some have actually been based on the evaluation of a large body of data [e.g., the EU new substance database (7)]. Overall, guidance on the application of these structural alerts in a regulatory setting remains insufficient.

Published structural alerts for the prediction of skin lesion potential were gathered by Hulzebos and her colleagues (23), and were assessed as alerts for irritation or corrosion or a combination of corrosion/irritation based on previously described mechanisms (24). Unfortunately, the compiled alerts (23) cannot be used directly for classification and labeling purposes because in many cases the predicted endpoints have been insufficiently defined. Some alerts are directly related to classification and labeling, while others are based e.g., on human patch tests or on expert judgment on chemical reactivity. In the original literature, often no distinction was made with respect to classification according to regulatory classification systems (12,20). Hulzebos and her colleagues defined each structural fragment within the categorized alerts as precisely as possible. This holds true not only for the structural alert itself, but also for adjacent structures that are not associated with skin irritation or skin corrosion. To describe these structural alerts more accurately, standardized wording is proposed, since this is crucial for computerized SAR systems.

It was decided to evaluate a number of these alerts in more detail using both literature data and similar chemicals from Annex I to EU Directive 67/548/EEC, the EU Dangerous Substance Directive (25), as an external training set. Whenever possible, their performance should be quantified using experimental data and, in general, a mechanistic basis should be established to explain why specific alerts have limitations that are defined by their (chemical) applicability domain. The selection of alerts is based on mechanism of action, in particular unspecific, electrophilic binding to biomolecules in the skin (26). In addition, the only alerts already accepted and applied in a regulatory setting—peroxides and hydroperoxides—have been evaluated for comparison with the results of the other evaluated alerts.

As a result of this work, it was found that several alerts, e.g., the activated alkyl/alkyne/benzyl alerts, provide more predictive potential for the classification of substances as skin irritant or corrosive than the (hydro)peroxide alerts. Some alerts, e.g., the ketone alert without any activating features, were found to be of little use; although frequently mentioned in the literature, they do not offer significant predictive potential for the classification of substances as skin irritants or corrosives. In addition, activated nitriles were evaluated, based on mechanistic considerations of their reactivity. These nitriles proved a valuable extension for the description of the activated alkyl (and potentially the alkyne and benzyl) alert.

The prevalidated structural alerts (9) are shown in Table 10 which gives information on the performance of the selected structural alerts as predictors for classification of a substance as irritant to skin (labeled R38) or corrosive (labeled R34 or R35), using data from the EU Annex I to Directive 67/548/EEC (25) and from literature. The performance is indicated as the percentage of the total number of substances containing the alert that are classified as either corrosive or irritant. The performances can be compared to the first structural alert—(hydro)peroxides—as this is an alert already incorporated in the EU Classification and Labelling Guideline (12).

These alerts are intended to be used for positive classification of chemicals causing skin irritation or skin corrosion according to regulatory guidelines and, therefore, are defined in an unambiguous way that can be used for both manual and computerized systems. The general domain of these prevalidated structural alerts is limited by the physicochemical property limit values of chemicals not causing skin irritation and corrosion. These physicochemical exclusion rules are higher in the hierarchy, because they were derived in such a way that, for all chemicals in the group, skin corrosion and/or irritation can be excluded. For some of the rules, those that cannot totally exclude skin lesions due to the limited size of the training set from which they were developed, both structural alerts and physicochemical limits, may be equally important. By defining the (structural) domain of the respective alert as strictly as possible, and thus lowering the false positive rate, a number of the alerts, most notably the alerts for allylic/propargylic/benzylic activation (including allylic

TABLE 10 Performance of Selected Structural Alerts as Predictors for Classification of a Substance as R38 (Irritant to Skin) or R34/35 (Corrosive)

Alert	Subclass	Structure	Total	Corrosive	Irritant	Non-irritant	Percent correct	R-group definitions
(Hydro)peroxides	a.	R1–O–O–H					71%	
	b.	R2–O–O–R2						
	a. Hydroperoxides		8	6	0	2	75%	R = –C, –P, –S, or –H
	b. Substituted peroxides		9	0	4	5	44%	R = –C, –P, –S
	excl. anhydrides		6	0	4	2	67%	R = –C, –P, –S, but NOT –C(=O)R
Activated unsaturated subst.	a.						93%	
	b.							
	c.							
	a. Allylic activation		17	3	13	1	94%	X = –Cl, –Br, –I, –OSO₂R, –OH, –CN
	b. Propargylic activation		4	0	3	1	75%	R = –H, –C-anything
	c. Benzylic activation		7	0	7	0	100%	
Aldehydes	a.						60%	
	b.							
	a. Aldehydes		57	2	32	23	60%	R = –H, –C-anything
	b. Allylic aldehydes		10	2	7	1	90%	R = –H, –C-anything
Heterocyclic 3-rings	a.						66%	
	b.							
	a. Epoxides		30	5	15	10	67%	R = –H, –C-anything
	b. Aziridines		2	1	0	1	50%	R = –H, –C-anything

(Continued)

TABLE 10 Performance of Selected Structural Alerts as Predictors for Classification of a Substance as R38 (Irritant to Skin) or R34/35 (Corrosive) (Continued)

Alert	Subclass	Total	Corrosive	Irritant	Non-irritant	Percent correct	R-group definitions
(Meth)acrylates						62%	
	(Meth)acrylic acids/esters	63	7	32	24	62%	R=−H, −C-anything double bond not part of ring
Quinones						100%	R1, R2=−H, −OH, −C or −O−C at least one R1 must be −H R1 is NOT −CN
	o- and p-quinones	2	0	2	0	100%	
Ketones						17%	
	Ketones	90	0	15	75	17%	R=−C-anything
Hydrazines						15%	
	Hydrazines	13	0	2	11	15%	R=−H, −C-anything

Source: From Ref. 9.

aldehydes), should become acceptable for regulatory purposes. In the last part of Chapter 29 ("Regulatory Needs for the Evaluation of (Q)SARs") it was demonstrated how regulators and industry can evaluate the (Q)SARs presented here in the same way as they evaluate results of current toxicological reports.

SUMMARY

The (Q)SAR rules to predict the absence of skin irritation potential of chemicals, presented in Table 8, have a high potential for regulatory acceptance. They are documented according to the OECD principles for the validation of (Q)SARs. External validation results of the rules show that for 98% of the chemicals the prediction is correct (8). The structural alerts listed in Table 10 have also been described in detail (9) and can be used for positive classification.

Prediction of skin irritation properties of a specific chemical can be performed easily and transparently. The applicability domain and the internal and external performance of the specific models allow assignment of a reliability score for each chemical (8,9) since both strong and weak rules have been assessed. However, it is strongly recommended that both the exclusion rules and the structural alerts are used and combined with other available information within an ITS, such as the SICRET tool (3) described in the Chapter 29.

ACKNOWLEDGMENTS

The authors wish to acknowledge the Dutch Organization for Health Research and Development, ZonM, ECB, and the Dutch Ministry of Housing and Spatial Planning for their financial contribution to the evaluation of (Q)SARs research. The authors are indebted Betty Hakkert and Maaike van Zijverden (RIVM) for critical comments on the manuscript.

REFERENCES

1. European Commission. White Paper on a Strategy for a Future Chemicals Policy. Brussels: Commission of the European Communities, 2003. (Accessed May 2006 at http://europa.eu. int/comm/environment/chemicals/whitepaper.htm)
2. Worth AP, Bassan A, Gallegos A, et al. The characterisation of (quantitative) structure–activity relationships: Preliminary guidance. ECB report, 2005. (Accessed August 2006 at http://ecb.jrc.it/QSAR/home.php?CONTENU=/QSAR/qsar_tools/sommaire.php)
3. Walker JD, Gerner I, Hulzebos ET, et al. The Skin Irritation Corrosion Rules Estimation Tool (SICRET). QSAR Comb Sci 2005; 24:378–84.
4. OECD. Guideline for Testing of Chemicals No. 404, Acute Dermal Irritation/Corrosion, OECD, Paris, 2002:1–13.
5. Gerner I, Walker JD, Hulzebos ET, et al. Use of physicochemical property limits to develop rules for identifying chemical substances with no skin irritation or corrosion potential. QSAR Comb Sci 2004; 23:726–33.
6. Hulzebos ET, Walker JD, Gerner I, et al. Use of structural alerts to develop rules for identifying chemical substances with skin irritation or skin corrosion potential. QSAR Comb Sci 2005; 24:332–42.
7. Gerner I, Zinke S, Graetschel G, et al. Development of a decision support system for the introduction of alternative methods into local irritancy/corrosivity testing strategies. Creation of fundamental rules for a decision support system. ATLA 2000; 28:665–98.

8. Rorije E, Hulzebos E. Evaluation of (Q)SARs for the prediction of skin irritation/corrosion potential. Physico-chemical exclusion rules. (Accessed September 2006 at http://ecb.jrc.it/QSAR/Documents/QSAR/EvaluationofSkinIrritationQSARs)

9. Rorije E, Herzler M, Hulzebos E, et al. Evaluation of structural alerts for skin irritation or corrosion—alerts for unspecific reactivity (in preparation).

10. European Commission. Commission Directive 2004/73/EC of 29 April 2004 adapting to technical progress for the twenty-ninth time Council Directive 67/548/EEC on the approximation of the laws, regulations and administrative provisions relating to the classification, packaging and labelling of dangerous substances. Official J Eur Union 2004; L152:1–311.

11. Gerner I, Graetschel G, Kahl J, et al. Development of a decision support system for the introduction of alternative methods into local irritation/corrosion testing strategies: development of a relational data base. ATLA 2000; 28:11–28.

12. European Commission. Annex VI of the Directive 67/548/EEC. General classification and labelling requirements for dangerous substances and preparations. Official Journal of the European Communities, L225, 2001:263–314

13. Roberts MS, Walters KA. The relationship between structure and barrier function of skin. In: Roberts MS, Walters KA, eds. Dermal Absorption and Toxicity Assessment. New York: Marcel Dekker, 1998:1–42.

14. Staab HA. Kohaesionseigenschaften. In: Staab HA, ed. Einfuehrung in Die Theoretische Organische Chemie. Germany: Verlag Chemie Weinheim, 1960:655–66.

15. Potts RO, Guy RH. Predicting skin permeability. Pharm Res 1992; 9:663–9.

16. Jackson JA, Diliberto JJ, Birnbaum LS. Estimation of octanol–water partition coefficients and correlation with dermal absorption for several polyhalogenated aromatic hydrocarbons. Fundam Appl Toxicol 1993; 21:334–44.

17. European Commission. Technical Guidance Document on risk assessment in support of Commission Directive 93/67/EEC on risk assessment for new notified substances and Commission Regulation (EC) No 1488/94 on risk assessment for existing substances and Directive 98/8/EC of the European Parliament and of the Council concerning the placing of biocidal products on the market, 2003:214.

18. Barratt M. Appendix A: Quantitative Structure activity relationships for skin corrosivity. In: Botham PA, Chamberlain M, Barratt MD, et al. A prevalidation study on in vitro skin corrosivity testing. The report and recommendation of ECVAM Workshop 6, ATLA 1995; 23:219–255.

19. OECD. Harmonised system for the classification of chemicals which cause skin irritation/corrosion. In: OECD, Harmonised Integrated Classification System for Human Health and Environmental Hazards of Chemical Substances and Mixtures. ENV/JM/MONO(2001)6, OECD, Paris, 2001:25–30.

20. United Nations. Globally Harmonized System of classification and labelling of chemicals, UN ST/SG/AC.10/30, United Nations Publications sales no. E.03.II.E.25. United Nations, New York/Geneva, 2003.

21. Walker JD. Chemical selection by the Interagency Testing Committee: use of computerized substructure searching to identify chemical groups for health effects, chemical fate and ecological effects testing. Sci Total Environ 1991; 109/110:691–700.

22. Aptula AO, Roberts DW. Mechanistic applicability domains for nonanimal-based prediction of toxicological end points: general principles and application to reactive toxicity. Chem Res Toxicol 2006; 19:1097–105.

23. Hulzebos EM, Maslankiewicz L, Walker JD. Verification of literature-derived SARs for skin irritancy by EU new chemicals. QSAR Comb Sci 2003; 22:351–63.

24. Walker JD, Gerner I, Hulzebos E, et al. (Q)SARs for predicting skin irritation and corrosion: mechanisms, transparency and applicability of predictions. QSAR Comb Sci 2004; 23:721–5.

25. European Commission. Annex I to EU Directive 67/548/EEC. List of dangerous substances. Latest update by ATP:29, Official Journal of the European Communities L152, 30/04/2004.

26. Verhaar HJM, vanLeeuwen CJ, Hermens JLM. Classifying environmental pollutants. Structure–activity relationships for predicting aquatic toxicity. Chemosphere 1995; 25:471–91.

31 Regulatory Assessment of Skin Sensitization

Winfried Steiling
Henkel KGaA, Corporate SHE and Product Safety—Human Safety Assessment, Düsseldorf, Germany

Hans-Werner Vohr
Department of Toxicology, Bayer HealthCare AG, Wuppertal, Germany

INTRODUCTION

Dermal contact to skin sensitizing substances (contact allergens) gives rise to an allergic contact dermatitis (ACD). Such exposure causes induction of contact allergy (sensitization). Reexposure of a sensitized individual to that contact allergen may cause an allergic reaction (elicitation) and become an ACD. The dose sufficient for induction is generally higher than the dose affecting the elicitation. To avoid ACD, the sensitized individual has to avoid further contact to this specific substance at levels causing elicitation.

One of the fundamental toxicological concerns with existing and new chemicals is their skin sensitization potential. Therefore, regulators require appropriate skin sensitization tests using either guinea pigs or the local lymph node assay (LLNA) in mice for hazard identification (1,2). Furthermore, proper risk assessment is necessary when either chemicals are intended for dermal contact, like cosmetic ingredients or likely to come into skin contact as with other consumer products.

A special form of skin sensitization is photoallergic skin reactions (photosensitization), observed with the diversity of skin reactions, and therefore not normally covered by routine testing. Such photoreactions (phototoxicity) with "photosensitive" (radiation-absorbing) substances occur after irradiation with sunlight, predominately with the UVA spectrum (320–400 nm) rather than with UVB or UVC. Generally, phototoxicity can be subdivided into different phenomena as described in the specific phototoxicity chapters of this book.

METHODS
Standard In Vivo Tests
Guinea Pig Maximization Test
The guinea pig maximization test (GPMT) is one of the most popular, but also internationally required and officially accepted, skin sensitization tests using guinea pigs. According to the protocol of Magnusson and Kligman (3,4) intradermal injections of the test substance, in combination with Freund's complete adjuvant (FCA) are applied during the induction phase. In such adjuvant assays, FCA stimulates nonspecifically the immune system of treated animals, enhancing their ability to respond to sensitizing chemicals.

The Organization for Economic Cooperation and Development (OECD) protocol (5) requires 20 animals in the test group and 10 naive control animals. For the induction, six intradermal injections are applied in the neck region, followed by one single topical application (epicutaneous induction) one week later. The six intradermal injections comprise two parallel applications each of the diluted test substance, of the diluted test substance in combination with FCA, or simply of FCA. Control animals are treated in the same way with the test substance replaced by the vehicle. The epicutaneous induction is achieved by applying an occlusive patch containing the test substance for 48 hours. Hypoallergenic patches are placed between and on the injection sites, covered with aluminum foil and held securely in place for 48 hours on the skin using self-adhesive tapes (occlusive application). For both induction phases, minimal irritating concentrations of the test substance are selected on the basis of dose range-finding studies.

Within the intradermal pilot study, irritating effects after intradermal injection have to be analyzed in the presence of previously injected FCA. Severe local effects such as redness and swelling around the injection areas are frequently observed even at the lowest concentrations. Such effects may be the result of inflammation due to non-sterile conditions, the injected FCA, as well as any chemical irritation potency per se.

A quite different situation is associated with the second pilot study, where doses are checked for the topical induction and elicitation phase in the GPMT. Any irritation effect at a specific test concentration is directly linked to the test chemical's compatibility. The scoring of these reactions and therefore the determination of the minimal irritating concentration for topical induction and the maximum nonirritating concentration for the challenge phase is predominately affected by the irritation potential of the test chemical.

Two weeks following the induction phase, the elicitation phase is started by applying 24 hours occlusive patches on the flanks of test and control animals. During this challenge, the maximal nonirritating concentration of the test chemical is applied. The severity of skin effects, such as the occurrence of erythema and edema, are scored 24 and 48 hours after patch removal using a four-point grading scale.

A skin sensitizer is characterized by a rate of responding animals during the challenge phase of at least 30% compared to the vehicle control group (6).

Occluded Patch Test

The standard test protocol according to the method of Buehler (7) describes a nonadjuvant guinea pig test that uses occluded topical patches for both the induction and elicitation phases of contact sensitization, without intradermal applications (8). Typically, this protocol requires 20 animals in the test group and 10 naive control animals (5).

For the induction phase, three patches (one per week) containing the test substance at minimal irritating concentration are applied topically for six hours to guinea pig flanks. Two weeks later, all animals receive patches with the maximal nonirritating concentration of the test substance for six hours under occlusive conditions to elicit possible immune responses. Both the minimal irritating and the maximal nonirritating concentrations are defined according to pilot study results. Severity of skin effects, such as erythema and edema, are subjectively scored 24 and 48 hours after patch removal according to a four-point grading scale.

The criterion for a skin sensitizer in this nonadjuvant test is given by a rate of skin reactions in at least 15% of the treated animals during the challenge phase compared to the vehicle control group (6).

Modern In Vivo Tests
Murine LLNA

In contrast to the standard skin sensitization tests in guinea pigs, this test analyses immune responses during the induction phase excluding elicitation. According to the standard LLNA protocol groups of four to five mice are topically exposed to various concentrations of the test chemical, or the chosen vehicle, on the dorsal part of both ears (9,10). This treatment is repeated on three consecutive days. Five days following the initial treatment, [^{3}H]-thymidine is intravenously injected to all mice via their tail vain. Mice are sacrificed five hours later and the draining (auricular) lymph nodes excised and eventually pooled for each group. A single cell suspension of lymph node cells is prepared and processed for γ-scintillation counting. Radioactivity is measured as the mean incorporation of [^{3}H]-thymidine per lymph node and represents stimulated DNA synthesis in the nodes.

According to this protocol, skin sensitizers are defined as those that induce a threefold or greater increase in isotope incorporation (at one or more test concentrations) compared with concurrent vehicle controls [effective concentration (EC3) threshold].

The validity of LLNA data in respect to human clinical data, specifically to the human repeated insult patch test (HRIPT) has been shown in several studies (11), but it may be oversensitive for some chemicals (12).

This LLNA protocol became officially accepted as a stand-alone alternative for the formerly required guinea pig adjuvant test and obtained the status of an OECD standard test (13). Furthermore, the U.S. Environmental Protection Agency (EPA) published a revised guideline in 2003 (14) which also accepts the LLNA as a stand-alone assay. Some important recommendations and comments in both (OECD, EPA) guidelines or the related report of the U.S. Interagency Coordinating Committee on the Validation of Alternative Methods (ICCVAM) (15) are not always at hand and should be specifically mentioned:

1. The LLNA is the preferred method but should not replace guinea pig methods in general. Properties of certain test materials may recommend guinea pig assays as the preferred test system for those chemicals in the future.
2. It must be ensured that the applied test material is in contact to exposed mice ears during the induction phase and does not immediately run off.
3. Although the standard protocol requires the measurement of DNA integrated radioactive labeled thymidine, other endpoints for the assessment of proliferation are accepted, if there is "justification and appropriate scientific support, including full citations and description of the methodology."
4. There is concern about the influence of irritating properties of test material that may cause nonspecific cell proliferation in the draining lymph node and thus could lead to false-positive test results.

With respect to the first comment there is so much enthusiasm about the advantages of the LLNA compared to guinea pig tests, such as refinement of animal tests, measurement of objective parameter, and the short-term protocol, that some advantages of guinea pig assays are often ignored. It needs some time to put guinea pig assays back in their deserved places.

Since 1996, alternative protocols to measure the proliferative activity of draining lymph node cell responses have been proposed (16–19), with alternatives to radiolabeled thymidine, either by characterization of draining lymph node cells using flow cytometry (20,21) or by determination of cytokines after in vitro restimulation (20,22). Only flow cytometry has been evaluated thoroughly in the context of interlaboratory trials (23,24).

Special In Vivo Tests (Photoreactions)
Several in vivo assays for the detection of phototoxic potential in guinea pigs, rats, and mice have been described in the literature. Some of these tests have acquired a degree of internationally acceptance, e.g., the guinea pig optimization test (25), the modified mouse ear swelling test (MEST) (26) introduced by Gerberick and Ryan (27), or the Photo Lymph Node Assay in rats (28) or mice (17).

It is of fundamental importance to consider, even for short-term assays, parameters to distinguish between photoallergy and photoirritancy. Photoirritating properties are much more common than photoallergic properties for several classes of compounds (29,30). Some anti-infective agents such as griseofulvin, tetracyclines, and fluoroquinolones are well-known photoirritants (31–33), rather than photo-sensitizers. The measurement of both photoallergy and the photoirritancy are dealt differently in the relevant European or U.S. guidelines (34,35).

In Vitro Alternatives
Driven by the principles of the three R's (i.e., Refinement, Reduction, and Replacement of animal tests), there is an urgent need to optimize currently accepted test methods. Specific parameters such as physical–chemical properties, calculated with intelligent computer programs may be employed, but the use of artificial skin models are also useful and promising activities for the future.

In Vitro Sensitization Testing in Cell Cultures
Specific human blood cells, such as immature dendritic cells derived from peripheral blood monocytes (36), or cell lines from human tumors (monocytic leukemia or histiocytic lymphoma) (36,37) are used as promising models for the prediction of skin sensitizing properties of substances. End points in these models are increased expression of cell surface marker molecules like CD54 or CD86, induction of interleukin-1β, or aquaporin $P3$ gene expression. Up to now, only few standard substances have been tested in such cell culture models, and correlation with in vivo findings (LLNA) was not always given. In comparison to in vivo, several parameters have to be taken into consideration for a reasonable assessment of the results. Skin penetration properties, vehicle diversity, cytotoxicity, or solubility of the compounds tested are major factors causing differences in both systems (36). Realistically, it will take years before such cell culture models may get any acceptable status for regulatory purposes.

Human Skin Models in Irritation/Sensitization Testing
Reconstituted human skin models (three-dimensional models, 3D) are commer-cially available and successfully used in routine testing for biological responses to chemicals. To date, such in vitro investigations are mainly used in determination of corrosive and irritating potential. To obtain scientific and official acceptance of these models, they have to be standardized and clearly defined in order to ensure reliable and reproducible data.

In contrast to cell cultures, the use of 3D skin models allows the application of insoluble chemicals and preparations under the intended use conditions and allows histological examination for further tissue analysis. Furthermore, such skin models are robust for test materials with extreme pH-values or even for the exposure of solids (38), as mentioned in the corresponding OECD protocol for in vitro testing of corrosivity (39).

Disadvantages of such 3D skin models are the limited number of commercially available systems (e.g., EpiDerm, SkinEthics, EPISKIN, and CellSystems), the lack of skin appendages such as hair follicles, sebaceous glands, or sweat glands in these reconstructions, and the lack of validation of these test systems.

Most of these aspects are not only restricted to in vitro determination of corrosion/irritation, but also important for use in in vitro sensitization studies.

Although it has been described for a reconstructed human epidermis (40), there is no convincing evidence to date that (photo)allergic reactions of compounds can be safely predicted by such skin models. Therefore, 3D skin models are promising alternatives, but not yet recommended by regulators even for screening (photo)sensitizing properties of chemicals or drugs.

Structure–Activity Relationships

Specific skin sensitization potential is related to physical–chemical parameters of the individual chemical. Today appropriate computer programs for structure–activity relationships (SARs) that group chemicals according to their complex physical–chemical attributes are available and could be used to simplify the complexity of sensitization tests (41). Recent studies have shown that within a selected chemical space of aromatic amines, phenols, and aldehydes, a set of three descriptors are successful for such SAR (42). These descriptors are as follows:

- Fractional positive atomic charge weighted per molecular surface area,
- Differences between partial positive and negative molecular surface areas, and
- Hydrophilicity given as $\log P_{o/w}$ (the distribution of a chemical between octanol/water).

Atomic charges can be calculated and projected via the solvent-water-accessible-surface specific for a chemical structure using appropriate computer programs. Using a decision tree, all three descriptors will contribute to the final estimation of skin sensitization potential.

The SAR is of supplementary value for the screening of new chemicals as well as for optimizing individual LLNA test protocols (refinement). The combination of SAR data with the corresponding LLNA test results is scientifically helpful in understanding the interaction of chemicals with the immune system and prospectively helps to reduce animal tests. Therefore, SAR is a valuable contribution to both the refinement and the reduction of animal tests (43).

Photosensitization

In recent years, several in vitro models have been developed to screen chemicals for photoreactivity, especially for photoirritation. The only current officially accepted method is the 3T3 neutral red uptake (NRU) Phototoxicity assay (34,44,45).

Apart from the 3T3 Assay, one of the most promising in vitro tests to screen for photo skin irritation potential is the photohemolysis test (46). Irradiated photo-sensitive chemicals are able to affect the membrane integrity of exposed human or animal erythrocytes. The photometric quantification of hemoglobin liberation is used as a marker for the photoirritation potential. This model seems to be sensitive and appropriate, not only for detecting water insoluble phototoxic chemicals that often generate false positives in the 3T3 photo cytotoxicity test (47,48).

There are no validated robust in vitro methods for the detection of photosensitizing chemicals, but it seems unlikely that chemicals will be photosensitizers if there is no photoirritation potential detected in the above mentioned in vitro tests.

REGULATION
Raw Chemicals
According to the current EU Directive 67/548/EEC (6), substances shall be classified as sensitizing and assigned the symbol "Xi," the indication of danger "Irritant" and the risk phrase R43 (*May cause sensitization by skin contact*) in accordance with the following criteria:

- If practical experience shows the substance to be capable of inducing a sensitization by skin contact in a substantial number of persons, or
- Where there are positive results from an appropriate animal test.

Comments Regarding the Use of R43: Human Evidence
The following evidence (practical experience) is sufficient to classify a substance with R43:

- Positive data from appropriate patch testing, normally in more than one dermatological clinic,
- Epidemiological studies showing allergic contacts dermatitis caused by the substance; situations in which a high proportion of those exposed exhibit characteristic symptoms are to be looked at with special concern, even if the number of cases is small, or
- Positive data from experimental studies in man.

The following is sufficient to classify a substance with R43 when there is supportive evidence:

- Isolated episodes of ACD, or
- Epidemiological studies where chance, bias, or confounders have not been ruled out fully with reasonable confidence.

Supportive evidence may include:

- Data from animal tests performed according to existing guidelines, with a result that does not meet the criteria given in the section on animal studies but is sufficiently close to the limit to be considered significant,
- Data from non-standard methods, or
- Appropriate SARs.

Positive results from appropriate animal tests are:

In the case of the adjuvant type test method for skin sensitization, a response of at least 30% of the animals is considered positive. For nonadjuvant guinea pig test methods a response of at least 15% of the animals is considered positive. With respect to lymph node assays performed in mice, such cut-off (threshold) value is defined by a fixed increase in cell proliferation compared to controls, i.e., increase in stimulation indices (SI). Similar to the situation in guinea pigs mentioned above, thresholds depend on the protocol used. If cell proliferation is measured by

[^{3}H]-thymidine incorporation, the threshold is defined as a threefold increase of SI compared to controls (EC3). If cell proliferation is determined by a nonradioactive method based on cell counting, this factor is for example 1.5-fold (EC1.5) (23,24).

Formulations/Mixtures/Products

According to the related EU Directives (6,49), formulations, mixtures and products shall be classified as sensitizing (R43, *May cause sensitization by skin contact*) and assigned the symbol "Xi" when containing a classified skin sensitizer, or in accordance with the following criteria:

- If practical experience shows the preparation to be capable of inducing a sensitization by skin contact in a substantial number of persons, or
- Where there are positive results from an appropriate animal test.

The default concentration value of a classified skin sensitizer for labeling of preparations with R43 is 1%. Preparations containing $>0.1\%$ of a classified sensitizer must have the warning phrase "Contains xxx (name of the sensitizing substance). May cause an allergic reaction."

Currently, 533 substances are classified with R43 an Annex I of Directive 67/548/EEC. A specific concentration limit for labeling with R43 below 1% has been set for 22 of these substances. Producers and importers are obliged to classify and label chemical substances not listed in this Annex I, if they fulfill the classification criteria already mentioned. Cosmetic products represent an exception in this sense because of different regulations according to the EU cosmetic directive.

Global Harmonization System

Activities started in 2002 to establish a globally harmonized chemical classification system (GHS) for hazardous chemicals according to their individual toxicological profile. According to the current status, it is proposed to have the same criteria for classifying a chemical as a skin sensitizer as within the current EU chemical regulation. For a skin sensitizer there will be a requirement to bring the signal word "Warning" and the hazard statement: "May cause an allergic skin reaction" on the package (50). Beside these similarities to the actual EU classification/labeling system, there is a proposal to have different skin sensitization categories in GHS that would take the sensitization potency into account.

Cosmetics

In regard to the European Cosmetic Directive (CD) (51), it is forbidden to put a cosmetic product on the market which causes damage to human health when applied under normal or reasonably foreseeable conditions of use. Based on this requirement and the intended skin contact of most of the cosmetic ingredients, sufficient data on skin sensitization potential of such chemicals are necessary. Beside the guinea pig tests and the LLNA, appropriate dermatological studies, such as the RIPT in volunteers are necessary. It should be mentioned that for ethical reasons, the latter is normally not performed to obtain toxicological safety data, but to approve the compatibility of final cosmetic products. With the 6th Amendment of the CD, cosmetic products have to contain information on the ingredients used (INCI declaration). Consumers are thereby informed on the presence of chemicals for which they may have a personal sensitivity.

Phototoxic Chemicals

In 2000, the European Commission issued the first guideline on an in vitro method for testing the phototoxic potential of chemicals (52). The "In vitro 3T3 NRU Phototoxicity Test" was the first alternative method that was fully validated and accepted by the regulators. However, from the very beginning it has been debatable if negative test results should be taken without any further in vivo validation.

In 2002, the European Medicines Agency published a Note for Guidance dealing with photosafety testing of medicinal products for human use, which came into effect in 2002 (34). The modified lymph node assay and the MEST are suggested as possible methods for in vivo screening test on the photoallergenicity of compounds.

Since the issue of this Guidance some controversial details have been in discussion. For example, one of the main criteria for initiating photosafety screening is the principle UV/light-absorption in the range of 290 to 700 nm, without defining limit values for relevance. All compounds absorbing light in this range have to be treated the same, irrespective of the quantity of absorption. This is in contrast to the OECD guideline (45), which states: "If the molar extinction/absorption coefficient is less than 10 L/mol/cm, the chemical has no photoreactive potential and does not need to be tested."

In 2003, the FDA published a guideline on photosafety testing for medical products (35) that was contradictory to the European guideline in several respects:

FDA. Animal testing endorsed, but use in vitro to plan in vivo; preclinical testing is not predictive of photoallergy. Testing should take place only if the drug is applied to the skin or the eye or is distributed to these tissues, and if skin or eye are exposed to sunlight.

EU. Stand-alone in vitro 3T3 NRU PT strongly endorsed, but guinea pig test or different "state-of-the-art" preclinical tests (like modified LLNA) may provide valuable information. Testing needed if drug absorbs light at 290 to 700 nm, if it reaches eye or skin after systemic administration, if it is photo-instable, or if SAR suggests adverse photoeffects.

QUALITATIVE RISK ASSESSMENT

Potency, the base for a qualitative risk assessment, is best defined as the inherent or intrinsic ability of a chemical to effect a biological change. With respect to skin sensitization and ACD, the relevant biological change is either: induction of skin sensitization in a previously not sensitized subject or elicitation of ACD in a previously sensitized subject (53).

When a substance has been classified as a skin sensitizer (R43) in accordance with current EU criteria, further categorization can be considered based on the sensitization potency. For the existence of clear evidence, it has to be assumed that the study (GPMT or LLNA) was conducted in full compliance with the specific OECD guideline, or with the related EU test method B6. The LLNA protocol is promising and the test results are less influenced by subjective criteria. It is crucial that the GPMT test is properly conducted (54) if it is to be used to obtain data supporting categorization based on sensitization potency.

The original grading and classification of skin sensitizers, based on the sensitization rate shown by challenge in the GPMT (3), is shown in Table 1.

TABLE 1 Classification of Skin Sensitizers after Challenge in the Guinea Pig Maximization Test

Sensitization rate (%)	Sensitization grade	Sensitization class
0–8	I	Weak
9–28	II	Mild
29–64	III	Moderate
65–80	IV	Strong
81–100	V	Extreme

It should be noted that according to this original scheme, the GPMT is not able to predict whether a substance is a nonsensitizer. This data interpretation is different to that used as a cut-off limit for categorization of skin sensitizers according to the EU chemical regulation and the GHS (6,55), which is a minimum of 30% responding animals during elicitation.

The dose sufficient for induction is generally higher than the dose affecting the elicitation. Searching for thresholds of elicitation seems to be challenging. There is no debate on the existence of such thresholds but, due to multiple influencing parameters (e.g., skin condition, exposed skin area, galenic, cross-sensitivity to other allergens) and the lack of sufficient methods for the quantification of their impact, any fixed value could not be generalized. The establishment of standard factors, based on measured values for the induction could be an option out of this dilemma.

Recognizing the complexity during the elicitation phase, the definition of threshold values for induction is much less difficult. The measurement of sensitization induction is well established and the use of standard tests like the LLNA is officially accepted and required (56). There is a considerable amount of LLNA data from different chemical groups e.g., pesticides, drugs, and consumer products and appropriate to compare this with human data (11).

In 2002, a task force at the European Centre for Ecotoxicology and Toxicology of Chemicals (ECETOC) started work on: *Chemical Sensitization: Classification According to Potency*. Within their final report, recommendations were made for a classification scheme based upon the use of data derived from OECD guideline methods for skin sensitization testing (57–59).

Parallel with activities at ECETOC, a similar task was undertaken by an Expert Working Group on sensitization commissioned by the European Chemicals Bureau (ECB). Both groups have worked on a refinement for the way, contact allergens are currently classified, based upon an appreciation that chemicals may differ substantially with regard to their potency to induce skin sensitization. The reports of both groups recommend the recognition of categories described as *Extreme*, *Strong*, and *Moderate* (59,60). The ECB is in favor of a cut-off EC3-value for the boundary between *Extreme* and *Strong* of 0.2%, and between *Strong* and *Moderate* of 2%. The ECETOC experts considered that chemicals of the latter group with an EC3-value of > 2% to 100% is too broad, and propose an additional category for weak sensitizers with a boundary set at 10%. There is supporting justification for such an extra category, as sensitizers with an LLNA EC3 value of 10% or above have only a very low potential to cause skin sensitization, even under conditions where the opportunities for exposure are significant. ECETOC focuses on the LLNA data for categorization of allergenic potential for two reasons: first, because it is this assay that will most commonly be used to provide data that are suitable for potency ranking and classification, and second, because the same principles apply to results derived from guinea pig tests (61).

It seems worthwhile to prevent induction of sensitization to avoid problems with the elicitation. Following such a track, which would offer an ideal ethical situation to run dermatological tests for individual measurement of elicitation in volunteers, there will be a need to differentiate the "power," the potency, of individual chemicals. The current data set of chemical specific sensitization potency is of obvious use to categorize chemicals according to their potency to induce sensitization. The recommended categorization as: *Weak, Moderate, Strong*, and *Extreme* sensitizers for properly tested chemicals, should have an impact on hazard identification, which is currently limited to labeling with the R43 phrase (*May cause sensitization by skin contact*), required by European legislation (6). The proposed categories could be given e.g., in the individual safety data sheet of the particular chemical. With this information on potency of chemicals to induce skin sensitization, an appropriate system has to be established (potency related threshold values) for the rule to label formulations/mixtures containing such sensitizer.

REFERENCES

1. Botham PA, Basketter DA, Maurer T, et al. Skin sensitisation—a critical review of predictive test methods in animal and man. Food Chem Toxicol 1991; 29:275–86.
2. Steiling W, Basketter D, Berthold K, et al. Skin sensitisation testing—new perspectives and recommendations. Food Chem Toxicol 2001; 39:293–301.
3. Magnusson B, Kligman AM. Allergic contact dermatitis in guinea pig. Identification of contact allergens. Springfield, IL: Charles C Thomas, 1970.
4. Magnusson B, Kligman AM. The identification of contact allergens by animal assay. The guinea pig maximization test. J Invest Dermatol 1969; 52:268–76.
5. OECD Guideline for the Testing of Chemicals. No. 406: Skin Sensitisation. Organisation for Economic Co-operation and Development, Paris, France, 1992.
6. Council Directive 67/548/EEC of 27 June 1967 on the approximation of laws, regulations and administrative provisions relating to the classification, packaging and labelling of dangerous substances. Official Journal 196, 16/08/1967, Annex VI, 2004/73/EC.
7. Buehler EV. Delayed contact hypersensitivity in the guinea pig. Arch Dermatol 1965; 91:171–7.
8. Robinson MK, Nusair TL, Fletcher ER, et al. A review of the Buehler guinea pig skin sensitization test and its use in a risk assessment process for human skin sensitization. Toxicology 1990; 61:91–107.
9. Kimber I, Basketter DA. The murine local lymph node assay: a commentary on collaborative studies and new directions. Food Chem Toxicol 1992; 30:165–9.
10. Kimber I, Dearman RJ, Scholes EW, et al. The local lymph node assay: developments and applications. Toxicology 1994; 93:13–31.
11. Basketter DA, Clapp C, Jefferies D, et al. Predictive identification of human skin sensitization thresholds. Contact Dermatitis 2005; 53:260–7.
12. Vohr H-W, Ahr HJ. The local lymph node assay being too sensitive? Arch Toxicol 2005; 79:721–8.
13. OECD Guideline for the Testing of Chemicals. No. 429: Skin Sensitisation: Local Lymph Node Assay. Organisation for Economic Co-operation and Development, Paris, France, 2002.
14. EPA, 2003 guideline OPPTS 870.2600, Skin Sensitization, March 2003.
15. ICCVAM (Interagency Coordinating Committee on the Validation of Alternative Methods). The murine local lymph node assay: a test for assessing the allergic contact

dermatitis potential of chemicals/compounds. The results of an independent peer review evaluation coordinated by the ICCVAM. NIH Publication No. 99-4494. National Institutes of Health, Bethesda, 1999. (http://iccvam.niehs.nih.gov)

16. Homey B, von Schilling Ch, Blumel J, et al. An integrated model for the differentiation of chemical-induced allergic and irritant skin reactions. Toxicol Appl Pharmacol 1998; 153:83–94.

17. Vohr H-W, Homey B, Schuppe H, et al. Photoreactions detected in a modified local lymph node assay in the mouse. Photodermatol Photoimmunol Photomed 1994; 10:57–64.

18. Vohr H-W, Blumel J, Blotz A, et al. An intra-laboratory validation of the integrated model for the differentiation of skin reaction (IMDS): discrimination between (photo)allergic and (photo)irritant skin reactions in mice. Arch Toxicol 2000; 73(10–11):501–9.

19. Sikorski EE, Gerberick GF, Ryan CA, et al. Phenotypic analysis of lymphocyte subpopulations in lymph nodes draining the ear following exposure to contact allergens and irritants. Fundam Appl Toxicol 1996; 34:25–35.

20. Ulrich P, Homey B, Vohr H-W. A modified murine local lymph node assay for the differentiation of contact photoallergy from phototoxicity by analysis of cytokine expression in skin-draining lymph node cells. Toxicology 1998; 125:149–68.

21. Gerberick GF, Cruse LW, Ryan CA, et al. Use of a B cell marker (B220) to discriminate between allergens and irritants in the local lymph node assay. Toxicol Sci 2002; 68(2):420–8.

22. Suda A, Yamashita M, Tabei M, et al. Local lymph node assay with non-radioactive endpoints. J Toxicol Sci 2001; 27:205–18.

23. Ehling G, Hecht M, Heusener A, et al. An European inter-laboratory validation of alternative endpoints of the murine local lymph node assay. First round. Toxicology 2005; 212(1):60–8.

24. Ehling G, Hecht M, Heusener A, et al. An European inter-laboratory validation of alternative endpoints of the murine local lymph node assay. 2nd round. Toxicology 2005; 212(1):69–79.

25. Maurer T, Thomann P, Weirich EG, et al. The optimization test in the guinea-pig. A method for the predictive evaluation of the contact allergenicity of chemicals. Agents Actions 1975; 5:174–9.

26. Gad SC, Dunn BJ, Dobbs DW, et al. Development and validation of an alternative dermal sensitisation test: the mouse ear swelling test (MEST). Toxicol Appl Pharmacol 1986; 84:93–114.

27. Gerberick GF, Ryan CA. A predictive mouse ear-swelling model for investigating topical phototoxicity. Food Chem Toxicol 1990; 28:361–8.

28. Schuppe H-C, Homey B, Ulrich P, et al. A local lymph node assay in rats for predicting chemical-induced contact and photocontact reactivity. Dermatosen (Occup Environ) 1999; 47:16–23.

29. Blotz A, Michel J, Moysan A, et al. Analyses of cutaneous fluoroquinolones photo-reactivity using the integrated model for the differentiation of skin reactions. J Photochem Photobiol 2000; 58:46–53.

30. Neumann NJ, Blotz A, Wasinska-Kempka G, et al. Evaluation of phototoxic and photoallergic potentials of 13 compounds by different in vitro and in vivo methods. J Photochem Photobiol 2005; 79:25–34.

31. Allen JE. Drug-induced photosensitivity. Clin Pharm 1993; 12:580–7.

32. Epstein JH, Wintroub BU. Photosensitivity due to drugs. Drugs 1985; 30:42–57.

33. Gould JW, Mercurino MG, Elemets CA. Cutaneous photosensisitivity diseases induced by exogenous agents. J Am Acad Dermatol 1995; 33:551–73.

34. The European Agency for the Evaluation of Medicinal Products (EMEA), Committee for Proprietary of Medicinal Products (CPMP): Note for Guidance on Photosafety Testing, CPMP/SWP/398/01, June 2002.

35. U.S. Department of Health and Human Services, Food and Drug Administration (FDA) Center for Drug Evaluation and Research (CDER), Guidance for Industry, Photosafety Testing, May 2003.

36. Aeby P, Wyss C, Beck H, et al. Characterization of the sensitising potential of chemicals by in vitro analysis of dendritic cell activation and skin penetration. J Invest Dermatol 2004; 122:1154–64.
37. Ashikaga T, Yoshida Y, Hirota M, et al. Development of an in vitro skin sensitisation test using human cell lines: the human cell line activation Test (h-CLAT). I. Optimization of the h-CLAT protocol. Toxicol In Vitro 2006; 20:767–73.
38. Kandárová H, Liebsch M, Spielmann H, et al. Assessment of the human epidermis model SkinEthic RHE for in vitro skin corrosion testing of chemicals according to new OECD TG 431. Toxicol In Vitro 2006; 20:547–59.
39. OECD Guideline for the Testing of Chemicals, No. 431: In vitro Skin Corrosion—Human Skin Model Test. Organisation for Economic Co-operation and Development, Paris, France, 2004.
40. Coquette A, Berna N, Vandenbosch A, et al. Analysis of interleukin-1alpha (IL-1alpha) and interleukin-8 (IL-8) expression and release in in vitro reconstructed human epidermis for the prediction of in vivo skin irritation and/or sensitization. Toxicol In Vitro 2003; 17:311–21.
41. Cronin M. Predicting Chemical Toxicity and Fate. Boca Raton, FL: CRC Press, 2004.
42. Steiling W, Ghosh R, Knübel G, et al. SAR meets LLNA—structure activity relationship triggers the local lymph node assay for testing the skin sensitisation potential. ALTEX 2005; 22:273.
43. Gerner I, Barratt MD, Zinke S, et al. Development and prevalidation of a list of structure–activity relationship rules to be used in expert systems for prediction of the skin-sensitising properties of chemicals. Altern Lab Anim 2004; 32:487–509.
44. Spielmann H, Balls M, Brand M, et al. First results of the EU/COLIPA project on in vitro phototoxicity testing: first results obtained with the Balb/c 3T3 cell phototoxicity assay. Toxicol In Vitro 1994; 8:793–6.
45. OECD Guidelines for Testing of Chemicals, 2004. Guideline No. 432. In vitro 3T3 NRU Phototoxicity Test. Organisation for Economic Co-operation and Development, Paris, France, 2004.
46. Kahn G, Fleischaker BI. Red blood cell hemolysis by photosensitising compounds. J Invest Dermatol 1971; 56(2):85–97.
47. Pape W, Hoppe U. In vitro methods for the assessment of primary local effects of topically applied preparations. Skin Pharmacol 1991; 4:205–12.
48. Pape WJ, Maurer T, Pfannenbecker U, et al. Red blood cell phototoxicity test (photo-haemolysis and haemoglobin oxidation): EU/COLIPA validation program on phototoxicity (phase II). Altern Lab Anim 2001; 29(2):145–62.
49. EU Directive 1999/45/EC of the European Parliament and of the Council of 31 May 1999 concerning the approximation of laws, regulations and administrative provisions of the Member States relating to restrictions on the marketing and use of certain dangerous substances and preparations. Official Journal L 166, 01/07/1999, 1999.
50. United Nations. Globally harmonized system of classification and labelling of chemicals (GHS). 1st revised edition, ST/SG/AC.10/30/Rev.1, 2005, Chapter 3.4, 151–8.
51. Council Directive 76/768/EEC of 27 July 1976 on the approximation of the laws of the Member States relating to cosmetic products. Official Journal L 262, 27/1/1976, 1976.
52. Commission Directive 2000/33/EC of 25 April 2000 adapting to technical progress for the 27th time Council Directive 67/548/EEC on the approximation of laws, regulations and administrative provisions relating to the classification, packaging and labelling of dangerous substances. Official Journal L 13, 08/06/2000, 2000.
53. Griem P, Goebel C, Scheffler H. Proposal for a risk assessment methodology for skin sensitisation based on sensitisation potency data. Regul Toxicol Pharmacol 2003; 38:269–90.
54. Schlede E, Eppler R. Testing for skin sensitization according to the notification procedure for new chemicals: the Magnusson and Kligman test. Contact Dermatitis 1995; 32:1–4.
55. United Nations Economic Commission for Europe (UNECE). Globally Harmonized System of Classification and Labelling of Chemicals (GHS) Part 3. Health and environmental hazards.

56. Gerberick GF, Ryan CA, Kimber I, et al. Local lymph node assay: validation assessment for regulatory purposes. Am J Contact Dermat 2000; 11:3–18.
57. Kimber I, Basketter DA, Butler M, et al. Contact Sensitisation: Classification According to Potency a Commentary. European Centre for Ecotoxicology and Toxicology of Chemicals (ECETOC) Document No. 43, 2003.
58. Kimber I, Basketter DA, Butler M, et al. Contact Sensitisation: Classification According to Potency. European Centre for Ecotoxicology and Toxicology of Chemicals (ECETOC) Technical Report No. 87, 2003.
59. Kimber I, Basketter DA, Butler M, et al. Classification of contact allergens according to potency: proposals. Food Chem Toxicol 2003; 41:1799–809.
60. European Chemical Bureau (ECB), Summary record of the Expert Group meeting on sensitisation (Potency), ENV/JM/HCL/M (2005)1, Paris 05-06 May, 2004, 2005, 1–12.
61. Basketter DA, Gerberick GF, Kimber I. Measurement of allergenic potency using the local lymph node assay. Trends Pharmacol Sci 2001; 22:264–5.

32

Assessment of Topical Bioequivalence Using Microdialysis and Other Techniques

Eva Benfeldt
Department of Dermatology, Gentofte Hospital, University of Copenhagen, Hellerup, Denmark

Edward D. Bashaw
Division III, Office of Clinical Pharmacology, U.S. Food and Drug Administration, Rockville, Maryland, U.S.A.

Vinod P. Shah
Pharmaceutical Consultant, North Potomac, Maryland, U.S.A.

INTRODUCTION
Background
In the Food and Drug Administration (FDA) criteria for evaluations of bioavailability (1), it is stated that for drugs not intended to be absorbed into the bloodstream, measurements should reflect the rate and extent to which the active molecule "becomes available at the site of action." The defined target tissue toward which topical drug therapy is aimed can be the stratum corneum (SC), the deeper epidermis or the dermis. Current FDA requirements for bioequivalence determination of topical drug products are dependent on the pharmacological class of the dosage form. For glucocorticoid dosage forms, a blanching assay procedure using a chromameter is recommended. For all other topical drug products, a draft guidance describing dermatopharmacokinetic methodology was published but later withdrawn by FDA. As a result, currently comparative clinical trials are required for bioequivalence determination between test and reference topical drug products.

With the emergence of microdialysis methodology, we now have a technique which enables us to sample in the skin as a target organ and obtain pharmacokinetics with real-time chronology. Microdialysis is a technique for sampling of endogenous and exogenous substances in the extracellular space in the living tissue. While the majority of microdialysis applications are preclinical studies on neurotransmitter release, microdialysis has rapidly been adopted for the clinical setting, initially with experiments on subcutaneous adipose tissue glucose levels in the mid-1980s. The first studies on human drug pharmacokinetics were published in the early 1990s. Today FDA and Conformité Européene-approved microdialysis catheters are available for use in humans and the sampling technique can be performed in virtually every given human tissue including myocardium, brain, lung, and also human tumors. For a review of microdialysis, see the recent American Association of Pharmaceutical Scientists (AAPS)/FDA Workshop Report on microdialysis (2).

The views expressed in this chapter are those of the authors and do not necessarily reflect the opinions of their companies/institutions or the official policy of the FDA. No official support or endorsement by the FDA is intended or should be inferred.

TABLE 1   Advantages and Limitations of Microdialysis and Dermatopharmacokinetic Methods

Advantages	Limitations
Microdialysis methodology	
Highly dynamic continuous sampling	Requires an initial investment in pumps
High-resolution real-time kinetics	Requires training of skills
Both drug and metabolites in one sample	Needs sensitive analysis
Minimally invasive	Drug-specific problems
Multiple sites in one animal/person	Lipophilic drugs
Purified samples (protein free)	High protein binding of drugs
Highly reproducible	Absolute tissue levels difficult to estimate
Allows simultaneous use of auxiliary techniques	Recovery is influenced by local blood flow
Tape-stripping methodology	
Requires minimal training	End point measurements only
Noninvasive	Samples need purification
Multiple sites in one animal/person	Uneven sample layer/depth
Few analytical problems	Variability between laboratories
Highly reproducible	Correlation with dermal concentration?

Cutaneous microdialysis sampling in the skin provides continuous real-time monitoring of biochemical events in the tissue, and it is performed under minimally invasive conditions in comparison with traditional and invasive methods (skin biopsy, skin stripping, and skin blisters) where chronological or dynamic studies are either not feasible or very difficult to conduct.

The present chapter aims to give an introduction to the principles of cutaneous microdialysis as well as the advantages and limitations of the technique. Similarly, the well-established dermatopharmacokinetic method or tape-stripping methodology will be described briefly before a study comparing the two methodologies (Table 1) is presented and discussed. Finally, the regulatory perspective on methodologies available for bioequivalence studies of topical formulations will be addressed.

METHODOLOGIES
Microdialysis Technique
The technique of microdialysis involves the implantation of a small probe into a specific region of a tissue or fluid-filled space. A variety of probe designs have been used, including linear, U-shaped, or concentric geometries. Semi-permeable membrane materials used in probe construction range from low- to high-molecular weight cut off. During microdialysis, a physiologically compatible perfusion fluid (perfusate) is delivered through the probe at a low and constant flow rate (e.g., 0.1–5.0 µL/min). Exchange of solutes occurs in both directions along the semi-permeable membrane of the probe, resulting in a dialysate solute concentration that is a fraction of the tissue extracellular diffusible (unbound) level. This fraction is referred to as the *relative recovery*. The recovery of a given compound closely reflects the concentration of unbound, i.e., pharmacologically active, compound in the intercellular fluid of the tissue surrounding the probe. The typical microdialysis membranes have low-molecular weight cut-off values (2–20 kDa) and samples will

thus be free from protein with no need for sample clean up and no enzymatic degradation of the substances collected.

The analysis of the samples can be one of the biggest challenges using microdialysis (3). Several technical issues in the analysis of microdialysis samples, in particular the limits of detection, required sample volume and analytical interferences need to be considered, and the sampling and analysis parts must be designed in conjunction with each other. The typical total micro-dialysate volumes of a few μL or less and analyte concentrations in the pM or μM range present a challenge for the analytical chemist. Thus, it is important to balance the flow rate and the analytical system. The method can be particularly challenging when used for sampling very lipophilic or very highly protein-bound drugs due to low recoveries of these compounds (4). It is possible to partially compensate for inadequate analytical sensitivity by employing long sampling intervals, low flow rates or by pooling dialysates from several probes. However, the experimental parameters are often determined by a compromise between the analytical sensitivity and the characteristics of the substance investigated.

Many experimental conditions affect probe recovery, including microdialysis flow rate (perfusion), temperature, probe membrane composition and surface area, nature of the dialyzed tissue, physicochemical properties of the analyte of interest, and other factors that alter molecular diffusion characteristics. In general, the higher the perfusion flow rate, the lower the relative recovery. Higher temperatures and greater probe membrane areas usually result in increased recovery.

Microdialysis as a sampling technique is volume-neutral, i.e., there is no net fluid volume loss from the animal or human subject in connection with sampling. A special feature of microdialysis is the possibility of sampling both prodrug and active drug in the same sample during drug metabolization in the body. This has been shown for the metabolism of famciclovir to penciclovir (5) and for the very rapid metabolism of orally ingested acetylsalicylic acid to salicylic acid, occurring in the plasma (6).

Since microdialysis is labor intensive and requires specialized skills, it is not suitable for high throughput screening of large numbers of compounds. Rather, it is used to address specific questions from early in discovery to compounds in development.

Clinical microdialysis has been shown to be a safe, reproducible, ethically acceptable and relatively inexpensive technique for studying tissue biochemistry and drug distribution in humans.

Microdialysis Methodology for Sampling in the Skin

The first reports on cutaneous microdialysis were published in 1991 (7), and since then the technique has developed into a very versatile tool for skin research. The dermal microdialysis method can provide very detailed chronological pharmaco-kinetic data and several sampling sites can be studied simultaneously in the same volunteer. Employing microdialysis sampling, diverse research areas such as basic physiology/endogenous substances as well as the pathophysiology of inflammation and allergic responses, pharmacokinetics and pharmacodynamics of topical and systemic drugs, skin barrier function and drug penetration into the skin have been investigated. The method is currently undergoing rapid development in topical drug penetration research. For a comprehensive review, which also includes theoretical/mathematical background and troubleshooting issues, see Ref. 8.

Microdialysis Methodology for Studies of Topical Formulations

The initial microdialysis study of percutaneous penetration concerned the penetration of ethanol applied to the skin surface (7). Since then, the research area has branched out to include transdermal medication such as the nicotine patch (9), topical versus oral administration of the same drug, e.g., ibuprofen (10), salicylic acid (11), or psoralen (12), and topical penetration of dermatological formulations (4,13). Benfeldt et al. (6) have studied the highly significant effect of barrier perturbation procedures on cutaneous penetration of salicylic acid. The effect of iontophoresis on topical drug delivery to the skin and subsequent systemic delivery has been studied by Stagni and coworkers (14,15).

For studies of topical drug administration, the influence of the probe depth (the distance from the surface of the skin to the microdialysis membrane inserted in the skin) on the drug concentration sampled has been debated. The depth of the probe in the skin can be measured by 20 MHz ultrasound scanning, e.g., using the Dermascan-C (Cortex, Hadsund, Denmark), which has an accuracy of around 0.02 mm in the measurement of skin thickness. It is recommended that skin thickness and probe depth is measured in three separate scans along the length of the probe in situ (near probe entry, middle, and near probe exit) and use the mean for calculations (8).

Some authors have shown that more superficial probe implantation results in higher dialysate concentrations (16), and this correlation is plausible from a theoretical point of view and can be appreciated in Figure 1. However, probes are usually inserted over a narrow range of depth (0.6–1.0 mm) in the dermis. Furthermore, the implantation depth becomes less variable with increasing investigator experience, reducing standard deviation in implantation depth to, e.g., ±0.16 mm (6). Most studies have been unable to demonstrate the correlation between probe depth and topical drug penetration (9,14,17,18).

A recent study investigated the relationship between in vitro permeation methodology and ex vivo microdialysis for percutaneous penetration of topically applied drugs (19) and in another ex vivo study, the effect of formulation on the topical penetration of a herbal remedy was investigated by microdialysis (20). The topical penetration of several different components in a topical analgesic solution has also been demonstrated by microdialysis (21).

Microdialysis methodology in the skin is easily combined with other methods such as Laser Doppler Flowmetry, Laser Doppler Perfusion Imaging, trans-epidermal water loss, colorimetry, high-resolution ultrasound scanning, or scoring of itch and pain.

Microdialysis for Topical Bioequivalence Studies

For assessment of bioequivalence of topical drug formulations, the technique has been considered promising, but in need of validation, by the regulatory authorities. In 2001, Kreilgaard and coworkers published the first human study demonstrating the potential of dermal microdialysis for bioequivalence studies of topical formulations (13). In this study, dermal microdialysis sampling and pharmacodynamic assessment of the pain-relieving effect of the formulations compared lidocaine delivery from two different vehicles. Recently, a study comparing microdialysis and dermatopharmacokinetic methodology was published (22), and the conclusions from this work will be reported in more detail later in the present chapter.

Similar to dermatopharmacokinetics, for bioequivalence studies dermal microdialysis also allows the testing of both T (test) and R (reference) product at

Microdialysis after topical drug administration

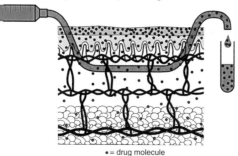

• = drug molecule

FIGURE 1 Principle of microdialysis sampling by a linear probe. The perfusate is pumped through the probe at a preset, low flow rate. During the passage through the membranaceous portion, small molecules diffuse across the membrane. The perfusate is now termed the dialysate.

the same time in the same individuals. Although dermal microdialysis is comparatively more invasive than dermatopharmacokinetics, it can be performed in barrier perturbed or diseased skin (Fig. 2).

The Dermatopharmacokinetic Methodology

In the determination of bioequivalence of topical products, the method of choice has been the tape-stripping technique, also called the dermatopharmacokinetic method (1,23). The method consists of a standardized protocol of repeated applications and removal of adhesive tape on the skin surface, whereby consecutive layers of SC cells are sampled (Fig. 3). Using analysis of each tape strip, it has been shown that the drug concentration in the SC decreases log linearly, and that about 90% of the concentration is found in the first 10 strips. The next 10 strips contributes less than 5% (24). Auxiliary techniques can be used to further determine the mass of SC cells or thickness removed by the sampling procedure (25,26), or by quantification of SC mass by protein analysis of strips (27). In order to further validate the sampling methodology, an evaluation of SC thickness by tape-stripping (28) could be undertaken prior to or preferably during the dermatopharmacokinetic experiment.

For assessment of drug penetration deeper than the cell layers of the SC, the predictive value of the method relies on the studies by Rougier and coworkers (29). For compounds with varying physicochemical characteristics, Rougier and coworkers showed a good correlation between the concentration in SC at 30 minutes and

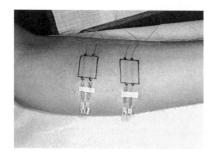

FIGURE 2 Linear microdialysis probes in situ in the dermis. The length accessible to microdialysis sampling is 3 cm. A microdialysis pump provides the perfusate flow of 1.25 µL/min. Samples of 25 µL are collected every 20 minutes for 5 hours. At $t=0$ the topical formulation is applied in a dose of 4 mg/cm^2 and left throughout the experiment. Markings for insertion of the guide cannula are circles in order to avoid the introduction of a tattoo.

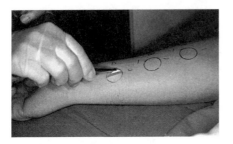

FIGURE 3   Black-white photo of tape-stripping practical procedure. Tape discs (D-Squame® Skin Sampling Discs; Cuderm Corp., Dallas, Texas, U.S.A.) were applied and removed by pincers following gentle pressure with the blunt end after application to assure good skin contact, and alternating strip removal directions (North, South, East, and West).

systemic absorption over four days (using radiolabeled compounds, excretion collection, and analysis).

This is particularly relevant for drugs aimed at an effect at a deeper level in the epidermis or in the dermis as a target organ.

The dermatopharmacokinetic method is concentration dependent when used for comparative studies of topical formulations, and has not been standardized for use in diseased skin. The weakness of the dermatopharmacokinetic approach is the end point nature of the data obtained and the lack of studies confirming the correlation between dermatopharmacokinetic data and clinical efficacy.

COMPARISON OF THE TWO METHODOLOGIES

In order to explore the performance of these two methods, we conducted a study designed to evaluate the relationship between dermatopharmacokinetic and dermal microdialysis methodology. We employed the dermatopharmacokinetic method (30) with simultaneous sampling in the dermis by microdialysis. The sampling matrix is thus essentially different, and the overall evaluation concerns the relationship between the results obtained with the two methodologies. Two formulations known to have different drug penetration profiles (cream and ointment with the same 5% active compound) were used.

Study Design

Topical lidocaine cream and ointment (both 5%) were investigated in eight healthy human volunteers (four male and four female). On one forearm microdialysis sampling was undertaken (four probes in two penetration areas sampled for five hours), and on the other arm tape stripping was performed (30 and 120 minutes after product application). Lidocaine content in the samples was determined using high-performance liquid chromatography–mass spectrometry.

Results of the Comparative Study

For dermal microdialysis: both cream and ointment formulation provided measurable dermal concentrations of lidocaine in the dialysates; the cream formulation provided rapid penetration with an almost fivefold higher area under the curve (AUC) than the ointment formulation (Fig. 4B). Pharmacokinetics for the whole group of subjects are shown for both formulations in Figure 4A. Measurements of probe depth demonstrated highly accurate placement horizontally within the dermis. Analyses of the influence of remaining covariables (actual dose applied,

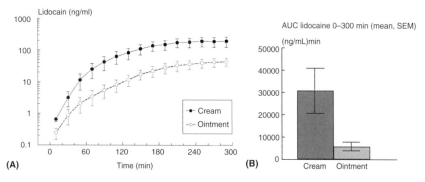

FIGURE 4   Different penetration from the two formulations: microdialysis sampling methodology. (A) Pharmacokinetics obtained by microdialysis, showing the dermal lidocaine penetration from the cream (solid black) and ointment (grey line) for all volunteers ($n=8$). Means with standard error of the mean (SEM) in log-scale. (B) Mean area under the curve with SEM for cream (dark grey) and ointment (light grey) formulation, sampled by microdialysis.

gender, age, room temperature, and humidity; 70 possible correlations) were without significant findings of any effect on lidocaine kinetics, sampled by microdialysis.

For the dermatopharmacokinetic method, the tape-stripping procedure robustly discriminated between cream and ointment formulations at both 30- and 120-minute sampling time (Fig. 5).

Overall, an excellent rank order correlation was found between the dermatopharmacokinetic result and the dermal microdialysis result: both methods provided the same overall result with the 5% cream formulation delivering 2.5- to 3-fold more lidocaine to the skin when investigated by the dermatopharmacokinetic method (significant difference; $p \leq 0.0001$) and a 4.8-fold difference when investigated by microdialysis methodology at the same time in the same volunteers (significant difference; $p=0.018$ and 0.030 for AUC and C_{max}, respectively).

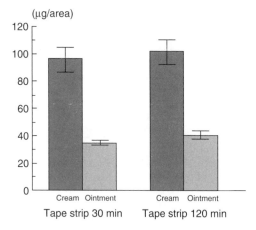

FIGURE 5   Different penetration from the two formulations: dermatopharmacokinetic methodology. Pharmacokinetics by tape-stripping methodology. The mean lidocaine content in cumulated tape strips is shown for cream (dark grey) and ointment (light grey) formulation ($n=8$), sampled at $t=30$ minutes and $t=120$ minutes. Error bars are standard error of the mean.

Correlation Between the Two Methods
Thus, correlations between the two methods were expected to exist, and pharmacokinetic parameters from dermal microdialysis were tested against dermatopharmacokinetic results for both 30- and 120-minute samples. Significant correlations were present only with ointment formulation tape strip 120 minutes and AUC, C_{max}, or their logarithms. For further details, please consult (22).

Bioequivalence Evaluation by the Two Methods
For microdialysis methodology. The two formulations were tested on two separate occasions in the same eight individuals. For each person, the difference in logAUC between cream and ointment was calculated. The mean difference in logAUC was 1.575 ± 0.515 (mean $\pm$ standard error of the mean, 90% CI 0.599–2.551), and the mean ratio for all subjects was 4.83. Thus, the bioavailability of lidocaine from the cream formulation, relative to the ointment, is 483% with a 90% confidence interval of 182% to 1282%. The two formulations are therefore not bioequivalent, and cannot be regarded as interchangeable.

For the dermatopharmacokinetic method. In a similar fashion, the dermatopharmacokinetic data obtained for the two formulations can be compared with bioequivalence evaluation methodology in order to reject bioequivalence.

For dermatopharmacokinetics 30 minutes: mean ratio for cream/ointment is 2.72, the confidence interval for the difference is 0.849 to 1.150 and the interval for the ratio is the antilog: 234% to 316%. This is outside of the 80% to 125% bioequivalence criteria.

At 120 minutes: mean ratio for cream/ointment is 2.48, the confidence interval for the difference is 0.671 to 1.146 and the interval for the ratio 196% to 315%.

Imagining that the two formulations had indeed been similar, and the ratio had been 1, then the above intervals for the ratio would have been (86–116%) and (79–127%), which would mean fulfillment of the bioequivalence criteria for dermatopharmacokinetics at 30 minutes, but not fulfillment for dermatopharmacokinetics at 120 minutes. Since cream and ointment are two different types of formulations, they should not be tested for bioequivalence. The above calculation simply illustrates that the two formulations are not bioequivalent.

Analysis of Variability Components in Microdialysis Sampling
The design of the study facilitated identification of the various components that are integrated in the overall variability of microdialysis sampling of topical drug penetration. The analysis by the variance component model demonstrates the intrasubject variability of 19% between probes and 20% between the two application sites. Thus, intersubject variability accounted for the remaining 61% of the variance observed.

Calculations of Sample Size for Topical Bioequivalence Studies by Microdialysis
Based on the analysis of variance above, the number of subjects necessary for a bioequivalence study of two formulations by microdialysis can be calculated (Table 2). The large difference in number of subjects needed, depending on whether the formulations are tested one at a time or simultaneously in the same subject reflects the impact of the interindividual differences in topical drug penetration, probably founded in differences in skin barrier function.

TABLE 2 Bioequivalence Study Size Estimates: Number of Subjects Required for Bioequivalence Determination of Topical Formulations in Healthy Human Volunteers

Probability (%)	Limits of variation (%)[a]	Two probes per area	Three probes per area
Bioequivalence study with two formulations in each subject			
80	<25 (80–125)	20	14
80	<33	13	9
90	<25	27	18
90	<33	17	12
95	<25	33	23
95	<33	21	15
Bioequivalence study with one formulation in each subject			
80	<25 (80–125)	711	695
80	<33	427	417
90	<25	985	962
90	<33	591	577
95	<25	1244	1215
95	<33	746	729

Based on intraindividual (upper) and interindividual (lower) variabilities.
[a] The limit of variation for equivalency determination described as "<25%" means less than factor 1.25 above and below the mean, thus between 125% and 100/1.25=80%. The third row in each bioequivalence study, with 90% probability and limitation of variability to between 80% and 125%, corresponds with current Food and Drug Administration criteria for bioequivalence determination.

CONCLUSIONS

A good rank order relationship between microdialysis and dermatopharmacokinetic methodologies was established in this study. Thus, the use of these methods in bioequivalence determination between test product and reference product has been established (22,31). The option of evaluating bioequivalence of topical formulations using microdialysis is in many ways better than embarking on expensive clinical trials, which is a current requirement for generic drug approvals. To gain adequate statistical power, clinical trials may require as many as 300 patients (23). Employing the dermatopharmacokinetic method, it has been estimated that between 40 and 50 subjects are needed for a bioequivalence study (31). Statistical calculations, based on the data from the lidocaine study, determine that using dermal microdialysis, bioequivalence studies with 90% CI and 80% to 125% bioequivalence limits can be conducted in 27 subjects, using two probes in each test area, or 18 subjects using three probes per formulation application site (Table 2).

REGULATORY ASPECTS

Bioavailability assessment is critical in early phases of drug development. As defined in United States Code of Federal Regulations [CFR, Title 21, section 320.1(a)] (1), bioavailability means the rate and extent to which the active ingredient or active moiety is absorbed from a drug product and becomes available at the site of action. Microdialysis has been used to measure in vivo tissue concentrations of endogenous compounds and to assess drug concentrations closest to the site of action in various human tissues, such as peripheral tissue or skin, in both healthy volunteers and patients. Consequently, the technique is gaining recognition as a tool in drug development to select an appropriate compound and to optimize dosing regimens.

Evidences to this are drug development plans using the technique in support of clinical data assessment.

The FDA is receptive to microdialysis data as part of an overall preclinical and clinical pharmacology package. The method has been used for formulation optimization programs and has been requested by the FDA, both in the pre- and post- approval setting, as an adjunct to in vivo bioavailability trials. In addition, microdialysis has been proposed by both the FDA and pharmaceutical companies as a way to address specific safety issues relating to systemic drug delivery of drugs intended for topical action.

Both dermatopharmacokinetic and microdialysis methods have a good potential for application in drug development and in regulatory assessments. However, for both methods the inter- and intra-laboratory reproducibility and validity will need to be established before the methods can be accepted as a regulatory tool for determining bioequivalence between the test and reference topical drug products.

Dermatopharmacokinetics is currently not accepted by the FDA as a method of in vivo bioavailability testing due to concerns about the technique's replication across study sites. While it may have a future role in the evaluation of cutaneous drug penetration, there is currently less confidence in the regulatory applicability of the results from a dermatopharmacokinetic study versus a microdialysis study.

In conclusion, microdialysis data are likely to become an important part of new drug submissions, and thus is expected to contribute to the FDA Critical Path Initiative (32) to facilitate innovation in drug development.

RECOMMENDATIONS

- Both microdialysis and dermatopharmacokinetic methods can be considered suitable in addressing various aspects of dermal drug delivery, specific to each method. Prior to embarking on either method, a pharmaceutical company should engage the appropriate regulatory body in discussions with regard to both method selection and how the results will be utilized in the development program.
- If a concentration difference exists between the formulations to be tested, microdialysis in the target tissue (dermis) should be considered most appropriate choice.
- If the site of action is the SC, dermatopharmacokinetic methodology can be considered the most appropriate choice.
- If the dermis is the site of action, microdialysis methodology should be preferred.
- If the drug of interest is very lipophilic, microdialysis sampling as well as dermatopharmacokinetic methodology may be necessary in order to characterize penetration into and subsequently through the upper layers of the skin.

REFERENCES

1. Food and Drug Cosmetics Act. 21 CFR 320, 2002.
2. Chaurasia CS, Müller M, Bashaw ED, et al. AAPS–FDA Workshop white paper: microdialysis principles, application and regulatory perspectives. J Clin Pharmacol 2007; 47:589–603.

3. Davies MI, Cooper JD, Desmond SS, et al. Analytical considerations for microdialysis sampling. Adv Drug Deliv Rev 2000; 45:169–88.
4. Benfeldt E, Groth L. Feasibility of measuring lipophilic or protein-bound drugs in the dermis by in vivo microdialysis after topical or systemic drug administration. Acta Derm Venereol 1998; 78(4):274–8.
5. Borg N, Gotharson E, Benfeldt E, et al. Distribution to the skin of penciclovir after oral famciclovir administration in healthy volunteers: comparison of the suction blister technique and cutaneous microdialysis. Acta Derm Venereol 1999; 79(4):274–7.
6. Benfeldt E, Serup J, Menne T. Microdialysis vs. suction blister technique for in vivo sampling of pharmacokinetics in the human dermis. Acta Derm Venereol 1999; 79(5): 338–42.
7. Anderson C, Andersson T, Molander M. Ethanol absorption across human skin measured by in vivo microdialysis technique. Acta Derm Venereol 1991; 71(5):389–93.
8. Groth L, García Ortiz P, Benfeldt E. Microdialysis methodology for sampling in the skin. In: Serup J, Jemec GBE, Grove G, eds. Handbook of Non-Invasive Methods and the Skin. 2nd ed. Boca Raton, FL: CRC Press, 2006:443–54.
9. Hegemann L, Forstinger C, Partsch B, et al. Microdialysis in cutaneous pharmacology: kinetic analysis of transdermally delivered nicotine. J Invest Dermatol 1995; 104(5): 839–43.
10. Tegeder I, Muth-Selbach U, Lotsch J, et al. Application of microdialysis for the determination of muscle and subcutaneous tissue concentrations after oral and topical ibuprofen administration. Clin Pharmacol Ther 1999; 65(4):357–68.
11. Benfeldt E. In vivo microdialysis for the investigation of drug levels in the dermis and the effect of barrier perturbation on cutaneous drug penetration. Studies in hairless rats and human subjects. Acta Derm Venereol Suppl 1999; 206:1–59.
12. Tegeder I, Brautigam L, Podda M, et al. Time course of 8-methoxypsoralen concentrations in skin and plasma after topical (bath and cream) and oral administration of 8-methoxypsoralen. Clin Pharmacol Ther 2002; 71(3):153–61.
13. Kreilgaard M, Kemme MJ, Burggraaf J, et al. Influence of a microemulsion vehicle on cutaneous bioequivalence of a lipophilic model drug assessed by microdialysis and pharmacodynamics. Pharm Res 2001; 18(5):593–9.
14. Benfeldt E, Serup J, Menne T. Effect of barrier perturbation on cutaneous salicylic acid penetration in human skin: in vivo pharmacokinetics using microdialysis and non-invasive quantification of barrier function. Br J Dermatol 1999; 140(4):739–48.
15. Stagni G, O'Donnell D, Liu YJ, et al. Iontophoretic current and intradermal microdialysis recovery in humans. J Pharmacol Toxicol Methods 1999; 41(1):49–54.
16. Benfeldt E, Serup J. Effect of barrier perturbation on cutaneous penetration of salicylic acid in hairless rats: in vivo pharmacokinetics using microdialysis and non-invasive quantification of barrier function. Arch Dermatol Res 1999; 291(9):517–26.
17. Muller M, Mascher H, Kikuta C, et al. Diclofenac concentrations in defined tissue layers after topical administration. Clin Pharmacol Ther 1997; 62(3):293–9.
18. Simonsen L, Jorgensen A, Benfeldt E, et al. Differentiated in vivo skin penetration of salicylic compounds in hairless rats measured by cutaneous microdialysis. Eur J Pharm Sci 2003; 21:379–88.
19. Leveque N, Makki S, Hadgraft J, et al. Comparison of Franz cells and microdialysis for assessing salicylic acid penetration through human skin. Int J Pharm 2004; 69(2):323–8.
20. Oberthur C, Heinemann C, Elsner P, et al. A comparative study on the skin penetration of pure tryptanthrin and tryptanthrin in Isatis tinctoria extract by dermal microdialysis coupled with isotope dilution ESI–LC–MS. Planta Med 2003; 69(5):385–9.
21. McDonald S, Lunte C. Determination of the dermal penetration of esterom components using microdialysis sampling. Pharm Res 2003; 20(11):1827–34.
22. Benfeldt E, Hansen SH, Volund A, et al. Bioequivalence of topical formulations in humans: evaluation by dermal microdialysis sampling and the dermatopharmacokinetic method. J Invest Dermatol 2007; 127(1):170–8.
23. Shah VP, Flynn GL, Yacobi A, et al. Bioequivalence of topical dermatological dosage forms—methods of evaluation of bioequivalence. Pharm Res 1998; 15(2):167–71.

24. Caron JC, Queille-Roussel C, Shah VP, et al. The correlation between the drug penetration and vasoconstriction of hydrocortisone creams in human. J Am Acad Dermatol 1990; 23:458–62.
25. Weigmann H, Lademann J, Pelchrzim R, et al. Bioavailability of clobetasol propionate-quantification of drug concentrations in the stratum corneum by dermatopharmacokinetics using tape stripping. Skin Pharmacol Appl Skin Physiol 1999; 12(1–2):46–53.
26. Weigmann H, Lademann J, Meffert H, et al. Determination of the horny layer profile by tape stripping in combination with optical spectroscopy in the visible range as a prerequisite to quantify percutaneous absorption. Skin Pharmacol Appl Skin Physiol 1999; 12(1–2):34–45.
27. Dreher F, Modjtahedi BS, Modjtahedi SP, et al. Quantification of stratum corneum removal by adhesive tape stripping by total protein assay in 96-well microplates. Skin Res Technol 2005; 11:97–101.
28. Kalia YN, Alberti I, Naik A, et al. Assessment of topical bioavailability in vivo: the importance of stratum corneum thickness. Skin Pharmacol Appl Skin Physiol 2001; 14(Suppl. 1):82–6.
29. Rougier A, Lotte C, Maibach HI. In vivo percutaneous penetration of some organic compounds related to anatomic site in humans: predictive assessment by the stripping method. J Pharm Sci 1987; 76(6):451–4.
30. Shah VP. Progress in methodologies for evaluating bioequivalence of topical formulations. Am J Clin Dermatol 2001; 2(5):275–80.
31. Pershing LK, Nelson JL, Corlett JL, et al. Assessment of dermatopharmacokinetic approach in the bioequivalence determination of topical tretinoin gel products. J Am Acad Dermatol 2003; 48(5):740–51.
32. FDA. Innovation or stagnation? Challenge and opportunity on the Critical Path to new medical products. U.S. Department of Health and Human Services, Food and Drug Administration, 2004. (Accessed September 9, 2007 at http://www.fda.gov/oc/initiatives/criticalpath/reports/generic.html)

33

An Industry Perspective of Topical Dermal Bioequivalence

Dawn McCleverty, Richard Lyons, and Brian Henry
Pfizer Global Research and Development, Sandwich, Kent, U.K.

INTRODUCTION

In the course of developing a topical dermatological product, the benefit and/or regulatory recommendation for the establishment of product bioequivalence presents at a number of key stages. Bioequivalence documentation is required to support New Drug Application (NDA) and abbreviated New Drug Application (ANDA) submissions (1). The data may be used to support changes between formulations used in clinical trials, to link formulations used in trials and stability studies (if different), and to support progression from clinical trial formulations to the proposed commercial product (2). All topical drug products intended for marketing under an abbreviated application are required to generate evidence of in vivo bioequivalence (3). In addition, if the inactive ingredients in an ANDA are not the same as the reference listed drug, the applicant should demonstrate to the agency that the change(s) do not affect the safety and/or efficacy of the proposed drug product. The Food and Drug Administration (FDA) guideline suggests that a comparative BA study could satisfy this recommendation.

In the case of post-approval changes, bioequivalence documentation is again required (4) to support level 3 changes (those likely to have a significant impact on formulation quality and performance). A full bioequivalence study on the highest strength is required and the guidance on study design states that "any appropriately validated study may be used for the topical dermatological drug product."

Classical bioequivalence studies to establish the equivalence of two solid oral dosage forms measure drug concentrations in biological fluids such as blood or urine following single or multiple administration (5). However, the lack of such accessible biological fluids in the case of some topically/locally applied agents presents a challenge. The FDA recommends a series of in vitro and in vivo methods, in order of preference, to assess bioequivalence in this circumstance (1,6):

1. Pharmacokinetic measurements based on measurement of an active drug and/or metabolite in blood, plasma, and/or urine
2. Pharmacodynamic effect studies
3. Comparative clinical trials
4. In vitro studies.

As mentioned, for products applied topically and intended to act without systemic absorption, the approach to determine bioequivalence based on systemic measurements is not applicable. In the absence of an appropriate pharmacodynamic endpoint, comparative clinical studies are in principle required. It has been reported that "clinical efficacy trials aimed at showing the bioequivalence of topical dermatological products are relatively insensitive, time-consuming and costly. To gain adequate statistical power required to make a clear bioequivalence determination, they may require as many as 300 patients" (7). There is therefore a clear need for a method which will allow a cost efficient determination of bioequivalence in a reasonable patient population. The minimally invasive technique of dermal microdialysis to establish bioequivalence of topically applied agents in humans by measuring local tissue concentrations with time, utilizing a dermato-pharmacokinetic (DPK) approach could fulfill these criteria. The DPK approach has been considered specifically for skin stripping (1) but should be applicable to any approach relating concentration in the skin to a drug's therapeutic action (7).

Microdialysis is a sampling technique that can be used to sample endogenous and exogenous solutes in the extracellular space of tissues by means of a dialysis membrane which is permeable to small molecules and water. The microdialysis membrane or probe is implanted in the tissue of interest and perfused, typically with a physiologically relevant media, setting up a concentration gradient along its length. Compounds can diffuse into or out of the probe depending on the direction of the concentration gradient. Data obtained from such studies may be presented in a variety of ways: relative recovery or loss, tissue concentration, area under the concentration curve (AUC), and C_{max}. The use of microdialysis to sample extracellular fluid was first described in 1966 (8), and since that time its use has increased and the technique has been extensively reviewed in the literature (9–13). Probes have been adapted, perfusion systems technically improved and with the coupling of the technique to analytical methodologies, e.g., high-performance liquid chromatography (HPLC), microdialysis has become one of the major tools for bioanalytical sampling. Alongside these technical advances, the variety of animal species incorporated has increased. With the advance to the introduction of microdialysis in man in the late 1980s, the extension to clinical pharmacological studies has opened a gateway to obtaining information regarding drug distribution processes to clinically relevant target sites. Microdialysis had been applied to the measurement of free tissue concentrations of endogenous compounds and also to the determination of the tissue distribution of drug molecules in a large number of human tissues [e.g., bone, lung, heart, brain, skin, neoplastic tissue, and soft tissues, such as skeletal muscle and blood (11,14,15)].

In the clinical setting, sampling techniques which could be used to demonstrate dermal bioequivalence of topically applied agents which are both minimally invasive and which also give an indication of tissue concentrations at a target site in the skin with time are limited. Techniques, such as skin stripping, suction blisters, tissue biopsy, and dermal imaging techniques, such as confocal laser scanning microscopy, have all been extensively reviewed in the literature and therefore will not be discussed here (7,9,16–18). These methods have their place, but are restrictive in the amount of information generated and require a large number of subjects or a large number of sampling sites on a particular subject to obtain a concentration/time profile, therefore increasing the cost of the study as well as the invasiveness involved. Concerns have been raised regarding the technique-sensitive nature of skin stripping and the variability associated with the data generated. The assessment of dermal bioequivalence of topical corticosteroids has successfully utilized a vasoconstriction protocol (19), however, this methodology is restricted to agents demonstrating this specific pharmacodynamic endpoint.

Dermal microdialysis has the potential to address the gap in available sampling techniques due to its minimally invasive nature and its ability to generate concentration/time profiles at a target site with good time resolution when a sufficiently sensitive analytical method is available. Recent publications have commented on the fact that dermal microdialysis is a technique which has utility in a clinical setting (14,20,21) but information is lacking on the manner in which this technique could be applied to a manageable patient population, in particular in the field of dermal bioequivalence testing.

In order to confidently use dermal microdialysis in a clinical setting, one must determine whether the degree of variability associated with the technique allows its practical application to the determination of dermal bioequivalence of topically applied agents with a reasonable number of subjects. A review of literature data was conducted to estimate the variances associated with the subject-to-subject variability and the probe-to-probe variability within the subjects to determine the degree to which such clinical studies must be powered to demonstrate dermal bioequivalence in line with regulatory requirements (1). In order to successfully utilize dermal microdialysis to establish bioequivalence of topically applied agents, particular care must be applied to study design. Steps to overcome the inherent variability between subjects and to maintain subject numbers at reasonable levels will be discussed.

MATERIALS AND METHODS
Statistical Analysis
The technique of Restricted Maximum Likelihood, as implemented in the SAS® V8.02 procedure MIXED, was used to estimate the variances associated with the subject-to-subject variability and the probe-to-probe variability within the subjects. Sample size calculations were performed using NQuery Adviser V4.0. Graphics have been produced using SPLUS® 2000 Release 3, StatGaphics® Plus V5, and Microsoft® Excel 2000.

Data Analysis
Raw data retrieval from the literature for inclusion in these analyses proved challenging. The parameter chosen for analysis was the AUC of the concentration/time profiles and/or C_{max} from as many subjects as possible. The greatest amount of data available to us was that generated by Dr. W Keene (22). The primary analysis has been conducted using this data and the degree of variability from this study is then compared to available literature (23–29).

In Vivo Study Design for Primary Data Set
The data set used in this analysis (Tables 1 and 2) was from an in vivo study on eight human volunteers (four males, four females aged 19–24) (22). The design of the trial required each subject to have a total of six microdialysis probes inserted, which were divided into three pairs (probe 1 and probe 2 for each pair) according to the perfusate to be used:

1. Ringers perfusate—application site unoccluded
2. Ringers and noradrenaline (5 μg/mL) perfusate—application site unoccluded
3. Ringers and noradrenaline (5 μg/mL) perfusate—application site occluded.

Noradrenaline was included in the perfusate to decrease dermal blood flow, allowing higher local tissue concentrations to be maintained. Occluding the

TABLE 1 Summary of Dialysate Methyl Salicylate Concentrations (μg/mL) for Each Probe and at Each Time Point

Subject	Perfusate	Pre-dose		0–1 hr		1–2 hrs		2–3 hrs		3–4 hrs		4–5 hrs	
		Probe 1	Probe 2	Probe 1	Probe 2	Probe 1	Probe 2	Probe 1	Probe 2	Probe 1	Probe 2	Probe 1	Probe 2
1	Ringers	ND	ND	0.82	1.13	0.22	0.44	ND	ND	ND	ND	ND	ND
	Ringers + NA	ND	ND	1.54	1.04	0.85	0.53	0.47	0.30	0.30	0.17	0.21	0.16
	Ringers + NA occluded	ND	ND	2.01	1.55	2.19	1.33	1.27	0.96	0.89	0.83	0.80	0.58
2	Ringers	ND	ND	0.63	—	0.49	—	0.45	—	0.45	—	0.52	—
	Ringers + NA	ND	ND	0.21	—	0.17	—	0.25	—	1.24	—	0.32	—
	Ringers + NA occluded	ND	ND	0.30	0.97	0.29	0.72	0.29	0.78	0.66	0.90	0.13	0.73
3	Ringers	ND	ND	0.22	—	0.21	—	ND	—	ND	—	ND	—
	Ringers + NA	ND	ND	0.36	—	0.19	—	ND	—	ND	—	ND	—
	Ringers + NA occluded	ND	ND	0.17	0.13	0.50	0.31	0.38	0.34	0.25	0.36	0.25	0.33
4	Ringers	ND	ND	0.63	0.54	0.47	0.12	0.15	ND	ND	ND	ND	ND
	Ringers + NA	ND	ND	0.96	1.27	0.50	0.50	0.17	0.16	0.11	0.11	0.10	ND
	Ringers + NA occluded	ND	ND	0.91	0.38	0.96	0.55	0.68	0.29	0.57	0.21	0.46	0.25
5	Ringers	ND	ND	0.63	—	ND	—	ND	—	ND	—	ND	—
	Ringers + NA	ND	ND	0.97	—	0.22	—	0.16	—	ND	—	ND	—
	Ringers + NA occluded	ND	ND	1.94	1.00	0.91	0.73	0.50	0.49	0.61	0.33	ND	ND
6	Ringers	ND	ND	0.39	1.04	0.35	0.41	ND	ND	0.17	ND	ND	ND
	Ringers + NA	ND	ND	0.50	2.95	0.48	0.87	0.28	0.23	0.20	0.23	ND	ND
	Ringers + NA occluded	ND	ND	1.13	1.12	1.15	1.40	0.50	0.69	0.48	0.47	ND	0.42
7	Ringers	ND	ND	0.30	0.30	0.10	0.09	ND	ND	ND	ND	ND	ND
	Ringers + NA	ND	ND	0.50	1.60	0.20	0.30	0.08	0.10	ND	0.07	ND	ND
	Ringers + NA occluded	ND	ND	1.00	0.30	0.60	0.30	0.40	0.20	0.20	0.10	0.10	0.08
8	Ringers	ND	ND	1.70	1.93	0.27	0.43	0.14	0.24	0.17	0.13	0.12	ND
	Ringers + NA	ND	ND	1.65	0.47	0.53	0.18	0.27	0.05	0.17	ND	ND	ND
	Ringers + NA occluded	ND	ND	0.65	0.48	0.64	0.34	0.34	0.21	0.21	0.16	0.09	0.05

Abbreviations: NA, noradrenaline; ND, none detected; —, not available due to analytical problems.
Source: From Ref. 22.

TABLE 2 Summary of Dialysate Salicylic Acid Concentrations (μg/mL) for Each Probe and at Each Time Point

Subject	Perfusate	Pre-dose Probe 1	Pre-dose Probe 2	0–1 hr Probe 1	0–1 hr Probe 2	1–2 hrs Probe 1	1–2 hrs Probe 2	2–3 hrs Probe 1	2–3 hrs Probe 2	3–4 hrs Probe 1	3–4 hrs Probe 2	4–5 hrs Probe 1	4–5 hrs Probe 2
1	Ringers	0.12	0.13	0.28	0.32	0.54	0.60	0.39	0.51	0.29	0.36	0.18	0.13
	Ringers + NA	0.14	0.11	0.25	0.04	0.41	0.36	0.50	0.43	0.72	0.37	0.48	0.37
	Ringers + NA occluded	0.12	0.13	0.37	0.32	0.83	0.53	1.02	0.84	1.23	0.70	1.31	0.94
2	Ringers	0.04	—	0.15	—	0.48	—	0.84	—	0.93	—	0.61	—
	Ringers + NA	0.10	—	0.20	—	0.39	—	0.48	—	0.50	—	0.47	—
	Ringers + NA occluded	0.09	0.06	0.21	0.14	0.47	0.22	0.44	0.27	1.17	0.46	0.99	0.47
3	Ringers	0.08	—	0.07	—	0.15	—	0.15	—	0.08	—	0.09	—
	Ringers + NA	ND	—	0.52	—	1.01	—	1.05	—	1.16	—	0.97	—
	Ringers + NA occluded	0.03	0.04	0.13	0.12	0.47	0.65	0.73	1.29	0.91	1.46	1.11	1.55
4	Ringers	ND	ND	0.11	0.05	0.45	0.16	0.47	0.17	0.31	0.09	0.21	0.07
	Ringers + NA	0.07	0.04	0.36	0.44	1.15	1.24	1.22	1.11	1.23	0.84	0.69	0.59
	Ringers + NA occluded	0.05	0.04	0.25	0.20	0.98	0.70	1.46	1.06	1.59	1.14	1.59	1.07
5	Ringers	ND	—	0.37	—	0.54	—	0.38	—	0.21	—	ND	—
	Ringers + NA	0.10	—	0.65	—	1.41	—	1.35	—	0.09	—	ND	—
	Ringers + NA occluded	0.05	ND	0.44	0.44	1.49	1.74	1.33	2.88	2.26	2.32	—	—
6	Ringers	ND	ND	0.07	0.30	0.20	0.28	0.11	0.13	0.09	0.14	0.06	0.07
	Ringers + NA	0.04	0.10	0.34	0.10	0.38	0.24	0.04	0.25	0.36	0.24	0.29	0.21
	Ringers + NA occluded	0.12	0.04	0.12	0.30	0.51	0.60	0.63	0.62	0.62	0.85	0.69	0.96
7	Ringers	ND	ND	0.19	0.20	0.23	0.24	0.14	0.13	0.06	0.03	ND	0.06
	Ringers + NA	ND	ND	0.61	1.31	1.46	2.08	1.28	1.37	0.82	0.99	ND	0.64
	Ringers + NA occluded	0.03	0.04	0.76	0.86	1.97	2.40	2.46	2.54	2.05	2.03	1.70	1.84
8	Ringers	ND	ND	0.36	0.62	0.45	1.02	0.53	0.82	0.19	0.55	0.13	0.33
	Ringers + NA	ND	0.02	0.54	0.80	1.29	1.77	1.17	1.71	0.81	1.36	0.48	0.86
	Ringers + NA occluded	ND	ND	0.52	0.54	1.44	1.26	1.82	1.61	1.83	1.52	1.66	1.17

Abbreviations: NA, noradrenaline; ND, none detected; —, not available due to analytical problems.
Source: From Ref. 22.

application site has the effect of further boosting local tissue concentrations. The 2 kDa probes were used, perfused at a rate of 0.4 mL/hr. The probes were positioned to a depth of 0.4 to 0.6 mm (verified using ultrasound) in the ventral forearm of the volunteers.

The topically applied vehicle contained methyl salicylate at saturation in a 50% propylene glycol/50% water vehicle. A 0.1 mL was pipetted into a drug well (Comfeel® Plus Ulcer Dressing; Coloplast Ltd., Peterborough, U.K.) secured over the application site. Where wells were occluded, a sheet of the dressing material was applied over the well immediately following vehicle application.

RESULTS AND DISCUSSION
Overview
The concentration of methyl salicylate and its metabolite salicylic acid was measured by HPLC hourly over a five-hour period (Tables 1 and 2). While methyl salicylate is a recognized rubefacient (30), it is the final tissue concentrations that are of interest in this analysis rather than the means by which they were achieved.

The purpose of the statistical analysis detailed below is to use the variation observed in this group of subjects to predict the numbers of subjects required in future two group comparative studies. The data show that there is significant variation in the concentration profiles across subjects within each of the perfusates. In some cases, variability in the profiles can be seen for the two probes within a subject/perfusate combination, in particular for methyl salicylate.

The main response of interest in terms of measuring dermal delivery is the AUC and this has been calculated for each curve using trapezoidal integration. It is usual for such areas to be transformed by taking logarithms and there is some evidence that this transformation would be beneficial for this analysis as can be seen in Figures 1 and 2 where areas are plotted on a log-scale. An analysis of the data to estimate the components of variance that can be attributed to variation between subjects and to variation between the probes within each subject has been conducted. The estimates, pooled across perfusates, are shown in Table 3. It can be seen from this data that the estimates of variance components are similar across the two compounds, particularly when one bears in mind the uncertainty in the individual estimates, as shown by the confidence limits (the width of the confidence intervals

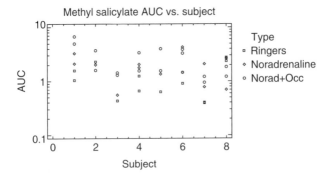

FIGURE 1 Methyl salicylate. Plot of AUC against subject showing variation between and within subjects. *Abbreviation*: AUC, area under the concentration curve.

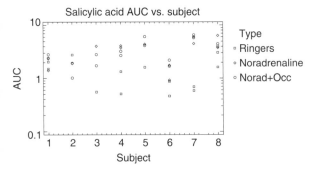

FIGURE 2 Salicylic acid. Plot of AUC against subject showing variation between and within subjects. *Abbreviation*: AUC, area under the concentration curve.

TABLE 3 Estimates of Variance Components

Compound	Source of variation	Variance component estimate	Approximately 95% confidence limits
Methyl salicylate	Subjects	0.20	0.09–0.89
	Probes	0.21	0.12–0.46
Salicylic acid	Subjects	0.26	0.13–0.67
	Probes	0.11	0.06–0.23

reflects the fact that there are relatively few subjects in this study). However, the between-probe variation is somewhat higher in the methyl salicylate group.

Number of Subjects Required for a Parallel Group Study

For a study comparing two treatments, if each subject is assigned to one or other of the two treatment groups then the subject-to-subject variability is important in the calculations of sample sizes. One can use these estimates of variability to predict what the variation will be in a future study with any number of repeat probes for each subject. Here the calculations have been made for up to four probes per subject and the results are presented in terms of the standard deviation (SD) (Table 4).

Sample Sizes Required to Detect Changes in Area

Given the variability estimates in Table 4, it is possible to calculate what level of change in AUC between two groups of subjects we might reasonably expect to detect using a two-sample t-test at the 5% level of significance. The change in AUC is measured in terms of a ratio (this is a consequence of using the log transform of

TABLE 4 Estimates of Standard Deviation

Compound	Number of probes per subject			
	1	2	3	4
Methyl salicylate	0.64	0.55	0.52	0.50
Salicylic acid	0.60	0.56	0.55	0.54

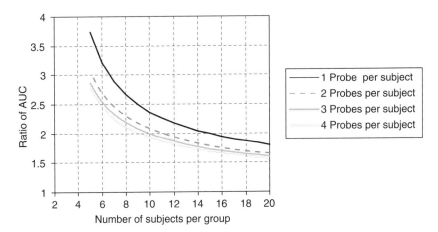

FIGURE 3   Relationship between the true ratio of areas under the concentration curve (AUC) that can be detected with 80% power and the number of subjects in each group based on the variance estimates from the methyl salicylate data.

the areas). A reasonable chance of detecting a given ratio is defined here as 80% (the power of the test). What level of ratio detected will depend on the number of subjects in each of the groups, Figure 3 shows this relationship for the methyl salicylate data. For example, with just five subjects in each group with only one probe we could only reasonably expect to detect areas that were about four times greater in one group than in the other. By increasing the number of probes to two, this ratio reduces to about three times. Increasing the number of probes per subject further results in smaller and smaller reductions in the ratio. By increasing the number of subjects, the ratio rapidly decreases and then flattens out. By using 20 subjects per group, each with two probes, one could expect to detect areas in one treatment group that were roughly half as big again as in the second treatment group.

Number of Subjects Required for a Within Patient Comparison Study

If each subject has both treatments applied then subject-to-subject variability is eliminated from the calculation of sample sizes. However, there could be an important source of variability due to a subject by treatment interaction which would mean that the true underlying difference between the treatments was not the same for each subject. No information is available as to whether this source of variability is likely to be important in a future study as clearly no treatment information is available in the background data so it is assumed that the individual subject reactions to the treatments would not alter the resulting absorption. This would have to be established on a compound by compound, or treatment by treatment, basis in any given study. If one assumes that the treatment by subject interaction is negligible, then one can use the probe variances in Table 4 to estimate the variability one would see from using two probes per treatment on a number of subjects in a paired t-test (or the corresponding equivalence test). Because of this assumption, the plots presented should be treated as a "best case scenario" in terms of the numbers of subjects required. Figure 4 illustrates that by removing the subject-to-subject variability one is able to detect much smaller changes in the areas

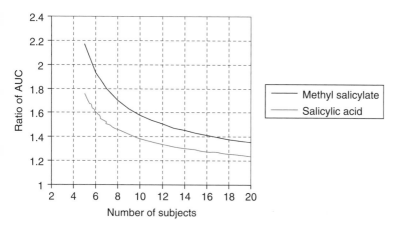

FIGURE 4 Relationship between the true ratio of areas under the concentration curve (AUC) that can be detected with 80% power and the total number of subjects in the study.

than was the case for the two-sample *t*-test. For example, with just five subjects in each group we could reasonably expect to detect areas that were about two times greater in one group than in the other.

Sample Sizes Required to Meet Bioequivalence Criteria

The FDA accepted bioequivalence criterion states that a 90% confidence interval for the ratio of the group means should lie within 80% to 125% for AUC (1). A standard requirement is that a sufficient number of subjects should be used in each group so that there is an 80% chance of declaring equivalence when there is no difference between the groups. In a parallel group study, to achieve this with one probe per subject we would need to have 147 subjects per group; with two probes per subject, this reduces to 105 subjects per group (Fig. 5). Such a study design therefore would require a very large number of subjects in order to establish the bioequivalence of

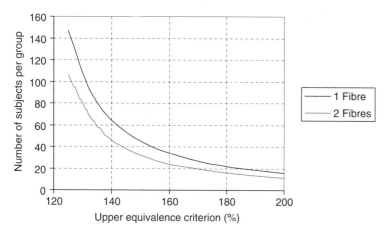

FIGURE 5 Relationship between the number of subjects required and the upper equivalence limit (1 and 2 fibers).

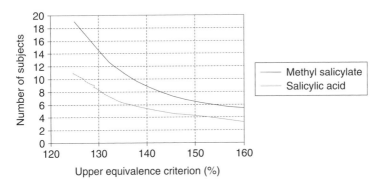

FIGURE 6   Relationship between the number of subjects required and the upper equivalence limit.

two topically applied agents. A reasonable number of subjects (e.g., 20 per group), using this design, would only establish bioequivalence if the equivalence limits were set at 56% to 180%, well outside the current criteria.

If, however, the study design is altered to a within-subject comparison study, each subject having both treatment groups applied to two probes, then the subject-to-subject variability is eliminated from the calculation of sample sizes. Assuming the treatment by subject interaction is negligible, then one can use the probe variances in Table 4 as estimates of the variability one would see from using two probes on a number of subjects in a paired t-test (or the corresponding equivalence test). Figure 6 shows the total number of subjects required to achieve 80% power for a range of upper equivalence limits (the lower limit is simply the reciprocal of the upper limit). So, in this case, with a total of 20 subjects there is a reasonable chance of meeting the 80% to 125% equivalence criterion.

Variability in Literature Data

The analyses discussed thus far have been based on results from eight volunteers and one study center (22). In order to determine if the degree of variability seen in these studies was representative of studies being conducted at other centers, a literature review was conducted. In general very few papers publish raw data in sufficient detail to conduct a full statistical analysis, however, the papers presented here (23–29) contained sufficient detail to allow us to convert their summary statistics to an estimate of the Coefficient of Variation (CV). This measure (also known as the Relative Standard Deviation) simply expresses the SD as a percentage of the mean. For this literature data, it is therefore not possible to look at the relative sizes of the between- and within-subject variation. In most cases, the published summary statistics are based on a single probe per subject and so the analysis reviews the sum of these two components of variation. This has therefore been used as the common measure of variation wherever possible and represents the variability observed from a study where only one probe per subject was used.

The studies cover a range of locations, probe types, and compounds analyzed with details summarized in Table 5. It would be expected that a large range of CV values between the various studies would be seen just by chance, especially given that some of the estimates of mean and SD are based on relatively small numbers of subjects. However, while it does appear that underlying CV is not the same in every

TABLE 5 Summary of Analysis of Literature Data

Reference	Probe	Tissue site	Number of subjects	Formulation	%CV AUC	%CV C_{max}/Tissue concentration
22	Gambro, 2 kDa, 30 mm	Dermis	8	Saturated methyl salicylate 50% propylene glycol/50% water (v/v)	71	
				Salicylic acid—levels measured following application of formulation above	67	
23	Gambro GFS + 12, 2 kDa, 30 mm	Dermis	8	Microemulsion containing 7.5% (w/w) lidocaine	93	
				Xylocain 5% (w/w) cream (lidocaine)	56	
24	CMA 10, 20 kDa, 16 mm	Superficial adipose tissue	7	Diclofenac gel (Emugel)	98	
		Deep subcutaneous tissue			150	
25	Gambro GFE 18, 2 kDa, 30 mm	Dermis	15	5% (w/v) salicylic acid in ethanol	32	
26	CMA 60, 20 kDa, 30 mm	Muscle	11	5% Ibuprofen gel	142	169
		Dermis			83	78
27	CMA 10, 20 kDa, 10 mm	Dermis	9	Nicotine patch		48
28	CMA 10, 20 kDa, 16 mm	Muscle	12	5% Diclofenac foam		104
29	CMA 70, 20 kDa	Dermis	3	20% Methylsalicylate		42
		Subcutaneous tissue		20% Methylsalicylate		75
		Dermis		7% Glycolsalicylate		90
Median					83	78

Abbreviation: AUC, area under the concentration curve.

study, there is still a measure of agreement between the studies. The variability associated with the primary study used to conduct this analysis falls within the variability range seen in the literature and it therefore appears we can reasonably apply the statistical approach used here to the wider use of microdialysis for dermal bioequivalence testing.

CONCLUSION

The development of novel treatments to be applied to the skin may be hindered by the lack of appropriate methods to determine the relative bioavailability of various formulations during the development program. The minimally invasive technique of dermal microdialysis can be utilized in order to evaluate bioequivalence of topically applied agents in humans by measuring local tissue concentrations with time. The study design must be optimized in order to ensure reasonable subject numbers for a given study. From the studies reviewed this would require a within-subject comparison study where at least two probes are used for both formulations tested, and both formulations are applied to each subject so that the subject-to-subject variability is eliminated from the comparison formulations (each subject acting as its own control). In this situation, it is then possible to demonstrate, with 80% power and a subject population of approximately 20, that two topically applied formulations deliver the same tissue AUC, within 80% to 125% equivalence limits.

ACKNOWLEDGMENTS

We gratefully acknowledge the helpful discussions and assistance provided by Dr. R Ogilvie, Pfizer Global R and D, Dr. WE Keene, and Professor AG Renwick OBE (Retired) formerly of The Faculty of Medicine, Health and Biological Sciences, Southampton University, U.K. In addition, we would like to thank Professor Renwick OBE for granting permission to use the raw data contained in these analyses.

This work has previously been published in the International Journal of Pharmaceutics 2006; 308:1–7.

REFERENCES

1. FDA Guidance for Industry. Draft Guidance, Topical Dermatological Drug Product NDAs and ANDAs—In Vivo Bioavailability, Bioequivalence, In Vitro Release and Associated Studies, June 1998 (withdrawn May 2002).
2. Chen M, Shah V, Patnaik R, et al. Bioavailability and bioequivalence: an FDA regulatory overview. Pharm Res 2001; 18:1645–50.
3. FDA, Title 21 Code of Federal Regulations (CFR) Part 320.21, April 2005.
4. FDA Guidance for Industry. Nonsterile Semisolid Dosage Forms, Scale-Up and Post-approval Changes: Chemistry, Manufacturing and Controls; In Vitro Release Testing and In Vivo Bioequivalence Documentation, May 1997.
5. FDA Guidance for Industry. Bioavailability and Bioequivalence Studies for Orally Administered Drug Products—General Considerations, March 2003.
6. FDA, Title 21 Code of Federal Regulations (CFR) Part 320.24, April 2005.
7. Shah V, Flynn G, Yacobi A, et al. Bioequivalence of topical dermatological dosage forms—methods of evaluation of bioequivalence. Pharm Res 1998; 15:167–71.
8. Bito L, Davson H, Levin E, et al. The concentrations of free amino acids and other electrolytes in cerebrospinal fluid, in vivo dialysate of brain and blood plasma of the dog. J Neurochem 1966; 13:1057–67.

9. Stahl M, Bouw B, Jackson A, et al. Human microdialysis. Curr Pharm Biotechnol 2002; 3:165–78.
10. Benveniste H, Hüttemeier P. Microdialysis—theory and application. Prog Neurobiol 1990; 3:195–215.
11. Elmquist W, Sawchuk R. Application of microdialysis in pharmacokinetic studies. Pharm Res 1997; 14:267–88.
12. Groth L. Cutaneous microdialysis—a new technique for the assessment of skin penetration. Curr Probl Dermatol 1998; 26:90–8.
13. Anderson C, Anderson T, Boman A. Cutaneous microdialysis of human in vivo dermal absorption studies. In: Robert MS, Walters KA, eds. Dermal Absorption and Toxicity Assessment. 1st ed. New York: Marcel Dekker Inc., 1998:231–44.
14. Müller M. Microdialysis in clinical drug delivery studies. Adv Drug Deliv Rev 2000; 45:255–69.
15. de la Peña A, Liu P, Derendorf H. Microdialysis in peripheral tissues. Adv Drug Deliv Rev 2000; 45:189–216.
16. Pershing L, Bakhtian S, Poncelet C, et al. Comparison of skin stripping, in vitro release and skin blanching response methods to measure dose response and similarity of triamcinolone acetonide cream strengths from two manufactured sources. J Pharm Sci 2002; 91:1312–23.
17. Weigmann H, Lademann J, Schanzer S, et al. Correlation of the local distribution of topically applied substances inside the stratum corneum determined by tape-stripping to differences in bioavailability. Skin Pharmacol Appl Skin Physiol 2001; 14(Suppl. 1):98–102.
18. Benfeldt E, Serup J, Menné T. Microdialysis vs. suction blister technique for in vivo sampling of pharmacokinetics in the human dermis. Acta Derm Venereol 1999; 79:338–42.
19. FDA Guidance for Industry. Topical Dermatologic Corticosteroids: In Vivo Bioequivalence, June 1995.
20. Müller M, Schmid R, Georgopoulos A, et al. Application of microdialysis to clinical pharmacokinetics in humans. Clin Pharmacol Ther 1995; 57:371–80.
21. Kreilgaard K. Assessment of cutaneous drug delivery using microdialysis. Adv Drug Deliv Rev 2002; 54:S99–121.
22. Keene W. Evaluation of microdialysis as a tool for studying percutaneous drug absorption and cutaneous metabolism. PhD Thesis, Faculty of Medicine, University of Southampton, 2002.
23. Kreilgaard M, Kemme M, Burggraaf J, et al. Influence of a microemulsion vehicle on cutaneous bioequivalence of a lipophilic model drug assessed by microdialysis and pharmacodynamics. Pharm Res 2001; 18:593–9.
24. Müller M, Mascher H, Kikuta C, et al. Diclofenac concentrations in defined tissue layers after topical administration. Clin Pharmacol Ther 1997; 62:293–9.
25. Benfeldt E, Serup J, Menné T. Effect of barrier perturbation on cutaneous salicylic acid penetration in human skin: in vivo pharmacokinetics using microdialysis and non-invasive quantification of barrier function. Br J Dermatol 1999; 140:739–48.
26. Tegeder I, Muth-Selbach U, Lötsch J, et al. Application of microdialysis for the determination of muscle and subcutaneous tissue concentrations after oral and topical ibuprofen administration. Clin Pharmacol Ther 1999; 65:357–68.
27. Hegemann L, Forstinger C, Partsch B, et al. Microdialysis in cutaneous pharmacology: kinetic analysis of transdermally delivered nicotine. J Invest Dermatol 1995; 104:839–43.
28. Müller M, Rastelli C, Ferri P, et al. Transdermal penetration of diclofenac after multiple epicutaneous administration. J Rheumatol 1998; 25:1833–6.
29. Cross S, Anderson C, Roberts M. Topical penetration of commercial salicylate esters and salts using human isolated skin and clinical microdialysis studies. Br J Clin Pharmacol 1998; 46:29–35.
30. Cross S, Megwa S, Benson H, et al. Self promotion of deep tissue penetration and distribution of methylsalicylate after topical application. Pharm Res 1999; 16:427–33.

34 Dermal Absorption of Chemical Contaminants from Soil

John C. Kissel
Department of Environmental and Occupational Health Sciences,
University of Washington, Seattle, Washington, U.S.A.

Elizabeth W. Spalt
Integral Consulting, Inc., Mercer Island, Washington, U.S.A.

Jeffry H. Shirai
Department of Environmental and Occupational Health Sciences,
University of Washington, Seattle, Washington, U.S.A.

Annette L. Bunge
Department of Chemical Engineering, Colorado School of Mines, Golden,
Colorado, U.S.A.

BACKGROUND

Recently, Spalt et al. (1) critically reviewed the available (English language) literature describing dermal absorption from soil. The earliest entry in that review is a paper by Swiss investigators concerning oral and dermal absorption of 2,3,7,8-tetrachlorodibenzo-*p*-dioxin (TCDD) in multiple formulations including soil (2). That investigation was inspired by dioxin contamination events in Germany and Italy in the 1970s. All but one of the subsequent studies identified in the review were conducted in the United States. Given the universality of English as the language of science, this observation presumably reflects research funding priorities stemming from political attention to hazardous waste sites and other contaminated lands, and the relative importance of quantitative risk assessment in the regulatory environment in the United States, rather than mere language bias. Regardless, the total body of research is quite limited [Spalt et al. (1) found fewer than 50 distinct studies] and represents the efforts of a relatively small group of investigators. In addition to its limited scope, significant shortcomings of the extant dermal-absorption-from-soil literature include (*i*) a lack of uniformity of methodology, which greatly hinders systematic comparison across compounds and laboratories, (*ii*) frequently inadequate reporting of experimental details, and (*iii*) obvious flaws in some experimental approaches.

As a consequence, commonly used procedures for estimation of dermal absorption of chemical contaminants from soil are not well developed. Current U.S. Environmental Protection Agency (USEPA) guidance for use in investigations of the worst uncontrolled and abandoned toxic waste sites in the United States, those designated Superfund sites, presents recommendations for estimation of absorption of contaminants from both soil and water (3). The soil protocol is

TABLE 1   Chemicals for Which Fractional Dermal Availabilities from Soil are Specified in Current U.S. Enviromental Protection Agency Guidance

Arsenic
Cadmium
Chlordane
2,4-Dichlorophenoxyacetic acid
DDT
2,3,7,8-Tetrachlorodibenzo-*p*-dioxin and other dioxins
Lindane
Benzo(*a*)pyrene and other polyaromatic hydrocarbons
Aroclors 1242/1254 and other polychlorinated biphenyls
Pentachlorophenol
Semivolatile organic compounds
Organic nitro compounds (12 values)

Source: From Ref. 3, as supplemented by Ref. 32.

relatively primitive and depends heavily upon literal acceptance of results, expressed as fraction of initial dose absorbed, for the limited number of chemicals (shown in Table 1) for which experimental results are available. In some cases, measurements made on one chemical were extended to the entire class of chemicals [e.g., benzo(*a*)pyrene as a surrogate for all polyaromatic hydrocarbons, TCDD for all dioxins, and Aroclor 1242 or 1254 for all polychlorinated biphenyls (PCBs)]. For contamination of soil by semivolatile organic compounds (SVOCs) not otherwise listed, a default availability of 10% is recommended. For unlisted chemicals that cannot be characterized as SVOCs, no default is stipulated and a qualitative approach is recommended.

In contrast, a relatively well-founded protocol for estimation of dermal absorption of chemicals from water is described in the same guidance. This disparity reflects the fact that many more studies with much greater uniformity of methodology are available for water. Specifically, data describing absorption from water obtained in vitro using human cadaver skin were available for about 90 organic compounds at the time the USEPA guidance was written,[a] whereas only about one-third as many compounds have been studied in experimental investigations of absorption from soil by all methods. A theoretically more rigorous approach for soil, based on the water permeation data, has been proposed by Bunge and Parks (4,5), but has not been adequately tested due to lack of suitable data and has not been widely adopted. In a limited comparison with results from a set of experiments that were sufficiently described (6), the Bunge and Parks approach (5) over-estimated dermal absorption of lindane and 2,4-dichlorphenoxyacetic acid (2,4-D) from two soils.

All soils have a limited capacity to interact with a given contaminant, which is essentially the saturation limit (7). If the amount of contaminant in soil exceeds this limit, neat chemical will be present. Based on rudimentary chemical and physical principles, an organic chemical sorbed to soil at a concentration less than saturation of the soil would be expected to be less available for dermal absorption than it would be in neat form. Sorption on soil should lower fugacity and hence reduce the thermodynamic driving force for dermal absorption and might also reasonably be expected to increase mass transfer resistance. In concert, these effects should reduce flux into skin. Recent results for two different soils

---

[a] There are now water data for approximately 150 compounds.

contaminated with methyl paraben (7,8), which included determinations of soil saturation, are consistent with the fugacity argument. The results reported in the early paper by Poiger and Schlatter (2) noted above are also generally in accord with this basic concept. In those experiments, TCDD was apparently less well absorbed from soil than from neat compound and even less well absorbed from activated carbon than from soil. However, the intervening literature is not consistent on even this fundamental point as several investigators have reported that they did not observe reduced availability from soil in the experiments they conducted. A sampling of those reports is described briefly below.

SELECTED EXAMPLES
Case 1
Wester et al. (9–13) have conducted in vivo experiments using rhesus monkeys in which absorption of radiolabeled chemicals [Aroclor 1242, benzo(*a*)pyrene, chlordane, 1,1,1-trichloro-2,2-bis(*p*-chlorophenyl)ethane (DDT), 2,4-D, and pentachlorophenol] was assessed after application in solvent and in soil to abdominal skin. Availability was assessed by collection of urine for several days to several weeks with adjustment for radiolabel recovery after intravenous administration. In four of six cases, Wester et al. found no statistical difference between availability (expressed as percent of initial dose) from soil and solvent. They summarized these results in the following manner (13):

> Absorption levels of pentachlorophenol, chlordane, PCBs, and … 2,4-D are the same from acetone and soil.

Note that Wester et al. do not conclude merely that their in vivo results do not show a difference between absorption from their soil and absorption from solvent deposition for the four compounds, a position that would be both accurate and appropriately cautious. Rather they assert that soil (and apparently not just their own rather artificial soil, which is described in more detail below) has no effect on transfer of these lipophilic compounds to skin. Strong empirical evidence exists that soils are sorbents for a broad range of non-ionized organic chemicals [e.g., (14)]. Because the quotation above is inconsistent with fundamental chemical principles, it is reasonable to question the adequacy of the experimental protocol on which it is based.

There are at least two explanations for the observed results. The first is that all four compounds were applied to the soil at concentrations exceeding the saturation limit. This does not appear to be the case in these experiments (1) (but cannot be absolutely ruled out as characteristics of the post-sieved soil were not reported). A second, more plausible explanation is that the methods used in the solvent deposition and soil application protocols were actually much more similar than might be first assumed. Wester et al. did not report the time elapsed between chemical addition to soil and application of amended soil to skin, suggesting that they considered this variable to be unimportant. They did routinely describe mixing under conditions that would permit solvent to dissipate (9–13), but acknowledge that they did not verify dissipation (12). Visual examination of soil is not an adequate test for the presence or absence of solvent residue and cannot provide assessment of whether an added chemical has reached equilibrium with (i.e., dissolved into) soil organic carbon. The Yolo County soil used in all studies by Wester et al. was prepared by sieving a soil with a relatively low organic carbon content (approximately 1% by weight) to exclude particles with diameters less than

180 μm or greater than 300 μm. The resulting soil would have consisted of fine to medium sand with unknown and probably lower organic carbon content than the whole soil. If the time elapsed between chemical amendment of the soil and application of that soil to the monkeys' abdomens was relatively short, the applied chemicals may have still been in solvent or present as neat chemical on the surface of the soil grains at the time of application. Spreading the soil on the skin could then have distributed chemical either alone or in residual solvent to the skin. This would make the initial chemical transfer substantial, and larger than from chemical sorbed to soil. Under those circumstances, similar dermal absorption from solvent and soil applications would be expected.

Direct transfer of chemical to skin, either in solvent or as neat chemical not yet adsorbed by the soil, would also explain why transfer from soil was apparently efficient even though complete coverage of the exposed skin may have lasted for only a brief period. Wester et al. applied their soil to the abdomens of anesthetized monkeys with the animals in a horizontal position. After the application site was covered with a water vapor permeable membrane sandwiched between a pair of concave aluminum eye guards, the monkeys were placed in an upright position in restraint chairs. Given the particle size range used, sloughing of the soil to the bottom of the cover device is likely. The fact that absorption from soil was statistically indistinguishable from absorption from solvent-deposited chemical suggests that transfer from soil to skin had already occurred prior to placement of the monkeys in the restraint chairs.

Case 2

Qiao and Riviere (15) examined absorption of 3,3',4,4'-tetrachlorobiphenyl (TCB) in an ex vivo pig model. They compared results following deposition in acetone, methylene chloride, a water–acetone mixture, and a soil–water–acetone mixture. Since acetone and methylene chloride would be expected to evaporate quickly (after application at μL/cm^2 solvent loadings), two of the experiments were actually tests of absorption from solvent-deposited pure compound. Radiolabel was counted in various compartments. Overall "penetration" was assessed as cumulative perfusion plus depot in tissues other than stratum corneum. The highest value was reported for the non-occluded soil–water–acetone mixture. Qiao and Riviere concluded that:

> The data indicate that PCB dermal risk can be much higher with exposure in soil than with exposure in liquid solutions.

The overall mass recovery (i.e., the sum of TCB found ultimately in all compartments expressed as a fraction of the initial mass applied) in the various versions of the study were both highly variable and generally low (mean recoveries ranged from 39% to 80% across vehicles). Under the circumstances, cautious interpretation would seem appropriate. A noticeable difference between the non-occluded soil–water–acetone experiments and the solvent deposition experiments (which provide the basis for the conclusion quoted above) is that in the solvent deposition experiments much larger portions of the initial dose were recovered from the dosing device (an adhesive template). A plausible partial explanation for the observed result is therefore that the soil matrix served to retard loss of TCB to the dosing device. More importantly, the TCB was added at about 3000 ppm of dry soil, an amount probably substantially in excess of its solubility in that phase

(1). In addition, the initial "soil" mixture was roughly 55% soil, 30% water, and 15% acetone. The manner in which the TCB was added was not described, but apparently occurred only "several hours" before the start of the experiment. Storage conditions in the interim were also not reported. Under these circumstances, it is unlikely that much of the TCB had partitioned to the soil. Therefore, transfer of TCB to skin during the course of the experiment was probably from phases other than soil, including neat compound. Qiao and Riviere cite the PCB work by Wester et al. (11) noted above as supportive of their finding.

Case 3

Abdel-Rahman and co-workers (16–18) have reported results of in vivo studies in which soils and radiolabeled volatile organic compounds (VOCs) were applied to rats. In these experiments, glass caps were fitted to the backs of the rats. Although the protocol is ambiguously described, it appears that soil was first applied under the cap and then benzene, toluene, or *m*-xylene was added to the soil. Soil–chemical contact time prior to chemical–skin contact in these experiments was therefore negligible. In addition, the chemicals were added to each of two soils at roughly 25% by weight, an amount greatly in excess of the likely sorption capacity of either. Results were assessed by monitoring radiolabel in blood, tissues, and excreta. Interpretation of these experiments is complicated by competition between volatilization and dermal absorption, and by the authors' decision to present results normalized by the non-volatilized fraction. Despite the presence of the glass caps, losses of benzene and toluene were very substantial (roughly 40–70% of initial dose). In the case of *m*-xylene, volatilization losses were apparently very minor, and absorption from soils, as represented by area under the plasma concentration versus time curve, was reported to be statistically indistinguishable from absorption from pure *m*-xylene. Cumulative excretion (urine, feces, and expired air) of radiolabel at 48 hours approached 100% of initial dose with or without soil. Given that the soils were supersaturated, this is not surprising. Application of *m*-xylene alone and *m*-xylene slurried with soil both led to dermal exposure to, and absorption of, *m*-xylene liquid. The value of these experiments with respect to understanding of dermal absorption from contaminated soils is unclear. Opportunity for significant dermal contact with soils saturated with solvents is limited at best. In readily accessible, near-surface soils, VOCs evaporate relatively rapidly, and are unlikely to be found at high concentrations. Solvent contamination of subsurface soils is a common problem, but cleanup of subsurface solvents does not routinely involve manual excavation.

DISCUSSION

The examples presented above are illustrative of the generally poor quality of the existing dermal-absorption-from-soil literature. Use of poorly designed protocols and uncritical acceptance of results are common. Many of the published studies display little understanding of conditions under which exposures to contaminated soils might occur, of relevant properties of soils, or of basic sorption/desorption phenomena. Spalt et al. (1) identified few studies without one or more significant flaws. Key shortcomings include the use of soil supersaturated with the target chemical, failure to appropriately consider the effects of multiple soil layers, and incomplete reporting of experimental details needed for interpretation of results. In at least 10 published studies, soil saturation was likely to have been

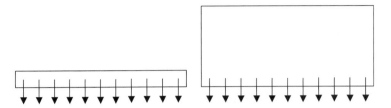

FIGURE 1   Schematic of initial flux from thin and thick soil loads.

exceeded (in some cases greatly exceeded) (1). Experiments in which exposure is to supersaturated soils, which contain free chemical, do not advance understanding of dermal absorption of chemicals sorbed on soil. Saturation should be evaluated in advance. A rough estimate of the saturation limit of a given chemical in soil can be generated from the following two equations:

$$K_d = f_{oc} K_{oc} \tag{1}$$

$$C_{soil,sat} = C_{w,sat} K_d \tag{2}$$

where K_d is the soil:water partition coefficient (mL/g), f_{oc} is the weight fraction of organic carbon in the soil, K_{oc} is the organic carbon:water partition coefficient (mL/g), $C_{soil,sat}$ is the saturation limit of the contaminant in soil (mg/kg), and $C_{w,sat}$ is the saturation limit of the contaminant in water or solubility (mg/L). Implicit in equation (1) is the assumption that sorption occurs in the organic carbon fraction and not on inorganic surfaces. It is therefore not applicable if the potential sorbate is ionized or if the soil has very low organic carbon or substantial clay mineral content. Even in the absence of such conditions, estimates of $C_{soil,sat}$ are uncertain because $C_{w,sat}$ and K_{oc} are uncertain. Estimates of $C_{w,sat}$ and K_{oc} should not be assumed to deviate less than a factor of 10 from actual values (19). Even if experimental values are available, differences in experimental conditions can render a given value substantially uncertain (19). Investigators wishing to examine absorption from soil should therefore conduct their experiments at concentrations well below estimated saturation limits.

Common reliance upon fractional absorption as the primary measure of dermal uptake from soil is an additional problem. Reduced fractional absorption with increased mass of applied soil (i.e., increased number of soil layers) is well documented (6,8,20–22). Arguments to the contrary (13,23–25) are based on demonstrable errors (1). The underlying concept is simple. Consider thin and thick layers of soil (shown schematically in Fig. 1). If coverage is complete in each case, and conditions other than soil loading, such as concentration of the contaminant in the soil (C_{soil}), are equivalent, initial fluxes from the thick and thin layers should also be equivalent, although the chemical load to the skin (mass of chemical/area) will be smaller for the thin layer. That is:

$$J_{thin} = J_{thick} \tag{3}$$

and

$$C_{soil} \left(\frac{M_{soil}}{A} \right)_{thin} < C_{soil} \left(\frac{M_{soil}}{A} \right)_{thick} \tag{4}$$

in which J is flux through skin (mass of chemical/area/time), M_{soil}/A is soil load (mass of soil/area), and C_{soil} (M_{soil}/A) is the chemical load. It follows then that the fractional rate of absorption (time^{-1}), defined as the ratio of the flux of chemical to the chemical load, must be greater for the thin layer as stated in equation (5):

$$\frac{J_{thin}}{C_{soil}\left(\frac{M_{soil}}{A}\right)_{thin}} > \frac{J_{thick}}{C_{soil}\left(\frac{M_{soil}}{A}\right)_{thick}} \tag{5}$$

Fractional absorption can therefore be artificially reduced by applying soil loads well in excess of the minimum required to cover the skin sample with a single layer of soil particles (i.e., the monolayer load). This phenomenon has long been recognized. Early USEPA guidance (26) contains an explicit, if imperfect (6), protocol for adjustment of fractional absorption for layering. Nevertheless, more recent guidance (3) still relies upon fixed values of fractional availabilities for a limited number of compounds.

Nominal estimation of monolayer loading is straightforward. Assuming face-centered packing of solid spherical soil particles of uniform diameter, the mass of soil required to provide monolayer coverage can be estimated (6) as:

$$\left(\frac{M_{soil}}{A}\right)_{monolayer} = \frac{\rho_{particle}(\pi d^3/6)}{d^2} = \rho_{particle}\frac{\pi d}{6} \tag{6}$$

where $(M_{soil}/A)_{monolayer}$ is the soil load (mg/cm^2) representing a monolayer, $\rho_{particle}$ is the particle density of the soil (mg/cm^3), and d is the particle diameter (cm), usually taken as the geometric mean of the range of particle diameters. Assuming a soil particle diameter of 10 μm and specific gravity of 2.65, equation (6) gives a value of 1.4 mg/cm^2 for $(M_{soil}/A)_{monolayer}$. Since soil particles are not actually uniformly sized spheres, the output from equation (6) is approximate.

Actual exposures to soil typically involve average skin loadings less than 1 mg/cm^2 (27–31). That means that normal exposures to most skin surfaces are probably at sub-monolayer loadings (although averages may reflect localized multilayer clumps). The potential therefore does exist for underestimation of dermal absorption if the value of fraction absorbed used in an exposure assessment is taken directly from experiments conducted with multiple soil layers (assuming that other factors, such as duration of exposure, are appropriate). For instance, consider the 3% dermal absorption of TCDD reported in the previously discussed work by Poiger and Schlatter (2), and taken as the current default estimate by the USEPA (3). Poiger and Schlatter's soil was sieved to less than 160 μm and then ground further with mortar and pestle to an unknown final particle size distribution. They applied the soil at a skin load of 13 to 17 mg/cm^2 (dry soil basis), which probably represents at least 5 to 10 layers of soil. Therefore, they could have reduced their soil load without impacting the flux of TCDD into skin in their experiments. Had they done so, they would have found greater apparent fractional uptake.

One way to avoid the layering effect is to conduct experiments at monolayer or lower loading. However, using low loadings may present significant experimental challenges related to achievement of uniform distribution of soil on the skin and/or adequate analytical sensitivity. For these reasons, experiments with multiple layers have advantages over sub-monolayer experiments as long as the results are interpreted appropriately. Data may be extracted as average flux over a specified interval of time. It is reasonable to expect that flux from sub-monolayer soil loads should not exceed determinations made with multiple soil layers. Given this expectation, an upper limit for the cumulative mass absorbed per unit area of skin $(M_{abs}/A)_{upper\ limit}$ from exposure to a sub-monolayer load of soil $(M_{soil}/A)_{sub}$ over the same time interval (t) as the flux determination in a multiple layer experiment $(J_{multi})_t$ can be estimated as follows:

$$\left(\frac{M_{abs}}{A}\right)_{upper\ limit} = (C_{soil})_{sub}\left(\frac{M_{soil}}{A}\right)_{sub}\left\{1-\exp\left[\frac{-t\frac{(J_{multi})_t}{C_{multi}}\frac{(C_{soil,sat})_{multi}}{(C_{soil,sat})_{sub}}}{\left(\frac{M_{soil}}{A}\right)_{sub}}\right]\right\} \quad (7)$$

in which $(C_{soil})_{sub}$ and $(C_{soil})_{multi}$ designate the contaminant concentrations on soil for the sub-monolayer and the multiple layer soils, respectively, and $(C_{soil,sat})_{sub}$ and $(C_{soil,sat})_{multi}$ represent the soil saturation concentrations for the sub-monolayer and multiple layer soils. Equation (7) was derived from a differential mass balance of the chemical on the soil with the assumptions that soil concentrations are less than saturation, flux measured in the multiple layer experiments is proportional to concentration, and that maximum flux occurs when the soil is saturated (7). The ratio of soil saturation concentrations is required to adjust the experimental determination from the multiple layer experiment to sub-monolayer coverage of the skin by a different soil. If the sub-monolayer soil in the absorption estimate is the same as the soil used in the multiple layer experiments, then $(C_{soil,sat})_{sub}/(C_{soil,sat})_{multi} = 1$. If the two soils are different, the saturation ratio for an organic compound can be approximated, per equations (1) and (2), by the ratio of the organic carbon mass fraction (f_{oc}) in each soil as given in equation (8):

$$\frac{(C_{soil,sat})_{sub}}{(C_{soil,sat})_{multi}} = \frac{(f_{oc})_{sub}}{(f_{oc})_{multi}} \quad (8)$$

Although equation (7) is based on a plausible assumption of thermodynamic activity as the driving force for mass transfer, additional data of suitable quality are required to test it and, if necessary, to guide development of an improved relationship. In particular, additional data are needed that elucidate the effects of soil load above and below monolayer, exposure time, and soil characteristics such as organic carbon content, particle size distribution, soil hydration, and mineral content. Data describing effects of key chemical properties are also needed, particularly of those properties that could determine soil saturation, soil-to-skin transfer, and transfer between soil layers (e.g., octanol–water partition coefficient, water saturation, and vapor pressure).

Provision of new data will require new experiments. As noted above, prediction of absorption from soil lags prediction of absorption from water, which has benefited from more systematic experimentation using relatively simple in vitro methods. In vivo experiments are frequently considered to be superior to in vitro investigations for physiological reasons, but implementation of in vivo experimentation requires tradeoffs. First, most compounds of interest cannot be tested in vivo in humans. This leads immediately to issues of interspecies extrapolation. In addition, in vivo dermal methodologies using non-human animals typically entail unrealistic exposure conditions, as movements of non-human subjects are not easily controlled. If an air gap develops and/or soil sloughs, mass transfer conditions will be altered from those intended and mathematical description may become very difficult. Experimental procedures should ensure that soil–skin contact is maintained. Because tight wrapping may cause occlusion, which is also undesirable, non-human in vivo studies of absorption from granular material are inherently problematic. Prevention

TABLE 2 Recommendations for Experimental Determination of Absorption from Soil

Particle size range	Fine fractions of soils should not be excluded, and coarse particles should not be included, unless particle size is an experimental variable. The currently most common limit of 150 μm is a reasonable cut point for coarse particles based on precedent, but lower upper limits can also be justified.
Soil load	Potential layering effects should be considered at the design stage. Results should not be reported as percent absorbed if applied loads exceed monolayer unless layering is an experimental variable. Because uniform distribution of soil on skin (especially over small areas) is difficult, experiments conducted above monolayer may be appropriate, or even preferred, but results from layered experiments should be reported in terms of flux only.
Soil saturation	Chemical concentrations in soil should not approach the estimated solubility of the compound of interest in the test soil. This can be demonstrated by measurements at several soil concentrations or by determination of soil saturation.
Soil–chemical contact	At a minimum, thorough blending of the chemical with the soil should be demonstrated. If the target chemical is added to soil by solvent deposition, methods that ensure solvent dissipation prior to application to skin should be employed. Additional time may be necessary to allow the chemical to equilibrate with the soil, which should be the goal. Time of soil–chemical contact prior to skin exposure should be uniform across experiments unless soil–chemical contact time is an experimental variable.
Soil–skin contact	Measurements describing absorption at times less than 24 hours and temporal patterns of absorption are critically lacking in the current literature.
In vitro methodologies	In vitro experiments should be designed such that potential for flux limitation is minimized. Relative capacities of donor and receptor compartments should be evaluated. Design considerations should include modification of experiment duration, soil load, and measurement point.
In vivo methodologies	In vivo experimental protocols should provide continuous contact of the soil with the skin site without occlusion. Assurance that exposure by ingestion or inhalation is negligible should be provided by explicitly substantiated argument or physical means.
Reporting	Complete reporting of methodological parameters should be provided including, but not limited to, characteristics of soil as applied (i.e., the minimum and maximum particle sizes, organic carbon content, level of hydration), soil–chemical and soil–skin contact times, chemical-to-soil and soil-to-skin application methods, postexposure washing methods, and mass recoveries in all compartments before and after any adjustments. If results are corrected for recovery in parallel intravenous or oral studies, parameters derived from those studies, including statistical variability, should be explicitly reported. Mass recovery calculations should be transparent.

Source: From Ref. 1.

of exposure from routes other than dermal absorption is also often difficult when using animals. A final limitation involving in vivo experimentation with certain animals is the inability to estimate overall recovery. When using humans or other primates in dermal studies, total recovery cannot be measured directly (unless short-term excretion approaches 100%), but must be estimated based on recovery observed following administration by another route.

In comparison to in vivo experimentation, the in vitro alternative offers several potential benefits including lower cost, greater rapidity, simpler experimentation, routine use of human tissue, and more easily implemented mass accounting. The most commonly mentioned shortcoming involves the potential for flux limitation because the skin is not vascularized. Flux limitation can occur if the rate of transport from the skin to the receptor fluid is slower than the rate of transport from soil to skin. However, studies can be designed in such a way that the layers of the skin beneath the epidermis do not limit flux (i.e., penetration is determined through the epidermis only) and that the capacity for the skin and receptor fluid to absorb contaminant is sufficiently large that the soil-to-skin concentration gradient is not artificially reduced.

RECOMMENDATIONS

The current body of interpretable experimental investigations of dermal absorption of chemical contaminants from soil is inadequate to permit rigorous evaluation of new modeling strategies, to confidently predict uptake of compounds that have not yet been investigated, or even to extend predictions of dermal absorption for contaminants that have been studied (under limited conditions) to alternative conditions. Additional, systematic effort is needed. Recommendations for future investigations have been compiled (1) and are summarized in Table 2.

ACKNOWLEDGMENTS

This work was funded in part via USEPA Cooperative Agreements R-82963201-0 and R-83043101-0. It has not been reviewed by the Agency and no endorsement should be inferred. ES was also partially supported via CDC/NIOSH Training Grant T42/CCT010418-11.

REFERENCES

1. Spalt E, Kissel JC, Shirai JH, et al. Dermal absorption of environmental contaminants from soil and sediment: a critical review. J Expo Sci Environ Epidemiol (in press).
2. Poiger H, Schlatter C. Influence of solvents and adsorbents on dermal and intestinal absorption of TCDD. Food Cosmet Toxicol 1980; 18(5):477–81.
3. USEPA. Risk Assessment Guidance for Superfund (RAGS), Volume I: Human Health Evaluation Manual (Part E, Supplemental Guidance for Dermal Risk Assessment), Final Report, EPA-540-R-99-005. Washington, DC: Office of Superfund Remediation and Technology Innovation, 2004.
4. Bunge AL, Parks JM. Predicting dermal absorption from contact with chemically contaminated soils. ASTM Spec Tech Publ, No. 1317, 1997:227–44.
5. Bunge AL, Parks JM. Soil contamination: theoretical descriptions. In: Roberts MS, Walters KA, eds. Dermal Absorption and Toxicity Assessment. New York: Marcel Dekker, Inc., 1998:669–96.
6. Duff RM, Kissel JC. Effect of soil loading on dermal absorption efficiency from contaminated soils. J Toxicol Environ Health 1996; 48:93–106.
7. Deglin, SE. Dermal absorption of nonvolatile organic chemicals from soils. PhD thesis, Colorado School of Mines, Golden, Colorado, 2007.
8. Deglin SE, Macalady DL, Bunge AL. Absorption from contaminated soil through skin and silicone rubber membrane: 2. Effect of soil concentration. Environ Sci Technol (submitted).
9. Wester RC, Maibach HI, Bucks DAW, et al. Percutaneous absorption of [14C]DDT and [14C]benzo(a)pyrene from soil. Fundam Appl Toxicol 1990; 15:510–6.
10. Wester RC, Maibach HI, Sedik L, et al. Percutaneous absorption of [14C] chlordane from soil. J Toxicol Environ Health 1992; 35:269–77.

11. Wester RC, Maibach HI, Sedik L, et al. Percutaneous absorption of PCBs from soil: in vivo rhesus monkey, in vitro human skin, and binding to powered human stratum corneum. J Toxicol Environ Health 1993; 39:375–82.
12. Wester RC, Maibach HI, Sedik L, et al. Percutaneous absorption of pentachlorophenol from soil. Fundam Appl Toxicol 1993; 20:68–71.
13. Wester RC, Melendres J, Logan F, et al. Percutaneous absorption of 2,4-dichlorophenoxyacetic acid from soil with respect to the soil load and skin contact time: in vivo absorption in rhesus monkey and in vitro absorption in human skin. J Toxicol Environ Health 1996; 47:335–44.
14. Alexander M. Aging, bioavailability, and overestimation of risk from environmental pollutants. Environ Sci Technol 2000; 34(20):4259–65.
15. Qiao GL, Riviere JE. Dermal absorption and tissue disposition of 3,3',4,4'-tetrachlorobiphenyl (TCB) in an ex vivo pig model: assessing the impact of dermal exposure variables. Int J Occup Environ Health 2000; 6(2):127–37.
16. Skowronski GA, Turkall RM, Abdel-Rahman MS. Soil absorption alters bioavailability of benzene in dermally exposed male rats. Am Ind Hyg Assoc J 1988; 49:506–11.
17. Skowronski GA, Turkall RM, Abdel-Rahman MS. Effects of soil on percutaneous absorption of toluene in male rats. J Toxicol Environ Health 1989; 26:373–84.
18. Skowronski GA, Turkall RM, Kadry RM, et al. Effects of soil on the dermal bioavailability of *m*-xylene in male rats. Environ Res 1990; 51:182–93.
19. Lyman WJ, Reeehl WF, Rosenblatt DH. Handbook of Chemical Property Estimation Methods. New York: McGraw-Hill, 1982.
20. Yang JJ, Roy TA, Krueger AJ, et al. In vitro and in vivo percutaneous absorption of benzo[*a*]pyrene from petroleum crude-fortified soil in the rat. Bull Environ Contam Toxicol 1989; 43:207–14.
21. Touraille GD, McCarley KD, Bunge AL, et al. Percutaneous absorption of 4-cyanophenol from freshly contaminated soil in vitro: effects of soil loading and contamination concentration. Environ Sci Technol 2005; 39:3723–31.
22. Deglin SE, Macalady DL, Bunge AL. Absorption from contaminated soil through skin and silicone rubber membrane: 1. Effect of soil loading. Environ Sci Technol (submitted).
23. Wester RC, Maibach HI. Percutaneous absorption of hazardous substances from water and soil. In: Roberts MS, Walters KA, eds. Dermal Absorption and Toxicity Assessment. New York: Marcel Dekker, Inc., 1998:697–707.
24. Wester RC, Maibach HI. Skin contamination and absorption of chemicals from water and soil. In: Bronaugh RL, Maibach HI, eds. Percutaneous Absorption: Drugs-Cosmetics-Mechanisms-Methodology. 3rd ed. New York: Marcel Dekker, Inc., 1999:133–48.
25. Wester RC, Maibach HI. Skin contamination and absorption of chemicals from water and soil. In: Bronaugh RL, Maibach HI, eds. Percutaneous Absorption: Drugs-Cosmetics-Mechanisms-Methodology. 4th ed. Boca Raton, FL: Taylor & Francis Group LLC, 2005:107–21.
26. USEPA. Dermal Exposure Assessment: Principles and Applications, Interim Report, EPA/600/8-91/011B. Washington, DC: Office of Health and Environmental Assessment, 1992.
27. Kissel JC, Richter KY, Fenske RA. Factors affecting soil adherence to skin in hand-press trials. Bull Environ Contam Toxicol 1996; 56:722–8.
28. Holmes K, Shirai J, Richter K, et al. Field measurement of dermal soil loadings in occupational and recreational activities. Environ Res 1999; 80:148–57.
29. Kissel J, Richter KY, Fenske RA. Field measurement of dermal soil loading attributed to various activities: implications for exposure assessment. Risk Anal 1996; 16:115–25.
30. Kissel JC, Shirai JH, Richter KY, et al. Investigation of dermal contact with soil in controlled trials. J Soil Contam 1998; 7:737–52.
31. Choate LM, Ranville JF, Bunge AL, et al. Dermally adhered soil: 1. Amount and particle-size distribution. Integr Environ Assess Manag 2006; 2(4):375–84.
32. USEPA. Risk Assessment Guidance for Superfund (RAGS), Volume I: Human Health Evaluation Manual (Part E, Supplemental Guidance for Dermal Risk Assessment) Interim. (Accessed October 1, 2007 at http://www.epa.gov/oswer/riskassessment/ragse/index.htm)

Percutaneous Absorption of Pesticides

Jon R. Heylings
Research and Investigative Toxicology, Syngenta Central Toxicology Laboratory, Macclesfield, Cheshire, U.K.

David J. Esdaile
LAB International Research Centre, Szabadságpuszta, Veszprém, Hungary

INTRODUCTION

The dermal route is the most likely exposure route for almost all pesticide-containing products. The assessment of percutaneous absorption is therefore an important part of the safety evaluation of pesticide products. Within the European Union (EU), data on the absorption of the active ingredient through the skin are obligatory for inclusion in Annex I of Directive 91/414 of the European Community (1). Inclusion of active substances in Annex I is only possible if the crop protection products containing them can be used with acceptable risk to humans. Evaluation of risk to populations who may be exposed to pesticides (e.g., manufacturers, workers, spray operators, bystanders) is essential in order to authorize the use of these products in the market.

Exposure to pesticides primarily occurs via occupational exposure during the handling and normal use of crop protection products. Following skin contact, the active ingredient has the potential to be absorbed through the skin and may become systemically available. As part of the overall risk assessment process, the toxicological profile of the active ingredient and the extent of exposure are determined. The assessment of percutaneous absorption under relevant field exposure conditions is then used to predict whether the amount of the active ingredient that could be absorbed has any likely adverse health consequences.

The systemic dose that is considered to be safe for exposed individuals is derived from the results of toxicological investigations, and the acceptable operator exposure level (AOEL) is established. The quantitative estimate for skin exposure for a particular type of application is derived from experimental data for the specific formulation or a similar type of application, or may be based on a theoretical model such as the European Predictive Operator Exposure Model (EUROPOEM) (2). The result of such an assessment is wide ranging. In many cases, the data generated in percutaneous absorption studies will determine whether the product can be registered for a specific application. It may determine that the risk from dermal contact is negligible even if the entire dose applied to the skin was systemically available, or the safety may depend on a low percentage skin absorption being demonstrated. Alternatively, it may determine that specific personal protective equipment or engineering controls are required in order to minimize or prevent dermal exposure. The assessment may determine that there is a significant risk for human health and the product will not be registered for the specific use.

Dermal absorption studies for pesticide products should be performed in accordance with the Organisation for Economic Cooperation and Development (OECD) test guidelines 427 (in vivo) and 428 (in vitro) and their associated Guidance Document No. 28 (3–5). Data from these studies allow the comparison of the external exposure, derived from separate operator exposure (OPEX) models, with the AOEL. The AOEL is the acceptable systemic dose, based on the toxicity of the active ingredient and is expressed in mg/kg per day. If the evaluations, including the dermal absorption value, exceed the AOEL, then the product would not be approved for the specific use under consideration.

The OECD guidelines for dermal absorption provide the basic framework for the practical methods used to assess the skin absorption of chemicals and the products that contain them. As such, the guidelines are not specific to a particular industry or regulatory area. They are intended to cover the general principles of the tests and to provide information on where additional guidance can be sought. For crop protection products, more specific guidance can be found in separate documents including EC SANCO 222/2000 rev. 7 (6). This describes the process for assessing dermal absorption of pesticides, based on the OECD guidelines, plus how the data are used in the risk assessment process for pesticide products. This guidance used in the EU has a tiered approach for occupational risk assessment in which dermal absorption and exposure assessment are integrated. Although the OECD includes as its members the U.S.A. and Canada, there are different approaches within North America's system for pesticide regulation. For example, U.S. Environmental Protection Agency (EPA) has a separate Health Effects Test Guideline OPPTS 870.7600 (7) for pesticides. This covers in vivo studies only.

In 1992, the intention was to provide OECD Member States with a single harmonized approach for the assessment of dermal absorption. This would include industrial chemicals, cosmetic products, and pesticides. The original proposal from the United Kingdom outlined an in vitro and in vivo test method. Over the next five years, a number of expert groups met, reviewed, and tried to resolve the issues that prevented the establishment of a new test guideline. These mainly centered round the in vitro method and the lack of formal validation. A number of Workshops and OECD Steering Committees and Expert Groups met and continued to work to resolve the issues on how the in vitro method should be used in risk assessment. In 1997, the Toxicology Group of the European Crop Protection Association (ECPA) volunteered to assist with the preparation of a draft OECD Guidance Document for dermal absorption, in addition to the revision of the draft OECD test guidelines. A subgroup of technical experts from ECPA was formed to undertake this task. Further versions of the draft test guideline emerged. In 2000, an OECD Expert Group was appointed to resolve the final few remaining issues. This group included experts from the U.S. EPA, Health Canada, the U.S. Food and Drug Administration, the ECPA, and the OECD Secretariat. Finally, in May 2001, a final consensus was reached by the Joint Meeting of the Chemicals Committee and Working Group on Chemicals, Pesticides and Biotechnology. The OECD test guidelines for dermal absorption were approved. A synopsis of the history of this particular test guideline was made by Herman Koeter (8).

Despite the existence of OECD test guidelines, there are still differences in the way in which dermal absorption of pesticides is both conducted and interpreted between North America and other OECD Member States. These differences, and the attempts to harmonize the approaches for dermal absorption and risk assessment, are the subject of ongoing discussions and workshops (9). One of the major issues is the reluctance of North America to accept in vitro dermal absorption studies in the regulation process due to lack of formal validation, despite the overwhelming evidence presented in various publications and reviews that in vitro data, as used in the EU for over 20 years for pesticide products, provide a useful approach to the prediction of dermal absorption in humans (4,9–11). Indeed, all areas of industry, with the exception of pesticides in North America, endorse the in vitro approach in OECD 428. For example, the in vitro approach, using non-viable human skin, is used in the human risk assessment process for industrial chemicals, as endorsed by the EPA (12). It therefore remains surprising that in North America the regulation of industrial chemicals and also personal care products, which are intended to be applied to the skin, utilize the in vitro dermal absorption approach, but the in vitro method is not deemed acceptable by other parts of the Agency that regulate pesticide-containing products.

Perhaps one of the difficulties for some regulatory authorities to accept the in vitro approach relates to the aspect of predictive accuracy. In conventional validation of a hazard-based test, the objective is to develop an in vitro model that is robust and predicts in vivo with an acceptable degree of accuracy. In the pesticide dermal absorption field, we are making a quantitative assessment of the likely systemic exposure of an active ingredient from a formulated product not the assessment of positive or negative result. Prediction of percutaneous absorption using in vitro approaches is not about the development of a like-for-like replacement model, but to provide a conservative approach where the in vitro study is unlikely to underestimate skin absorption compared with an in vivo approach. Furthermore, skin absorption is one area of the toxicological sciences where human models are accepted practice. Therefore, the key scientific aspect of any "validation" is the prediction of human absorption from human skin models. Providing the in vitro human model does not underestimate absorption in human, it should have a role in the regulatory process.

A flow diagram is provided (Fig. 1), which shows the various steps in a tiered approach required to demonstrate safety as related to skin exposure to an agrochemical product. This diagram is a proposed scheme, based on the principal current regulatory requirements and the experience of the authors; but it must be noted that different regulatory authorities have different opinions on which studies are acceptable in the regulatory process.

The focus of the rest of this chapter is to provide information on the current issues relating to dermal absorption of pesticides and to cover the various theoretical and practical aspects that relate to the overall registration process. Since much of the detailed methodology of the in vitro and in vivo models is dealt with elsewhere in this book, we will focus on the elements of the test models that are important for pesticides, as well as data interpretation and how it is used in human risk assessment.

PREDICTION, THEORETICAL FORMULATION CONCEPTS, AND PRACTICAL APPROACHES BEFORE TESTING
Quantitative Structure–Activity Relationships
It is evident that the physicochemistry of a molecule will control its diffusion through a membrane. The best known predictive quantitative structure–activity relationship (QSAR) model in dermal absorption is that of Potts and Guy (15). This shows that a combination of molecular size (described by molecular weight) and

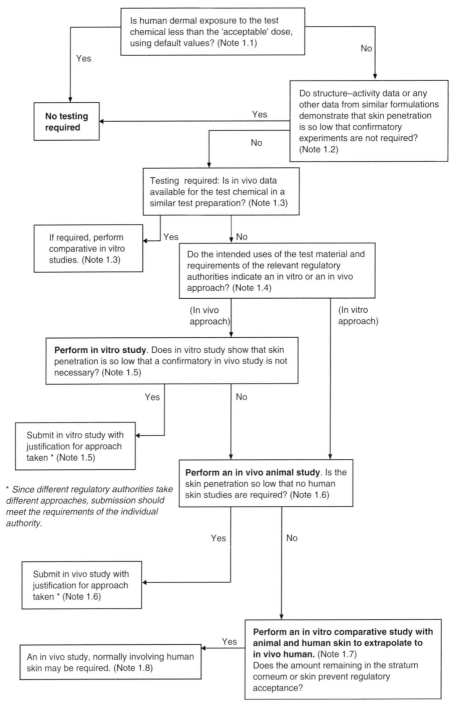

FIGURE 1 A proposed decision tree for performance of in vivo/in vitro studies for a pesticide of unknown dermal absorption.

Notes for Figure 1

1.1. The theoretical maximum dermal exposure to the test chemical in a specified time period should be estimated. This will rely on the default absorption percentage, which is often 100% unless a lower value can be justified. Exposure = dermal dose per individual × default percentage absorption/body weight as mg/kg per day or mg/kg per hour. If this value is lower than the "acceptable" exposure limit and the regulatory authority accepts the calculations, then no percutaneous absorption testing should be required.

1.2. In some cases, it is possible to demonstrate that the skin penetration of a chemical will be near zero. Examples include large molecules such as polymers, large charged ions, or chemicals in a physical form such as large insoluble crystal structures. In other cases, it may be possible to make appropriate structure–activity predictions by mathematical calculation, based on the physicochemical characteristics. Where a robust prediction can be made that is sufficiently conservative or where the safety margin is sufficiently large, the evaluation should be acceptable to regulatory authorities. Evaluations of this nature should be justified on a case-by-case basis, but acceptability will be affected by the knowledgeability of the individual regulatory authority. It is recognized that predictions of penetration from multicomponent formulations are more complex than predictions for pure chemicals or simple solutions.

In some cases, there will be existing information about the penetration characteristics for a similar formulation. Where the formulations are adequately similar, it can be assumed that the penetration characteristics will be similar, and hence if the margins of safety are large enough, no further experimental work should be required.

1.3. In cases where adequate in vivo data exist for a similar formulation but that the differences between the formulation may influence the penetration characteristics, the usual approach will be to perform bridging studies. Evaluation of skin penetration in vitro can be used to assess relative penetration between similar formulations or similar chemicals (as flux, percentage absorption, or K_p values). In vitro studies can also be used to predict relative penetration for the same formulation between different exposure conditions on similar skin. For example, skin penetration of a test chemical from formulation A in vivo in humans is known to be 10% of the applied dose per 24 hours. In an in vitro study, formulation A gave 30% penetration at 24 hours, formulation B gave 15% penetration at 24 hours. Hence, the extrapolated in vivo human skin penetration over 24 hours for formulation B is $(10\% \times 15/30) = 5\%$.

1.4. Certain regulatory authorities have specific requirements to avoid in vivo experimentation whenever an alternative can be justified. Other authorities prefer the use of live animals in safety evaluation studies. Hence, although the choice of study type should include an ethical approach with a reduction of animal use wherever possible, the regulatory bodies do have the right to specify certain studies for inclusion in regulatory submissions.

1.5. In vitro evaluation under correct conditions can give a conservative estimate of in vivo skin penetration of a chemical from a dermal exposure, normally as mg/cm^2 per hour (or per day). If this evaluation shows that the potential systemic exposure would not exceed the acceptable dose, then in vivo experimentation will not be required. It should be noted that in vitro studies using rat skin give absorption characteristics higher (often 5 to 10 times higher) than the in vivo human absorption values.

1.6. Evaluation of skin penetration in vivo can be used to assess skin penetration in the test species, under the specific conditions of exposure used in the study. The rat is the species of choice for many regulatory authorities. It must be noted that the rat has relatively permeable skin compared with that of humans. The protective external layer of the rat against its normal environment is the layer of hair, for humans it is the SC, hence in the rat the SC is relatively permeable. Some species (such as the pig) have skin permeability characteristics close to that of human; where a more accurate prediction of human skin penetration is required, consideration should be given to use of such models. A correctly performed in vivo skin penetration study will give a conservative estimate of the amount of chemical which could become systemically available from dermal exposure, normally on a 24-hour basis. Where the in vivo data show an adequate safety margin, no further experimentation should be required.

1.7. In many cases, an in vivo rat dermal absorption study will be required for a new chemical or active ingredient. Where a better estimate of absorption through human skin is required, a common approach is to perform a comparative assay of in vitro absorption in animal versus human skin. When these data are combined with animal in vivo data, they allow the prediction of in vivo human absorption, provided that the exposure conditions were adequately similar (1,10,13), i.e., skin penetration in vivo in human is extrapolated from:

$$\frac{\text{Rat in vivo} \times \text{Human in vitro}}{\text{Rat in vitro}}$$

1.8. Human volunteer studies or worker exposure studies with markers of exposure may be scientifically justified if they can be performed with full ethical approval; however, a number of regulatory authorities discourage or refuse to accept human volunteer studies for political reasons. A study with human skin grafted onto nude mice [HuSki model as described in (14)] is likely to provide good quality data with human skin to justify the lack of systemic absorption of chemical from the skin compartment. In some cases, it may be possible to demonstrate the lack of absorption from the skin over time with a rat in vivo model. Although, since the relatively high permeability of rat skin can make this difficult, in vivo studies in other species such as the pig may be more appropriate.

the stratum corneum (SC)—aqueous vehicle partition coefficient [estimated from the octanol–water partition coefficient (P_{ow})] is able to predict maximum flux from a saturated aqueous solution through skin. Small improvements to this QSAR model have included the use of molecular characteristics such as strength of crystal forces (melting point) and hydrogen bonding. However, there is no publicly available QSAR model that is adequately reliable for use in predicting absorption from finite doses or from nonaqueous products or complex multicomponent formulations. Hence, at his stage, QSAR is not an available tool for avoiding experimental work to measure skin absorption for most agrochemical products, although there is a good theoretical case that such a model is feasible.

Common Practices in Skin Penetration Evaluation

The current regulatory procedure for evaluating human in vivo skin absorption within Europe is well documented (6). As a first step, the potential human exposure is assessed, then if the theoretical total amount present on skin were absorbed, and the AOEL were not exceeded, then no further evaluation is needed. The physicochemistry of the active ingredient (AI) may be taken into account to justify less than 100% absorption as the default absorption factor. However current European regulations do not account for realistic absorption percentages without experimental evidence. The traditional approach to provide experimental evidence involves the performance of an in vivo rat skin absorption study with the agrochemical formulation, commonly of the commercial concentrate formulation and of the typical in-use spray dilution. Rat skin is generally far more permeable than human skin (10,11,14). To make an assessment of the equivalent human in vivo absorption, in vitro studies performed with the same formulations in both rat and human skin allow a correction factor to be applied to the rat in vivo result. Thus, a prediction of the human in vivo percentage absorption can be made (see Fig. 1, footnote 1.7).

This procedure is commonly performed for a representative formulation. It is well known that changes to formulations can have effects on skin absorption. For example, adjuvants can enhance absorption and other components can reduce absorption. Agrochemical companies sometimes have a range of similar formulations that are adapted for specific pests, local climates, or specific use patterns. Therefore, it is a common practice to use in vitro tests to compare such formulations with the "reference" formulation, which was tested in vivo, such that a correction factor can be derived to produce an estimate of human in vivo absorption for a range of relatively similar formulations.

Test Formulations

The applied dose of the test preparation of agrochemical formulations for skin absorption studies should mimic the "in-use" conditions (4). Normally the preparation will be made with a radiolabeled active ingredient in order to trace the absorption. Some agrochemical formulations are complex mixtures; it is critical that the added radiolabeled chemical is in the same form and compartment as the cold active ingredient. This can require specialist formulation knowledge for certain formulations types; for example, for oil-in-water or water-in-oil emulsions, granules, and powders, it can be difficult to ensure that the radiolabeled material is correctly distributed.

Skin Types Used in In Vitro Studies

The most common skin types used are from rat, pig, and human. Other types of skin are rarely used. Rat skin is used because rats are used for the full range of safety evaluation studies on systemic toxicity and metabolism as well as for in vivo skin absorption studies. Pig skin has characteristics much nearer to human skin, since rat skin tends to be highly permeable for many chemicals; there are good ethical reasons to use pig skin, since it is obtained from animals being killed for food and not specifically bred for tissue donation. Human skin is ideal for use in vitro but there are drawbacks; it can be difficult to obtain in adequate quality and quantity, there are risks of human pathogenic viruses such as HIV, which make handling the tissues technically difficult. Human skin can be prepared as a full-thickness sample, dermatomed to a few hundred microns, or as epidermal membranes (essentially the SC and the epidermal layers). Thicker skin samples can result in a delay in the diffusion of chemical into the receptor fluid (RF), so the thinner membranes are preferable (5).

The following section deals specifically with human skin, but the principles apply equally to methods using skin from other species.

PRACTICAL METHODS: ISSUES RELATING TO PESTICIDES
Human Skin Models
Tissue Quality and Barrier Integrity Measurement

Human skin is the preferred model for the assessment of dermal absorption of pesticide products. Indeed, it is regarded as the "gold standard" for such assessments (9). The OECD 428 test guideline (4) is quite specific about the need for measurement of the skin barrier integrity prior to studies. Skin tissue from humans is procured, transported, stored, prepared, and handled in potentially so many different ways that some uniform assessment of the quality of each specimen is very important. Surprisingly, over the many years of operation of the in vitro percutaneous absorption method, there have been only a few systematic evaluations of the skin barrier integrity across species, skin preparation type (e.g., epidermal membranes, dermatomed skin), and the integrity method being used (16,17). Traditionally, tritiated water flux was used as the primary method to determine skin integrity and particularly to check if any gross physical damage had been caused to the specimen such as may be caused by instruments during dissection and preparation. More recently, the electrical resistance (ER) and, in some cases, transepidermal water loss (TEWL) have largely replaced the tritiated water flux approach, largely due to the gains in efficiency, cost, and safety (17). The ER and TEWL methods are just as useful as tritiated water for measuring barrier damage and the former is very simple and allows damaged specimens to be identified and replaced quickly. One of the key considerations here is what actually constitutes "normal" skin when determining values by these simple barrier integrity checks. This is particularly important with human skin. Obviously, specimens that appear grossly abnormal or are physically damaged during preparation should not be used. However, values of tritiated water flux, ER, or TEWL have their own broad distributions across human donors and within donors. This inherent variability can be controlled to a certain extent by the use of skin from the same anatomical site. Abdominal skin is generally regarded as the most useful and widely used anatomical site for human skin studies and is recommended in various guidance documents in this field (6,9–11). It has an intermediate SC thickness and follicle density. Other factors, as mentioned above, can broaden the distribution of skin integrity values in human skin beyond just biological variability. Indeed, certain skin tissue banks that provide skin sometimes have whole batches with "abnormal" integrity values and others, perhaps with more careful adherence to preparation, storage, and shipping have consistently better integrity values. This is obviously not due to inherent variability across the population but due to quality control. These features are only easy to detect and monitor in laboratories that have a high turnover of in vitro percutaneous absorption studies, maintain skin integrity databases, and utilize multiple skin banks. Poor quality tissues would be more difficult to identify in small one-off operations, particularly in less experienced laboratories.

If we make the assumption that quality control of human skin specimens from procurement to point of use is satisfactory, we still have the issue of intrinsic biological variability and what constitutes acceptable values of tritiated water, ER, and TEWL for in vitro skin absorption experiments. It is recognized that the dermal absorption of chemicals will vary across a group of replicates, more so in the diverse target human than in the relatively homogeneous animal skin taken from the same strain, sex, body weight, etc. Therefore, we must not narrow down "acceptable" human skin specimens to, for example, those of very low permeability to water. Specimens must be of acceptable quality and representative of the population.

The methods for assessing skin integrity in OECD 428 (4) are described but no suggested cutoff values for normal skin are specified in the OECD guidance. The paper by Davies et al. (17), published after the OECD test guideline, has studied a wide range of species and skin preparation types comparing tritiated water and ER as skin integrity measures. In this paper, there are suggested cutoff values that this specific laboratory recommends to accept/reject specimens mounted in static diffusion cells for use in percutaneous absorption studies (Table 1). It is critical that new laboratories entering into the field of in vitro percutaneous absorption understand these potential issues relating to the barrier integrity of their skin samples. Since the SC is the most important component of these studies, its function must be representative of in vivo conditions. Otherwise the interpretation of the dermal absorption potential of the test chemical can be compromised.

TABLE 1 Acceptance Values for Tritiated Water (T_2O) Permeability Coefficient and Electrical Resistance (ER) Using Standard Diffusion Cells for Various Skin Preparations

Species	Skin type	T_2O permeability (cm/hr)	ER ($k\Omega/cm^2$)	ER ($k\Omega$)[a]
Human	Epidermis	<1.5	3.94	>10
	Whole	<1.5	3.94	>10
Rat	Epidermis	<2.5	0.98	>2.5
	Whole	<2.5	1.18	>3.0
Pig	Epidermis	<4.5	1.18	>3.0
	Whole	<4.5	1.57	>4.0
Mouse	Whole	<1.2	6.33	>5.0
Rabbit	Whole	<13	0.35	>0.8
Guinea pig	Whole	<2.0	1.97	>5.0

[a] Static diffusion cells – Skin area $=2.54\ cm^2$, with the exception of mouse where area $=0.79\ cm^2$.
Source: From Ref. 17.

Receptor Fluid and Solubilization of the Test Substance

The OECD test guideline 428 (4) permits a range of RFs that can be used for in vitro percutaneous absorption studies. The primary reason for this is the wide-ranging physicochemical properties of the test substances that are being measured. The key principle here is that the test substance must be soluble in the chosen RF. If the solution concentration of the test substance exceeds 10% of its saturated concentration in the RF during a study, then the diffusion (and therefore the quantity of material in the receptor) may be underestimated since sink conditions have not been maintained. This is stated in the OECD Guidance Document (5) and is a key element relating to the interpretation of these studies. For example, if a lipophilic test substance is used with an aqueous receptor, then it is likely that the test substance with a poor aqueous solubility will partition into the skin tissue rather than into the RF. Hence, measurements of the chemical in the RF would underestimate the absorption, due to improper test conditions related to RF solubility. This effect can have a greater impact when full-thickness skin is used, compared with epidermal membranes. If the RF does not adequately solubilize the test substance, then a proportion of the dose applied to the skin surface that remains in the tissue following surface decontamination at the end of the exposure period, should then be included as absorbed.

The authors consider that many laboratories pay insufficient attention to the skin:receptor partitioning effects that are key to the in vitro method. Where test substances are freely water soluble, there is not much of a problem and saline-based receptors are acceptable. However, when test substances are less water soluble, investigators often incorporate surfactants or other additives to the aqueous receptor to "improve" the solubility of the chemical under study. It clearly states in the OECD guidance that the solubility in the receptor should be established and that it is not a rate-limiting step (5). For the more lipophilic test substances, even those that penetrate the skin relatively easily, the addition of "solubilizers" such as polyethylene glycol and albumin to the receptor may not be adequate to maintain the sink conditions. Rather than supplement a physiological medium with solubilizers, another option is to select an appropriate solvent system which ensures that partitioning from skin to receptor is not rate limiting. Many laboratories use ethanol:water mixtures that are permitted in OECD 428 as a universal receptor approach to achieve this (18,19). Skin absorption is a passive process and does not rely on active biochemical processes. The rate and extent of absorption is determined by the ability of the test substance to diffuse through the skin barrier, the SC, which is a non-living tissue. Clearly, if the objective of the study involves assessment of skin metabolism and not just diffusion, then only a physiological receptor can be used. This is carefully spelled out in the OECD Test Guideline 428. It is important to recognize that the OECD guideline is primarily designed to assess the risk from systemic exposure to the chemical in question by measuring the quantity of the chemical that can diffuse from the surface of the skin and into the RF. When a solvent-based receptor is used, that invariably aids the partitioning of the test material from skin to receptor, and it is unlikely that the amount of test substance absorbed will be underestimated. There are other advantages of the universal receptor approach when it comes to measurement of the test substance. Specific cold analytical methods are compatible with ethanol:water mixtures, whereas other solubilizing additives can interfere with a number of non-radio-labeled methods of analysis.

OECD guidance on the in vitro method for percutaneous absorption also states that the choice of receptor medium should not affect skin preparation integrity. Guidance is given elsewhere in this chapter and in other published reports about the various methods for assessing skin integrity and the advantages/disadvantages of each approach (17). Naturally, if a simple physiological receptor solution of isotonic saline is used, then this is less likely to cause any changes to the tissue which could indirectly affect dermal absorption. However, use of solubilizers and solvents are more likely to act as absorption enhancers and increase the absorption of the test chemical. Therefore, in the context of risk assessment, any increase in overall skin absorption caused by a solvent system would be deemed as conservative. It should be pointed out that studies comparing in vitro and in vivo absorption which have utilized solvent receptors have shown that the in vitro approach generally over-predicts in vivo absorption (11,18,19). If the effect of the receptor on the skin barrier is an important aspect of the study, the skin integrity can also be measured following exposure to the test chemical. This is useful in the context of study performance or where potentially irritant adjuvants are used in products (20). Skin integrity checks in untreated controls undertaken at the end of the exposure period can also be used to demonstrate that the receptor medium does not cause barrier disruption in its own right.

Assessment of Solid, Granular, or Volatile Products
The dermal absorption of pesticide test substances (or formulated products containing the test substance) that are in a solid form at the temperature of the skin surface normally require a vehicle or carrier to allow it to interact with the SC. Dry solid large particles or granules are very poor platforms for dermal absorption. Fine particles and dusts (depending on the actual particle size) will absorb any surrounding moisture on the skin surface and will therefore have more surface contact and a greater ability to penetrate the tissue. When in vitro or in vivo dermal absorption studies are designed to assess the risk from contact with solids, it is important to examine the actual real-life exposure scenario. This includes a number of aspects such as the particle size and the potential exposure period. For example, if the material at the top of a container is a lumpy granule but is a fine dust at the bottom of the same container due to settling, it is prudent to test the finer dust material since it is likely to have a greater opportunity to release and deliver the

active onto and into the skin. The OECD guideline suggests that moistening of the solid should be undertaken for in vitro and in vivo dermal absorption studies. In order to better simulate typical exposure, it would be more useful and relevant to compare the neat material with a simulated sweat type of application. This would involve preparing a ground down version of the solid in this sweat medium that is then applied to the skin as a paste. This would provide a conservative assessment of dermal absorption relative to the neat solid and represents a worst-case scenario that may occur during handling of the chemical or product.

For products that are volatile at room temperature, or likely to be lost from the skin via evaporation during their normal use, it is important to measure the amount of the applied dose that is lost during in vitro and in vivo studies. This is a key element of the mass balance and in situations where this has not been quantified by trapping the test substance in the void above the skin surface, the study is compromised and the "missing" fraction of the dose would therefore be assumed to have been absorbed. The usual procedure for studies with volatile test substances is to place a charcoal filter above the donor chamber (in vitro) or skin device (in vivo), and to extract the compound from the matrix at the end of the exposure period. With some of the more volatile pesticide products, such as soil fumigants, a significant proportion of the applied dose may be lost from the skin surface by evaporation.

REFERENCE CHEMICALS AND REPRODUCIBILITY OF THE IN VITRO METHOD

There are numerous literature references on in vitro percutaneous absorption. The consensus is that the method can predict in vivo absorption, when evaluating the potential systemic exposure of chemicals and formulated products, following dermal application (5,9). However, since the in vitro method was not subjected to a formal validation program, there are still a number of key issues relating to the methodology which do not have sufficient published scientific evidence to make the method universally acceptable to all regulatory authorities dealing with pesticide registration. The OECD guidance directs any new laboratory to demonstrate their competency with the in vitro technique by providing data on specific reference chemicals. The reference chemicals named in the OECD guidance are benzoic acid, caffeine, and testosterone. These widely studied compounds cover a range of polarities, since this particular physicochemical property can have a major influence on skin absorption. In one such exercise, the skin integrity characteristics of human skin that was sourced, prepared, and stored in different laboratories (Syngenta CTL in the United Kingdom and TNO in The Netherlands) was compared. The permeability coefficient for tritiated water was very similar in the two labs with values of 1.0×10^{-3} cm/hr (CTL) and 1.1×10^{-3} cm/hr (TNO) for a group of six normal human skin samples. This study determined how transferable two independent methods of measuring in vitro percutaneous absorption was, by comparing data for tritiated water flux and that of the three reference chemicals, benzoic acid, caffeine, and testosterone. A standard protocol was used to study the reference chemicals under Good Laboratory Practice (GLP) in the two laboratories using different diffusion skin cell equipment. The chemicals were applied in a universal application vehicle (1 mg/mL in a 50% ethanol in physiological saline). The application rate was 100 µL/cm² ($\equiv$ 100 µg penetrant per cm²) and the donor

TABLE 2　Inter-Laboratory Comparison of Reference Chemicals Using Human
Epidermal Membranes

	Absorption after 24 hr (%)		Maximum absorption rate (μg/cm^2/hr)	
Test chemical	TNO	CTL	TNO	CTL
Caffeine	6 ± 1.1	8 ± 1.3	0.3 ± 0.04	0.5 ± 0.08
Testosterone	36 ± 3.7	21 ± 4.7	1.7 ± 0.19	1.2 ± 0.27
Benzoic acid	63 ± 1.8	69 ± 3.0	5.3 ± 0.45	3.4 ± 0.15

Mean values ($\pm$ SEM) for $n = 10$ observations in each case.
Abbreviations: CTL, Syngenta Central Toxicology Laboratory; TNO, TNO Nutrition and Food Research Institute.

chambers were occluded for the entire exposure period (24 hours) to maximize
absorption of the test penetrants.

The two laboratories routinely use the in vitro method and have many years
experience of it. As shown in Table 2, the permeability to the three test chemicals
was also very similar in the two labs indicating robustness of the method. A wider
study (21) involving many labs who had less experience with in vitro percutaneous
absorption showed where the potential pitfalls that can lead to variability are, but
nevertheless there was reasonable concordance across labs.

INTERPRETATION OF DATA

Generally for pesticide skin absorption studies, the application is finite (low
volume) rather than infinite (high volume), and the results of the study are
presented as percent dose absorbed, rather than flux. The reason for this type of
data presentation is that the majority of the regulatory authorities prefer this format;
it is more readily applicable to their safety calculation procedures.

Following both in vivo and in vitro studies, there is sometimes a high proportion of test chemical remaining in the SC and/or underlying skin at the end of
the study. This is particularly the case with more highly lipophilic substances or
with chemicals that bind to skin components (e.g., amines). This fraction is not
classed as absorbed [the OECD definition of absorbed dose is the test substance
reaching the RF or systemic circulation within a specified period of time (4)].
However, in the interpretation of data by regulatory authorities, the SC/skin
fraction may be included as potentially absorbable unless there is good evidence
that it is not (6). The reason for this approach is to ensure a conservative risk
assessment.

In cases where the risk assessment is not acceptable following this conservative approach, it is important to have more information about the fate of the
chemical found in the skin layers.

Fate of Chemical in the Skin Layers

The diffusion of a chemical through skin is a complex, dynamic process. Although
the processes are governed by the physicochemistry of the test substance and the
structure of the skin layers, it is difficult to describe the whole process in
mathematical terms. Many mathematical models do exist and relate to various
aspects of conditions of skin absorption (see Section QSAR), but there are no useful
universal models to cover the most common exposure scenarios.

During in vivo and in vitro studies, a non-volatile pesticide will be in one or more of these compartments.

1. Dislodgeable from the skin surface at the end of exposure
2. Remain associated with the application or protection system or as contamination on the surface of the skin outside the treated area
3. Remain bound to the skin surface at the treatment site (difficult to remove)
4. Remain in the SC
5. Remain in the epidermis
6. Remain in the dermis or deeper tissue layers
7. Be absorbed (present in the RF or in systemic circulation)

The fractions (1), (2), and (3) are clearly not absorbed, and the fraction (7) is clearly absorbed. For the other fractions the question is, what would be the fate of the fraction if the study duration was beyond the exposure period being studied? If it would be sloughed off the skin surface by the normal desquamation of the skin layers, then it would not be absorbed. If it diffuses into the dermis, then it would be absorbed. In most cases, there is no experimental evidence for the specific test chemical. However, in studies with human volunteers, it is common to find that the majority of the residue in the SC is lost by desquamation (22). Similarly in rodent studies on pesticide products, where rats have been carefully bandaged daily to trap desquamated skin, it is common to find a significant portion of the SC fraction is lost and not absorbed. In a model with human skin grafted onto nude mice (HuSki), it was shown that even with a highly lipophilic molecule (lindane), the majority of the SC fraction was lost by desquamation (14).

In the case of in vitro studies, the study is commonly terminated at 24 hours (due to the slow degeneration of skin integrity in vitro). Therefore, it is more difficult to be certain of the potential fate of chemical remaining at the treated site because the time profile over several days can only be studied in vivo. The solubility of the test chemical in the RF is an important factor affecting the amount of residue in the skin. For materials of low lipophilicity, the partitioning of the test chemical into the RF from the skin is not a problem. In these cases, the amount of test chemical remaining in the SC/skin is generally relatively small, except when chemicals bind to the skin layers. For more lipophilic chemicals, the use of a more lipophilic RF will favor partitioning into the RF from the skin. This is designed to model the physiological situation of the capillary circulation in vivo which would remove chemicals reaching the epidermis–dermis interface by diffusion into the circulating blood. Therefore, for more lipophilic chemicals, either a more lipophilic RF must be used or the skin fraction must be included as the absorbable dose.

For in vivo studies, the daily measurements of excreted test chemical gives an estimate of the elimination profile with time. When this shows that all, or almost all elimination is complete, then we can be confident that no, or almost no more chemical is being absorbed from the application site. However, if the elimination process is slow, then this demonstrates that either the chemical is still becoming available to the systemic circulation at the application site, or that the elimination characteristics from the various physiological compartments, is slow. Data from the elimination characteristics following administration via another route can help clarify which of these factors are relevant.

Agencies regulating pesticide products will take a conservative approach, often including the SC/skin fraction into the absorbable dose. Therefore, the study design should allow for this and where a significant skin residue remains, appropriate data should be produced to show the likely fate of the skin dose. An example of this would be for an amine chemical structure that binds to skin: The performance of a rat in vivo study can show that after the exposure period no further chemical becomes available systemically and that a significant percentage of the amount in the SC is lost by desquamation daily. This evidence can be sufficient to exclude the SC/skin residue in the absorbable dose in the regulatory calculations.

Where only a relatively small fraction of chemical becomes truly available to the systemic circulation, and a much larger fraction remains in the SC/skin compartments, the fate of the skin residue can be important in the regulatory process. In these cases, it can be critical to demonstrate that this residual fraction is not absorbable. When it is critical to show the fate of the SC fraction over time, the most suitable model for this is probably the HuSki where the fate of the chemical can be traced for more than 10 days after exposure (14).

DEVELOPMENT AND SAFETY TESTING OF NEW PESTICIDE PRODUCTS

The safety testing that is required for a new pesticide formulation of an existing product is usually limited to a small number of acute toxicity studies to establish that the hazard characteristics of the product, in combination with all the ingredients within the formulation, are similar to registered products containing this chemical. This toxicology work involves specific end points that include oral and dermal toxicity, skin and eye irritation, and skin sensitization. In addition, a key end point that is a requirement for registration of any new formulation is the assessment of the systemic exposure following dermal contact with the product concentrate and the in-use spray dilutions. This forms part of the OPEX risk assessment. Here, the key study that is used by regulatory authorities, under the protocol defined in the test guideline OECD 428, is the determination of human skin absorption in vitro. This absorption parameter ties together the toxicology hazard data that have determined the no adverse effect level in experimental animals with the human exposure that is expected (or has been determined) in the field. If the skin absorption is determined to be above a critical value in the risk assessment, and does not meet the margin of safety required, then this can prevent the use of the product in the intended market.

During the development of new agrochemical products, the adjuvants incorporated into formulations are often designed to get the active into the target organisms, normally through a lipid barrier, as effectively as possible. Human skin has evolved to keep chemicals out of the systemic circulation by having a highly compacted lipid structure as the external layer of the epidermis, known as the SC. This kinetic dilemma, i.e., uptake (plant/insect) and exclusion (animal) between cuticle and skin, is depicted in Figure 2 for an herbicide. The problem is that the same adjuvants designed to improve bioefficacy often act as skin absorption enhancers, or they can cause skin toxicity themselves.

The pesticide industry often makes assumptions that the development of a new formulation will have minimal effects on dermal absorption and the existing risk assessment for the product will be acceptable for registration. Even during the development of a new active, there can be unforeseen toxicology problems that were not identified until the complete formulation is tested. This can involve considerable effort, and delay, to get the new product through the registration

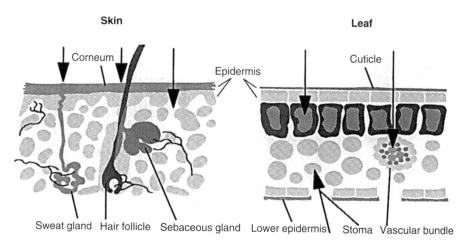

FIGURE 2   Points of entry into animal and plant cell external membrane barriers.

process. Likewise, where new formulations or mixtures are being developed for use in home and garden markets, the margins of safety are often more stringent than for professional crop protection use and often lower skin absorption is required to meet risk assessments. In these areas of the market, the skin hazard notation can also restrict or even totally prevent the use of products, due to potential skin exposure to the more sensitive members of the population.

There is a natural tendency in the pesticide industry to play safe and use registered "inerts" (i.e., formulation components other than the active ingredient) in new agrochemical formulations. However, this stifles innovation and development of even safer formulations because acceptable adjuvants not only have a lower business risk but also provide a lower gain without a competitive edge. Likewise, emerging formulation technologies such as nanoparticles are an area of particular importance in the dermal absorption field and are coming under increasing regulatory scrutiny (9). Safety of these new platforms in relation to potential systemic exposure from skin contact needs careful consideration before such new technologies are put into full-scale product development. By bringing the safety issues involved with the major route of human exposure, the skin, into the early stages of R&D and understanding the formulation chemistry that results in effective but safe formulations makes good business sense. Pesticide organizations that have wide-ranging formulation science and technology expertise and also have experts in toxicology who understand the science, methodology, and registration require- ments associated with dermal absorption and dermal toxicity are in a unique position to bring their mutual expertise closer and to develop safe innovative products.

A new challenge is therefore to build new pesticide formulations that have differential actions on human skin and the intended biological target. This would ideally involve research to characterize the absorption process across membranes to understand the thermodynamic, toxicological, and kinetic aspects of adjuvant chemistry on uptake of the active chemical across different lipid membrane barriers. This approach to formulation development has a common thread across herbicides, fungicides, and insecticides. The outcome of a more integrated formulation and dermal research approach should be the identification and development of better and more innovative formulations that have improved safety profiles. This has the potential to lead to a new generation of even safer pesticide products.

REFERENCES

1. European Community. Commission Directive 94/79/EC amending Council Directive 91/414/EEC concerning the placing of plant protection products on the market. Off J Eur Commun 1994; L354:21.
2. van Hemmen JJ. EUROPOEM, a predictive occupational exposure database for registration purposes of pesticides. Appl Occup Environ Hyg 2001; 16:246–50. (http://www.enduser.co.uk/europoem/)
3. OECD guideline for the testing of chemicals. Skin absorption: in vivo method. 427. Adopted: 13 April 2004:1–8.
4. OECD guideline for the testing of chemicals. Skin absorption: in vitro method. 428. Adopted: 13 April 2004:1–8.
5. OECD Guidance Document for the Conduct of Skin Absorption Studies. OECD series on testing and assessment. Number 28. ENV/JM/MONO 2004; 2:1–31. (http://appli1.oecd.org/olis/2004doc.nsf/linkto/env-jm-mono(2004)2)
6. EC Guidance Document on Dermal Absorption. European Commission, SANCO/222/2000 rev. 2004; 7:1–15.
7. U.S. EPA Health Effects Test Guidelines. U.S. Environmental Protection Agency, OPPTS 870.7600. Dermal Penetration 1998:1–12.
8. Koeter HBWM. Dialogue and collaboration: a personal view on laboratory animal welfare developments in general, and on ECVAM's first decade in particular. Altern Lab Anim 2002; 30(Suppl. 2):207–10.
9. IPCS Dermal Absorption. World Health Organization, International Programme on Chemical Safety. Environmental Health Criteria 2006:235. (http://www.who.int/ipcs/publications/ehc/en/index.html)
10. Howes D, Guy R, Hadgraft J, et al. Methods for assessing percutaneous absorption, report and recommendations of ECVAM Workshop 13. Altern Lab Anim 1996; 24:81–106.
11. ECETOC Percutaneous Absorption. European Centre for Ecotoxicology and Toxicology of Chemicals, Brussels, Monograph No. 20 1993:1–80.
12. U.S. Environmental Protection Agency. Proposed test rule for in vitro dermal absorption rate testing of certain chemicals of interest to occupational safety and health administration; proposed rule. Fed Regist 1999; 64:31073–90.
13. Scott RC, Carmichael NG, Huckle KR, et al. Methods for measuring dermal penetration of pesticides. Food Chem Toxicol 1993; 31:523–9.
14. Capt A, Luzy AP, Esdaile D, et al. Comparison of the human skin grafted onto nude mouse model with in vivo and in vitro models in the prediction of percutaneous penetration of three lipophilic pesticides. Regul Toxicol Pharmacol 2007; 47:274–87.
15. Potts RO, Guy RH. Predicting skin permeability. Pharm Res 1992; 9:663–9.
16. Fasano WJ, Manning LA. Rapid integrity assessment of rat and human epidermal membranes for in vitro dermal regulatory testing: correlation of electrical resistance with tritiated water permeability. Toxicol In Vitro 2002; 16:731–40.
17. Davies DJ, Ward RJ, Heylings JR. Multi-species assessment of electrical resistance as a skin integrity marker for in vitro percutaneous absorption studies. Toxicol In Vitro 2004; 18:351–8.
18. Scott RC, Batten PL, Clowes HM, et al. Further validation of an in vitro method to reduce the need for in vivo studies for measuring the absorption of chemicals through rat skin. Fundam Appl Toxicol 1992; 19:484–92.
19. Ramsey JD, Woollen BH, Auton TR, et al. The predictive accuracy of in vitro measurements for the dermal absorption of a lipophilic penetrant (fluazifop-butyl) through rat and human skin. Fundam Appl Toxicol 1994; 23:230–6.

20. Heylings JR, Diot S, Esdaile DJ, et al. A prevalidation study on the in vitro skin irritation function test (SIFT) for prediction of acute skin irritation in vivo: results and evaluation of ECVAM phase III. Toxicol In Vitro 2003; 17:123–38.
21. Williams FM. EDETOX. Evaluations and predictions of dermal absorption of toxic chemicals. Int Arch Occup Environ Health 2004; 77:150–1.
22. Ramsey JD, Woollen BH, Auton TR, et al. Pharmacokinetics of fluazifop-butyl in human volunteers II: dermal dosing. Hum Exp Toxicol 1992; 11:247–54.

36 Bathing Water: Percutaneous Absorption of Water Contaminants

Richard P. Moody
Healthy Environments and Consumer Safety Branch, Environmental Health Centre, Ottawa, Canada

INTRODUCTION

Aquatic pollutants may be absorbed into the skin by swimmers and bathers, leading to the risk of exposure via the dermal route to a wide array of potentially toxic pollutants. Many noxious pollutants [e.g., polyaromatic hydrocarbons (PAHs), polychlorinated biphenyls, dioxins] are very lipophilic and are expected to partition extensively into the stratum corneum lipids of human skin (1). In the past, concerns about exposure to these fat-soluble water contaminants have been ignored since it was thought that their low water solubility [e.g., water solubility of dichlorodiphenyltrichloroethane (DDT) is 1.2 ppb] limited their maximum concentration to only trace levels in water. However, lipophilic compounds are known to readily adsorb to organic matter suspended in or floating on lake water. All natural aquatic bodies have a thin film of floating oil (the surface slick, usually a mixture of natural oils exuded from aquatic biota, decomposition products of biota, and natural seepage of petroleum hydrocarbons) and lipophilic pollutants will partition into this phase and reach concentrations far surpassing those in the subsurface water. Marine and fresh water spills of crude oil from shipping as well as the effluent from power engines used in boating and pleasure craft add to this oil slick. When bathers immerse themselves in the water, their entire body surface would at once receive total body coverage by this oil film along with its adherent floating sediment. A bather is thus rapidly exposed over the entire skin surface to lipophilic environmental contaminants dissolved and/or suspended in the slick. The rate of transdermal absorption of these compounds is affected by the anatomic site exposed, the chemical nature of the compound, environmental factors (water temperature, pH, etc.), the use of commercial sun tan oils and other "cosmetics," and by the presence of dermal abrasions and other skin ailments (1,2).

Lipophilic compounds may partition into the skin and attain relatively high concentrations and form reservoirs. Work in our laboratory [reviewed in Ref. (3)] has indicated that washing the skin with soap, 24 hours after exposure, may liberate this reservoir, washing the compound into the skin. We concluded that bathers may acquire a dermal reservoir of environmental contaminants while swimming and that this reservoir could be made bioavailable and hence be of concern in the event of post-bathing soap washing. Other researchers have shown that soap washing may increase the amount of absorption of these compounds, especially if the time of the wash onset is delayed (1,4).

In this chapter, we present some of our data in context with swimming and bathing exposure to water contaminants, and discuss the significance of the wash-in effect. Although the discussion will pertain mainly to swimming exposure, it should be evident that such exposure is also relevant to the case of a person showering or having a bath. We focus on lipophile partitioning and the slick dermal exposure hypothesis. The introduction and majority of the text are based on our original chapter (3) with an update at the end of the text.

CONCEPTUAL FRAMEWORK OF SWIMMING/BATHING EXPOSURE

Earlier reviews of basic factors concerning dermal absorption of water contaminants by swimmers/bathers are available (1,5,6). Octanol–water partition coefficients (K_{ow}) have been widely used in attempts to predict the rate of dermal absorption of compounds. The optimum lipophilicity for skin permeation has been reported to be about log K_{ow} of 1, but some researchers have placed the peak of the parabolic correlation at a log K_{ow} of 2 to 3 [e.g., (7)]. We examined the partitioning of pesticide compounds from water into a floating surface layer of octanol (8). This concept is being introduced here in order to conceptualize chemical partitioning in the context of naturally occurring slicks and bathing water.

The "Slick" Concept

Maguire et al. (9) investigated the concentration of inorganic tin and several organic tin species in the surface microlayer of water samples from a marina in Toronto, Canada. They reported levels of three tin species up to 10^4 times greater than those in the subsurface water. Platford et al. (10) reported that the concentration of the pesticides DDT and hexachlorobenzene in octanol films was much greater than concentrations achieved in bulk water subphase. If one considers an oily film of octanol floating on top of a body of water (Fig. 1), a lipophilic compound dissolved in the water will partition preferentially into the octanol layer. In the case where the octanol–water volume ratio is small (e.g., an octanol slick), further concentration by the lipophile occurs because the partition coefficient of a solute is independent of the octanol and water volumes used at low solute concentrations. At equilibrium, the concentration of the lipophile will be much greater in the octanol than that it would have been for a bulk phase (equal volume) octanol–water partition system. If the octanol volume is initially reduced, then the resultant lipophile concentration in the octanol will be greater as long as phase saturation does not occur. Saturation of the water and/or oil slick phases is improbable in aquatic habitats, given the low levels of water contaminants normally present. In the case of a swimmer exposed to an infinite volume of water, lipophile partitioning would be expected to result in high skin lipid concentrations of the water contaminants. The skin of the swimmer can be viewed as an octanol layer floating on the water surface and a similar partitioning process should ensue. Of course, the skin concentration of a compound may not necessarily relate directly to systemic availability since the compound may reside as a non-bioavailable dermal reservoir.

The "Wash-In" Effect

PAHs are ubiquitous contaminants of both marine and fresh water habitats (11). Up to 43% of an applied dose of benzo[a]pyrene was absorbed through skin (12) with 8.4 µg/cm^2 being absorbed in vitro by human skin (13). Of this calculated absorbed dose, however, only 1.5% was observed to permeate into the receiver solution, the remainder being present as a dermal reservoir. This reservoir was considered to be potentially bioavailable for the purposes of conducting a conservative health hazard exposure assessment. Consistent with this assumption

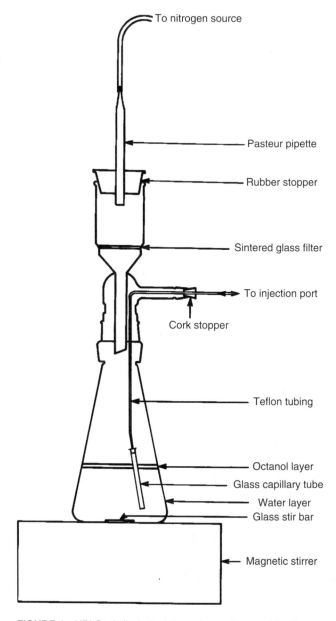

FIGURE 1 HPLC stir flask depicting a layer of octanol floating on water. If the water contained a mixture of pesticides, the more lipophilic compounds would partition preferentially into the upper octanol phase and attain concentrations in the octanol far surpassing the original water concentrations. If at equilibrium one were to dip a finger into the water through the octanol and then remove the finger with its now adherent octanol film, one would receive a much higher dose of the lipophilic pesticides than if octanol had not been present since the octanol "slick" together with the extracted contaminants would adhere to the skin. *Source*: From Ref. 8.

was our observation that a wash-in effect occurred (13) and it is quite possible that subsequent washing could have liberated more of this dermal reservoir.

The insect repellent N,N-diethyl-m-toluamide (DEET) is a lipophilic compound [log K_{ow}=2.0; (8)] that is in common use by cottagers, boaters, and others engaged in aquatic activities. We examined the dermal absorption of DEET, from three commercially available formulations, using rat, hairless guinea pig, and human skin in vitro, and the data were compared with in vivo studies with rats (14). In this study, a wash-in effect was reported since the 24-hour soap wash was associated with a profound increase in the % absorption observed post-washing in all three species tested in vitro (Figs. 2–4). The study also revealed that the in vivo rat study underestimated the dermal absorption of DEET assessed in vitro. We question, therefore, the applicability of in vivo tests conducted on animals for examining bathing exposure.

Other Environmental Factors
The swimming/bathing exposure environment is extremely variable. Water temperature ranges from the near freezing marine temperatures encountered in northern locations to the relatively warm water used in hot tubs and spas. The suspended sediment (silt, algae, microbiota) load in natural waters is highly variable hence the potential exposure to sediment-associated water contaminants would differ (2). The aqueous bathing environment would serve to hydrate the skin and enhance the absorption of water contaminants (1,15). An important factor with unusual relevance to swimming exposure is the effect of solar radiation on dermal absorption of water contaminants (16,17). A further important factor not usually considered in dermal absorption studies is the effect of physical exercise (18).

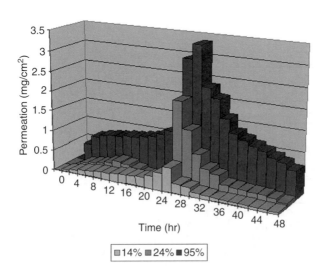

FIGURE 2 In vitro analysis of ^{14}C-DEET permeating rat skin from three commercial DEET formulations. The percentage of DEET in each formulation is shown. The mean (n=4) DEET permeation (mg/cm^2) in the receiver solution is shown versus time. The skin was washed with Radiacwash® (Biodex Medical Systems Inc., Shirley, New York, U.S.A.) and water at 24-hour postexposure. *Source*: From Ref. 14.

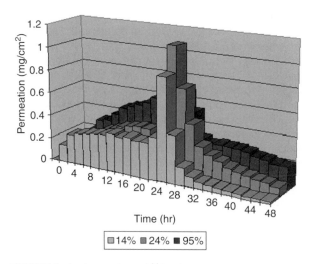

FIGURE 3 In vitro analysis of ^{14}C-DEET permeating hairless guinea pig skin from three commercial DEET formulations. The percentage of DEET in each formulation is shown. The mean ($n=4$) DEET permeation (mg/cm^2) in the receiver solution is shown versus time. The skin was washed with Radiacwash® (Biodex Medical Systems Inc., Shirley, New York, U.S.A.) water at 24-hour post-exposure. *Source*: From Ref. 14.

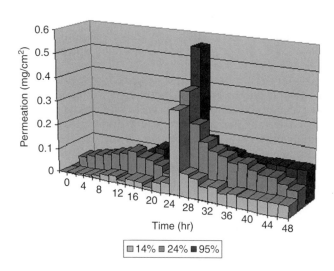

FIGURE 4 In vitro analysis of ^{14}C-DEET permeating human skin from three commercial DEET formulations. The percentage of DEET in each formulation is shown. The mean ($n=4$) DEET permeation (mg/cm^2) in the receiver solution is shown versus time. The skin was washed with Radiacwash® (Biodex Medical Systems Inc., Shirley, New York, U.S.A.) and water at 24-hour postexposure. *Source*: From Ref. 14.

Mixture Effects and Transdermal Accelerants

It has been well established that some chemicals can exert an accelerant effect upon the skin absorption of another compound applied topically. The insect repellent DEET, commonly used by bathers, may act as a skin permeation enhancer (19). In our studies with the herbicide 2,4-dichlorophenoxyacetic acid (2,4-D) amine, we did not discern a significant DEET-associated enhancing effect when the herbicide was applied in water to the palmar surface (20). However, we did find evidence of a DEET-associated effect on the dermal absorption of the insecticide fenitrothion (21). Given the extensive use of DEET by people engaged in aquatic activities, the possibility of a DEET enhancement effect warrants further investigation under conditions comparable to its use by the public before and/or after swimming and bathing exposure.

It is also important to consider the effect of barrier creams because it is a common practice for marathon swimmers to apply petroleum jelly liberally prior to swimming for leech control. This practice may actually serve to protect the swimmer from dermal uptake of water contaminants. The barrier properties of petrolatum have been reported albeit not in context with swimming/bathing exposure (22). Conversely petrolatum may increase the hydration of the stratum corneum thereby increasing its permeability (23).

Absorption of Hydrophilic Water Contaminants

It is important to appreciate that smaller dermal flux rates for hydrophilic solutes do not necessarily preclude the risk of a toxic dose being absorbed. Wester and Maibach (1) have reported significant dermal absorption of metals dissolved in water in their salt form. Cadmium and arsenic were shown to be absorbed through human skin in vitro. Rahman et al. (24) reported a linear increase in arsenic absorption with dose and a maximum absorption of 62% of the applied dose using an aqueous vehicle and with mouse skin in vitro. Conversely, in a well-controlled in vivo study with human subjects, exposed to lithium (40 ppm) in spa/tub water, no significant elevation in blood serum levels was detected above pre-exposure levels (25).

The extraordinary variety of environmental factors that come into play when trying to evaluate the literature data within a swimming/bathing exposure context necessitates the development of a rapid screening test to provide the data required for a proper hazard/risk evaluation of the degree of health problem inherent in modern day swimming/bathing practices. We have developed such a rapid in vitro skin bioassay procedure (automated in vitro dermal absorption, AIVDA) that involves the use of very small skin permeation tubes (SPTs) (Fig. 5) and was described in detail in our earlier chapter (3).

FUTURE RESEARCH

Further studies should be conducted to determine the importance of the surface slick hypothesis. Although of major consequence in highly polluted waters, the health impact of the concept of surface slick exposure for bathers using relatively clean city tap water will need to be determined. Furthermore, a number of tests are required to examine the effect of environmental factors (e.g., water sediment load, water temperature and pH, solar irradiation) and endogenous factors (e.g., skin age, anatomic site, mixture effects, presence of cosmetics) on dermal absorption

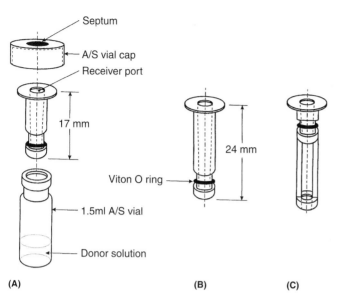

FIGURE 5 SPT method of measuring swimming/bathing exposure to water contaminants. Short (17 mm) (**A**) and long (24 mm) SPTs (**B**) for measuring absorption from different depths in the donor solution. (**C**) A vertically slotted SPT used for diffusion studies with dialysis membrane tubes. The tubes were machined from Teflon to fit into standard HPLC glass A/S vials. The septum in the vial cap prevents loss of volatiles. The septum is pierced by an A/S needle and the receiver solution inside the SPT is removed for HPLC analysis. The donor solution can contain a small magnetic stir bar. The Viton O-ring (B&N Transmission, Ottawa, Ontario, Canada) holds the skin specimen sandwiched between dialysis membrane to prevent tissue debris from entering the receiver/donor solutions. *Abbreviations*: A/S, autosampler; SPT, skin permeation tube.

following swimming/bathing exposure. Validation of in vitro tests with data acquired from tests conducted in vivo is necessary in order to provide an alternative to animal testing.

UPDATE FOR DERMAL ABSORPTION AND TOXICITY ASSESSMENT, 2ND EDITION

Since initially preparing this review for the first edition of *Dermal Absorption and Toxicity Assessment* (3), there have been surprisingly few further advances made in the swimming/bathing dermal absorption research area. Wester and Maibach (26) have recently reviewed the percutaneous absorption of contaminants from drinking water and considered the ability of skin to act as a "lipid sink." Bunge and McDougal (1999) have reviewed the dermal absorption of drinking water contaminants, including dermal vapor exposure to volatiles such as chloroform at elevated levels in hot showers. Bunge and McDougal (27) also briefly consider the effect of soaps and surfactants, this being relevant to the wash-in effect recently reviewed by Moody and Maibach (28). Of particular interest was the still unknown nature of the specific wash-in mechanism(s) involved. We concluded (ibid) that the potential mechanisms involve surfactant effects (e.g., skin surface delipidation), hydration (e.g., stratum corneum swelling), acid–base effects (e.g., ionization, pK_a), friction effects (e.g., rub off), and/or an unknown effect of the soap wash skin cleansing method used in vitro. We recommended that further well-controlled studies were needed.

Most literature reports in the swimming/bathing dermal absorption research area, published after our review, are concerned with dermal exposure to volatile trihalomethanes such as chloroform. Islam et al. (29) reported dermal absorption of chloroform in hairless rats tested in vivo after a 30-minute bath. Studies from our own laboratories reported the absorption of chloroform, trichloroethylene, and tetrachloroethylene in human skin using the AIVDA aluminum flow-through cell (30). Of note was the effect of the bathing water temperature in vitro for human skin wherein a two- to threefold increase in chloroform skin permeability was obtained when the bath temperature was elevated from 11°C to 50°C. Gordon et al. (31) reported 30-fold higher exhaled breath levels of chloroform in human subjects wearing face masks supplying pure air and for bathing at the highest water temperatures in studies conducted from 30°C to 40°C. Corley et al. (32) reported temperature-related increased dermal absorption of chloroform in humans tested in vivo using physiological pharmacokinetic modeling. Xu and Weisel (33) reported human dermal absorption of chloroform and haloketones after measuring breath samples for subjects following a 30-minute bath.

Volatile chemicals other than chloroform have also been reported to be absorbed through skin during bathing. For example, elevated toluene levels were reported in exhaled breath of human volunteers in warm hydrotherapy baths, where the inhalation exposure route was excluded by supplying pure breathing air (34). Similar data have been obtained for xylene (35). Nakai et al. (36) reported the effect of environmental conditions on benzene absorption in human skin using the AIVDA flow-through cell to model swimming/bathing exposure. This study showed increased skin permeability of benzene with water temperature. It also reported a potential permeation enhancing effect on benzene by a commercial sunscreen product, although no significant effect of the same brand of sunscreen was observed for chloroform (30). The permeation rates for both benzene and chloroform were not affected by the presence of a commercial skin moisturizer or a baby oil formulation (30,36). More recently, Pont et al. (37) reported that several active ingredients of sunscreen products, including DEET, enhanced the absorption of the herbicide 2,4-D in hairless mouse skin and human skin in vitro. In contrast, our study conducted with a more hydrophilic dimethylamine salt of 2,4-D indicated that DEET did not enhance the percutaneous absorption of 2,4-D dimethylamine in human volunteers (20). It is interesting that Pont et al. (37) observed DEET-enhanced dermal absorption of 2,4-D [log $K_{ow} = 2.62$ (estimated by KowWin, Syracuse Research Corporation, Syracuse, New York, U.S.A.)] in vitro but we found no such enhancement for the more hydrophilic 2,4-D dimethylamine salt (log $K_{ow} = 0.84$, K_{ow}Win estimate). This is consistent with our earlier supposition that DEET may preferentially enhance lipophiles. Obviously further research is needed in this area. For recent reviews of mixture effects on percutaneous absorption, see (38,39).

Since reporting an alternative to animal testing using our AIVDA method with Teflon SPTs made in-house, our laboratory proceeded to develop SPTs made from aluminum at the Science and Technology Centre at Carleton University in Ottawa, Ontario, Canada using a "twin tube design" and reported their use for both finite (40) and infinite dose studies (41). A disposable form of flow-through cell using commercially available polymer chambers was reported by Moody and

Akram (42). As well as in vitro models, we have also developed alternative in silico dermal quantitative structure–activity relationship (QSAR) quantitative structure–property relationship (QSPR) models based on the Flynn in vitro database (43,44).

To clarify the development of our slick hypothesis (3), we note that since the partition coefficient is independent of the *relative* volumes of octanol and water used (45) but the concentration of a lipophile in octanol can be highly dependent on the octanol volume if the water volume stays constant (46) suggests that the octanol concentration of a lipophile may increase markedly in cases where a low octanol–water volume ratio exists such as that in a surface slick. Since developing the slick concept, it has been challenged by colleagues in that the oil slick concentration of lipophilic water contaminants may increase at small oil volumes, but since toxicity depends on both concentration and dose volume, the dermal exposure may not increase appreciably since the oil slick volume is relatively small. However, we note that since only a small volume of the surface slick film should remain adhering to the skin per unit surface area after the swimmer/bather leaves the water, this possibility may not be applicable, at least for post-swimming/bathing dermal absorption. In the case of post-swimming exposure, the volume of slick/cm^2 left adhering to skin would be small irrespective of the thickness or volume of the slick layer. Hence, a smaller volume of slick floating on the water surface overall would not necessarily affect the final volume remaining on the skin and the resulting increased dose/exposure due to a higher slick concentration of a lipophile may not be compensated for by the reduction in slick volume in situ. Since the volume of oil slick film retained on skin will vary, however, due to oil viscosity and temperature, the importance of such factors needs to be determined experimentally. Our SPT technique provides a good method to study this since the tube can be positioned to hold the skin in the oil slick or deeper in the water phase for comparison. Another aspect to consider is that at small oil-to-water volume ratios as in a slick situation where the water volume of a lake, for example, can be considered infinite, the time required to reach equilibrium increases. In such a case when oil is recently introduced, for example, in the common use of bath/spa oil products, there may not be sufficient time for lipophilic water contaminants to concentrate in the oil layer. Still, these exposure scenarios require testing under well-controlled environmental conditions.

Given the particular complexity of swimming/bathing exposure, the effect of less explored environmental conditions such as solar ultraviolet irradiation, the concentration of lipophiles by surface slicks, or that post-swimming soap washing/showering may cause wash-in effects, the need for the development of cost-effective, rapid methods specialized in modeling this particular exposure appears evident. The rapidly growing list of "natural" herbal chemicals such as phytochemicals used in bathing/spa products will likely expedite such method development.

SUMMARY AND CONCLUSIONS

We have outlined the basic factors expected to play important roles in determining the degree of exposure to water contaminants for individuals engaged in swimming/bathing activity and briefly reviewed recent data in this field. The importance of surface slick exposure and lipophile partitioning has been emphasized. Future research is necessary to examine the wide variety of factors known to affect dermal absorption from swimming/bathing exposure so that the degree of health risk to the public can be assessed.

ACKNOWLEDGMENTS

We wish to thank Ms. Brita Nadeau and Mr. Eric Nicholson for technical assistance in our laboratory studies, and Mr. Jack Kelly for machining the SPT cells and for help with their design. We are grateful to Dr. Ih Chu for many helpful discussions and to Dr. Chu, Dr. D. Clapin, and Ms. S. Gupta for reviewing the manuscript. We also thank our Audio/Visual Department for assistance with the graphics. We wish to thank Mr. Hart MacPherson and Dr. Jamie Nakai for internal review of the update.

REFERENCES

1. Wester RC, Maibach HI. Percutaneous absorption of chemicals from water simulating swimming and bathing and from vapor exposure. In: Wang RGM, ed. Environmental Science and Pollution Control Series 9. Water Contamination and Health: Integration of Exposure Assessment, Toxicology, and Risk Assessment. New York: Marcel Dekker Inc., 1994:149–65.
2. Moody RP, Chu I. Dermal exposure to environmental contaminants in the Great Lakes. Environ Health Perspect 1995; 103(9):103–14.
3. Moody RP. Bathing water: percutaneous absorption of water contaminants. In: Roberts MS, Walters KA, eds. Dermal Absorption and Toxicity Assessment. New York: Marcel Dekker, 1998:709–25.
4. Lange M, Nitzsche K, Zesch A. Percutaneous absorption of lindane in healthy volunteers and scabies patients. Dependency of penetration kinetics in serum upon frequency of application, time and mode of washing. Arch Dermatol Res 1981; 271:387–99.
5. Wester RC, Maibach HI, Sedik L, et al. In vitro percutaneous absorption of cadmium from water and soil into human skin. Fundam Appl Toxicol 1992; 19:1–5.
6. EPA Report. Interim Guidance for Dermal Exposure Assessment. Exposure Assessment Group, U.S. Environmental Protection Agency, Washington, D.C., Report #OHEA-E-367, Chapter 5, 1990:11–3.
7. Singh P, Roberts MS. Skin permeability and local tissue concentrations of nonsteroidal anti-inflammatory drugs after topical application. J Pharmacol Exp Ther 1994; 268:144–51.
8. Moody RP, Carroll JM, Kresta AME. Automated high performance liquid chromatography and liquid scintillation counting determination of pesticide mixture octanol/water partition rates. Toxicol Ind Health 1987; 3:479–90.
9. Maguire RJ, Chau YK, Bengert GA, et al. Occurrence of organotin in Ontario lakes and rivers. Environ Sci Technol 1982; 16(10):698–702.
10. Platford RF, Carey JH, Hale EJ. The environmental significance of surface films. Part 1: Octanol–water partition coefficients for DDT and hexachlorobenzene. Environ Pollut Ser B 1982; 3:125–8.
11. Andelman JB, Snodgrass JE. Incidence and significance of polynuclear aromatic hydrocarbons in the water environment. CRC Crit Rev Envir Control 1974; 4:69–83.
12. Ng KME, Chu I, Bronaugh RL, et al. Percutaneous absorption and metabolism of pyrene, benzo[a]pyrene, and di(2-ethylhexyl) phthalate: comparison of in vitro and in vivo results in the hairless guinea pig. Toxicol Appl Pharmacol 1992; 115:216–23.
13. Moody RP, Nadeau B, Chu I. In vivo and in vitro dermal absorption of benzo[a]pyrene in rat, guinea pig, human and tissue-cultured skin. J Dermatol Sci 1995; 9:48–58.
14. Moody RP, Nadeau B, Chu I. In vitro dermal absorption of N,N-diethyl-m-toluamide (DEET) in rat, guinea pig and human skin. In Vitro Toxicol 1995; 8(3):263–75.

15. Roberts MS, Walker M. Water the most natural penetration enhancer. In: Walters KA, Hadgraft J, eds. Pharmaceutical Skin Penetration Enhancement. New York: Marcel Dekker Inc., 1993:1–30.
16. McAuliffe DJ, Blank IH. Effects of UVA (320–400 nm) on the barrier characteristics of the skin. J Invest Dermatol 1991; 96(5):758–62.
17. Lehman P, Melnik B, Holzle E, et al. The effect of UV-A and UV-B irradiation on the skin barrier. Skin physiologic, electron microscopy and lipid biochemistry studies. Hautarzt 1992; 43:344–51.
18. Levesque B, Ayotte P, LeBlanc A, et al. Evaluation of dermal and respiratory chloroform exposure in humans. Environ Health Perspect 1994; 102(12):1082–7.
19. Windheuser JJ, Haslam JL, Caldwell L, et al. The use of N,N-diethyl-m-toluamide to enhance dermal and transdermal delivery of drugs. J Pharm Sci 1982; 17(11):1211–3.
20. Moody RP, Wester R, Maibach HI. Dermal absorption of the phenoxy herbicide 2,4-D dimethylamine in humans: effect of DEET and anatomic site. J Toxicol Environ Health 1992; 36:241–50.
21. Moody RP, Riedel D, Ritter L, et al. The effect of DEET (N,N-diethyl-m-toluamide) on dermal persistence and absorption of the insecticide, fenitrothion, in rats and rhesus monkeys. J Toxicol Environ Health 1987; 22(4):5159.
22. Treffel P, Gabard B, Juch R. Evaluation of barrier creams: an in vitro technique on human skin. Acta Derm Venereol (Stockh) 1994; 74:7–11.
23. Shani J, Barak S, Levi D, et al. Skin penetration of minerals in psoriatics and guinea-pigs bathing in hypertonic salt solutions. Pharmacol Res Commun 1985; 17:501–12.
24. Rahman MS, Hall LL, Hughes MF. In vitro percutaneous absorption of sodium arsenate in B6C3F$_1$ mice. Toxic In Vitro 1994; 8(3):441–8.
25. McCarty JD, Carter SP, Fletcher MJ, et al. Study of the lithium absorption by users of spas treated with lithium ion. Human Exp Toxicol 1994; 13:315–9.
26. Wester RC, Maibach HI. Skin contamination and absorption of chemicals from water and soil. In: Bronaugh RL, Maibach HI, eds. Percutaneous Absorption Drugs–Cosmetics–Mechanisms–Methodology. 4th ed. New York: Taylor & Francis, 2005:107–21.
27. Bunge AL, McDougal JN. Dermal uptake. In: Olin SS, ed. Exposure to Contaminants in Drinking Water. Boca Raton: CRC Press, 1999:137–81.
28. Moody RP, Maibach, HI. Skin decontamination: importance of the wash-in effect. Food Chem Toxicol 2006; 44:1783–8.
29. Islam MS, Zhao L, Zhou J, et al. Systemic uptake and clearance of chloroform by hairless rats following dermal exposure. I. Brief exposure to aqueous solutions. Risk Anal 1996; 16(3):349–57.
30. Nakai JS, Stathpoulos PB, Cambell GL, et al. Penetration of chloroform, trichloroethylene, and tetrachloroethylene through human skin. J Toxicol Environ Health A 1999; 58:157–70.
31. Gordon SM, Wallace LA, Callahan PJ, et al. Effect of water temperature on dermal exposure to chloroform. Environ Health Perspect 1998; 106(6):337–45.
32. Corley RA, Gordon SM, Wallace LA. Physiologically based pharmacokinetic modelling of the temperature-dependent dermal absorption of chloroform by humans following bath water exposures. Toxicol Sci 2000; 53(1):13–23.
33. Xu X, Weisel CP. Dermal uptake of chloroform and haloketones during bathing. J Expo Anal Environ Epidemiol 2005; 15(4):289–96.
34. Thrall KD, Weitz KK, Woodstock AD. Use of real-time breath analysis and physiologically based pharmacokinetic modeling to evaluate dermal absorption of aqueous toluene in human volunteers. Toxicol Sci 2002; 68(2):280–7.
35. Thrall KD, Woodstock AD. Evaluation of the dermal bioavailability of aqueous xylene in F344 rats and human volunteers. J Toxicol Environ Health A 2003; 66:1267–81.
36. Nakai JS, Chu I, Li-Muller A, et al. Effect of environmental conditions on the penetration of benzene through human skin. J Toxicol Environ Health 1997; 51:447–62.
37. Pont AR, Charron AR, Brand RM. Active ingredients in sunscreens act as topical penetration enhancers for the herbicide 2-4-dichlorophenoxyacetic acid. Toxicol Appl Pharmacol 2004; 195:348–54.

38. Riviere JE, Brooks JD. Predicting skin permeability from complex chemical mixtures. Toxicol Appl Pharmacol 2005; 208:99–110.
39. Riviere JE. Chemical mixtures. In: Riviere JE, ed. Dermal Absorption. Models in Toxicology and Pharmacology. New York: Taylor & Francis, 2006:283–304.
40. Moody RP. Automated in vitro dermal absorption (AIVDA): a new in vitro method for investigating transdermal flux. ATLA 1997; 25:347–57.
41. Moody RP. Automated in vitro dermal absorption (AIVDA): predicting skin permeation of atrazine with finite and infinite (swimming/bathing) exposure models. Toxicol In Vitro 2000; 14:467–74.
42. Moody RP, Akram M. Automated in vitro dermal absorption (AIDA): development of a cost-effective diffusion cell. Toxicol Mech Method 2004; 14:361–6.
43. Kirchner LA, Moody RP, Doyle E, et al. The prediction of skin permeability using physicochemical data. ATLA 1997; 25:359–70.
44. Moody RP, MacPherson H. Determination of dermal QSAR/QSPRs by brute force regression: multi-parameter model development with Molsuite 2000. J Toxicol Environ Health A 2003; 66:1927–42.
45. Leo A, Hansch C, Elkin D. Partition coefficients and their uses. Chem Rev 1971; 71(6):525–616.
46. Moody RP. Algicidal activity of formulated fenitrothion: the effect of the co-solvent, Aerotex 3470, on unicellular freshwater algae. PhD Thesis, University of Ottawa, 1982 (Appendix viii, 145–53).

37

Percutaneous Absorption of Prodrugs and Soft Drugs

Kenneth B. Sloan and Scott C. Wasdo
Department of Medicinal Chemistry, University of Florida, Gainesville, Florida, U.S.A.

INTRODUCTION

In the search for ways to improve the topical delivery of drugs for local or systemic effects, two approaches have received the most attention recently: devices and penetration enhancers (1). Lost in the attention paid to those two approaches has been the prodrug approach that could be an attractive alternative to devices and penetration enhancers (2). A prodrug is a transient, inactive chemical derivative of a known parent drug, which improves some physicochemical property such as low solubility, metabolic instability, or other problematic properties of the drug, so that the active drug is delivered more effectively to the target tissue. One reason that the prodrug approach has not been explored as extensively as it might have been, based on its theoretical promise, may be that many of the reported improvements in transdermal delivery by prodrug approaches were modest, at best only two- to fourfold (3). However, since an increase in transdermal delivery is linked to an increase in dermal delivery, an improvement in transdermal delivery of two- to fourfold, and hence in dermal delivery for a local effect, can make the difference between a successful product or not. Similar improvements in oral delivery have made a difference in the success of oral products (4). On the other hand, transdermal delivery through a relatively small surface area, but for a systemic effect, will require a much larger improvement because a much larger dose is required for a systemic effect. Thus, a prodrug approach may be more ideally suited to solving local rather than systemic delivery problems, while possibly too much emphasis has been placed on using prodrugs topically to improve systemic delivery in the past. In this chapter, we will discuss the development of design directives to optimize the physicochemical properties of the prodrug to optimize the delivery of the active drug, discuss the results of the application of the design directives to model drugs, give examples of prodrugs that have been approved for topical use, and give examples of soft drugs that have been approved for topical use.

Soft drugs are the opposite of prodrugs. Soft drugs are initially active and are chemically or enzymatically converted to inactive metabolites. This inactive metabolite approach is represented by most of the currently marketed soft drugs. Since both prodrugs and soft drugs rely on chemical or enzymatic reactions to either activate or inactivate them, respectively, it is appropriate to discuss the two together: the design directives for improving their physicochemical properties and hence their topical delivery will be the same.

DESIGN DIRECTIVES

Since there has not been any systematic study of the trends in the physicochemical properties of soft drugs that enhance their topical delivery, we will focus only on the design directives that have been deduced from analyses of the effect of changes in the physicochemical properties of prodrugs, relative to their respective active parents, that result in increased topical delivery. We assume that changes in the physicochemical properties of prodrugs that result in increased topical delivery, if used as the basis for change in the properties of soft drugs and new drug candidates, will also result in their increased topical delivery.

For some time it has been known that, for a homologous series of more lipophilic prodrugs, the members of the series that were more hydrophilic gave the highest permeation through hairless mouse skin in vitro (5–7). However, since many of the series of those prodrugs were hydrolytically unstable, a nonprotic lipid vehicle, typically isopropyl myristate (IPM), was used as the vehicle, and since the available mathematical models for topical delivery were developed from data using only the delivery of drugs from water (AQ) (8,9) and propylene glycol (PG) (10) or selected prodrugs from PG (11), a new mathematical model for the delivery of active drugs by their prodrugs from IPM was developed.

Fick's first law is the starting point for the development of most mathematical models for topical delivery. Here we will briefly review the development of the new model using Fick's law

$$J_V = (D/L)(C_{M1} - C_{Mn}) \tag{1}$$

where J_V is the flux from a specific vehicle, D is the diffusion coefficient, L is the effective thickness of the membrane, C_{M1} is the concentration of the permeant in the first few layers of the stratum corneum (SC), and C_{Mn} is the concentration of the permeant in the last layer of the SC. C_{Mn} is assumed to approach zero at steady state under sink conditions. L is assumed to be a constant for the same species of skin (hairless mouse, human, etc.), for the same experimental conditions used for the preparation of the membrane (heat separated epidermis, dermatomed full-thickness skin, isolated SC) and for whether in vitro or in vivo. D can be calculated from $D = D_0 \exp(-\beta MV)$ or $\log D = \log D_0 - \beta MV$ where D_0 is the diffusion coefficient of a hypothetical molecule of zero molecular volume (also a constant) and molecular weight (MW) can be substituted for molecular volume (MV) (12). Since it is difficult to measure experimentally, C_{M1} is usually calculated from the product of the concentration of the permeant in the vehicle, C_V, and the partition coefficient between the vehicle and the first few layers of the SC, $K_{M1:V}$. This gives

$$\log J_V = \log D_0/L - \beta MW + \log K_{M1:V} + \log C_V \tag{2}$$

When a lipid such as IPM is used as the vehicle, there is a problem with analyzing the results starting with equation (2). It is impossible to directly measure $\log K_{M1:V}$, or its surrogate partition coefficient between another lipid (LIPID) and a vehicle $(K_{LIPID:V})^y$ constant (c), because the lipid surrogate for the membrane and the vehicle tend to be at least very soluble in each other or miscible. This obstacle was overcome by using the following identity when $V = $ IPM (13).

$$K_{M1:V} = K_{M1:IPM} = \frac{K_{M1:AQ}}{K_{IPM:AQ}}$$

Since

$$K_{M1:AQ} = (K_{IPM:AQ})^y c$$

then,

$$K_{M1:IPM} = \frac{(K_{IPM:AQ})^y c}{K_{IPM:AQ}} \tag{3}$$

Substitution of equation (3) into equation (2), but where IPM is the vehicle, $\log D_0/L + \log c$ is a constant (x), and β is z gives

$$\log J_{IPM} = x - z\,MW + y\log K_{IPM:AQ} - \log K_{IPM:AQ} + \log C_{IPM}$$

When a saturated solution of the permeant in IPM is used (J_{IPM} becomes maximum flux, J_{MIPM}), the partition coefficient terms are expanded to solubility terms ($y\log S_{IPM} - y\log S_{AQ} - \log S_{IPM} + \log S_{AQ}$) and the terms are collected, equation (4) results

$$\log J_{MIPM} = x - z\,MW + y\log S_{IPM} + (1-y)\log S_{AQ} \tag{4}$$

When other lipids are used as the vehicle, $y\log S_{IPM}$ becomes $y\log S_{LIPID}$.

On the other hand, when the vehicle is water, octanol (OCT) (or another lipid) is substituted for M1 in $K_{M1:V}$ and a saturated solution is used, equation (2) first becomes

$$\log J_{MAQ} = x - z\,MW + y\log K_{OCT:AQ} + \log S_{AQ} \tag{5}$$

and then after expansion of K to solubility terms and collection of those terms, equation (5) becomes

$$\log J_{MAQ} = x - z\,MW + y\log S_{OCT} + (1-y)\log S_{AQ} \tag{6}$$

equations (6) and (4) are identical to each other, except for the lipid used.

On the other hand, if $\log S_{AQ}$ is subtracted from both sides of equation (5), equation (7) results. Equation (7) is in the form of the Potts–Guy equation (12), which is the equation most often used to model data from the delivery of drugs from water through human skin in vitro.

$$\log J_{MAQ} - \log S_{AQ} = \log P_{AQ} = x - z\,MW + y\log K_{OCT:AQ} \tag{7}$$

Obviously, equation (7) will give as good a fit to data as equation (5). However, what are the design directives from equations (6) and (4) compared to equation (5)? The design directives are clear for equations (6) and (4): optimize lipid and aqueous solubility to optimize flux regardless of the vehicle. The design directives based on equation (5) [and (7)] are not nearly as clear, especially if the vehicle is a lipid, as has been discussed in great detail elsewhere (14).

APPLICATION OF DESIGN DIRECTIVES TO PRODRUGS

There are two different general types of prodrugs, based on the promoiety and enabling group, which have been used for topical delivery: acyl and acylheteroalkyl. Examples of these types of prodrugs and their mechanisms of hydrolysis have been discussed in great detail elsewhere (2,6,7). Selected, representative examples are given in Tables 1 and 2 for both types of prodrugs but for two different types of parent, active drugs: small (relatively more hydrophilic) and large (relatively more lipophilic). Based on the physicochemical data from these selected

TABLE 1 Topical Delivery of 5-Fluorouracil (5-FU) by its Alkylcarbonyl (1-AC-5-FU), Alkyloxy-carbonyl (1-AOC-5-FU), and Alkylcarbonyloxymethyl (3-ACOM-5-FU) Prodrugs from Isopropyl Myristate (IPM) and Water Through Hairless Mouse Skin In Vitro

	S_{IPM}[a]	$\log K_{IPM:4.0}$[b]	$eS_{4.0}$[a]	J_{MIPM}[c,d]	C_s[e]	J_{MAQ}[c,f]
1-AC-5-FU,R=						
1, C1[g]	22.1	-0.73	120	9.3	68	—
2, C2	36.4	-0.12	47.6	4.3	69	—
3, C3	17.4	0.43	6.50	1.3	8.2	—
4, C4	39.2	1.05	3.48	1.0	16	—
5, C5	112.7	1.58	2.94	1.1	11	—
6, C7	110.7	2.88	0.15	0.60	12	—
1-AOC-5-FU						
7, C1	2.13	-1.72	112	2.62	8.3	—
8, C2	13.1	-1.12	175	5.92	18.0	—
9, C3	15.2	-0.44	42.2	2.31	5.0	—
10, C4	33.8	0.15	24.1	2.23	4.2	—
11, C6	153	1.49	4.94	1.54	11.0	—
12, C8	36.2	2.45	0.13	0.29	3.2	—
3-ACOM-5-FU						
13, C1	1.22	-1.62	51.3	0.60	5.4	0.017
14, C2	15.9	-1.03	171	2.18	5.8	0.039
15, C3	26.4	-0.45	74.1	2.87	11.8	0.074
16, C4	29.8	0.13	21.9	1.32	5.6	0.037
17, C5	42.8	0.74	7.74	1.01	4.9	0.039
18, C7	40.2	1.90	0.51	0.17	1.8	0.014
5-FU	0.049	-3.24	85.4	0.24	3.7	0.011

[a] Solubilities in mM.
[b] Partition coefficient between IPM and pH 4.0 buffer.
[c] Maximum flux from IPM.
[d] Flux in $\mu mol/cm^2/hr$.
[e] Concentration of total species leached from skin in 24 hours after donor phase removed.
[f] Maximum flux from water.
[g] C1,C2, etc. refer to the number of carbons in the alkyl chain.

examples of types of promoieties combined with two different types of parent drug, it is apparent that the design directives from equations (4) and (6) are useful in optimizing topical delivery of prodrugs (analogs and new drugs as well), while equations (5) and (7) are not.

5-Fluorouracil

Table 1 shows the physicochemical and permeation data obtained from three homologous series of prodrugs of 5-fluorouracil (5-FU; a small, relatively hydro-philic drug) which have been selected based on their different rates of hydrolysis and the fact that a different member of each series gives the greatest enhancement of flux (15–17). In each of the three series, the solubility of the prodrug in IPM (S_{IPM}) increases with increasing alkyl chain length until the C5 or C6 member, and then decreases with further elongation of the chain. This is not unusual for such homologous series (2). On the other hand, the $K_{IPM:4.0}$ values increase in a regular manner throughout each series: the methylene π value for the difference between the $\log K_{IPM:4.0}$ values for successive members of the series is a constant regardless of what the absolute values of S_{IPM} (and $S_{4.0}$) are. Thus, $K_{IPM:4.0}$ (or for that matter $K_{OCT:AQ}$) are not good surrogates for absolute lipid solubilities.

TABLE 2 Topical Delivery of Natrexone (NTX) by its Alkylcarbonyl (3-AC-NTX), Alkyloxycarbonyl (3-AOC-NTX), and Alkylaminocarbonyl (3-AAC-NTX) Prodrugs from Mineral Oil (MO) Through Human Skin In Vitro

	MW	Log S_{MO}[a]	Log $S_{7.4}$[a]	Log J_{MMO}[b,c]	Log $SR_{MO:7.4}$[d]	Δ log J_{MMO}[e]
3-AC-NTX, R=						
19, C1[f]	383	0.31	0.29	−1.81	0.02	0.33
20, C2	397	0.64	0.10	−1.95	0.54	0.14
21, C3	411	0.62	0.02	−2.25	0.60	0.08
22, C4	425	0.98	−0.23	−2.17	1.21	0.03
23, C5	439	0.84	−0.55	−2.07	1.39	0.34
24, C6	453	0.88	−0.74	−2.15	1.62	0.36
25, C4,(CH$_3$)$_3$C–	425	0.51	−0.92	−2.89	1.43	0.16
26, C4,(CH$_3$)$_2$CHCH$_2$	425	0.12	−0.85	−3.07	0.97	0.18
27, C5,(C$_2$H$_5$)$_2$CH–	439	0.75	−0.57	−2.71	1.32	0.25
28, C3,(CH$_3$)$_2$CH–	411	0.07	−0.49	−2.65	0.56	0.05
3-AOC-NTX						
29, 0C1	399	−0.48	0.48	−2.16	−0.96	0.28
30, 0C2	413	−0.23	−0.20	−2.47	−0.03	0.23
31, 0C3	427	0.26	−0.01	−2.96	0.27	0.57
32, 0C4	441	0.85	−0.20	−2.44	1.05	0.23
33, 0C5	455	0.53	−0.77	−2.59	1.30	0.10
34, 0C3,(CH$_3$)$_2$CH–	427	−0.06	−0.59	−2.92	0.53	0.09
35, 0C4,(CH$_3$)$_3$C–	441	0.20	0.21	−2.43	0.41	0.11
3-AAC-NTX						
36, NHC2	412	0.00	1.15	−1.81	−1.15	0.07
37, NC2,(CH$_3$)$_2$N–	412	−0.70	0.48	−2.54	−1.18	0.03
NTX	341	−0.62	0.75	−2.54	−1.37	0.25

a Solubilities in mM.
b Maximum flux from MO.
c Flux in μmol/cm²/hr.
d Solubility ratio between MO and pH 7.4 buffer.
e Average absolute difference between experimental and calculated log J_{MMO}.
f C1, C2, etc. refer to the number of carbons in the alkyl chain.

The maximum estimated solubility in pH 4.0 buffer ($eS_{4.0}$; $S_{IPM}/K_{IPM:4.0}$) was reached by the first one or two members of these series, then decreased with increasing alkyl chain length. The fact that at least one member of these series was more soluble in pH 4.0 buffer than the parent, polar drug is due to the fact that in these series the crystal lattice energy is decreased by masking one of the highly polar N–H functional groups that is capable of forming strong intermolecular hydrogen bonds. The $S_{4.0}$ values for hydrolytically stable prodrugs, that were measured directly, followed the same trends and were generally quite close to $eS_{4.0}$ values (18).

In each series either the most, or the second most, water-soluble ($eS_{4.0}$) member of these more lipophilic series gave the highest flux value from IPM (J_{MIPM}). On the other hand, members exhibiting higher S_{IPM} (or S_{VEH}) and $K_{IPM:4.0}$ values gave the lowest flux values. Qualitatively, these results are representative of every series of prodrugs for which S_{IPM}, $eS_{4.0}$ (or $S_{4.0}$ or S_{AQ}), $K_{IPM:4.0}$ (or $K_{IPM:AQ}$), and J_{MIPM} data have been obtained ($n = 61$) (2,18). When the $n = 61$ data were fit to equation (4), the Roberts–Sloan (RS) model, the following coefficients for the independent variables were obtained: $\log J_{MIPM} = -0.49 + 0.52 \, \log S_{IPM} + 0.48 \, \log S_{e4.0} - 0.00271 \, MW$. The average absolute difference between the experimental $\log J_{MIPM}$ and the calculated $\log J_{MIPM}$ ($\Delta \log J_{MIPM}$) was 0.15 log units. Thus, for the delivery of total species containing the parent drug (prodrug + drug) through hairless mouse in vitro from IPM, there was a dependence on a balance between S_{IPM} and solubility in water ($eS_{4.0}$ or S_{AQ}) but not on $K_{IPM:4.0}$. $K_{IPM:4.0}$ and S_{IPM} trend in the opposite direction of J_{MIPM}.

The prodrugs giving the highest and lowest values for J_{MIPM} for delivery of total species were predicted correctly by equation (4) regardless of whether the prodrugs completely hydrolyzed during permeation or permeated partially intact. The series **1** to **6** (Table 1; Fig. 1) exhibited chemical half-lives of three to five minutes, so no trace of intact **1** to **6** was observed in the receptor phases (15). The series **7** to **12** (Table 1; Fig. 1) exhibited chemical half-lives of about 200 to 500 minutes and permeated mostly intact: 42%, 90%, 78%, 73%, and 74% intact, respectively (16). On the other hand, the series **13** to **18** (Table 1; Fig. 1) was even more stable chemically (half-lives > 100 hours) but were more completely hydro-lyzed during their permeation than **7** to **12**: 20%, 31%, 22%, 6%, 6%, and 6% intact, respectively (17). Several conclusions can be drawn from these results. First, stability toward chemical hydrolysis is not a good predictor of stability toward enzymatic hydrolysis. Second, the longer chain, more lipophilic members of each series were more completely converted to their more water-soluble parent drug: 5-FU. Thus, the poor performance of the more lipophilic members is not due to their lack of hydrolysis during permeation, which would have caused greater resistance to their permeation by the higher concentration of water in the dermis. Nor is their relative lack of performance due to their lack of solubility in the vehicle since they are the more lipid-soluble members of the series and they are being delivered from a lipid vehicle. Instead, their poor performance is due to their lack of solubility in the first layers of the SC, which is the driving force for permeation [equation (1)] and which depends on a balance of lipid and aqueous solubilities.

The delivery of the **13** to **18** series from water through hairless mouse skin gave the same qualitative results (19). The J_{MAQ} data in Table 1 were also part of a somewhat larger database ($n = 17$) obtained under the same conditions (19). When the J_{MAQ}, S_{IPM}, and S_{AQ} data from the $n = 17$ database were fit to equation (4), the following coefficients for the independent variables were

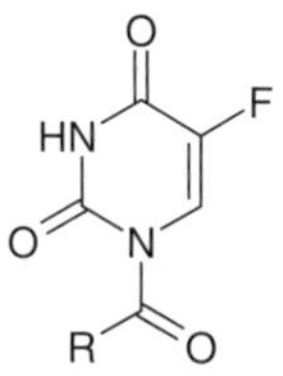

FIGURE 1 Prodrugs.

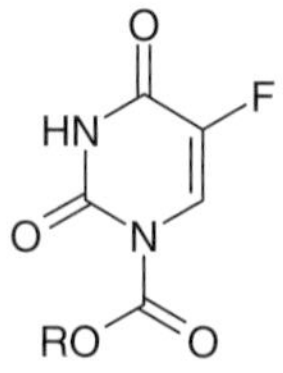

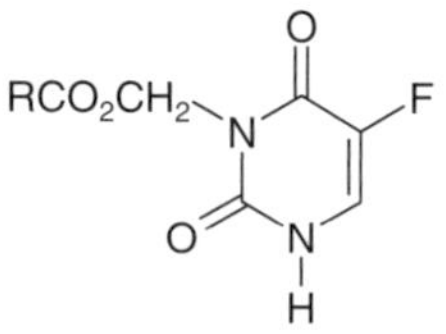

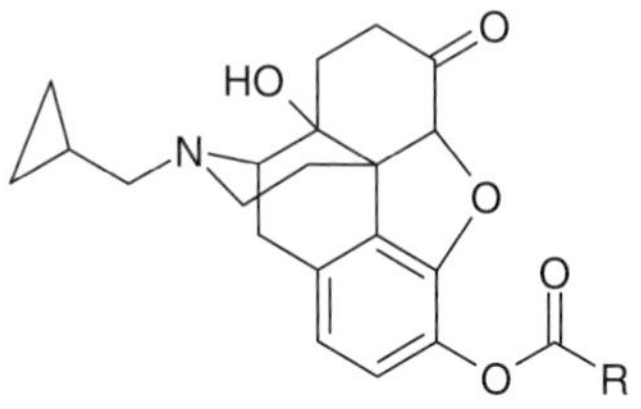

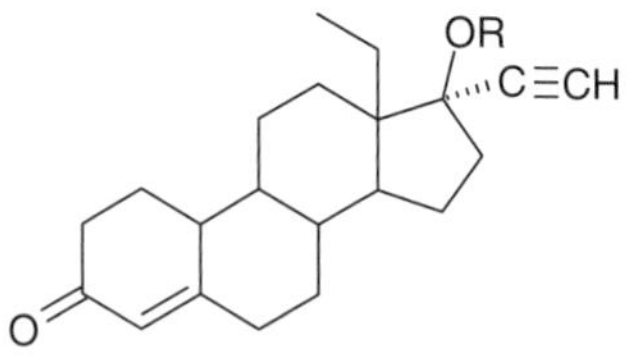

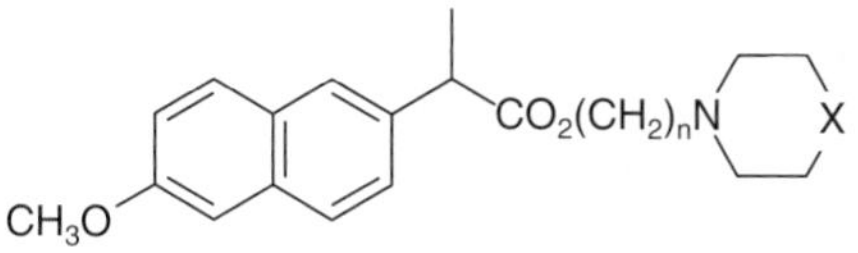

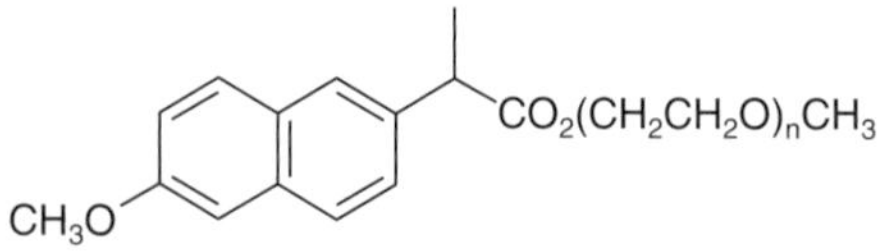

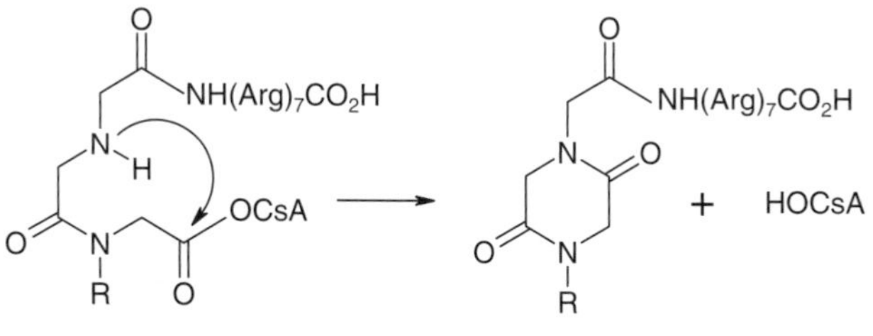

obtained: $\log J_{MAQ} = -1.497 + 0.66 \log S_{IPM} + 0.34 \log S_{AQ} - 0.00469$ MW. The rank order of delivery of the **13** to **18** series from water was the same as delivery from IPM (except for the C5 member) and again there was a dependence of flux on a balance of the S_{IPM} and S_{AQ} solubilities of the permeants. The big difference is the absolute values of J_{MIPM} were on average about 50 times greater than J_{MAQ}. This difference has been attributed to IPM causing an irreversible decrease in the resistance of the skin. This effect has proved to be reproducible when assessed by second application studies (20,21). The difference in flux values from different vehicles illustrate the point that *x*, *y*, and *z* values in equation (4) [or equation (6)] can only be expected to be relatively constant when the same vehicle and skin from the same species and prepared in the same manner are used in the experiments.

Naltrexone

The physicochemical and permeation data obtained from the three series of prodrugs of naltrexone (NTX; a large, relatively more lipophilic drug) (22–25) are given in Table 2. These have been selected because they represent three different types of acyl derivatives all reported by the same investigators, and delivered from the same lipid vehicle [mineral oil, (MO)] through human skin in vitro. This is in contrast to the data for the 5-FU prodrugs (Table 1) which was reported by Sloan and coworkers and used mouse skin.

In each of the series, the lipid solubilities (Table 2, S_{MO}) for the straight chain members increased with increasing chain length until C5, then decreased. This is similar to the S_{IPM} values for the 5-FU prodrugs. The trend in solubilities in pH 7.4 buffer ($S_{7.4}$) are also similar to those reported in Table 1 for the 5-FU prodrugs, except that in the NTX series the first member of each series was always more water soluble. Although no partition coefficients were measured experimentally, solubility ratios between the lipid (MO) and aqueous solubility (7.4) values ($SR_{MO:7.4}$) can be calculated from the S_{MO} and $S_{7.4}$ values (Table 2). As expected, the $SR_{MO:7.4}$ values increased with increasing alkyl chain length regardless of any decrease in experimentally measured S_{MO}. Although from Table 1, $SR_{IPM:4.0}$ values (data not given) were very similar to the measured $K_{IPM:4.0}$ values and those SR values gave consistent methylene π values, the $SR_{MO:7.4}$ values in Table 2 did not give consistent methylene π values.

The J_{MMO} values reported for the NTX prodrugs (Fig. 1, **19** to **37**) were qualitatively very similar to the J_{MIPM} values for 5-FU: the more water-soluble members of the more lipophilic series gave the higher flux values and the flux values generally decreased with increased lipophilicity. Thus, $SR_{MO:7.4}$ and S_{MO} trend in the opposite direction of J_{MMO}, while a balance of S_{MO} and $S_{7.4}$ lead to apparent optimization of J_{MMO} values. It should also be noted that delivery of another large, more lipophilic drug, buprenorphine, by its acyl prodrugs from MO through human skin gave results similar to those in Table 2: the acetyl member of the series which exhibited the lowest $K_{OCT:6.4}$ value gave the highest flux, while the member exhibiting the highest $K_{OCT:6.4}$ gave the lowest (26). No water solubilities were given for that series, so no further comparisons are possible.

When the S_{MO}, $S_{7.4}$, and MW data (Table 2) as independent variables and J_{MMO} as the dependent variable were fitted to equation (4), the following coefficients for the independent variable were obtained: $\log J_{MMO} = -1.86 + 0.48 \log S_{MO} + 0.52 \log S_{7.4} - 0.00151$ MW. Although the Δ $\log J_{MMO}$ values were very acceptable ($\Delta \log J_{MMO} = 0.194$ log units or $\pm 56\%$) for data from human skin obtained from different donors (some previously frozen, some fresh), the r^2 value was poor ($r^2 = 0.59$) probably because n was low ($n = 20$). There was only one apparent outlier in the data (**31**), and if that was removed $\Delta \log J_{MMO} = 0.162 \log$ units. Thus, regardless of the species of skin (mouse or human) and whether lipid or aqueous vehicles, the maximum flux of prodrugs can be optimized by designing a balance of increased S_{LIPID} and S_{AQ} into the promoiety.

Incorporation of Water-Solubilizing Groups into Promoieties

In view of the trend in maximum fluxes versus S_{LIPID}, S_{AQ}, and $K_{LIPID:AQ}$ observed for series of simple alkyl homologous series of acyl and acylheteroalkyl prodrugs, it was logical to determine the effect of incorporation of water-solubilizing groups into the promoiety. There are many examples of the syntheses and characterization of prodrugs designed to increase topical delivery which incorporate such water-solubilizing groups into the promoiety. Here we will discuss three types where each solubilizing group represents a different approach.

Levonorgestrel

One of the best examples of the effect that incorporation of a water-solubilizing group into a promoiety has on flux is the 17-acyl derivative of levonorgestrel (**38**, R = H) in Table 3 and Figure 1 (27). Here the solubilizing group is a dihydroxyalkyl (diol) type group (**41** and **42**), which is similar to the PG ester of nonsteroidal anti-inflammatory drugs suggested later by Guy and Hadgraft (28). For comparison purposes, the data for two alkyl chain prodrugs are also presented (**39** and **40**). Although **39** and **40** are more soluble in ethanol:water mixtures ($\log S_V = 2.78$ and 1.45 mM for **39** and **40**, respectively) than levonorgestrel in ethanol (1.28 mM), as the ratio of ethanol:water decreases and the vehicle becomes more water like, their S_V values should decrease relative to their ethanol solubilities. In the example given, $\log S_V$ for **39** decreases from 2.78 (95%) to 1.11 mM (62% ethanol). Thus, all the derivatives in the series are more soluble in ethanol than **38** and hence more lipid soluble. **41** and **42** are also more water soluble since they are more soluble in 40% ethanol than **38**, **39**, or **40** are in mixtures containing more ethanol. In fact, **39** and **40** were so insoluble in water that their $\log K_{OCT:AQ}$ could not be determined.

TABLE 3 Topical Delivery of Levonorgestrel (**38**)-Containing Species by its Alkylcarbonyl (**39** and **40**) and Alkyloxycarbonyl (**41** and **42**) Prodrugs Through Rat Skin from Ethanol:Water Mixtures In Vitro

R	Log S_V[a]	Log $K_{OCT:AQ}$[b]	Log J[c]
38, H	1.28 (100)	3.70	0–3.72
39, (C=O)C$_5$H$_{11}$	2.78 (95)		
	1.11 (62)		−3.24
40, (C=O)C$_4$H$_9$	1.45 (95)		−3.59
41, (C=O)OCH$_2$CH(OH)CH$_2$OH	1.48 (40)	3.22	−2.20
42, (C=O)O(CH$_2$)$_4$CH(OH)CH$_2$OH	2.60 (40)	3.75	−2.52

[a] Solubilities in mixtures of ethanol:water in mM where the value in parentheses is % ethanol in mixtures.
[b] Partition coefficient between octanol and water.
[c] Flux in $\mu mol/cm^2/hr$ from suspensions in mixtures of ethanol:water given in parentheses in log S_V column.

The flux values for **38** delivered from ethanol:water mixtures that were 40% to 100% ethanol did not vary substantially so that the delivery of total levonorgestrel-containing species by the derivatives from vehicles containing different amounts of ethanol are easily compared with those of **38**. The alkyl-substituted acyl derivatives **39** and **40** increased delivery of total levonorgestrel-containing species by 3- and 1.3-fold, respectively. **39** and **40** also delivered only **38**, effectively functioning as prodrugs. On the other hand, although **41** and **42** delivered 33- and 16-fold more levonorgestrel-containing species than **38** (because they were the more water-soluble derivatives), **41** and **42** permeated mainly intact. Thus, **41** and **42** are good examples of designing the correct solubility properties into the promoiety but not the correct hydrolytic stability so that they did not effectively function as prodrugs locally. These results also illustrate that topical delivery of a drug can often be improved only by making a more lipophilic prodrug, but in order to optimize flux a more hydrophilic as well as more lipophilic prodrug should be the design directive.

Naproxen
A second example of the use of a water-solubilizing functional group in the promoiety to increase flux is alkylaminoalkyl prodrugs. An alkylaminoalkyl ester of indomethacin (30) and an alkylaminoalkylcarbonyl ester of testosterone (29) were reported to substantially increase the flux of large, more lipophilic parent drugs. However, only recently a more systematic approach to evaluating this class of prodrugs has been undertaken. The characterization and evaluation of alkyl esters of naproxen (NAP) containing a basic alkyl amino group in the promoiety (31) are given in Table 4. Only two of the prodrugs are more soluble in OCT than the parent drug and none are more water soluble at the pH of their applied suspensions. However, they are all more soluble in pH 7.4 buffer than simple alkyl esters. The more water-soluble prodrugs (in the order of $S_{7.4}$ **46** > **44** > **43**) (Fig. 1) gave the highest $J_{M7.4}$ values where **44** gave about nine times and **46** about four times higher flux than NAP. By contrast the two derivatives exhibiting the higher log $K_{OCT:7.4}$ values gave the lowest flux values.

When the S_{OCT}, S_{AQ}, and MW data from an edited and extended Flynn database ($n = 103$) were fitted to equation (4) as the independent variables, and J_{MAQ} was the dependent variable, the following coefficients for the independent variables were obtained: $\log J_{MAQ} = -2.569 + 0.559 \log S_{OCT} + 0.441 \log S_{AQ} - 0.0041 \, MW$ where $r^2 = 0.90$ and $\Delta \log J_{MAQ} = 0.438$ log units (32). The NAP esters (Table 4) were not included in this analysis but their fit to the coefficients were only slightly worse than the average fit of the entire database: $\Delta \log J_{MAQ} = 0.52$ log units. Thus, the better performance by the more water-soluble members of the lipid-soluble members of this series is predicted qualitatively and quantitatively by their fit to the RS model [equation (4)].

The third example of the use of a water-solubilizing functional group in the promoiety to increase flux is polyoxyethylene (PEG) prodrugs. PEG esters, and their ability to increase S_{AQ}, have been known for some time. However, it was only recently that PEG esters have been evaluated for their ability to increase topical delivery. Bonina and coworkers have described the synthesis and evaluation of PEG esters to enhance the topical delivery of a number of large, relatively more lipophilic molecules where a carboxylic acid group has been masked (33,34). For comparison with the alkylaminoalkyl esters of NAP (Table 4), the physicochemical and flux data for a series of PEG esters of NAP (Fig. 1) are given in Table 5 (34). Of these

TABLE 4 Topical Delivery of Naproxen-Containing Species by Its Alkylaminoalkyl Prodrugs Through Human Skin from pH 7.4 Buffer In Vitro

	MW	$S_{7.4}{}^{a}$	Log $K_{OCT:7.4}$	$S_{OCT}{}^{a,b}$	Log $J_{M7.4}{}^{c}$	Δ log $J_{M7.4}{}^{c}$
Naproxen	230	102	0.30	204	−2.18 (0.00661)	−0.85
43, C2^{d},NH	342	30.2	0.74	166	−2.29 (0.00513)	−0.11
44, C2,N−CH$_3$	356	32.4	2.29	6310	−1.23 (0.0589)	0.12
45, C4,0	371	0.85	2.60	79.4	−2.82 (0.00151)	0.64
46, C4,N−CH$_3$	384	51.3	2.44	14,125	−1.56 (0.0275)	−0.37
47, C6,N−CH$_3$	412	0.006	3.92	50.1	−3.40 (0.000398)	1.02

[a] Solubilities in mM.
[b] Calculated from $(K_{OCT:7.4})(S_{7.4})$.
[c] Flux in µmol/cm^2/hr. Values in parentheses are $J_{M7.4}$.
[d] The numbers 2, 4, and 6 represent the value for n in the structure and the next notation represents X.

TABLE 5   Topical Delivery of Naproxen-Containing Species by Its Polyoxyethylene Ester Prodrugs Through Human Skin In Vitro from a Thin Film

	Log $K_{OCT:AQ}$	Log $S_{AQ}^{a,b}$	Log $S_{OCT}^{a,c}$	Log $J_M^{d,e}$	MW
Naproxen	3.0	−2.509	0.491	−2.648 (0.00225)	230
48, $n=1^f$	3.9	−2.553	1.347	−2.836 (0.00146)	318
49, $n=2$	3.7	−2.357	1.343	−2.664 (0.00217)	362
50, $n=3$	3.5	−2.051	1.449	−2.737 (0.00183)	406
51, $n=4$	3.2	−1.796	1.404	−2.351 (0.00446)	450
52, $n=5$	2.9	−1.513	1.387	−2.290 (0.00513)	494

[a] Solubilities in mM.
[b] Calculated from log $S_{AQ} = -1.07$ log $K_{OCT:7.4} + 0.672$.
[c] Calculated from log $K_{OCT:7.4} +$ log S_{AQ}.
[d] Flux in μmol/cm^2/hr. Values in parentheses are J_M.
[e] Calculated from (amount permeated at 24 hours)/(cm^2) (24 hours).
[f] n, number of oxyethylene units in ester.

physicochemical properties (Table 5), only the log $K_{OCT:7.4}$ values were determined experimentally. The log S_{AQ} values were estimated from log $S_{AQ} = -1.072$ log $K_{OCT:7.4} + 0.672$ and the S_{OCT} values were estimated from log $K_{OCT:7.4} +$ log S_{AQ}. Regardless of the origin of the S_{AQ} values, the trend of increased S_{AQ} with increased number of oxyethylene units was expected. The method of measuring the log J values was different from previous methods used to measuring log J_{MIPM}, J_{MMO}, or J_{MAQ} values reported in Tables 1–4. The PEG esters were applied in an ethanol solution and the ethanol evaporated to give a thin layer of the ester on the skin, so no vehicle was used. It was assumed that the oil on the surface of the skin was at its maximum thermodynamic activity. Only one measurement of amount permeated was taken at 24 hours. The log J values (Table 5) were obtained from the reported amount permeated at 24 hours divided by the surface area and time to give J in μmol/cm^2/hr. Thus, the log J values in Table 5 can be compared with those in Table 4. The J value for NAP itself (Table 5) is only 0.33 times $J_{M7.4}$ of NAP in Table 4; and the best prodrug in Table 5, **52**, is only about 2.5-fold better than NAP in Table 5, but only 0.1 times the best prodrug in Table 4, **44**. Taking into account the different fluxes of NAP in the two studies, the PEG prodrugs appear to be only 0.33 times as effective as the alkylaminoalkyl prodrugs. The PEG esters may be less effective because a large increase in MW is needed to increase the S_{AQ} of the PEG esters. Since MW is inversely related to flux, the increased MW required for the PEG esters is a disadvantage. On the other hand, the well-known lack of toxicity of the PEGs is an advantage.

Cyclosporin
Although the examples given above for increasing S_{AQ} are unionizable promoieties (**41** and **42, 48–52**) or they contain promoieties that are in equilibrium with a substantial % of unionized species, there are examples of promoieties that are permanently charged or are so highly charged as to be effectively permanently charged (and hence exhibit increased S_{AQ}) that have been reported to substantially increase the topical delivery of drugs. There are two different types of cyclosporine (CsA) derivative which exemplify this approach. The first example is of trialkylaminoalkylcarbonyl derivatives of the secondary hydroxyl group in CsA. Although no S_{AQ} values were given, the fact that the derivatives contained a

quaternary nitrogen suggests they are more water soluble than CsA (35). The two derivatives evaluated increased flux by 110 to 200 times. Unfortunately, only the intact prodrug was found in the skin or in the receptor phase. The design directive gave the correct physicochemical properties to increase flux but not to allow hydrolysis to CsA. The latter was attributed to steric hindrance to enzymatic hydrolysis.

The second example is an arginine-based molecular transporter where passive absorption is probably not the major route of permeation. Briefly, an oligomer of seven l-arginines was attached via a spacer to the secondary hydroxyl group in CsA (36). The spacer was designed so that it would undergo chemical (see Fig. 1, **53**) not enzymatic hydrolysis. Again no quantitative physicochemical data were given but the chemical hydrolysis was found to have a $t_{1/2}$ of about 90 minutes at pH 7.4. Using a mouse model for contact dermatitis, application of the prodrug reduced inflammation of the treated ear in a dose–response manner: 1%, 74%; 0.1%, 65%; 0.01%, 41% reduction. There was no reduction in inflammation from the application of CsA at up to twice the highest dose of prodrug. Topical application of a fluorinated corticosteroid was used as a positive control: 34% reduction. Thus, water-soluble prodrugs will increase the topical delivery of large lipophilic drugs and chemical-mediated hydrolysis must be another design directive to ensure the derivative performs as a prodrug.

EXAMPLES OF COMMERCIAL PRODRUGS

Prodrugs have been used for the topical delivery of glucocorticosteroids to treat various inflammatory conditions for about 50 years. The 21-esters in particular function primarily as delivery forms. For instance, it has been shown that the 21-esters of betamethasone bind less tightly to glucocorticoid receptors than betamethasone (37). Yet the 21-esters of betamethasone are up to 150 times more potent than betamethasone when tested in vivo using the vasoconstrictor assay (38). In addition, topical formulations of betamethasone are generally not much more effective than hydrocortisone formulations regardless of the presence of a 9α-fluoro in betamethasone. Thus, betamethasone formulations are generally classed as low potency and the 21-esters as high potency (39). The greatest contribution to earnings from topical prodrugs is by these glucocorticoid esters.

There are several other classes of drugs that are used topically which are not usually considered prodrugs because these are molecules to which structural groups must be added to activate them. The first of these are those based on the antimetabolite approach to treating proliferative disease states. For example, 5-FU is not intrinsically active and must be converted in vivo to the active species, 2′-deoxy-5-fluorouridine monophosphate (FdUMP). FdUMP is the species responsible for preferentially inhibiting thymidine synthetase in proliferating (cancer) cells (40). Although 2% to 5% 5-FU formulations are indicated for the topical treatment of premalignant keratoses and superficial basal cell carcinomas, the delivery of 5-FU is far from optimal. A broader range of indications could possibly be obtained for a prodrug of 5-FU with improved physicochemical properties: a prodrug of a prodrug. Two such prodrugs of 5-FU are already marketed but they are not indicated for topical use: tegafur and capecitabine (Fig. 2).

Acyclovir and penciclovir are both indicated for topical use in the treatment of herpes simplex virus (HSV-1) and -2, at 5% and 10% concentration, respectively (41). In each case, the molecule is activated by phosphorylation to the triphosphate

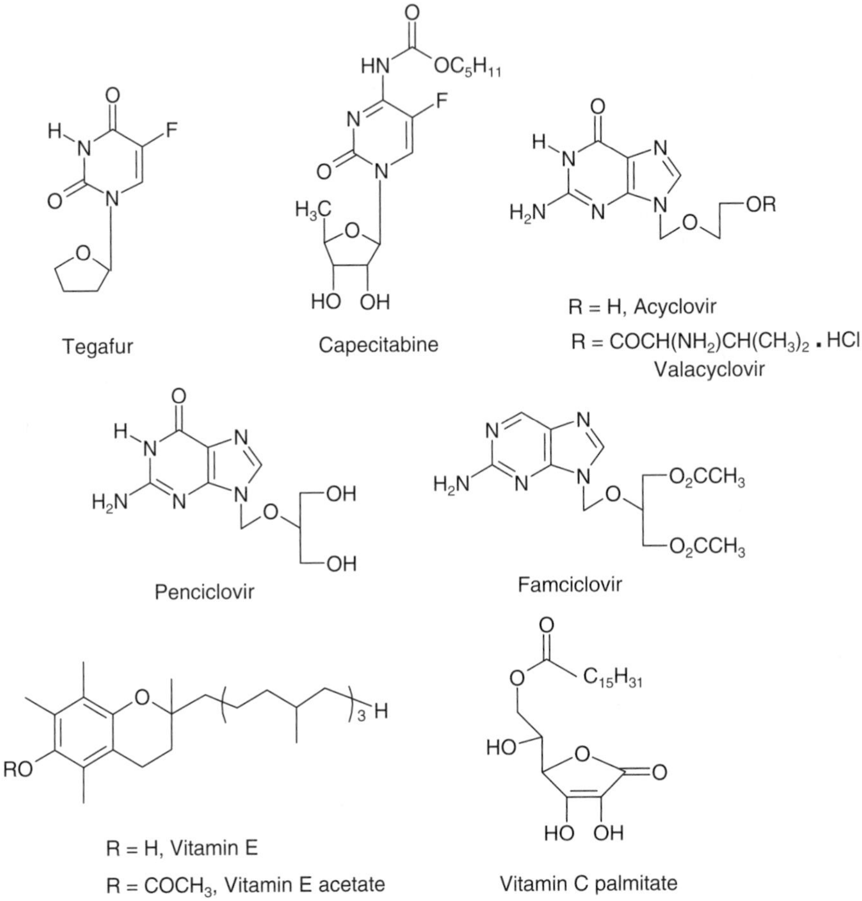

FIGURE 2 Commercial prodrugs.

level on the pseudo 5'-position where it inhibits DNA polymerase and causes chain termination. Two prodrugs of acyclovir and penciclovir are marketed: valacyclovir and famciclovir, respectively (Fig. 2). Based on the success of the aminoalkyl ester of testosterone enhancing topical delivery, valacyclovir may also be more effective at delivering acyclovir. Similarly, famciclovir exhibits potentially much better physicochemical properties than penciclovir (mp 102°C, soluble in water and sparingly soluble in ethanol vs. mp 275°C, soluble in water and insoluble in ethanol). The balance of lipid and aqueous solubility of famciclovir is much better than that of penciclovir.

Other examples are prodrugs of vitamins E and C (Fig. 2), which are both used in cosmetic formulations because of their antioxidant properties. Vitamin E is unstable toward oxidation on the phenol group, which ultimately leads to vitamin E quinone. The vitamin E phenol group is usually protected by acylation, most often acetylation, to give vitamin E acetate. However, since vitamin E acetate does not revert completely to vitamin E following topical application, less vitamin E is delivered by the prodrug than vitamin E itself (42). Vitamin C palmitate is a more stable derivative of vitamin C and is used in cosmetic formulations. The palmitate does not revert completely to vitamin C nor does it increase topical delivery of vitamin C (43). There are reports that vitamin C palmitate promotes ultraviolet-B-induced lipid peroxidation and cytotoxicity in keratinocytes (44). Thus, although prodrugs of vitamins E and C are used topically because they improve stability, the prodrugs do not deliver increased amounts of the parent vitamins. Rationally designed topical vitamin prodrugs could lead to improved topical delivery.

EXAMPLES OF TOPICAL SOFT DRUGS

There are few soft drugs approved for topical use and most are glucocorticoids. Here we discuss briefly examples of two such esters that are used commercially and one example of another soft steroid that has interesting potential use in reversing aging of the skin. Soft glucocorticoids, for treating inflammatory conditions, were first described in 1974 by two groups but based on the same general design (45). As far as we are aware, neither group categorized their approach as soft drug technology. However, the esters, fluocortin butyl and fluticasone propionate (Fig. 3), were designed to be initially active but to metabolize to the inactive substituted pregnan-21-oic and androstan-17-oic acids, respectively: a classic inactive metabolite approach. Thus, the potential exists for the esters to be active locally and become inactivated systemically following metabolism.

The other example is of a steroid that exhibits an entirely different pharmacological profile. It has recently been reported that 17β-estradiol may improve the function of aged skin by inhibiting the expression of extracellular matrix protein and upregulating type 1 procollagen, among other effects (46). The overall result is

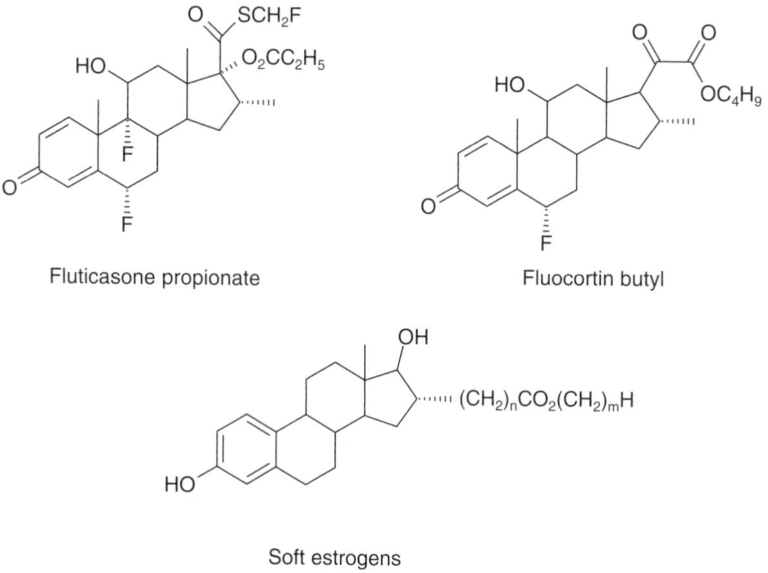

Fluticasone propionate   Fluocortin butyl

Soft estrogens

FIGURE 3   Soft commercial drugs.

a decrease in wrinkles and an increase in skin elasticity. However, topical 17β-estradiol is used for hormone replacement therapy and permeates the skin into systemic circulation where it can cause effects other than decreased wrinkles. On the other hand, although Hochberg and coworkers have reported that 17β-estradiol 16α-carboxylic acid esters (soft estrogen) show local estrogenic activity, several members of the series are inactive systemically because they have been metabolized to the inactive carboxylic acid (47). Thus, much broader indications for cosmetic applications may be possible for soft estrogens.

Since there is no solubility or flux data available for series of either the soft glucocorticoids or the soft estrogen, it is impossible to predict the effect of water and lipid solubilities on flux. However, it seems likely, considering the levonorgestrel example, that implementation of the same design directives would lead to the same successes.

CONCLUSION

The evidence suggests that, for prodrugs, not only increased lipid solubility but also increased water solubility is important for optimizing flux. There are a number of promoieties that have been shown to be useful for incorporating water solubility into the prodrug, which should facilitate the design of better topical prodrugs. It can be assumed that the same design principles should be successful in guiding the selection of soft drugs and new drug entities.

REFERENCES

1. Prausnitz MR, Mitragotri S, Langer R. Current status and future potential of transdermal drug delivery. Nat Rev Drug Discov 2004; 3:115–24.
2. Sloan KB, Wasdo S. Designing for topical delivery: prodrugs can make the difference. Med Res Rev 2003; 23:763–93.
3. Potts RO. The effect of partitioning and enzymatic hydrolysis on the percutaneous transport of lipophilic prodrugs. In: Sloan KB, ed. Prodrugs: Topical and Ocular Drug Delivery. New York: Marcel Dekker, Inc., 1992:205–20.
4. Beaumont K, Webster R, Gardner I, et al. Design of ester prodrugs to enhance oral absorption of poorly permeable compounds: challenges to the discovery scientist. Curr Drug Metab 2003; 4:461–85.
5. Sloan KB, Koch SAM, Siver KG. Mannich base derivatives of theophylline and 5-fluorouracil: syntheses, properties and topical delivery characteristics. Int J Pharm Sci 1984; 21:251–64.
6. Sloan KB. Prodrugs for dermal delivery. Adv Drug Deliv Rev 1989; 3:67–101.
7. Sloan KB. Functional group considerations in the development of prodrug approaches to solving topical delivery problem. In: Sloan KB, ed. Prodrugs: Topical and Ocular Drug Delivery. New York: Marcel Dekker, Inc., 1992:17–116.
8. Michaels AS, Chandrasekaran SK, Shaw JE. Drug permeation through human skin: theory and in vitro experimental measurement. AIChE J 1975; 21:985–96.
9. Anderson BD, Raykar PV. Solute structure–permeability relationships in human stratum corneum. J Invest Dermatol 1989; 93:280–6.
10. Kasting GB, Smith RL, Cooper ER. Effect of lipid solubility and molecular size on percutaneous absorption. In: Shroot B, Schaefer H, eds. Pharmacology and the Skin. Vol. 1. Basel: Karger, 1987:138–53.
11. Kasting GB, Smith RL, Anderson BD. Prodrugs for dermal delivery: solubility, molecular size and functional group effects. In: Sloan KB, ed. Prodrugs: Topical and Ocular Drug Delivery. New York: Marcel Dekker, Inc., 1992:117–61.

12. Potts RO, Guy RH. Predicting skin permeability. Pharm Res 1992; 9:663–9.
13. Roberts WJ, Sloan KB. Correlation of aqueous and lipid solubilities with flux for prodrugs of 5-fluorouracil, theophylline and 6-mercaptopurine: a Potts–Guy approach. J Pharm Sci 1999; 88:515–22.
14. Sloan KB, Wasdo SC, Rautio J. Design for optimized topical delivery: prodrugs and a paradigm change. Pharm Res 2006; 23:2729–47.
15. Beall HD, Sloan KB. Transdermal delivery of 5-fluorouracil (5-FU) by 1-alkylcarbonyl-5-FU prodrugs. Int J Pharm 1996; 129:203–10.
16. Beall HD, Prankerd R, Sloan KB. Transdermal delivery of 5-fluorouracil (5-FU) through hairless mouse skin by 1-alkyloxycarbonyl-5-FU prodrugs: physicochemical characterization of prodrugs and correlations with transdermal delivery. Int J Pharm 1994; 111:223–33.
17. Roberts WJ, Sloan KB. Topical delivery of 5-fluorouracil (5-FU) by 3-alkylcarbonyloxymethyl-5-FU prodrugs. J Pharm Sci 2003; 92:1028–36.
18. Wasdo SC, Sloan KB. Topical delivery of a model phenolic drug: alkyloxycarbonyl prodrugs of acetaminophen. Pharm Res 2004; 21:940–6.
19. Sloan KB, Wasdo SC, Ezike-Mkparu U, et al. Topical delivery of 5-fluorouracil (5-FU) and 6-mercaptopurine (6-MP) by their alkylcarbonyloxymethyl (ACOM) prodrugs from water: vehicle effects on design of prodrugs. Pharm Res 2003; 20:639–45.
20. Sloan KB, Koch SAM, Siver KG, et al. The use of solubility parameters of drug and vehicles to predict flux. J Invest Dermatol 1986; 87:244–52.
21. Sloan KB, Beall HD, Villanueva R, et al. The effect of receptor phase composition on the permeability of hairless mouse skin in diffusion cell experiments. Int J Pharm 1991; 73:97–104.
22. Stinchcomb AL, Swaan PW, Ekabo O, et al. Straight-chain naltrexone ester prodrugs: diffusion and concurrent esterase biotransformation in human skin. J Pharm Sci 2002; 91:2571–8.
23. Pillai O, Hamad MO, Crooks PA, Stinchcomb AL. Physicochemical evaluation, in vitro human skin diffusion, and concurrent biotransformation of 3-O-alkyl carbonate prodrugs of naltrexone. Pharm Res 2004; 21:1146–52.
24. Vaddi HK, Hamad MO, Chen J, et al. Human skin permeation of branched chain 3-O-alkyl ester and carbonate prodrugs of naltrexone. Pharm Res 2005; 22:758–65.
25. Valiveti S, Paudel KS, Hammell DC, et al. In vitro/in vivo correlation of transdermal naltrexone prodrugs in hairless guinea pigs. Pharm Res 2005; 22:981–9.
26. Stinchcomb AL, Paliwal A, Dua R, et al. Permeation of buprenorphine and its 3-alkyl-ester prodrugs through human skin. Pharm Res 1996; 13:1519–23.
27. Friend D, Catz P, Heller J, et al. Transdermal delivery of levonorgestrel II: effect of prodrug structure on skin permeability in vitro. J Control Release 1988; 7:251–61.
28. Guy RH, Hadgraft J. Percutaneous penetration enhancement: physicochemical considerations and implications for prodrug design. In: Sloan KB, ed. Prodrugs: Topical and Ocular Drug Delivery. New York: Marcel Dekker, Inc., 1992:1–16.
29. Milosovich S, Hussain A, Dittert L, et al. Testosteronyl-4-dimethylbutyrate-HCl: a prodrug with improved penetration rate. J Pharm Sci 1993; 82:227–8.
30. Jona JA, Dittert L, Crooks PA, et al. Design of novel prodrugs for the enhancement of the transdermal penetration of indomethacin. Int J Pharm 1995; 123:127–36.
31. Rautio J, Nevalainen T, Taipale H, et al. Piperazinylalkyl prodrugs of naproxen improve in vitro skin permeation. Eur J Pharm Sci 2000; 11:157–63.
32. Majumdar S, Thomas J, Wasdo SC, et al. The effect of water solubility of solutes on their flux through human skin: extended and edited Flynn database. AAPS J 2004; 6(S1):W4250.
33. Bonina FP, Montenegro L, DeCaprariis P, et al. In vitro and in vivo evaluation of polyoxyethylene indomethacin esters as dermal prodrugs. J Control Release 1995; 34:223–32.
34. Bonina FP, Puglia C, Barbuzzi T, et al. In vitro and in vivo evaluation of polyoxyethylene esters as dermal prodrugs of ketoprofen, naproxen and diclofenac. Eur J Pharm Sci 2001; 14:123–34.

35. Billich A, Vyplel H, Grassberger M, et al. Novel cyclosporine derivatives featuring enhanced skin penetration despite increased molecular weight. Bioorg Med Chem 2005; 13:3157–67.
36. Rothbard JB, Garlington S, Lin Q, et al. Conjugation of arginine oligomers to cyclosporine A facilitates topical delivery and inhibition of inflammation. Nat Med 2000; 6:1253–7.
37. Ponec M, Kempencar J, Shroot B, et al. Glucocorticoids: binding affinity and lipophilicity. J Pharm Sci 1986; 75:973–5.
38. McKenzie AW, Atkinson RM. Topical activities of betamethasone esters in man. Arch Dermatol 1964; 89:741–6.
39. Sloan KB, Araujo O, Flowers FP. Topical corticosteroid therapy. In: Arndt K, LeBoit PE, Robinson JK, Wintraub BU, eds. Cutaneous Medicine and Surgery: An Integrated Program in Dermatology. Philadelphia: WB Saunders Co., 1996:160–6.
40. Remers WA. Antineoplastic agents. In: Block JH, Beale JM, eds. Organic Medicinal and Pharmaceutical Chemistry. Philadelphia: Lippincott Williams and Wilkins, 2004:390–453.
41. Beale JM. Antiviral agents. In: Block JH, Beale JM, eds. Organic Medicinal and Pharmaceutical Chemistry. Philadelphia: Lippincott Williams and Wilkins, 2004:367–89.
42. Nakayama S, Katoh EM, Tsuzuki T, et al. Protective effect of α-tocopherol-6-O-phosphate against ultraviolet B-induced damage in cultured mouse skin. J Invest Dermatol 2003; 121:406–11.
43. Pinnell SR, Yang H, Omar M, et al. Topical L-ascorbic acid: percutaneous absorption studies. Dermatol Surg 2001; 27:137–42.
44. Meves A, Stock SN, Beyerle A, et al. Vitamin C derivative ascorbyl palmitate promotes ultraviolet-B-induced lipid peroxidation and cytotoxicity in keratinocytes. J Invest Dermatol 2002; 119:1103–8.
45. Phillipps GH. Locally active corticosteroids: structure activity relationships. In: Wilson L, Marks R, eds. Mechanisms of Topical Corticosteroids Activity. London: Churchill Livingstone, 1976:1–18.
46. Son ED, Lee JY, Lee S, et al. Topical application of 17β-estradiol increases extracellular matrix protein by stimulating TGF-β signaling in aged human skin in vivo. J Invest Dermatol 2005; 124:1149–61.
47. Labaree DC, Reynolds TY, Hochberg RB. Estradiol 16α-carboxylic acid esters as locally active estrogens. J Med Chem 2001; 44:1802–14.

38

Skin Penetration of Cosmetic Ingredients and Contaminants

Keith R. Brain
An-eX Analytical Services Ltd., and Cardiff University, Cardiff, U.K.

Kenneth A. Walters
An-eX Analytical Services Ltd., Cardiff, U.K.

INTRODUCTION

There is an increasing demand for data that quantify the rates of penetration and permeation of diverse chemical entities across human skin and can be used to estimate the potential systemic load following exposure. These estimates can subsequently be used for risk assessment purposes where the implications of the everyday use of a wide range of cosmetic products may be determined and appropriate steps taken to minimize any possible hazard. Risk assessment is the process by which the probability that a harmful effect may occur is determined (1). There are four steps involved in risk assessment: hazard assessment, dose–response assessment, exposure assessment, and risk characterization. It is evident that before any risk assessment may be made it is necessary to determine whether the compound under investigation is indeed harmful following systemic exposure (hazard) and this is usually obtained from studies in laboratory rodents, which provide a "no observed adverse effect level" (NOAEL), following oral or intravenous administration, which may be subsequently used, in combination with exposure assessment and skin permeability data, to assess dermal safety margins. While the NOAEL is obtained from a pragmatic experimental procedure performed using well established and validated protocols, the assessment of exposure and determination of skin permeability often leads to values that can be somewhat variable depending on the precise models and methods used (2–5).

Risk is principally a function of usage or exposure and any form of assessment should only be based on experimental protocols that reproduce demographic use of the product in question. In dermal risk assessment, it is important that any estimation or determination of skin absorption takes into consideration the likely amount, extent, and duration of exposure that would actually occur in use (6). Furthermore, there is a considerable amount of unequivocal data suggesting that no universal rule has presently been established regarding the calculation of the total "absorbed dose" for use in calculating safety margins in dermal risk assessment. Data must be generated for each compound and the results should be carefully analyzed before assessing the risk.

THE USE OF SKIN PENETRATION DATA IN DERMAL RISK ASSESSMENT OF COSMETICS

The European Union Cosmetics Directive targets the prohibition of animal testing of cosmetic ingredients and finished cosmetic products. The generation of margins of safety for cosmetic ingredients must be, therefore, solely dependent on in vitro evaluation. In many respects, risk assessment for components of cosmetic formulations should be a more straightforward task than, for example, that for environmental contaminants (7). Exposure periods and amounts of product applied to the skin can usually be more readily defined, the concentration of the component of interest within the product is usually known, and the content of other components that may affect skin permeation can be controlled, if necessary. There is also a more thorough understanding of the frequency of application, which can be established by demographic studies (6). The selected studies described below, from our laboratory and others, illustrate the potential use of experimentally derived in vitro skin permeation data in risk assessment for some cosmetic ingredients and contaminants.

Sunscreen Agents
The available data on the skin permeation of sunscreen actives have been reviewed (8) with new data appearing on a regular basis (9). An understanding of the potential for human systemic exposure is an integral part of the safety assessment of sunscreen actives used in consumer products (10) and an example is given below using data obtained for octyl salicylate. Other issues with respect to the use of sunscreen agents are their ability to modulate skin permeation (11) and the implications of this finding to the risk assessment of coadministered products (12).

Use of In Vitro Skin Permeation in Margin of Safety Estimation for Octyl Salicylate
The in vitro human skin permeation of a commonly used sunscreen active, octyl salicylate (2-ethylhexyl salicylate), was determined from two vehicles that were representative of typical commercial sunscreen products (13). The data showed that the percutaneous penetration of octyl salicylate from typical sunscreen vehicles was low (<1% over 48 hours) and that cumulative percutaneous penetration of ^{14}C-labeled material was very similar for both vehicles. From the values determined for the percutaneous penetration of octyl salicylate under in vitro conditions, predicted in vivo human exposure and safety margins can be calculated (using typical values for body weight and application amounts) as follows:

Typical adult body weight :   60 kg

Average amount of sunscreen applied per day   16 g

Maximum allowable concentration in sunscreen products :   5%

Maximum (in vitro) percutaneous absorption :   0.65%

Human exposure is calculated as : $\dfrac{16 \text{ g} \times 0.65\% \times 5\%}{60 \text{ kg}} = 0.087 \text{ mg/kg}$

Margin of safety may be calculated as : $\dfrac{250 \text{ mg/kg}}{0.087 \text{ mg/kg}} = 2900$

using the ratio of the lowest dose resulting in no observable toxicity (NOAEL 250 mg/kg) (14) to the estimated human dose.

Skin Penetration Enhancement Activity of Sunscreen Agents

The skin penetration enhancement potential of sunscreens has been recognized as a benefit in facilitating therapeutic action of topically applied drugs (11). For example, octyl salicylate was reported to increase skin permeation of testosterone 6.3-fold whereas padimate O increased that of testosterone, estradiol, and progesterone by 2.4-, 3.5-, and 9.3-fold, respectively, relative to controls (15). Although this observation has obvious significance in transdermal therapy, given the excellent safety profiles of the sunscreen agents evaluated, a greater concern associated with the use of sunscreens is their potential to enhance the absorption of other applied compounds, especially for those sunscreens included in barrier products. Sunscreens have been shown to promote the skin penetration of some potentially hazardous agents applied to the skin. Brand and colleagues (12,16) showed that the application of sunscreen formulations 30 minutes prior to application of the herbicide 2,4-dichlorophenoxyacetic acid significantly increased the penetration of the herbicide from six of nine commercially available products through hairless mouse skin. However, recognizing the unique sensitivity to enhancement of hairless mouse skin and the innate variability in human skin, it is questionable whether this reported enhancement will prove to be of any greater concern than that already associated with topical exposure to 2,4-dichlorophenoxyacetic acid. Similarly, concurrent administration of oxybenzone and the insect repellent N,N-diethyl-m-toluamide led to synergistic enhancement of the permeation of both compounds across pig skin in vitro (17).

Preservatives

All cosmetic products can support the growth of microorganisms. Preservatives are ingredients that prevent or retard microbial growth and thus protect cosmetic products from spoilage. The use of preservatives is required to prevent product damage caused by microorganisms during manufacture, storage, and inadvertent contamination by the consumer during use. Similarly, preservatives serve to protect consumers from possible infection from contaminated products. It is often necessary to use a preservative system containing more than one individual preservative. It is also important to appreciate that preservatives are intrinsically toxic materials and that a balance must be found between antimicrobial efficacy and toxicity. One of the most important recent issues regarding the safety of these systems is the suggestion that some compounds used as preservatives may possess estrogenic activity.

The Parabens Paradox

Short-chain alkyl esters of p-hydroxybenzoic acids (the parabens) are widely used for the preservation of cosmetic and personal care products. Recent reports have suggested a possible link between these compounds and breast cancer (18,19). Although there have been questions raised regarding the rationale, experimental design, and interpretation of these studies (20), it is clear that any potential risk associated with parabens use will ultimately be related to exposure, which is dependent upon usage patterns of the product and the rate and extent of their percutaneous absorption (21,22).

Earlier literature on the skin permeation of parabens was reviewed (23) and it was concluded that, although these compounds could permeate readily, the rate and extent of absorption was markedly dependent on the vehicle of application.

Further studies have confirmed this vehicle effect (24), evaluated the effect of skin permeation enhancers on parabens absorption (25), and have reported attempts to reduce the penetration of the preservatives (26).

Although several studies have evaluated the safety of parabens [reviewed in (27)], there appears to be no published data concerning or estimating margins of safety for these compounds. NOAEL of 5.7 g/kg/day for methyl paraben and 5.5 g/kg/day for propyl paraben have been suggested (28,29). Using data from Cross and Roberts (24), the amount of methyl and propyl parabens crossing human epidermal membranes, applied as a finite dose in a commercial allergy test ointment (5 mg/cm^2), amounted to 27.0 and 78.0 µg/cm^2, respectively, over a 10-hour period. Recognizing that such test ointments contain artificially high concentrations of the parabens (3% of each) and assuming that permeation continues in a linear fashion (unlikely), total daily percutaneous absorption amounts to approximately 65 µg/cm^2 for methyl paraben and 187 µg/cm^2 for propyl paraben. Further assuming continuous application over a total body area of 1.8 m^2, the maximum total daily intake would amount to 1.17 g methyl paraben and 3.37 g propyl paraben. Based on the NOAEL identified above, this results in margins of safety of 292 for methyl paraben and 98 for propyl paraben. These values should be considered extremely conservative and treated with caution as they are clearly based on the worst-case scenario of total body application of a formulation containing artificially high concentrations of the preservatives (approximately 10-fold higher than marketed preparations).

Fragrance Materials

Before use in any cosmetic, personal care, or household product, fragrance materials undergo extensive safety evaluations including risk assessments. As part of this process, it is essential to obtain reliable human skin permeation data in order to calculate margins of safety. For example, Hawkins et al. (30) determined the in vivo skin absorption of radiolabeled musk ambrette, musk ketone, and musk xylene, three compounds with a long history of use as fragrance ingredients (although musk ambrette is no longer used in fragrances). Musk ambrette, musk ketone, and musk xylene were applied to 100 cm^2 of dorsal skin of healthy human volunteers at a dose level of 10 to 20 µg/cm^2 and excess material was removed at six hours. Based on measurements of urine and feces over five days, 2.0% musk ambrette, 0.5% musk ketone, and 0.3% musk xylene were absorbed. Most of the material was excreted in the urine with less than 10% of the amount excreted being found in feces. Interestingly, no radioactivity was detected in plasma samples or in skin strips taken at five days.

The human skin permeation of another widely used fragrance material, methyl-3,4-methylene-dioxy-hydrocinnamic aldehyde (MMDHCA), was determined in vitro using ^{14}C-MMDHCA (31). Twenty microliters of a 1% solution of MMDHCA in ethanol were applied to the surface of diffusion cell–mounted epidermal membranes. Receptor fluid samples were taken at intervals over 48 hours and analyzed by liquid scintillation counting. At 24 and 48 hours, respectively, 42% and 50% of the applied dose of MMDHCA had permeated human skin in vitro. Only 67% of the applied dose was recovered by 48 hours, presumably due to concurrent loss by evaporation. A subchronic toxicity study, in which MMDHCA was applied dermally once daily to male and female rats at dose levels of 50, 150, or 300 mg/kg/day for at least 90 consecutive days showed that no test article–related mortalities or effects on estrous cycles, ophthalmic, body weights, absolute or relative organ weights, or male reproductive morphology/ function were observed. MMDHCA-related dermal irritation was observed across all dose levels with increased incidence and severity at 300 mg/kg/day. Irritation improved during a four-week recovery phase. The authors concluded that (*i*) MMDHCA exhibited moderately high human skin permeation, (*ii*) the NOAEL for dermal irritation was below 50 mg/kg/day when applied, and (*iii*) the NOAEL for systemic toxicity was greater than 300 mg/kg/day.

Finally, Brain et al. (32) determined the skin permeation of geranyl nitrile (GN) using human epidermal membranes in vitro following application (5 μL/cm^2) in 70% ethanol, under nonocclusive conditions, at the maximum in-use concentration of 1%. Permeation was measured over 24 hours using 6% (w/v) oleth-20 in pH 7.4 phosphate-buffered saline as the receptor medium. Permeation of a reference material (benzoic acid) was assessed using the same skin donors. Overall recovery of GN at 24 hours was low (approximately 14%) due to evaporation. Evaporative loss of GN from polytetrafluoroethylene sheets under the same conditions was rapid (93% over 24 hours), although this overestimated loss during permeation where evaporation competed with uptake. At 24 hours, 1.89 μg/cm^2 GN (representing 3.74% of the applied dose) had permeated. Following rapid initial permeation, the absorption plateaued, due to depletion. Levels of GN in the epidermis (plus any remaining stratum corneum after tape stripping) and receptor fluid were combined to produce a total absorbed dose value of 4.72%. The authors concluded that systemic exposure resulting from the use of GN as a fragrance ingredient, under unoccluded conditions, would be low based on the currently reported use levels.

Hair Dyes

Human poisoning by hair dyes is extremely rare and has only been reported following oral ingestion (33,34). Although there have been several reports that suggest a link between hair dye use and bladder cancer in both users and hair care professionals (35,36), conservative risk assessments and genotoxicity studies suggest that there is no, or negligible, cancer risk to consumers for ingredients that were found to be positive in rodent oral carcinogenicity studies (37,38).

Garrique and colleagues (39) investigated in vitro genotoxic properties of *p*-phenylenediamine (PPD) and its metabolites, N-monoacetylated-PPD (MAPPD), and N,N'-diacetylated-PPD (DAPPD) in the Ames test, the micronucleus test in human lymphocytes, and the mouse lymphoma assay (Hprt locus, PPD only). Since a considerable amount of metabolism of PPD occurs in the skin (40), the metabolites, MAPPD, and DAPPD represent the substances to which humans are systemically exposed following dermal absorption. In the Ames test, PPD was slightly mutagenic but MAPPD and DAPPD were negative in all tested strains. PPD did not induce mutation at the Hprt locus of L5178Y mouse lymphoma cells, which suggested that PPD is nonmutagenic in mammalian cells. In the in vitro micronucleus test, PPD induced micronuclei in cultured human peripheral blood lymphocytes but MAPPD and DAPPD did not, when tested up to 10 mM concentrations or to their limit of solubility. They concluded that the results of the Ames and micronucleus tests confirmed that PPD had a slight genotoxic potential in vitro, although it was nonmutagenic in mammalian cells. MAPPD and DAPPD were negative in both the Ames and the micronucleus tests indicating that these acetylated conversion products were detoxified metabolites and that they are biologically less reactive than the parent molecule PPD.

Hueber-Becker et al. (41) determined the absorption of radiolabeled PPD from a commercial oxidative hair dye in vivo (human) and in vitro (human and pig skin). Hair of eight male volunteers was dyed, cut, and collected. Blood, urine, and feces were analyzed for five days after hair dyeing. Human and pig ear skin in vitro were exposed to the same hair dye for 0.5 hour, and radioactivity distribution was measured at 24 hours. The recovery rate in the human volunteer study was about 96% of the applied dose. Washing water, cut hair, gloves, paper towels, caps, or scalp wash contained a total of 95.2% of the applied label and the amount of radioactivity absorbed was 0.50% (urine) and 0.04% (feces), which corresponded to 7.0 mg PPD absorbed. Most of the radioactivity was excreted within 24 hours. The total absorbed amounts in vitro were of 2.4% (human skin) or 3.4% (pig skin). The data indicated that hair dyeing with oxidative hair dyes would result in minimal systemic exposure and would be unlikely to pose a risk to human health.

The same group monitored the exposure of hairdressers to oxidative hair dyes for six working days under controlled conditions (42). Professional hairdressers colored natural human hair for six hours with an oxidative hair dye containing 2% ^{14}C-p-PPD. Three phases of hair dyeing were monitored: (i) dye preparation/hair dyeing, (ii) rinsing/shampooing/conditioning, and (iii) cutting/drying/styling. Urine and blood samples were collected from all exposed subjects. All biological samples and study materials were monitored and a ^{14}C-mass balance was performed daily. The hair wash contained about 45.5% of the applied radioactivity and the hair + scalp 53.5%. Plasma levels were below the limit of quantification. Excretion of [^{14}C] over 48 hours was variable and ranged from <2 to 18 μg PPD. The mass balance of [^{14}C] across the six study days was excellent at 102.5%. Overall, the mean, total systemic exposure of hairdressers to oxidative hair dyes over a working day including six dyeing processes was estimated at <0.36 μg PPD/kg body weight. Once again, the authors concluded that current safety precautions in the handling of hair dyes offered sufficient protection against local and systemic exposure and that professional exposure to oxidative hair dyes did not pose a risk to human health.

In conclusion, it is well known that the actives used in hair dye formulations can penetrate into and permeate across the skin (43). The rate and total cumulative amount of dye that has been shown to be absorbed, however, is small, variable, and can be dependent on the study protocol. Where similar protocols have been used in inter- and intra-laboratory studies variability is considerably reduced (44). Calculation of safety margins for hair dyes using in vitro skin permeation values is somewhat more complex than that illustrated above for a sunscreen agent. Whereas a typical sunscreen agent is applied as a leave-on product over a large area of the body, hair dye products are applied to the hair over a relatively small area of skin and remain in place for a short period of time. Typical margins of safety for hair dyes have been calculated to be in the multiple thousands (43).

Diethanolamine

Many cosmetic and personal care formulations contain alkanolamides [condensates of diethanolamine (DEA) with various fatty acids], which function as viscosity-increasing agents and foam boosters and are primarily used in rinse-off formulations. The available commercial condensates contain varying amounts of free DEA. Commercial triethanolamine, which may also contain a small amount of DEA, is also sometimes used in leave-on formulations such as creams and lotions. The toxicities of DEA condensates as cosmetic ingredients have been comprehensively reviewed (45,46) and it was concluded that they are safe as used. However, more recent studies by the National Toxicology Program (NTP) (47–49) suggested that there was "clear evidence" that DEA and cocamide DEA caused liver tumors in mice and "some evidence" that lauramide DEA acted similarly. The NTP concluded in their draft technical report that these findings were likely to be attributable to the free DEA present in the condensates. It is important to note that the NTP studies were conducted using an ethanol vehicle, which could facilitate skin absorption of DEA, and there is also evidence to suggest that dermal application of lauramide DEA in mice can result in significant oral ingestion if the treatment sites remain unprotected (50). The permeation of DEA through isolated skin of a variety of species, including man, has been assessed from neat DEA and aqueous DEA solutions applied at infinite dose (51). The data indicated that permeation was greater from the aqueous solution than from the neat chemical and that absorption through human skin was less than that through laboratory animal skin. These data, however, appear to have been generated to identify potential hazards during the manufacture and processing of DEA and its condensates and were obtained using conditions that are unlikely to be experienced by the end user of cosmetic products containing condensates.

Kraeling et al. (52) measured DEA absorption in human skin following exposures in shampoos, hair dyes, and body lotions. Radiolabeled ^{14}C-DEA was added to commercial products from each class and applied to excised viable and nonviable human skin in flow-through diffusion cells. The products remained in contact with the skin for 5 minutes, 30 minutes, and 24 hours for shampoos, hair dyes, and body lotions, respectively. At 24 hours most of the absorbed dose was found in skin: 2.8% for shampoos, 2.9% for hair dyes, and 10.0% for body lotions. Only small amounts had permeated through the skin and into the receptor fluid: 0.08%, 0.09%, and 0.9% for shampoos, hair dyes, and body lotions, respectively. In 72-hour daily-repeat dose studies with a lotion, DEA accumulated in the skin (29.2%) with little diffusing out into the receptor fluid. The authors concluded that permeation through the skin was low and that skin levels of DEA should not be included in estimates of systemic absorption used in exposure assessments.

Similarly, Brain et al. (53) generated skin penetration and permeation data for DEA applied in a range of typical formulations under in-use conditions. Seven rinse-off formulations and a leave-on emulsion, representing prototype cosmetic formulations and containing representative levels of DEA, were prepared. Target levels of DEA were attained by inclusion of DEA as either ^{14}C-DEA or a combination of ^{14}C-DEA and unlabeled DEA. Skin permeation and distribution were evaluated using human skin in vitro mounted on static diffusion cells. At least 12 replicate epidermal membranes were prepared from a minimum of four donors for each test group. Receptor phase samples were taken at appropriate time intervals. At the end of the test period, radioactivity remaining on the skin surface and on the diffusion cell donor cap was determined before the skin samples were tape stripped. The remaining tissue was solubilized and radioactivity determined. Permeation was very low from all vehicles applied under in-use conditions (range 1–48 ng/cm^2 over 24 hours). Comparison was also made between permeation and distribution of DEA from an infinite dose of a simple aqueous solution and the leave-on formulation through paired samples of fresh and frozen full-thickness skin from the same donors. When applied as an infinite dose in aqueous solution, DEA permeation at 24 hours was greater through frozen than through fresh skin. From the leave-on formulation, permeation was similar and very low for both fresh and frozen skin. Recovery of DEA after application of the aqueous solution to fresh human skin and subsequent aqueous and organic extraction of the epidermal and dermal tissue indicated that the majority ($>98\%$) of DEA was in the aqueous extract, suggesting that DEA was in the free state and not associated with the lipid fraction. These data provide a basis for the estimation of the potential systemic exposure and safety margins for DEA in representative cosmetic formulations.

It is important to appreciate that, for risk assessment purposes, the most appropriate measure in terms of dermal exposure is the amount of a particular compound that may cross the skin from a defined formulation under in-use conditions. With this in mind, the application vehicles used by Brain et al. (53) (representative of shampoo, bubble bath, and hair dye products) were applied either neat or with aqueous dilution and rinsed from the skin following an appropriate interval. As would be expected for those vehicles that were rinsed from the skin after short exposure periods, permeation was flat between 12 and 24 hours. On the other hand, the leave-on emulsion formulation remained in contact with the skin for the duration of the experiment and permeation continued to rise over the entire exposure period. Permeation data for all cosmetic vehicles studied are summarized in Table 1 where, for comparative purposes, only the 24 hours time point has been illustrated. Permeation of DEA from a simple aqueous solution at 24 hours was greater through frozen than fresh skin. In vitro measurements using nonviable skin are therefore more likely to provide overestimates, rather than underestimates, of in vivo human exposure to DEA. It was possible to calculate permeability coefficients for DEA from the simple aqueous solution across fresh and frozen skin. Values obtained for fresh (0.10×10^{-4} and 0.24×10^{-4} cm/hr) and frozen (0.51×10^{-4} cm/hr) skin compare

TABLE 1   Summary of Diethanolamine (DEA) Permeation Data from Cosmetic Vehicles

Vehicle	% DEA in vehicle	% DEA applied to skin[a]	24 Hour permeation (ng/cm^2)	24 Hour permeation (% applied dose)	Skin	N
Shampoo	0.98	0.098	18 ± 6	0.018 ± 0.006	Frozen	12
Shampoo	0.98	0.098	25 ± 6	0.025 ± 0.007	Frozen	12
Shampoo	0.25	0.025	8.5 ± 2.7	0.034 ± 0.011	Frozen	12
Shampoo	0.25	0.025	2.7 ± 1.3	0.011 ± 0.005	Frozen	12
Bubble bath	0.25	0.00083	4.2 ± 2.2	0.508 ± 0.265	Frozen	12
Moisturizing cream	0.008	0.008	1.3 ± 0.3	0.336 ± 0.080	Fresh	26
Moisturizing cream	0.008	0.008	0.6 ± 0.1	0.165 ± 0.032	Frozen	27
Semi-permanent hair dye	0.075	0.075	48 ± 11	0.063 ± 0.014	Frozen	10
Oxidative hair dye	0.249	0.125	28 ± 5	0.024 ± 0.004	Frozen	12

[a] Concentration of DEA applied to skin following vehicle dilution.

favorably with those obtained by Sun et al. (51) for DEA absorption from aqueous solution across human skin (0.34×10^{-4} cm/hr).

CONCLUDING REMARKS

The evolution of the Internet and the World Wide Web has probably been the greatest advancement in communications and the dissemination of information. Scientists can gain immediate access to research literature and the general public is able to gather information on topics of interest in all levels of detail. Unfortunately, there is a downside in that unsubstantiated rumors can spread like a forest fire. Among the many such rumors are those implicating cosmetic ingredients and actives as health hazards. While many of these rumors can be debunked on the basis of rational science, there remains a considerable body of work to be done to convince the doubters of the safety of cosmetics and their ingredients when the products are used correctly. The risk assessment process is much more accurate when based on real experimental data, rather than mathematical predictions, but only if the relevant experiments are logically designed and performed correctly. It is clear, therefore, that the selection of an appropriate experimental model that is based upon anticipated exposure conditions during actual product use is the most important aspect of the design of in vitro skin penetration studies, and will have a direct impact on the applicability of resultant data for use in cosmetic risk assessment. Careful consideration of individual protocol elements will greatly enhance the quality of results, their usefulness in the prediction of skin penetration in vivo, and the assessment of risk following actual human exposure.

Anticipated human exposure conditions should always dictate the choice of in vitro exposure conditions and how to interpret the data obtained. Thus, for cosmetics, the skin is normally exposed to very small amounts of vehicle and finite dose applications of the test substance are most relevant to human exposure assessment, especially for those materials that may be present at low levels or as trace contaminants in cosmetic formulations. Typically, such materials will be deposited at low levels on the skin following exposure.

In summary, useful information on the prediction of skin penetration of cosmetic ingredients can be obtained using in vitro methods. However, even data obtained under in vitro finite dose experimental conditions should be interpreted cautiously. For example, permeant volatility can complicate the conduct and interpretation of such experiments. In addition, in normal use the deposited material is often reduced by mechanical processes (e.g., abrasion by clothing, perspiration, sebum secretion) and normal activities (e.g., washing, bathing, skin cleansing), which are difficult to reproduce using in vitro models. Each of these factors should be carefully considered when using the data generated from skin penetration experiments for actual risk assessment purposes.

REFERENCES

1. Walters KA, Brain KR. How dermal absorption estimates are used in risk assessment. In: Riviere JE, ed. Dermal Absorption Models in Toxicology and Pharmacology. Boca Raton: Taylor & Francis, 2006:135–57.
2. Schneider T, Vermeulen R, Brouwer DH, et al. Conceptual model for assessment for dermal exposure. Occup Environ Med 1999; 56:765–73.

3. McDougal JN, Boeniger MF. Methods for assessing risks of dermal exposures in the workplace. Crit Rev Toxicol 2002; 32:291–327.
4. Marquart J, Brouwer DH, Gijsbers JH, et al. Determinants of dermal exposure relevant for exposure modeling in regulatory risk assessment. Ann Occup Hyg 2003; 47:599–607.
5. van de Sandt JJM. In vitro predictions of skin absorption: robustness and critical factors. In: Brain KR, Walters KA, eds. Perspectives in Percutaneous Penetration. Vol. 9a. Cardiff: STS Publishing, 2004:7.
6. Loretz L, Api AM, Barraj L, et al. Exposure data for personal care products: hairspray, spray perfume, liquid foundation, shampoo, body wash, and solid antiperspirant. Food Chem Toxicol 2006; 44:2008–18.
7. Yourick JJ, Bronaugh RL. Percutaneous penetration as it relates to the safety evaluation of cosmetic ingredients. In: Bronaugh RL, Maibach HI, eds. Percutaneous Absorption. 4th ed. New York: Taylor & Francis, 2005:595–604.
8. Walters KA, Roberts MS. Percutaneous absorption of sunscreens. In: Bronaugh RL, Maibach HI, eds. Percutaneous Absorption. 4th ed. New York: Taylor & Francis, 2005:681–700.
9. Gonzalez H, Farbrot A, Larko O, et al. Percutaneous absorption of the sunscreen benzophenone-3 after repeated whole-body applications, with and without ultraviolet irradiation. Br J Dermatol 2005; 154:337–40.
10. Food and Drug Administration. Sunscreen drug products for over-the-counter human use; final monograph. Fed Regist 1999; 64:27666.
11. Finnin BC, Morgan TM. Transdermal penetration enhancers: applications, limitations, and potential. J Pharm Sci 1999; 88:955–8.
12. Pont AR, Charron AR, Brand RM. Active ingredients in sunscreens act as topical penetration enhancers for the herbicide 2,4-dichlorophenoxyacetic acid. Toxicol Appl Pharmacol 2004; 195:348–54.
13. Walters KA, Brain KR, Howes D, et al. Percutaneous penetration of octyl salicylate from representative sunscreen formulations through human skin in vitro. Food Chem Toxicol 1997; 35:1219–25.
14. CTFA. Octyl salicylate: 13 week oral (dietary) subchronic toxicity study in rats (unpublished data).
15. Morgan TM, Reed BL, Finnin BC. Enhanced skin permeation of sex hormones with novel topical spray vehicles. J Pharm Sci 1998; 87:1213–8.
16. Brand RM, Spaulding M, Mueller C. Sunscreens can increase dermal penetration of 2,4-dichlorophenoxyacetic acid. J Toxicol Clin Toxicol 2002; 40:827–32.
17. Gu X, Wang T, Collins DM, et al. In vitro evaluation of concurrent use of commercially available insect repellent and sunscreen preparations. Br J Dermatol 2005; 152:1263–7.
18. Pugazhendhi D, Pope GS, Darbre PD. Oestrogenic activity of p-hydroxybenzoic acid (common metabolite of paraben esters) and methylparaben in human breast cancer cell lines. J Appl Toxicol 2005; 25:301–9.
19. Darbre PD. Environmental oestrogens, cosmetics and breast cancer. Best Pract Res Clin Endocrinol Metab 2006; 20:121–43.
20. Godfrey D. Parabens—a safe bet! 2006. (www.health-report.co.uk/parabens_industry_view.htm)
21. Harvey PW, Darbre P. Endocrine disrupters and human health: could oestrogenic chemicals in body care cosmetics adversely affect breast cancer incidence in women? A review of evidence and call for further research. J Appl Toxicol 2004; 24:167–76.
22. Golden R, Gandy J, Vollmer G. A review of the endocrine activity of parabens and implications for potential risks to human health. Crit Rev Toxicol 2005; 35:435–58.
23. Gettings SD, Howes D, Walters KA. Experimental design considerations and use of in vitro skin penetration data in cosmetic risk assessment. In Roberts MS, Walters, KA, eds. Dermal Absorption and Toxicity Assessment. New York: Marcel Dekker, 1998: 459–87.
24. Cross SE, Roberts MS. The effects of occlusion on epidermal penetration of parabens from a commercial allergy test ointment, acetone and ethanol vehicles. J Invest Dermatol 2000; 115:914–8.

25. Nanayakkara GR, Bartlett A, Forbes B, et al. The effect of unsaturated fatty acids in benzyl alcohol on the percutaneous permeation of three model permeants. Int J Pharm 2005; 301:129–39.

26. Hasegawa T, Kim S, Tsuchida M, et al. Decrease in skin permeation and antibacterial effect of parabens by a polymeric additive, poly(2-methacryloyl-oxyethyl phosphorylcholine-*co*-butylmetacrylate). Chem Pharm Bull 2005; 53:271–6.

27. Soni MG, Carabin IG, Burdock GA. Safety assessment of esters of *p*-hydroxybenzoic acid (parabens). Food Chem Toxicol 2005; 43:985–1015.

28. Soni MG, Taylor SL, Greenberg NA, et al. Evaluation of the health aspects of methyl paraben: a review of the published literature. Food Chem Toxicol 2002; 40:1335–73.

29. Soni MG, Burdock GA, Taylor SL, et al. Safety assessment of propyl paraben: a review of the published literature. Food Chem Toxicol 2001; 39:513–32.

30. Hawkins DR, Elsom LF, Kirkpatrick D, et al. Dermal absorption and disposition of musk ambrette, musk ketone and musk xylene in human subjects. Toxicol Lett 2002; 131:147–51.

31. Api AM, Lapczynski A, Isola DA, et al. In vitro penetration and subchronic toxicity of a-methyl-1,3-benzodioxole-5-propionaldehyde. Food Chem Toxicol 2006; 45:702–7.

32. Brain KR, Green DM, Lalko J, et al. In-vitro human skin penetration of the fragrance material geranyl nitrile. Toxicol in Vitro 2007; 21:133–8.

33. Suliman SM, Homeida M, Aboud OI. Paraphenylenediamine induced acute tubular necrosis following hair dye ingestion. Hum Toxicol 1983; 2:633–5.

34. Nohynek GJ, Fautz R, Benech-Kieffer F, et al. Toxicity and human health risk of hair dyes. Food Chem Toxicol 2004; 42:517–43.

35. Gago-Dominguez M, Castelao JE, Yuan JM, et al. Use of permanent hair dyes and bladder-cancer risk. Int J Cancer 2001; 94:903–6.

36. Czene K, Tiikkaja S, Hemminki K. Cancer risks in hairdressers: assessment of carcinogenicity of hair dyes and gels. Int J Cancer 2003; 105:108–12.

37. Kirkland D, Marzin D. An assessment of the genotoxicity of 2-hydroxy-1,4-naphthoquinone, the natural dye ingredient of Henna. Mutat Res 2003; 537:183–99.

38. Andrew AS, Schned AR, Heaney JA, et al. Bladder cancer risk and personal hair dye use. Int J Cancer 2004; 109:581–6.

39. Garrique JL, Ballantyne M, Kumaravel T, et al. In vitro genotoxicity of *para*-phenylenediamine and its *N*-monoacetyl or *N,N'*-diacetyl metabolites. Mutat Res 2006; 608:58–71.

40. Dressler WE, Appelqvist T. Plasma/blood pharmacokinetics and metabolism after dermal exposure to p-aminophenol or p-phenylenediamine. Food Chem Toxicol 2006; 44:371–9.

41. Hueber-Becker F, Nohynek GD, Meuling WJ, et al. Human systemic exposure to a [14]C-*p*-phenylenediamine-containing oxidative hair dye and correlation with in vitro percutaneous absorption in human or pig skin. Food Chem Toxicol 2004; 42:1227–36.

42. Hueber-Becker F, Nohynek GD, Dufour EK, et al. Occupational exposure to [14]C-*p*-phenylenediamine-containing oxidative hair dyes: a mass balance study. Food Chem Toxicol 2007; 45:160–9.

43. Dressler WE. Percutaneous absorption of hair dyes. In: Roberts MS, Walters KA, eds. Dermal Absorption and Toxicity Assessment. 2nd ed. New York: Informa Healthcare, 2008:619–34.

44. Beck H, Brain K, Dressler W, et al. An interlaboratory/interspecies comparison of percutaneous penetration of [14]C-*p*-phenylenediamine (PPD) from a hair dye formulation in vitro. In: Brain KR, Walters KA, eds. Perspectives in Percutaneous Penetration. Vol. 7a. Cardiff: STS Publishing, 2000:27.

45. CIR. Cosmetic Ingredient Review—final report on the safety assessment of cocamide DEA, lauramide DEA, linoleamide DEA, and oleamide DEA. J Am Coll Toxicol 1986; 5:415–54.

46. CIR. Cosmetic Ingredient Review—amended final report on the safety assessment of cocamide DEA. J Am Coll Toxicol 1996; 15(6):527–42.

47. National Toxicology Program. Technical Report 478, Toxicology and carcinogenesis studies of diethanolamine (CAS No. 111-42-2) in F344/N rats and B6C3F$_1$ mice (dermal studies), 1999.

48. National Toxicology Program. Technical Report 480, Toxicology and carcinogenesis studies of lauric acid diethanolamine condensate (CAS No. 120-40-1) in F344/N rats and B6C3F$_1$ mice (dermal studies), 1999.

49. National Toxicology Program. Technical Report 479, Toxicology and carcinogenesis studies of coconut oil acid diethanolamine condensate (CAS No. 68603-42-9) in F344/N rats and B6C3F$_1$ mice (dermal studies), 2001.

50. Mathews JM, Decosta K, Thomas BF. Lauramide diethanolamine absorption, metabolism, and disposition in rats and mice after oral, intravenous, and dermal administration. Drug Metab Dispos 1996; 24:702–10.

51. Sun JD, Beskitt JL, Tallant MJ, et al. In vitro skin penetration of monoethanolamine and diethanolamine using excised skin from rats, mice, rabbits, and humans. J Toxicol Cutan Ocul Toxicol 1996; 15:131–46.

52. Kraeling ME, Yourick JJ, Bronaugh RL. In vitro human skin penetration of diethanolamine. Food Chem Toxicol 2004; 42:1553–61.

53. Brain KR, Walters KA, Green DM, et al. Percutaneous penetration of diethanolamine through human skin in vitro: application from cosmetic vehicles. Food Chem Toxicol 2005; 43:681–90.

William E. Dressler
Independent Consultant, Huntington, Connecticut, U.S.A.

INTRODUCTION

Hair dyes represent an important class of cosmetic ingredients for consideration of their percutaneous absorption. In part, this is because of their widespread usage among women and increasing popularity among men. Further, the utility of chemicals from the aromatic or nitro-aromatic classes as hair dyes has drawn attention to their potential for toxicological effects associated with some members of the class.

In addition to toxicological tests ranging from mutagenicity to carcinogenicity conducted on hair dyes, usage is often captured among lifestyle factors and other chemical exposures in human epidemiological studies on a variety of health outcomes. While the weight of the evidence from both preclinical and human health studies supports the safety of hair dyes, responsible product stewardship in conjunction with regulatory oversight requires comprehensive toxicological evaluation. This includes continuing reassessment as improved toxicological testing methods and risk assessment principles evolve.

Integral to this safety assessment is the determination of the potential and extent of systemic exposure to hair dyes under use conditions. Percutaneous absorption studies, therefore, play a key role in helping to put the potential risks from hazard identification studies into proper perspective. Urine discoloration and observations that certain hair dyes induce allergic contact dermatitis provided indirect evidence of systemic exposure during normal use. This prompted early investigations, some using ^{14}C-ring-labeled hair dyes, which demonstrated acceptably low levels of systemic exposure associated with typical products and usage. These historical human data, taken as the "gold-standard," facilitated the development of reliable in vitro percutaneous absorption methods and protocols. This afforded a more practical opportunity for the systematic study of variables that may influence the extent of hair dye absorption as well as for the evaluation of novel dyes (or chemical reaction products) for which toxicological information may be limited. This chapter reviews hair dye chemistry relevant to understanding hair dye absorption, historical, and contemporary in vivo human data, and in vivo/in vitro data on the influence of metabolism and reactive dye chemistry on the nature of systemic exposures to hair dyes. The implications of this information for risk assessment are discussed.

HAIR DYE CLASSIFICATION AND CHEMISTRY

Chemical classification of hair dyes as either "oxidative" or "direct" provides the most relevant distinction between dye types. Oxidative hair dyeing involves chemical complexation of lower molecular weight precursor materials (primary intermediates and couplers) into colored polynuclear (polymeric) species within the hair fiber. The increased molecular size resulting from such complexation serves to trap the colored species within the hair shaft, imparting permanence. Oxidative hair dyes are mixed with a developer, typically hydrogen peroxide, prior to application. This serves to facilitate the chemical reactions and to bleach the natural melanin in the hair, allowing colors lighter than the natural shade to be produced.

In contrast, direct dyes are preformed colors that deposit on the hair cuticle and are therefore susceptible to fading over time caused by leaching of dye from the hair fiber during wear and shampooing. Chemically, the presence of a nitro group on a single (nitrobenzene) or double (nitro-diphenylamine) aromatic ring confers visible color. Azo- or hydroxyl-substituted anthraquinone molecules are also colored. Direct dyes can be further divided into "semipermanent" or "temporary" classes depending on their relative shampoo resistance. Semipermanents would typically maintain vibrancy through six to eight shampoos while the larger molecular weight temporary dyes would rinse out after one or two shampoos.

Some ambiguity derives from descriptors of formulated product performance. So-called "long-lasting semipermanent" or "demi-permanent" products utilize oxidative hair dye technology. Further, direct dyes are sometimes use as "toners" in oxidative dye formulations, though they do not participate in oxidative color formation. Leaching of these dyes from the hair could cause the oxidative shade to go "off-tone" over time.

Because of the highly desirable performance characteristics of oxidative dyes (both their permanence and ability to lighten), they account for the preponderance (80–90%) of hair dye usage in the United States and Europe. Commonly used oxidative and direct hair dyes are shown in Table 1.

Hair Dye Chemistry
Oxidative Dyes
Oxidative hair dyeing typically involves coupling of amino and hydroxyaromatic primary intermediates (referred to as the "precursors" in Europe) with hydroxy-benzenes (e.g., resorcinol), *m*-aminophenol, or *m*-diaminobenzenes (e.g., 2,4-diaminophenoxyethanol) couplers. The rate-limiting step, which is catalyzed by alkaline (pH 9.5–10.5) peroxide conditions, leads to the formation of a transient quinone di-imine, which rapidly combines with the coupler to produce a leuco dye. The leuco dye is then further oxidized to the basic indo dye chromophore. Couplers with one free position para to the hydroxyl- or amino-activating group (e.g., 4-amino-2-hydroxytoluene) will couple 1:1 with the primary intermediate; those with both para positions free (e.g., *m*-aminophenol) will couple in a 2:1 (primary intermediate:coupler) ratio forming a trimer. The rate of the addition of a secondary primary intermediate to form a trimer varies depending on the coupler. In the absence or deficiency of alternative couplers, certain primary intermediates can self-couple. For example, *p*-phenylenediamine (PPD) can form the trimer Bandrowski's base. This is relevant, therefore, to percutaneous absorption studies involving PPD alone where the reaction kinetics as well as the resulting reaction product is different in the absence of couplers than that formed with couplers.

The science and art of hair color technology is to formulate with one or more primary intermediates and an array of couplers such that their monochromatic reaction products blend to produce the desired shade(s). The associated complexity is apparent from Figure 1, showing a mix of dimeric and trimeric species that may

TABLE 1 Some Commonly Used Hair Dyes (and Selected Abbreviations Used in Text and Tables)

Oxidative dyes	Direct dyes
Primary intermediates	
PPD	HC Blue No. 2
p-Toluenediamine	HC Red No. 1
p-Aminophenol	HC Red No. 3
N,*N*-bis-(2-hydroxyethyl) PPD (*N*,*N*-bis)	HC Red No. 10/HC Red No. 11
1-Hydroxyethyl 4,5-diaminopyrazole	HC Yellow No. 2
4-Amino-*m*-cresol (4-a-MC)	HC Yellow No. 4
	HC Orange No. 1
Couplers	HC Violet No. 2
Resorcinol	Basic Blue 7
3-Methyl resorcinol	Basic Blue 99
4-Chlororesorcinol	Basic Red 76
1-Napthol	Basic Brown 17
2,7-Napthylenediol	Disperse Black 9
m-Aminophenol	Disperse Blue 3
p-Methylaminophenol	Disperse Violet 1
2,4-Diaminophenoxy ethanol	3-Nitro-*p*-hydroxyethylaminophenol
2-Methyl-5-hydroxyethylaminophenol	2-Amino-6-chloronitrophenol
4-Amino-2-hydroxytoluene	4-Hydroxypropylamino-3-nitrophenol
Phenylmethylpyrazolone	2-Nitro-5-glycerylmethylaniline
2,4,5,6-Tetraaminopyridine	Hydroxethyl-2-nitro-*p*-toluidine
1,3-Bis-(2,4-diaminophenoxy) propane	
2-Amino-4-hydroxyethylaminoanisole	
Hydroxyethyl-PPD sulfate	

Abbreviation: PPD, *p*-phenylenediamine.

be produced in a representative hair dye formulation containing PPD and several couplers. The concentrations of these reaction products will be dependent on the ratios of precursors selected to produce an individual shade and their relative reaction affinities. Thus the potential skin permeants available during the exposure period include progressively diminishing concentrations of precursor dyes and corresponding increasing concentrations of colored reaction products. Unreacted dye precursors may be available at the end of the exposure periods since excess couplers are often employed to prevent self-coupling of the primary intermediate.

Direct Dyes

When formulated in oxidative products, direct dyes would not participate in the oxidative reactions described above. In semipermanent products, varying shades are produced by combining different colored dyes, with blue dyes being important to the overall depth of color. In order to promote even dye uptake in the worn cuticle along the length and near the tip of the hair fiber, and the new-growth virgin cuticle near the scalp, different molecular weight dyes of the same color family are often employed (e.g., HC Red 1 and HC Red 3).

EXPOSURE CONSIDERATIONS

The chemistry and mode of use of hair dye products, taken together, pose a rather unique set of circumstances, different from other cosmetic materials with regard to exposure to the scalp and the potential for systemic availability of dye materials.

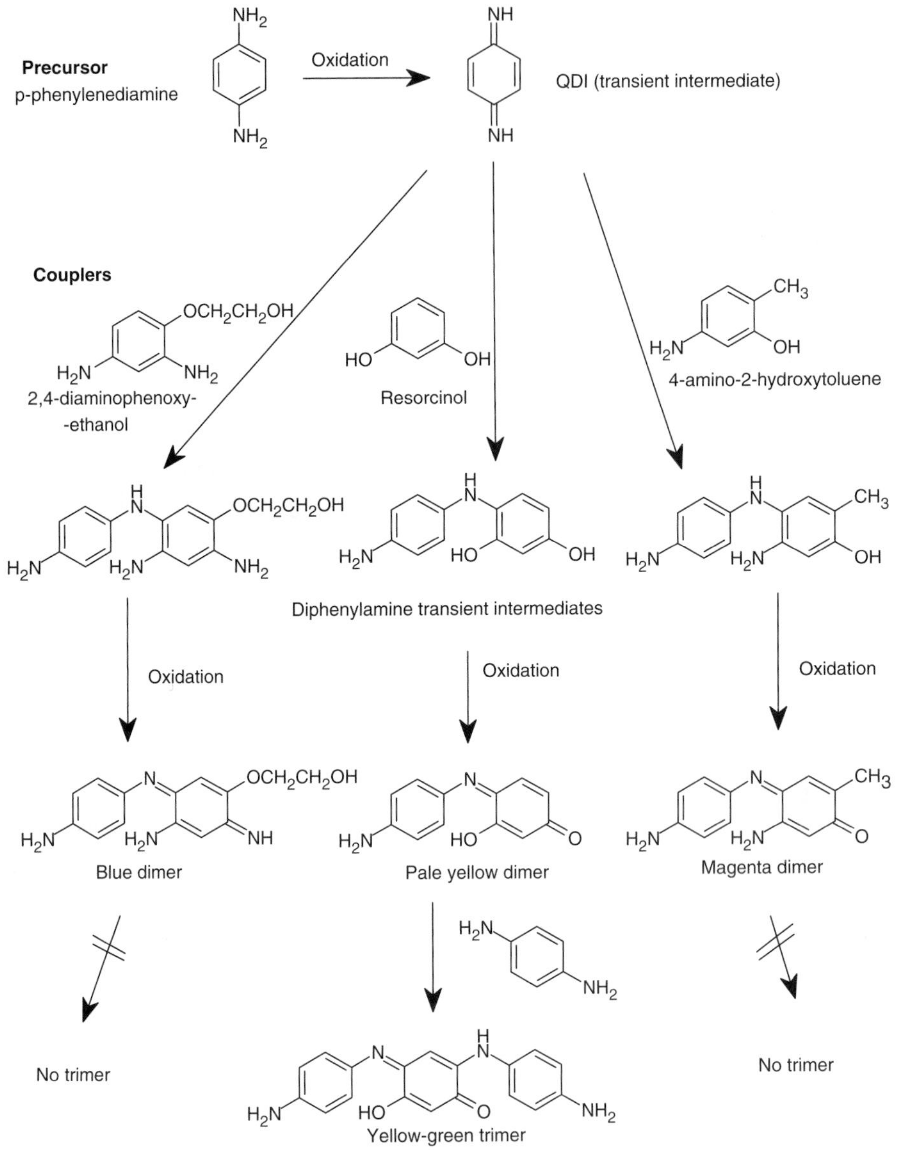

FIGURE 1 Reaction of PPD with various couplers to produce colored dimers and trimers. *Abbreviations*: PPD, *p*-phenylenediamine; QDI, quinonediimine.

Importantly, for oxidative dyes the potential permeants are continuously changing during the course of the exposure. Direct dyes may form a reservoir in the hair with continuing exposure of the scalp due to leaching.

The abundance of hair allows for larger apparent loading doses of formulation ($165 \, mg/cm^2$ for $100 \, g$ formulation applied to $600 \, cm^2$ of scalp) than could be achieved on non-hairy skin. Most of the applied material would be in contact with hair rather than scalp per se. Further, the hair provides a large surface area competing with scalp for dye uptake. Surface area estimates of medium length hair are in the range of 50,000 cm^2 (1). The intended targeting of dye for keratin in the hair may serve to limit dye penetration to the upper epidermis via skin binding. Dye bound in the upper epidermis may be lost through desquamation before penetration.

There are substantial shade-related variations in the concentration of dyes or precursors in formulated products with a sharp fall off in dye loads below black and dark brown shades. Thus the majority of users may experience exposures well below that of dark shades often used for percutaneous absorption studies.

Hair dye products are used on a discontinuous basis, typically every four to six weeks for oxidative dyes and two to four weeks for direct dyes. With oxidative dyes, hair recoloring often involves application of about one-third of the mixed material to the root (and scalp) area for 20 to 30 minutes, followed by application of the balance to the rest of the hair for the final 5 to 10 minutes.

IN VIVO DATA
Hair Dyeing in Humans

The earliest definitive studies on hair dye absorption in humans were performed by Maibach and Wolfram (2,3). These studies employed ^{14}C-ring-labeled oxidative precursors and/or direct dyes incorporated into representative products. Two of the direct dyes studied were included in oxidative formulations as toners and two were evaluated in conventional semipermanent products. After first mixing with peroxide, approximately 100 g was applied and worked into dry hair for five to eight minutes and left for an additional 20 minutes prior to rinsing with water. With direct dye formulations, approximately 88 g of material was applied in a similar manner after which the hair was wrapped in a plastic turban for the additional 30 minutes exposure. After rinsing, towel blotting, and drying, the hair was either left in place to simulate "application and wear" or, in some experiments ("application only") immediately clipped. Three or four subjects received each formulation. Percutaneous absorption was assessed by determining ^{14}C levels in urine and values were corrected for incomplete excretion using oral or parenteral data. Data, for PPD, shown in Table 2 would be most appropriately characterized as reflecting "^{14}C PPD-equivalent" levels since counts would include parent compounds and metabolic or chemical conversion products.

More recently Hueber-Becker et al. (4) conducted a similar study using eight volunteers, but restricted their evaluation to a single dye, ^{14}C-PPD. A dark shade containing 2% PPD and 1% *m*-aminophenol (after mixing) was applied in a manner similar to that described above, with shampoo added to the water rinse. The hair, previously cut to a standard length of about 2 cm, was completely removed after dyeing. A non-occlusive cap was used to collect shed epithelium and removed on day 2, followed by a shampoo wash. Radioactivity was measured in urine, feces, and plasma as well as hair, rinse water, and blotting materials. The mean (SD) absorption was equivalent to 7.0 ($\pm$3.4) mg or about 10 µg/cm^2 (Table 2). This was roughly proportional to the amounts reported in the original study that used a lower applied concentration of PPD.

Results for the other dye materials evaluated in the initial studies by Maibach and Wolfram are shown in Table 2. Oxidative dye couplers were tested in "application only" experiments and cumulative four-day absorption values were equivalent to 0.46 µg/cm^2 for resorcinol and 0.21 µg/cm^2 for 2,4-diaminoanisole.

TABLE 2 Human Volunteer Studies Using Radiolabeled Dyes Applied Under Actual
Use Conditions

			Mean cumulative absorption (μg/cm^2)		
	% Dye	Application	Application and wear		
Dye classification	(after mixing)	only	Day 1	Day 10	Day 30
Oxidative dyes					
Primary intermediates					
PPD	1.35	4.47	4.35	7.12	7.81
	2.00	10.00	–	–	–
Couplers					
2,4-Diaminoanisole	0.87	0.21	–	–	–
Resorcinol	0.61	0.46	–	–	–
Direct dyes					
4-Amino-2-nitrophenol	0.21[a]	0.67	–	–	–
2-Nitro-PPD	1.68[a]	1.33	2.20	4.86	8.68
HC Blue No. 1	1.48	1.55	2.81	5.26	9.38
HC Blue No. 2	1.77	–	0.23	1.57	2.00

Absorption values based on four-day (1.35% PPD) or 60-hour (2.00% PPD) urinary recoveries and estimated
700 cm^2 scalp area.
[a] Used as toner in oxidative formulation.
Abbreviations: –, not available; PPD, *p*-phenylenediamine.
Source: From Refs. 2–4.

Respectively, these values were about 10- and 20-fold lower than that seen
with PPD.

For the two direct dyes contained in oxidative formulations, the corresponding absorption values were 0.67 μg/cm^2 for 4-amino-2-nitrophenol and
1.33 μg/cm^2 for 2-nitro-PPD. For 2-nitro-PPD evaluated in "application and
wear" studies, cumulative absorption increased about fourfold from 2.2 to
8.7 μg/cm^2 from day 1 to 30.

With the HC Blue dyes contained in semipermanent formulations, a similar
pattern of incremental absorption was seen over time. This increment was about
3-fold for HC Blue 1 and 10-fold for HC Blue 2 (which had about 10-fold less initial
absorption). That such incremental absorption resulted from leaching of dye from
the hair over time was also apparent from an approximate twofold difference
between exposures from "application-only" versus "application and wear" studies
for 2-nitro-PPD and HC Blue 1.

In contrast, corresponding day 1 values for PPD from these differing exposure
scenarios were similar. Intermediate data between days 1 and 10 from the
"application and wear" studies were not provided (other than noting that most
absorption had occurred by day 2) to explain the approximate 1.6-fold increase over
this interval. In any event, essentially no further incremental absorption was seen
with PPD between days 20 and 30.

In addition to the radiolabel studies, there appear to be only two other
published human hair dye studies. Goetz et al. (5) applied products containing
between 0.28% and 1.26% PPD (after mixing) to five subjects evaluated on one to six
occasions. Using flash hydrolysis in a GC port to cleave PPD from its acetylated and
conjugated metabolites, they found absorption amounts corresponding to about 0.5
to 1 μg/cm^2 using GC-MS. Thus, absorption values were somewhat lower as would

be anticipated from formulas typically containing less PPD than those used in the other human studies.

For, *p*-toluenediamine a primary intermediate used widely in Europe, usually in place of PPD, Keise and Raucher (6) reported absorption from a hair color base containing an equivalent concentration (1.25% after mixing) of the single coupler, resorcinol, equivalent to about 6.6 $\mu g/cm^2$. According to Corbett (7), the cold analytical method used to measure the *N,N*-diacetyl derivative, isolated via thin layer chromatography, may have overestimated exposure, but the value was similar to that reported for similar concentrations of PPD. The results of other published studies conducted with multiple or single hair dyes in vivo using primates or rodents, compiled, and summarized elsewhere (8,9), showed absorption values clearly in the ranges of those reported above and following (for the direct dyes).

Pharmacokinetic and Metabolism Studies

The human plasma pharmacokinetic parameters calculated from the data of Hueber-Becker et al. (4) were as follows: C_{max} 0.087 µg eq/mL, T_{max} 2 hours, and AUC (0–12 hours) 0.67 µg eq hr/mL. Urinary excretion was essentially complete after 60 hours.

To determine the in vivo pharmacokinetics and metabolism of the two key primary intermediates, PPD and *p*-aminophenol (PAP), after dermal exposure, a minipig and/or groups of rats were treated over 10% to 20% of their body area under occlusion for periods of 4 to 24 hours (10). Blood and plasma were measured for radioactivity and the presence of metabolites. Only *N*-acetylated compounds, and not the parent dyes, were detected in plasma. PPD was converted to a single *N,N*-diacetyl metabolite, whereas PAP was mono-acetylated to *N*-acetyl-PAP (APAP, a widely used analgesic drug) and conjugated as the *O*-glucuronide or sulfate. Relevant pharmacokinetic parameters for PAP are shown in Table 3.

For comparison, the AUC (0–12 hours) after an oral dose of 500 mg APAP has been reported to be 31.8 µg hr/mL (11). This level is about 10- and 60-fold higher than values seen after exaggerated exposures to rat and minipig, respectively.

For PPD, mean (SD) four hours plasma levels were 1412 ($\pm$342) ng ^{14}C-PPD eq/mL in males and 7401 ($\pm$1831) ng ^{14}C-PPD eq/mL in females following a topical dose of 50 mg/kg applied to approximately 50 cm^2 (1 mg/cm^2) of body surface in this exaggerated exposure. Genotyping of the human subjects showed that the acetylation of PPD was most likely due to metabolism by epidermal *N*-acetyltransferase-1 (12). Similar metabolism of PAP and PPD to their

TABLE 3 Plasma Pharmacokinetic Data Following 24 Hours Occlusive Dermal Exposure to PAP in Female Rats and a Minipig

	14C-PAP	
Parameter (unit)	Rats (12 mg/kg)	Minipig (4.7 mg/kg)
t_{max} (hours)	4	12
$t_{1/2}$ (hours)	5.95	31.3
C_{max} (ng eq/mL)	498	11.7
AUC (ng eq hr/mL)	7038 (0–24 hours)	389 (0–72 hours)
	9271 (0–∞)	490 (0–∞)

Abbreviation: PAP, *p*-aminophenol.
Source: From Ref. 10.

N-monoacetyl and *N*-diacetyl derivitives was found by Nohynek et al. (13) using reconstituted human epidermis.

IN VITRO DATA

Because of constraints in routinely testing non-therapeutic radiolabeled materials in human volunteers and due to the complexity of cold analytical techniques, in vitro approaches provide a useful and practical strategy to evaluate the potential penetration of hair dyes. This is particularly important in that estimates of percutaneous absorption for hair dyes are routinely requested or required by international regulatory groups (Europe—SCCP: Scientific Committee on Consumer Products) or advisory bodies (United States—CIR: Cosmetic Ingredient Review). For novel compounds it may be useful to obtain such information early in the development process to aid in dosage selection for toxicology studies. Most recently, regulatory attention in Europe has focused on the potential systemic availability of the novel reaction products formed in the oxidative hair coloring process. Estimation of the potential exposure from properly conducted in vitro studies can be used to determine the necessity for toxicological testing and/or to aid in its design.

Emphasis is given here to those in vitro studies involving human skin, as the preferred tissue, or pig skin, considered as an acceptable non-human alternative. In this regard, it is useful to first examine the agreement between reported in vivo data obtained in humans under actual hair dyeing conditions and data obtained, using human or pig skin, in protocols designed to simulate human usage. Table 4 compares results from the two human in vivo studies described earlier with in vitro data obtained with the identical formulations in human and pig skin.

For the 1.3% PPD (after mixing) formulation, in vitro data were obtained in two independent laboratories using heat-separated human epidermal membranes, each lab using three to four donors with 12 to 20 total replicates, and in four independent labs using dermatomed or full thickness pig or minipig skin

TABLE 4 Comparison of Percutaneous Absorption Data on PPD from Identical Oxidative Formulations Under Actual (Human Volunteers) or Simulated (Human and Pig Skin, In Vitro) Use Conditions

% PPD (after mixing)	In vivo	Absorption ($\mu g/cm^2$)		
		In vitro		
		Compartment	Human skin	Pig skin
1.35	**4.47**	A. Stratum corneum	0.41–6.06	2.93–8.46
		B. Residual epidermis	0.04–2.04	–
		C. Dermis	(not present)	0.56–2.20
		D. Receptor fluid	**1.00–1.08**	**0.29–1.28**
		Total (B+C+D)	1.17–4.20	1.85–4.49
2.00	**10.0**	A. Stratum corneum	5.57	7.31
		B./C. Residual epidermis/dermis	5.65	13.19
		D. Receptor fluid	**4.92**	**1.43**
		Total (B+C+D)	10.57	14.62

In vivo absorption values are based on four-day (1.35% PPD) or 60-hour (2.00% PPD) urinary recoveries and an estimated 700 cm^2 scalp area. In vitro values are the ranges of mean values for two labs (human epidermal membranes) or four labs (pig skin). Bold text indicates key receptor fluid values.
Abbreviations: –, not available; PPD, *p*-phenylenediamine.
Source: From Refs. 2–4, 14.

(two to three donors; 10 to 12 total replicates) (14). For the 2.0% PPD (after mixing) formulation, in vitro data were obtained using four donors (two replicates each), in dermatomed human skin and in full thickness pig ear skin (4).

In vivo, 24-hour absorption with the 1.35% PPD formulation was equivalent to 4.47 $\mu g/cm^2$ and corresponding in vitro receptor fluid values among the test laboratories ranged from 1.0 to 1.1 $\mu g/cm^2$ in human skin and 0.29 to 1.28 $\mu g/cm^2$ for pig skin. Receptor fluid values for the 2.0% PPD formula were equivalent to 10 $\mu g/cm^2$ in volunteers and 4.92 and 1.43 $\mu g/cm^2$, respectively, in dermatomed human skin and full thickness pig ear skin.

Because of species-specific tissue processing issues and individual lab difference in skin handling techniques, it was not always possible to directly compare amounts found in each skin compartment (stratum corneum, residual epidermis, and, if present, dermis). In any event, these values were much more variable among individual labs than were receptor fluid values. Amounts remaining in or on the skin could have varied due to differences in the 30-minute postexposure rinsing efficiencies as determined from mass balance calculations (not shown). Varying amounts in residual epidermis and dermis could have resulted from differences in skin thickness. Full thickness pig ear skin data showed the highest dermal levels, despite comparable receptor fluid values.

It may be tempting to consider adding amounts in epidermal fractions to the receptor fluid values to improve comparability between in vivo and in vitro data. However, as discussed by Yourick et al. (15), this requires consideration of kinetic data to ascertain the mobility of these skin amounts. In the in vitro studies, receptor fluid values had peaked within 4 to 24 hours, indicating no continued mobility of remaining skin amounts.

In Vitro Data on Oxidative Dyes

Table 5 shows in vitro results reported for a number of oxidative dye couplers in representative formulations evaluated by Beck et al. (16,17). Receptor fluid values ranged about 10-fold from 0.25 to 2.46 $\mu g/cm^2$.

In Vitro Data on Colored Reaction Products of Oxidative Dyes

Although hair dye safety is already supported by lifetime skin painting studies with oxidative formulations providing exposures to relevant hair dye reaction products, the hair color industry has responded to recent EU regulatory concerns

TABLE 5 In Vitro Percutaneous Absorption Data for Several Oxidative Dye Precursors (Couplers) from Typical Formulations in Pig Skin

	% Dye (after mixing)	Absorption ($\mu g/cm^2$)
4-Amino-2-hydroxymethylphenol HCl	0.95–1.9	0.14
3,5-Diamino-2,6-dimethoxypyridine HCl	0.50	0.25
2-Amino-*p*-aminophenol HCl	3.0	0.52
N-(2-hydroxyethyl)-3,4-methylenedioxyaniline[a]	1.0	1.21
4-Chlororesorcinol	0.3–0.9	1.60
3,4-Diaminobenzoic acid HCl	2.0	1.96
2-Amino-6-methylphenol HCl	2.0	2.46

Absorption based on 72 hours receptor fluid values [calculated from data supplied by H. Beck (personal communication, 1996)]. HCl salts would disassociate to free bases at alkaline formulation pH.
[a] Not mixed.
Source: From Refs. 16, 17.

TABLE 6 In Vitro Percutaneous Absorption Data for Preformed Polymeric Reaction Products of Oxidative Dye Precursors

Coupler	Primary intermediate	Reaction product[a]-%	Skin preparation	Peroxide $(+/-)$	Absorption ($\mu g/cm^2$) mean (range)
4-Amino-2-	PPD	Dimer-1%	Human	+	(n.d.–0.01)
hydroxy-	p-Toluenediamine	Dimer-2%	Pig	−	(0.03–0.16)
toluene	p-Aminophenol	Dimer-1%	Human	+	(0.03–0.27)
	4-a-MC	Dimer-1%	Pig	−	0.20 (NA)
	HEDAP	Dimer-1%	Pig	−	0.009 (0.006–0.04)
Resorcinol	PPD	Trimer-1%	Human	−	0.09 (0.02–0.22)
				+	0.08 (0.04–0.14)
	N,N-bis	Trimer-1%	Human	+	0.03 (0.01–0.02)
m-AP	N,N-bis	Trimer-1%	Human	+	0.08 (0.02–0.18)
	HEDAP	Dimer-1%	Pig	−	0.006 (0.002–0.01)

Absorption values include epidermis, dermis, and receptor fluid.
[a] Percent of reaction product adjusted for peroxide dilution, where applicable.
Abbreviations: AP, Aminophenol; HEDAP, 1-hydroxyethyl 4,5-diaminopyrazole; NA, not available; PPD, p-phenylenediamine.
Source: From Refs. 19, 20.

regarding the potential exposure to and toxicity of these materials. The stable colored reaction products of selected combinations of primary intermediates and couplers were first isolated and characterized chemically. Percutaneous penetration studies were subsequently performed with several ^{14}C-ring-labeled reaction products. Table 6 summarizes the publicly available data (20). Values shown are both means and ranges since the SCCP is currently advocating the use of the maximum observed values as a "worse case" risk assessment scenario (18,19). Notably, those larger molecular weight species studied to date penetrate in the ng/cm^2 range, almost two or three orders of magnitude lower than the dye precursors. Interindividual variability appears to be as much as 10-fold, not surprising for such very low-level permeants.

The data shown conservatively includes amounts found in the residual epidermis (exclusive of the stratum corneum), which may have limited mobility for exposure to the systemic circulation. This is illustrated by further in vitro human skin data previously reported for PPD and PAP applied alone and in combination with other dye precursors in the presence of hair and/or hydrogen peroxide and obtained using heat-separated epidermal membranes (9).

Although absorption into receptor fluid was monitored for 48 hours, peak levels occurred within four hours. As shown for PPD in Table 7, there was an approximate 10-fold difference in the amount of material remaining on/in the skin through 48 hours in the absence and presence of hair, other dyes, and peroxide (0.69 $\mu g/cm^2$ vs. 6.39 $\mu g/cm^2$). However, receptor fluid values were comparable (1.96 and 1.87 $\mu g/cm^2$). For PAP (Table 7), there was an incremental increase in receptor fluid values between 24 and 48 hours when PAP was applied alone. When it was applied in combination with other dye precursors, receptor fluid values were about one-third of the "alone" values and the dye showed little further mobility from the epidermis between 24 and 48 hours.

In Vitro Data on Direct Dyes

Representative data from two survey type studies are shown in Table 8. In the first study (21), dyes were applied singly to human epidermal membranes, usually at

TABLE 7   In Vitro Percutaneous Data in Heat-Separated Human Epidermal Membranes for PPD and PAP Alone and in Combination with Other Dye Precursors, Hair, and/or Hydrogen Peroxide

No. replicates		Absorption ($\mu g/cm^2$)	
(No. donors)	Condition	Epidermis	Receptor fluid (hours)
PPD			
17(3)	PPD alone (1.35%)	0.69	1.96 (4-peak)
12(3)	PPD/precursors/H_2O_2	2.83	2.36 (4-peak)
14(4)	PPD/precursors/H_2O_2	3.42	2.28 (4-peak)
15(4)	PPD/precursors/H_2O_2/hair[a]	6.39	1.87 (4-peak)
PAP			
13(2)	PAP alone (0.42%)	2.21	0.32 (24)
			0.46 (48)
	PAP/precursors/H_2O_2	1.40	0.12 (24)
			0.13 (48)

Epidermal values include stratum corneum.
[a] Finely minced hair added to epidermal surface.
Abbreviations: PAP, *p*-aminophenol; PPD, *p*-phenylenediamine.
Source: From Ref. 9.

a 1.0% concentration. Receptor fluid values ranged from 0.04 to 1.57 $\mu g/cm^2$ for representative azo, nitrobenzene, and diphenylamine structures. The lowest absorption value was seen with an azo dye whose cleavage products would be PPD and another oxidative primary intermediate. It is possible that absorption might have been higher in viable skin with intact enzymatic azoreductase activity (in addition to any azoreduction that may be induced by skin flora). It is noteworthy that dyes with the highest skin amounts regularly displayed the least absorption, again suggesting limited mobility of these preformed colors from the skin reservoir. This is supported by the fact that the kinetic data (not given) had clearly plateaued by 24 hours for each dye with the exception of HC Yellow 4, which was among the most poorly absorbed.

In order to evaluate the potential influence of other chemically nonreactive dyes on penetration characteristics, a follow-up study was conducted with HC Yellow 4 (9). This dye was applied at a typical use level of 0.28% alone and in combination with seven other dyes for a total product dye load of 1.0%. Absorption of HC Yellow 4 by itself into receptor fluid at this concentration (lower than that discussed earlier) was about 0.08 $\mu g/cm^2$. However, the receptor fluid achieved only about 37% of this value when applied in combination with the other dyes. This reduction may have been caused by dye association through hydrogen bonding, which could increase the apparent molecular volume and reduce the mobility of the dye. Thus, percutaneous penetration studies conducted with some direct dyes evaluated alone may overestimate amounts available from typical formulated products.

Beck et al. (16,17) evaluated the percutaneous absorption of several other direct hair dyes at typical use levels in representative formulations using pig skin. As shown in Table 8, the range of receptor fluid values (0.04–1.14 $\mu g/cm^2$) for these dyes was clearly in the range of those described earlier from studies using human skin.

Similarly, absorption for other individual direct dyes, reported in numerous published studies focused on individual dyes, is almost invariably within the

TABLE 8 In Vitro Percutaneous Absorption of Direct Dyes from Hair Dye Bases Containing a Single Dye (Heat-Separated Human Epidermal Membranes) and Typical Formulations Containing Dye Mixtures (Pig Skin)

	Dyes alone				Dye mixtures		
% Dye		Skin (%)	Receptor fluid (μg/cm^2-48 hours)			% Dye	Receptor fluid (μg/cm^2-72 hours)
1.0	Disperse Black 9	0.42	0.04		4-Nitrophenylaminoethyl urea	0.25	0.04
1.0	HC Yellow No. 15	5.70	0.04		HC Blue No. 10	2.0	0.09
1.0	HC Yellow No. 4	2.23	0.12		HC Blue No. 9	1–2.0	0.10
1.5	HC Red No. 3	0.81	0.24		HC Violet No. 2	1–2.0	0.11
1.0	HC Yellow No. 2	0.27	1.36		HC Red No. 10/11 mixture	0.5–1	0.27
1.0	HC Red No. 14	0.71	1.47		Mixture[a]	2.0	0.36
1.0	HC Orange No. 1	0.44	1.49		HC Yellow No. 12	0.5	0.39
1.0	HC Red No. 1	0.37	1.57		2-Cl-5-nitro-hydroxyethyl PPD	2.0	1.14

Receptor fluid values for dye mixtures [calculated from data supplied by H. Beck (personal communication, 1996)].
[a] Mixture contained 1-amino-4-di(2-hydroxyethyl)-amino-2-nitrobenzene (76%) and HC Blue No. 2 (16%).
Abbreviation: PPD, *p*-phenylenediamine.
Source: From Refs. 16, 17, 21.

ranges shown here when data from experiments simulating actual human use are expressed on a μg/cm^2 basis (see Ref. 8 for details).

EXPOSURE ESTIMATION AND RISK ASSESSMENT

Integral to the risk assessment process is the determination of both the qualitative and the quantitative nature of the systemic exposure following application of (exposure to) the permeant of interest. As illustrated by the preceding data, dermal metabolism and, in the case of oxidative hair dyes, chemical complexation can influence the nature of the permeant and the extent of absorption. In the case of PPD and PAP, two primary intermediates used widely in hair dye formulations, dermal N-acetylation would result in exposure to the di- and mono-acetyl metabolites rather than the parent compounds. Therefore, the potential toxicities of the conversion products would be more relevant for risk assessment. This becomes increasingly important when toxicological data is obtained using a route of administration different than that for human exposure where the metabolism may also be different.

For oxidative dyes, exposure to the colored polymeric species formed on or in the skin needs to be considered. Available data, obtained by applying fixed concentrations of relatively high levels of preformed reaction products for the entire exposure period, indicate low levels (ng range) of availability. These data show interindividual variability characteristic of very poorly absorbed permeants.

Percutaneous absorption studies conducted using radiolabeled oxidative dye precursors provide data reflecting net exposure to precursor "equivalents." This may be adequate within chemical groupings, particularly to estimate exposure relative to well-studied benchmarks. For direct dyes, it may be useful to determine percutaneous absorption with individual compounds in order to provide more generalized information not restricted to a specific shade. Because of possible dye association by hydrogen bonding, this may overestimate exposures to the dye from formulated products that always contain a blend of colors to produce the desired shade.

Available in vivo and in vitro data on oxidative and direct dyes indicate that absorption occurs in a relatively narrow "dynamic range." This appears to be approximately 100-fold (e.g., 0.1–10 μg/cm^2) for the oxidative precursors and direct dyes and, for the combinations studied to date, in the ng/cm^2 range for dimeric and trimeric colored reaction products.

Traditional risk assessment employs uncertainty factors to account for both interspecies and intersubject variability (due to pharmacokinetic and pharmacodynamic factors). For threshold effects, factors of 10-fold are applied for each these variables resulting in a required safety factor of at least 100. Using the dynamic range of hair dye absorption described above, and no-observed-adverse-effect levels (NOAELs) of 10 to 100 mg/kg, representative of values seen with these types of materials, hypothetical safety margins are calculated in Table 9. For convenience, calculations are based on a scalp surface area of 700 cm^2 and a body weight of 70 kg. Under these assumptions calculated safety margins would range from 100 to 100,000 based on a single application and 30-fold higher considering once-a-month usage.

For materials such as the colored polymeric dimers and trimers showing absorption in the 0.01 to 0.001 μg/cm^2 range, each of the tabulated safety factors would be increased by one to two orders of magnitude assuming similar NOAELs.

TABLE 9   Hypothetical Safety Margins of a Range of Representative Cumulative Absorption Values for Hair Dyes and NOAELs

A	×	B	=	C	×	1/D	=	E	
								Safety margins	
Cumulative absorption, $\mu g/cm^2$		700 cm^2 scalp/70 kg BW		Estimated exposure (mg/kg/application)		NOAEL (mg/kg/day)		Single application	30-Day use
0.01				0.0001		10		100,000	3,000,000
				100		1,000,000		30,000,000	
0.1				0.001		10		10,000	300,000
				100		100,000		3,000,000	
1.0				0.01		10		1,000	30,000
				100		10,000		300,000	
10				0.1		10		100	3,000
				100		1,000		30,000	

Abbreviations: BW, body weight; NOAEL, no-observed adverse effect level.

In some circumstances, exposures may be below the Threshold for Toxicologic Concern (TTC) (22) employed for other types of risk assessment. The TTC is based on the premise that no discrete toxicological data are required to substantiate safety if exposure can be demonstrated to fall below predefined thresholds based on structural alerts. This may obviate the need for, or at least limit the scope of, further toxicological testing of certain of the polymeric compounds. Indeed, for certain hair dye materials that have produced carcinogenic effects in oral feeding studies conducted in rodents, calculations using accepted mathematical models assuming no threshold have indicated de minimus risk for exposures associated with hair dye use (see Ref. 8 for examples).

Exposure and risk assessments employ a series of conservative assumptions applied at each step in the calculations. Caution needs to be exercised so that the overall result is not overly conservative. In vitro percutaneous absorption experiments are often conducted at the highest proposed use levels, which may exceed levels in actual use. For direct dyes, more generalized studies conducted with single dyes may overestimate exposures from combinations of dyes actually used because of dye associations that may reduce mobility in the skin. Preformed oxidative dye precursor conversion products applied for the usual hair dye use period at relatively high concentrations (often needed to improve sensitivity in detecting low-level penetration) represent exaggerated exposures. Routine inclusion of amounts found in epidermal or dermal skin compartments may not be justified if supported by kinetic data showing limited skin mobility. At the least, the exposure estimation needs to consider the number of days over which incremental absorption occurs in the calculation of safety factors based on no-observed-adverse-effect levels expressed as mass (mg, μg, etc.)/kg body weight/day.

Percutaneous absorption studies with hair dyes tested at maximal use levels provide exposure estimates that reflect only the relatively small proportion (less than 10%) of the population using the darkest shades (black, dark brown). Particularly, for key primary intermediates used across the whole shade range including the lightest blondes, exposure may be substantially less for the majority of the exposed population.

Finally, dermal metabolic pathways may alter the permeant in a manner qualitatively or quantitatively different from alternate routes of administration (e.g., oral gavage) used for toxicological evaluations. It is therefore important that such differential metabolism be considered in overall safety assessment.

REFERENCES

1. Kalopissis G. Toxicology and hair dyes. In: Zivak C, ed. The Science of Hair Care. New York: Marcel Dekker, 1981:287–308.
2. Maibach HI, Wolfram LJ. Percutaneous penetration of hair dyes. J Soc Cosmet Chem 1981; 32:223–9.
3. Wolfram LJ, Maibach HI. Percutaneous penetration of hair dyes. Arch Dermatol Res 1985; 277:235–41.
4. Hueber-Becker F, Nohynek GJ, Meuling WJA, et al. Human systemic exposure to a ^{14}C-*para*-phenylenediamine-containing oxidative hair dye and correlation with in vitro percutaneous absorption in human or pig skin. Food Chem Toxicol 2004; 42:1227–36.
5. Goetz N, Lasserre P, Bore P, et al. Percutaneous absorption of *p*-phenylenediamine during actual hair dying procedure. Int J Cosmet Sci 1998; 10:63–73.
6. Keise M, Raucher E. The absorption of *p*-toluenediamine through human skin in hair dying. Toxicol Appl Pharmacol 1968; 12:495–507.
7. Corbett JF. Application of oxidative coupling reactions to the assay of *p*-phenylene-diamines and phenols. Anal Chem 1975; 47(2):308–13.
8. Dressler WE. Percutaneous absorption of hair dyes. In: Roberts MS, Walters KA, eds. Dermal Absorption and Toxicity Assessment. New York: Marcel Deckker, 1998:489–536.
9. Dressler WE. Hair dye absorption. In: Bronaugh RL, Maibach HI, eds. Percutaneous Absorption. 3rd ed. New York: Marcel Dekker, Inc., 1999:685–716.
10. Dressler WE, Appleqvist T. Plasma/blood pharmacokinetics and metabolism after dermal exposure to *para*-aminophenol or *para*-phenylenediamine. Food Chem Toxicol 2006; 44:371–9.
11. Walter-Sack I, Lucknow V, Guserle R, et al. Untersuchungen der relativen bioverfug-barkeit von paracetamol nach gabe von sformen. Arzneimittelforsch 1989; 39(1):719–42.
12. Nohynek GJ, Skare JA, Meuling WJA, et al. Urinary acetylated metabolites and N-acetyltransferase-2 genotype in human subjects treated with a *para*-phenylenedia-mine-containing oxidative hair dye. Food Chem Toxicol 2004; 42:1885–91.
13. Nohynek GJ, Duche D, Garrigues A, et al. Under the skin: biotransformation of *para*-aminophenol and *para*-phenylendiamine in reconstructed human epidermis and human hepatocytes. Toxicol Lett 2005; 158:196–212.
14. Beck H, Brain K, Dressler W, et al. An interlaboratory/interspecies comparison of the percutaneous penetration of ^{14}C-*p*-phenylenediamine (PPD) from a hair dye formu-lation, in vitro. In: Brain K, Walters K, eds. Perspectives in Percutaneous Penetration. Vol. 7a. Cardiff: STS Publishing, 2000:27.
15. Yourick JJ, Koenig ML, Yourick DL, et al. Fate of chemicals in the skin after dermal application: does the in vitro skin reservoir affect the estimate of systemic absorption. Toxicol Appl Pharmacol 2004; 195:309–20.
16. Beck H, Bracher M, Faller C, et al. Comparison of in vivo and in vitro skin permeation of hair dye. In: Scott RC, Guy RH, Hadgraft J et al, eds. Prediction of Percutaneous Penetration. Vol. 2. London: IBC Technical Services, 1991:441–50.
17. Beck H, Bracher M, Faller C, et al. Comparison of in vitro and in vivo skin permeation of hair dyes. Cosmet Toiletries 1993; 108:76–83.
18. Scientific Committee on Consumer Products. Basic criteria for the in vitro assessment of dermal absorption of cosmetic ingredients. SCCP/0970/06. (Adopted March 28, 2006 at http://europa.eu.int/comm/food/fs/sc/sccp/outcome_em.html)
19. Scientific Committee on Consumer Products. Opinion on exposure to reactants and reac-tion products of oxidative hair dye formulations. SCCP/0941/05. (Adopted December 13, 2005 at http://europa.eu.int/comm/food/fs/sc/sccp/outcome_em.html)

20. Scientific Committee on Consumer Products. Update of the annex to the opinion on exposure to reactants and reaction products of oxidative hair dye formulations (SCCP/ 0941/05). SCCP/1004/06. (Adopted June 20, 2006 at http://europa.eu.int/comm/food/ fs/sc/sccp/outcome_em.html)

21. Azri-Meehan S, Dressler WE, Grabarz R. Percutaneous penetration of semi-permanent (direct) hair dyes determined in vitro using human cadaver skin. Toxicologist 1996; 30:125.

22. Kroes R, Renwick AG, Cheeseman M, et al. Structure-based thresholds of toxicological concern (TTC): guidance to application to substances present at low levels in the diet. Food Chem Toxicol 2004; 42:65–83.

Dermal Absorption of Fragrance Materials

Keith R. Brain
An-eX Analytical Services, Ltd., and Cardiff University, Cardiff, U.K.

Jon Lalko
Research Institute for Fragrance Materials, Woodcliff Lake, New Jersey, U.S.A.

INTRODUCTION

The contents of this chapter are solely a consideration of dermal absorption of fragrance materials. It has been assumed that readers of this chapter will be well aware of the basics of skin permeation that are dealt with more than adequately elsewhere in this volume. Literature coverage has been focused on the scientific studies that are particularly relevant to consumer exposure to fragrance materials under in-use conditions.

According to the "Indicative Non-Exhaustive List," more than 2600 different materials have been reported to be used in the manufacture of fragrances (1), with annual volumes of use ranging from less than 1 kg to several thousand tons. Concentrations of fragrance materials in consumer products varies over five orders of magnitude, dependent on their function in the product and, although the largest volume of fragrance (~60%) is used in household products, such as soaps, detergents, and cleaners, these contain only relatively low levels of fragrance (2).

For over 30 years, the fragrance industry has adhered to a strict system of safety assurance. The Research Institute for Fragrance Materials (RIFM) was formed in 1966, as an independent nonprofit institute, charged with the task of obtaining and evaluating safety data on fragrance ingredients. Although fragrance chemicals have a long history of safe use, reevaluation of their safety is undertaken by RIFM to incorporate new data or usage patterns. Evaluations are based on a structurally related group approach with priorities being set based on volume of use, consumer exposure, and structural alerts for toxicity (2). RIFM maintains a comprehensive toxicological database of fragrance materials (3). Group safety evaluations are based on data gathered from both published and unpublished literature sources. In cases were data gaps exist RIFM conducts testing to fill those gaps. These data are evaluated by the RIFM Expert Panel (REXPAN), an independent, international group of scientists (4). The REXPAN includes experts in dermatology, pharmacokinetics, toxicokinetics, toxicology, pathology, and environmental science. Additional expertise is added to REXPAN by including adjunct members as necessary. REXPAN's findings and conclusions are published in peer-reviewed journals. This process results in transparent and well-documented conclusions that are provided to the International Fragrance Association (IFRA) for the purpose of human health risk management. IFRA publishes fragrance material standards that govern the use of fragrance materials (i.e., place use restrictions, set quality specifications, etc.).

Despite the use of fragrance materials for their olfactory properties, deposition on the skin is the primary route of exposure with the greatest coming from alcohol-based products (5). When assessing a fragrance ingredient, it is initially assumed that 100% of the material remaining on the skin is absorbed into the systemic circulation. In most cases the actual "in use" exposure scenario results in less absorption, though the extent of absorption is very much dependent on a variety of factors including evaporation, product matrix, application site, and degree of occlusion. For systemic effects, a refined assessment is often warranted based on this in use exposure. For this purpose, in vitro or in vivo studies may be required. The effect of skin penetration and disposition on local dermal effects, such as contact sensitization, is a complex topic and an area of considerable research and debate (6). Currently, Quantitative Risk Assessments for dermal sensitization seek to account for this variability by applying sensitization assessment factors (analogous to the safety assessment factors of traditional toxicology) (7).

Accurate estimation of dermal exposure to fragrance chemicals requires consideration of a number of factors (5). The quantity of product applied and the percentage of fragrance in the product, together with the retention factor (low for wash off products), gives the quantity of fragrance remaining on the skin. The type of product will define the total body area which is exposed, hence allowing calculation of the acute dose of fragrance applied per unit area.

During skin permeation of volatile materials, such as solvents and fragrances, there can often be considerable competition between partition of the permeant into the skin and evaporation from the skin, with air flow as an important factor. A linear relationship was reported between the amount of benzyl acetate applied to rat skin in vitro under occluded conditions (1660–33,130 $\mu g/cm^2$) and amount permeated at 24 hours (660 $\pm$ 40–10,270 $\pm$ 510 $\mu g/cm^2$) (8). When benzyl alcohol was applied unoccluded at nine dose levels (0.9–10,600 $\mu g/cm^2$) to human cadaver skin in vitro in a fume hood (9), penetration at 24 hours was found to increase with dose slowly, from 19.8 $\pm$ 2.9% to 29.2 $\pm$ 3.0%, with less than 4% of applied dose remaining on the surface, due to evaporation. It is common practice to attach absorptive traps above the donor chambers to retain evaporating material, improving mass balance (10). However, the presence of such traps can produce significant occlusion which has a very marked effect on skin permeation (11,12). In addition, trap absorption of the volatile material may be affected by competitive absorption of water vapor so that initially trapped material is subsequently lost. Less occlusive traps often use high skin surface air flow, leading to evaporative loss which is unrepresentative of actual exposure conditions. Experimental conditions should alter the evaporation as little as possible compared to in-use unoccluded conditions (13).

Mathematical approaches to modeling permeation and evaporation of volatile chemicals applied to skin have been developed (14–16) and are reviewed by Kasting (17). It is claimed that the method allows estimation of percentage absorption and absorption rate to within a factor of two for commonly encountered fragrance materials although the dataset used to validate this model to date is still limited in scope. An alternative approach is to include a procedure for the real time simultaneous determination of evaporative loss under the actual experimental conditions (7,18).

Rats have routinely been used for acute and chronic dermal toxicity studies. While such studies give useful basic data, they do not produce data directly relevant to in-use consumer exposure. In addition, unpredictable and substantial differences in not only absorption but also metabolism of fragrance materials have been reported.

A comparison between dermal absorption of cinnamic acid, cinnamyl alcohol, cinnamyl anthranilate, and safrole through monkey skin in vivo and human skin in vitro was reported (19). Under unoccluded conditions, permeation of cinnamic acid was significantly lower (17.8±4.9%) than through monkey skin (38.6±8.3%), but there was no significant difference for cinnamic alcohol or cinnamyl anthranilate. Comparison of skin absorption of diethyl maleate under occluded conditions in monkeys and humans gave similar data (69% and 54% at 24 hours, respectively; 20) and it was concluded that the monkey was a good model for human skin penetration. Further comparison of absorption of six benzyl derivatives (benzamide, benzoin, benzophenone, benzyl acetate, benzyl alcohol, and benzyl benzoate) in the monkey under occluded conditions showed similar absorption for all (~70% at 24 hours) and no correlation between skin penetration and octanol–water partition coefficient. However, under unoccluded conditions there was great variability between compounds that was attrributed to differences in volatility of the compounds.

It has long been known that the application vehicle can have a very significant influence on both peneration into and permeation through the skin (21). In vitro comparison of N,N-diethyl-m-toluamide (DEET) absorption from commercial formulations using human skin (22) showed that the total amount permeated was higher from 30% to 45% ethanolic solutions than from 60% to 90% ethanolic solutions or pure DEET. Jacobi et al. (23) studied absorption of vanillin into human skin in vivo from ethanol and oil in water emulsion vehicles using tape stripping and found that different amounts of tissue were removed per tape strip, demonstrating that the vehicle affected cohesion. Comparison of absorption of diethanolamine through human skin in vitro showed large differences in permeation and distribution from five representative cosmetic vehicles (24). Lalko et al. (25) demonstrated that the application vehicle had a marked effect on skin-sensitizing potential of allergens in the murine local lymph node assay. Politano et al. (26) studied the effects of three vehicles (diethyl phthalate, 3:1 diethyl phthalate:ethanol, and 1:3 diethyl phthalate:ethanol) on the human dermal irritation of a series of allyl esters and demonstrated a trend for lower concentration thresholds for irritation induction with increasing ethanol concentration.

The penetration enhancing effect of many terpenes moderated through disturbance of lipid organization is well-known and, particularly where fragrance materials are used at high levels, the potential exists for them to modulate the skin absorption of other molecules. Nielsen (27) reported in vitro data demonstrating that eucalyptus oil, tea tree oil, and peppermint oil, applied at concentrations of 0.1%, 1.0%, or 5.0%, modified the barrier function of human skin, assessed using permeation of tritiated water and benzoic acid, dose dependently. In a further study, Nielsen and Nielsen (28) showed that tea tree oil also modified the dermal uptake of the pesticide methiocarb.

DATA ON SPECIFIC FRAGRANCE MATERIALS

Information is presented below on materials of particular interest where robust literature data on percutaneous absorption exists.

Acetyl Cedrene

The dermal penetration of acetyl cedrene was reported from an in vitro study under unoccluded conditions. Briefly, 12 active dosed diffusion cells (Franz-type) were prepared plus two control cells. Epidermal membranes were used and their integrity was assessed by measuring the permeation rate of tritiated water over a period of one hour. Permeation of acetyl cedrene, from a 20 μL/cm^2 target dose of a 1% (w/v) solution in ethanol, was then measured at five time-points over 48 hours. At 48 hours, the epidermal membranes were wiped, tape stripped 10 times and the acetyl cedrene content of the wipes, strips, and remaining epidermis determined. The filter paper skin supports were extracted and the diffusion cell donor chambers washed and wiped. Potential evaporative loss of acetyl cedrene was estimated by measuring the loss from polytetrafluoroethylene (PTFE) sheets under the same experimental conditions. Following 48 hours of exposure, 22.65 ± 8.01 μg/cm^2 acetyl cedrene corresponding to $11.33 \pm 1.15\%$ of the applied dose had permeated. Overall recovery, including all compartments, of the applied acetyl cedrene at 48 hours was $68.1 \pm 1.7\%$. Evaporative loss was measured from the PTFE sheets to be 13% of the applied dose at 48 hours (29).

Acetyl Eugenol

Penetration of acetyl eugenol through human epidermal membranes, in vitro under occlusion, at infinite dose was reported as $0.175 \pm 0.056\%$ at 72 hours (30).

α-Amylcinnamic Alcohol

Penetration of α-amylcinnamic alcohol through human epidermal membranes, in vitro under occlusion, at infinite dose was first reported as $0.012 \pm 0.002\%$ at 72 hours (30).

α-Amylcinnamaldehyde

Penetration of α-amylcinnamaldehyde through human epidermal membranes, in vitro under occlusion, at infinite dose was reported as $0.002 \pm 0.001\%$ at 72 hours (30).

7-Acetyl-1,1,3,4,4,6-Hexamethyl-1,2,3,4-Tetrahydronaphthalene

Dermal studies in rats using alcoholic solutions under occlusion for six hours showed a total absorptions of ~19% for 7-acetyl-1,1,3,4,4,6-hexamethyl-1,2,3,4-tetrahydronaphthalene (AHTN) (31). However, human in vivo data using a alcoholic solution modeling a typical cologne product showed that the total absorbed dose was only ~1.0% for AHTN. Furthermore, over the 5-day experimental time period 14.5% was recovered from dressings over the application site indicating that material initially penetrating the skin was lost by desorption and/or desquamation before systemic uptake. In vitro human permeation rate and distribution of AHTN was determined after application in ethanol under in-use non-occlusive conditions to epidermal membranes (32). At 24 hours, $0.379 \pm 0.060\%$ of the applied AHTN had permeated. Overall recovery was $92.5 \pm 0.7\%$. Levels of fragrance material in the epidermis (plus any remaining stratum corneum after removal of 10 surface tape strips), filter paper skin support, and receptor fluid were combined to produce total absorbed doses of $4.06 \pm 0.38\%$.

Benzyl Acetate
Penetration of benzyl acetate through human epidermal membranes, in vitro under occlusion, at infinite dose was reported as $1.276 \pm 0.227\%$ at 72 hours (30).

Benzyl Benzoate
Penetration of benzyl acetate through human epidermal membranes, in vitro under occlusion, at infinite dose was reported as $0.018 \pm 0.002\%$ at 72 hours (30).

Benzyl Propionate
Penetration of benzyl propionate through human epidermal membranes, in vitro under occlusion, at infinite dose was reported as $0.392 \pm 0.036\%$ at 72 hours (30).

Benzyl Salicylate
Penetration of benzyl salicylate through human epidermal membranes, in vitro under occlusion, at infinite dose was reported as $0.031 \pm 0.004\%$ at 72 hours (30). In another in vitro study, a single application of $12\ \mu L/cm^2$ radiolabeled benzyl salicylate was applied to a $5\ cm^2$ area of excised naked rat skin. The material was applied as either 1%, 3%, or 10% in ethanol. Radioactivity was measured in skin washings, skin strippings, the skin itself and the receptor fluid. At 24 hours for the 1% dose group, 27.7% of the applied dose was found in skin wash, 0.4% in skin stripping, 9.3% in stripped skin, and 62.7% in receptor fluid at 24 hours. For the 3% dose group, 27.5% in skin wash, 1.6% in skin stripping, 12.0% in stripped skin, and 58.8% in receptor fluid. For the 10% dose group, 38.0% in skin wash, 4.0% in skin stripping, 17.7% in stripped skin, and 40.3% in receptor fluid (33).

Benzyl Derivatives—Comparative Absorption
Comparison of absorption of benzamide, benzoin, benzophenone, benzyl acetate, benzyl alcohol, and benzyl benzoate in the monkey under occluded conditions showed similar absorption for all ($\sim 70\%$ at 24 hours) with no correlation between skin penetration and octanol–water partition coefficient. Under unoccluded conditions there was great variability between compounds, which was attrributed to volatility differences (20). Absorption of neat benzyl acetate and benzyl acetate in ethanol through occluded rat skin was $\sim 49\%$ after 48 hours. Permeation of benzyl acetate from phenylethanol:benzyl acetate of 1:1 was $56.3 \pm 4.9\%$ and from dimethyl sulfoxide:benzyl acetate of 1:1 was $59.3 \pm 3.7\%$ (34). Penetration of benzyl acetate through rat and human skin was evaluated in vitro following application of neat benzyl acetate ($33.1\ mg/cm^2$) and occlusion (35). Absorption through rat skin was rapid and extensive ($34.3 \pm 3.9\%$ of dose at 24 hours and $55.8 \pm 5.0\%$ of dose at 72 hours). Absorption was significantly ($P < 0.05$) less rapid and extensive through human skin ($5.5 \pm 0.1\%$ of dose and $17.8 \pm 3.3\%$ of dose at 72 hours).

Cinnamic Acid
Percutaneous absorption of cinnamic acid in the rhesus monkey, from $4\ \mu g/cm^2$ [14C]-cinnamic acid in acetone was $38.6 \pm 8.3\%$ absorption from non-occluded skin and $83.9 \pm 2.7\%$ from occluded skin (36). In vitro absorption of cinnamic acid

through human skin was studied in vitro. The amount of cinnamic acid absorbed was $17.8 \pm 4.9\%$ for non-occluded and $60.8 \pm 10.2\%$ for occluded skin (36).

Cinnamic Alcohol
In an in vivo study using monkeys, in which the active was applied in acetone $25.4 \pm 4.4\%$ and $74.6 \pm 7.2\%$ was absorbed under unoccluded and occluded conditions, respectively (36). Data obtained in vitro using human skin (36) produced comparable data ($33.9 \pm 7.3\%$ and $65.9 \pm 7.9\%$ under unoccluded and occluded conditions, respectively). A more recent in vitro study under occlusion using conditions designed to maintain enzyme activity (37) reported that only 1.9% of the applied dose permeated with a further 3.5% recovered within the skin. Furthermore, significant amounts of the recovery within the skin and receptor medium was as cinnamic acid.

Cinnamaldehyde
Penetration of cinnamaldehyde through human epidermal membranes, in vitro under occlusion, at infinite dose was reported as $0.175 \pm 0.056\%$ at 72 hours (30). In vitro penetration from 200 mg/mL cinnamaldehyde in ethanol through full-thickness human skin was studied by Weibel and Hansen (38) who found that cinnamyl alcohol and cinnamic acid were present in the receptor phase in higher concentrations than cinnamaldehyde. In fresh human skin samples, 52% of the label from radiolabeled cinnamaldehyde was absorbed under occlusion but only 24% under unoccluded conditions (8,34). Full-thickness fresh skin sample were placed under conditions designed to maintain enzyme activity and 10 µL neat cinnamaldehyde applied (37). After 24 hours, the receptor phase contained 9.4% of the dose (2.6% cinnamaldehyde, 2.4% cinnamyl alcohol, and 4.4% cinnamic acid), the skin contained 6.6% of the dose (3.3% cinnamaldehyde, 0.4% cinnamyl alcohol, and 2.9% cinnamic acid) and 65.9% of the dose was recovered as unabsorbed cinnamic compounds (55.3% cinnamaldehyde and 10.6% cinnamic acid).

Coumarin
Absorption of coumarin from oil in water emulsion and ethanol vehicles through human and rat skin in vitro under conditions designed to maintain enzyme activity (39) showed that skin absorption was greater from the emulsion vehicle in both cases ($86.8 \pm 5.4\%$ vs. $54.9 \pm 0.63\%$ and $98.0 \pm 5.3\%$ vs. $64.4 \pm 0.29\%$ for rat and human, respectively). No evidence of metabolism was found. In vivo dermal absorption and metabolism of coumarin applied in 70% aqueous ethanol in rats and humans (40) showed rapid permeation with total absorption of 72% and 60%, respectively. In human subjects, coumarin was mainly metabolized to glucuronide and sulfate conjugates, whereas numerous unidentified metabolites were found in rat studies, demonstrating that rat metabolism data could not be extrapolated to humans.

Diphenyl Ether
Penetration of diphenyl ether through rat skin, in vitro under both occluded and unoccluded conditions was reported to be 0.3% of the applied dose at 72 hours (41). In a human in vitro study, it was reported that at 72 hours 0.2% of the applied dose had been absorbed under both occluded and unoccluded conditions (41).

Estragole

The dermal penetration of estragole was reported from an in vitro study under unoccluded conditions. Briefly, 12 active dosed diffusion cells (Franz-type) were prepared plus two control cells. Epidermal membranes were used and their integrity was assessed by measuring the permeation rate of tritiated water over a period of one hour. Permeation of estragole, from a 20 $\mu L/cm^2$ target dose of a 1% (w/v) solution in ethanol, was then measured at five time-points over 48 hours. At 48 hours, the epidermal membranes were wiped, tape stripped 10 times and the estragole content of the wipes, strips, and remaining epidermis determined. The filter paper skin supports were extracted and the diffusion cell donor chambers washed and wiped. Potential evaporative loss of estragole was estimated by measuring the loss from PTFE sheets under the same experimental conditions. Following 48 hours of exposure, 32.74 ± 3.10 $\mu g/cm^2$ estragole corresponding to $16.34 \pm 1.56\%$ of the applied dose had permeated. Overall recovery, including all compartments, of the applied estragole at 48 hours was $22.4 \pm 1.3\%$. Evaporative loss was high, as measured from the PTFE sheets to be 93.7% of the applied dose at 48 hours (29).

Eugenol

Penetration of eugenol through human epidermal membranes, in vitro under occlusion, at infinite dose was as $1.653 \pm 0.201\%$ at 72 hours (30). In fresh human skin samples 40% of the label from radiolabeled eugenol was absorbed in vitro under occlusion but only 34% under unoccluded conditions (8,34).

Eugenyl Acetate

Penetration of acetyl eugenol through human epidermal membranes, in vitro under occlusion, at infinite dose was $0.175 \pm 0.056\%$ at 72 hours (30).

Geranyl Nitrile

The dermal penetration of geranyl nitrile was reported from an in vitro study under unoccluded conditions. Briefly, 12 active dosed diffusion cells were prepared (using four donors) plus three control cells. Epidermal membranes were used and their integrity was assessed by measuring the permeation rate of tritiated water over a period of one hour. Permeation of geranyl nitrile, from a 5 $\mu L/cm^2$ target dose of a 1% (w/v) solution in 70/30 (v/v) ethanol/water, was then measured at 12 time-points over 24 hours, using a 6% buffered saline receptor phase. At 24 hours, the epidermal membranes were wiped, tape stripped 10 times and the geranyl nitrile content of the wipes, strips, and remaining epidermis determined. The filter paper skin supports were extracted and the diffusion cell donor chambers washed and wiped. Analysis of these samples allowed mass balance to be performed. Potential evaporative loss of geranyl nitrile was estimated by measuring the loss from PTFE sheets under the same experimental conditions. Following 24 hours of exposure, 1.89 ± 0.15 $\mu g/cm^2$ geranyl nitrile corresponding to $3.74 \pm 0.30\%$ of the applied dose had permeated. Following rapid initial permeation, the rate began to plateau due to rapid depletion of the donor phase through evaporation. The 24 hours surface wipe and donor chamber wash/wipe contained $6.23 \pm 0.16\%$ and $1.84 \pm 0.22\%$ of the applied dose, respectively. The stratum corneum tape strips contained $1.33 \pm 0.16\%$ of the applied dose and the epidermis, plus any remaining stratum corneum after tape stripping, contained $0.416 \pm 0.050\%$ of the applied dose. Overall recovery of the applied geranyl nitrile at 24 hours was low at $14.1 \pm 0.4\%$ due to evaporation of superficial geranyl nitrile (18).

α-Hexylcinnamaldehyde
Penetration of α-hexylcinnamaldehyde through human epidermal membranes, in vitro under occlusion, at infinite dose was 0.002% at 72 hours (30).

1,3,4,6,7,8-Hexahydro-4,6,6,7,8,8-Hexamethyl Cyclopenta-γ-2-Benzopyran
Dermal studies in rats using alcoholic solutions under occlusion for six hours showed total absorption of 14% for 1,3,4,6,7,8-hexahydro-4,6,6,7,8,8-hexamethyl cyclopenta-γ-2-benzopyran (HHCB) (31). However, human in vivo data using a alcoholic solution modeling a typical cologne product showed that the total absorbed dose was only 0.1% HHCB. Furthermore, over the 5-day experimental time period 19.5% of HHCB was recovered from dressings over the application site indicating that material initially penetrating the skin was lost by desorption and/or desquamation before systemic uptake. In vitro human permeation rate and distribution of HHCB was determined after application in ethanol under in-use non-occlusive conditions to epidermal membranes (42). At 24 hours, $0.397 \pm 0.057\%$ of the applied HHCB had permeated. Overall recovery was $92.1 \pm 0.8\%$. Levels of fragrance materials in the epidermis (plus any remaining stratum corneum after removal of 10 surface tape strips), filter paper skin support and receptor fluid were combined to produce total absorbed doses of $5.16 \pm 0.59\%$.

Isoamyl Salicylate
Penetration of isoamyl salicylate through human epidermal membranes, in vitro under occlusion, at infinite dose was $0.008 \pm 0.001\%$ at 72 hours (30).

Isoeugenol
Penetration of isoeugenol through human epidermal membranes, in vitro under occlusion, at infinite dose was $0.489 \pm 0.029\%$ at 72 hours (30).

Isoeugenol Methyl Ether
Penetration of isoeugenol methyl ether through human epidermal membranes, in vitro under occlusion, at infinite dose was $0.327 \pm 0.021\%$. at 72 hours (30).

D-Limonene
Penetration of D-Limonene through rat skin, in vitro under both occluded and unoccluded conditions was reported to be 6% of the applied dose at 72 hours (41). In a human in vitro study, it was reported that at 72 hours 3% of the applied dose had been absorbed under occluded conditions and 5% under unoccluded conditions (41).

Linalool
Blood levels of linalool and linalyl acetate were followed in a human subject for 90 minutes after the use of massage oil which contained lavender oil (containing 24.79% linalool and 29.59% linalyl acetate) and peanut oil in a 2:98 ratio. Linalool

and linalyl acetate were absorbed quickly and trace amounts were detected in the blood five minutes after finishing the massage. Mean plasma concentrations were 100 and 121 mg/mL and biological half-lives 13.76 and 14.3, respectively, (43).

2-Methoxy-4-Propylphenol
Penetration of 2-methoxy-4-propylphenol through human epidermal membranes, in vitro under occlusion, at infinite dose was $1.364 \pm 0.109\%$ at 72 hours (30).

Methyl Atrarate
The dermal penetration of methyl atrarate was reported from an in vitro study under unoccluded conditions. Briefly, 12 active dosed diffusion cells (Franz-type) were prepared plus two control cells. Epidermal membranes were used and their integrity was assessed by measuring the permeation rate of tritiated water over a period of one hour. Permeation of methyl atrarate, from a 20 $\mu L/cm^2$ target dose of a 1% (w/v) solution in ethanol, was then measured at five time-points over 48 hours. At 48 hours, the epidermal membranes were wiped, tape stripped 10 times and the methyl atrarate content of the wipes, strips, and remaining epidermis determined. The filter paper skin supports were extracted and the diffusion cell donor chambers washed and wiped. Potential evaporative loss of methyl atrarate was estimated by measuring the loss from PTFE sheets under the same experimental conditions. Following 48 hours of exposure, 40.53 ± 4.80 $\mu g/cm^2$ methyl atrarate corresponding to $20.29 \pm 2.42\%$ of the applied dose had permeated. Overall recovery, including all compartments, of the applied methyl atrarate at 48 hours was $94.7 \pm 0.6\%$. Evaporative loss was low, as measured from the PTFE sheets to be -4% of the applied dose at 48 hours (44).

α-Methylcinnamaldehyde
Penetration of α-Methylcinnamaldehyde through human epidermal membranes, in vitro under occlusion, at infinite dose was $0.149 \pm 0.016\%$ at 72 hours (30).

Methyl Eugenol
Penetration of methyl eugenol through human epidermal membranes, in vitro under occlusion, at infinite dose was $0.511 \pm 0.038\%$ at 72 hours (30). In another study, the dermal penetration of methyl eugenol was reported from an in vitro study under unoccluded conditions. Briefly, 12 active dosed diffusion cells (Franz-type) were prepared plus two control cells. Epidermal membranes were used and their integrity was assessed by measuring the permeation rate of tritiated water over a period of one hour. Permeation of methyl eugenol, from a 20 $\mu L/cm^2$ target dose of 1% (w/v) solution in ethanol, was then measured at five time-points over 48 hours. At 48 hours, the epidermal membranes were wiped, tape stripped 10 times, and the methyl eugenol content of the wipes, strips, and remaining epidermis determined. The filter paper skin supports were extracted and the diffusion cell donor chambers washed and wiped. Potential evaporative loss of estragole was estimated by measuring the loss from PTFE sheets under the same experimental conditions. Following 48 hours of exposure, 6.93 ± 4.87 $\mu g/cm^2$ methyl eugenol corresponding to $33.59 \pm 2.32\%$ of the applied dose had permeated. Overall recovery, including all compartments, of the applied methyl eugenol at

48 hours was $35.9 \pm 2.3\%$. Evaporative loss was high, as measured from the PTFE sheets to be 98.1% of the applied dose at 48 hours (29).

Methyl Dihydrojasmonate

The dermal penetration of methyl dihydrojasmonate was reported from an in vitro study under unoccluded conditions. Briefly, 12 active dosed diffusion cells (Franz-type) were prepared plus two control cells. Epidermal membranes were used and their integrity was assessed by measuring the permeation rate of tritiated water over a period of one hour. Permeation of methyl dihydrojasmonate, from 20 µL/cm^2 target dose of 1% (w/v) solution in ethanol, was then measured at five time-points over 48 hours. At 48 hours, the epidermal membranes were wiped, tape stripped 10 times and the methyl dihydrojasmonate content of the wipes, strips, and remaining epidermis determined. The filter paper skin supports were extracted and the diffusion cell donor chambers washed and wiped. Potential evaporative loss of methyl dihydrojasmonate was estimated by measuring the loss from PTFE sheets under the same experimental conditions. Following 48 hours of exposure, 92.17 ± 7.34 µg/cm^2 methyl dihydrojasmonate corresponding to $45.93 \pm 3.48\%$ of the applied dose had permeated. Overall recovery, including all compartments, of the applied methyl dihydrojasmonate at 48 hours was $94.7 \pm 0.6\%$. Evaporative loss was low, as measured from the PTFE sheets to be 86% of the applied dose at 48 hours (44).

α-Methyl-1,3-Benzodioxole-5-Propionaldehyde

The dermal penetration of α-methyl-1,3-benzodioxole-5-propionaldehyde (MMDHCA) was reported from an in vitro study under unoccluded conditions. Briefly, 12 active dosed diffusion cells (Franz-type) were prepared plus two control cells. Epidermal membranes were used and their integrity was assessed by measuring the permeation rate of tritiated water over a period of one hour. Permeation of MMDHCA, from a 20 µL/cm^2 target dose of a 1% (w/v) solution in ethanol, was then measured at five time-points over 48 hours. At 48 hours, the epidermal membranes were wiped, tape stripped 10 times and the methyl atrarate content of the wipes, strips, and remaining epidermis determined. The filter paper skin supports were extracted and the diffusion cell donor chambers washed and wiped. Potential evaporative loss of MMDHCA was estimated by measuring the loss from PTFE sheets under the same experimental conditions. Following 48 hours of exposure, 98.72 ± 5.78 µg/cm^2 methyl atrarate corresponding to $50.08 \pm 3.21\%$ of the applied dose had permeated. Overall recovery, including all compartments, of the applied MMDHCA at 48 hours was $94.7 \pm 0.6\%$. Evaporative loss was low, as measured from the PTFE sheets to be 19% of the applied dose at 48 hours (7,44).

Musk Ambrette

Due to both its photosenitization and neurotoxic potential, musk ambrette is no longer used as a fragrance ingredient (45). For comparative purposes, the availiable skin absorption data are included here. In vivo dermal absorption of musk ambrette in rats (46) at a dose of 11 µg/cm^2 showed absorption of ~40%. However, in vivo dermal absorption and disposition of musk ambrette in human subjects at a nominal dose of 10 to 20 µg/cm^2 (47) showed only 2.0% based on amounts excreted in the urine and feces over five days. Excretion was mainly as glucuronide conjugates, but these differed between rat and human subjects.

Musk Ketone

In vivo dermal absorption of musk ketone in rats (46) at a dose of 11 µg/cm^2 showed absorption of 31%. However, in vivo dermal absorption and disposition of musk ketone in human subjects at a nominal dose of 10 to 20 µg/cm^2 (47) showed only 0.5% was absorbed, based on amounts excreted in the urine and feces over five days. Excretion was mainly as glucuronide conjugates, but these differed between rat and human subjects.

Musk Xylene

In vivo dermal absorption of musk xylene in rats (46) at a dose of 11 µg/cm^2 showed absorption of 19%. However, in vivo dermal absorption and disposition of musk xylene in human subjects at a nominal dose of 10 to 20 µg/cm^2 (47) showed only 0.3%, based on amounts excreted in the urine and feces over five days. Excretion was mainly as glucuronide conjugates, but these differed between rat and human subjects. In vitro percutaneous absorption of musk xylene through human and guinea pig skin from two vehicles was reported (48). While total absorption from oil in water emulsion and methanol through guinea pig skin differed (55% and 45%, respectively) from human skin produced equivalent absorption (22%) from both vehicles.

1-(1,2,3,4,5,6,7,8-Octahydro-2,3,8,8-Tetramethyl-2-Naphthyl)Ethan-1-One

The dermal penetration of 1-(1,2,3,4,5,6,7,8-octahydro-2,3,8,8-tetramethyl-2-naphthyl)ethan-1-one (OTNE) was reported from an in vitro study under unoccluded conditions. Briefly, 12 active dosed diffusion cells (Franz-type) were prepared plus two control cells. Epidermal membranes were used and their integrity was assessed by measuring the permeation rate of tritiated water over a period of one hour. Permeation of OTNE, from 20 µL/cm^2 target dose of 1% (w/v) solution in ethanol, was then measured at five time-points over 48 hours. At 48 hours, the epidermal membranes were wiped, tape stripped 10 times and the OTNE content of the wipes, strips, and remaining epidermis determined. The filter paper skin supports were extracted and the diffusion cell donor chambers washed and wiped. Potential evaporative loss of geranyl nitrile was estimated by measuring the loss from PTFE sheets under the same experimental conditions. Following 48 hours of exposure, 8.08 ± 2.33 µg/cm^2 OTNE corresponding to 15.9 ± 1.19% of the applied dose had permeated. Overall recovery, including all compartments, of the applied OTNE at 48 hours was 53.3 ± 1.4%. Evaporative loss was measured from the PTFE sheets to be 43% of the applied dose at 48 hours (29).

2-Phenoxyethyl Isobutyrate

Penetration of 2-Phenoxyethyl isobutyrate through rat skin, in vitro under both occluded and unoccluded conditions was reported to be 46% of the applied dose at 72 hours under occlusive conditions and 41% unoccluded (41). In a human in vitro study, it was reported that at 72 hours 5% of the applied dose had been absorbed under both occluded and unocculded conditions (41).

Tea Tree Oil

An in vitro study using human epidermal membranes compared permeation of terpinen-4-ol (the main component of tea tree oil) from infinite doses of several formulations (39). Flux was highest from neat tea tree oil (0.262 ± 0.019 µL/cm^2), followed by the semisolid O/W emulsion (0.067 ± 0.001 µL/cm^2), ointment (0.051 ± 0.002 µL/cm^2), and cream (0.022 ± 0.001 µL/cm^2).

REFERENCES

1. European Commission, Commission Decision of 8 May 1996 establishing an inventory and a common nomenclature of ingredients employed in cosmetic products. Section II. Perfume and Aromatic Raw Materials. Directive 96/335/EC. Official J Eur Communities 1996; 39:526–679.
2. Ford RA, Domeyer B, Easterday O, Maier K, Middleton J. Criteria for development of a database for safety evaluation of fragrance ingredients. Regul Toxicol Pharmacol 2000; 31:166–81.
3. RIFM (Research Institute for Fragrance Materials Inc.) The Research Institute for Fragrance Materials - About Us. (Accessed October 1, 2007 at http://www.rifm.org/about.asp).
4. Bickers D, Calow P, Greim H, et al. A toxicologic and dermatologic assessment of linalool and related esters when used as fragrance ingredients. Food Chem Toxicol 2003; 41:919–42.
5. Cadby PA, Troy WR, Vey MG. Consumer exposure to fragrance ingredients: providing estimates for safety evaluation. Regul Toxicol Pharmacol 2002; 36:246–52.
6. Basketter D, Pease C, Kasting G, et al. Skin sensitisation and epidermal disposition: the relevance of epidermal disposition for sensitisation hazard identification and risk assessment. ATLA 2007; 35:137–54.
7. Api AM, Lapczynski A, Isola DA, Glenn Sipes I. In vitro penetration and subchronic toxicity of alpha-methyl-1,3-benzodioxole-5-propionaldehyde. Food Chem Toxicol 2007; 45:702–7.
8. Hotchkiss SA, Chidgey MA, Rose S, Caldwell J. Percutaneous absorption of benzyl acetate through rat skin in vitro. 1. Validation of an in vitro model against in vivo data. Food Chem Toxicol 1990; 28:443–7.
9. Miller MA, Bhatt V, Kasting GB. Dose and airflow dependence of benzyl alcohol disposition on skin. J Pharm Sci 2006; 95:281–91.
10. Reifenrath WG, Robinson PB. In vitro skin evaporation and penetration characteristics of mosquito repellents. J Pharm Sci 1982; 71:1014–8.
11. Frantz SW, Ballantyne B, Beskitt JL, Tallant MJ, Greco R. Pharmacokinetics of 2-ethyl-1, 3-hexanediol III in vitro skin penetration comparisons using the excised skin of humans, rats and rabbits. Fundam Appl Toxicol 1995; 28:1–8.
12. Lockley DJ, Howes D, Williams FM. Percutaneous penetration and metabolism of 2-ethoxyethanol. Toxicol Appl Pharmacol 2002; 180:74–82.
13. Yourick JJ, Hood HL, Bronaugh RL. Percutaneous absorption of fragrances. In: Bronaugh RL, Maibach HI, eds. Percutaneous Absorption. 3rd ed. New York: Marcel Dekker, 1999:673–84.
14. Saiyasombati P, Kasting GB. Disposition of benzyl alcohol after topical application to human skin in vitro. J Pharm Sci 2003; 92:2128–39.
15. Saiyasombati P, Kasting GB. Disposition of benzyl alcohol after topical application to human skin in vitro. J Pharm Sci 2003; 92(12):2534.
16. Saiyasombati P, Kasting GB. In vivo evaporation rate of benzyl alcohol from human skin. J Pharm Sci 2004; 93:515–20.
17. Kasting GB. Estimating the absorption of volatile compounds applied to skin. In: Riviere JE, ed. Dermal Absorption Models in Toxicology and Pharmacology. Boca Raton: Taylor & Francis, 2005:177–90.
18. Brain KR, Green DM, Lalko J, Api AM. In-vitro human skin penetration of the fragrance material geranyl nitrile. Toxicol In Vitro 2007; 21:133–8.

19. Bronaugh RL, Stewart RF, Wester RC, Bucks D, Mailbach HI, Anderson J. Comparison of percutaneous absorption of fragrances by humans and monkeys. Food Chem Toxicol 1985; 23:111–4.
20. Bronaugh RL, Wester RC, Bucks D, Maibach HI, Sarason R. In vivo percutaneous absorption of fragrance ingredients in rhesus monkeys and humans. Food Chem Toxicol 1990; 28:369–73.
21. Bronaugh RL, Franz TJ. Vehicle effects on percutaneous absorption: in vivo and in vitro comparisons with human skin. Br J Dermatol 1986; 115:1–11.
22. Stinecipher J, Shah J. Percutaneous permeation of N,N-diethyl-m-toluamide (DEET) from commercial mosquito repellents and the effect of solvent. J Toxicol Environ Health 1997; 52:119–35.
23. Jacobi U, Meykadeh N, Sterry W, Lademann J. Effect of the vehicle on the amount of stratum corneum removed by tape stripping. J Dtsch Dermatol Ges 2003; 1:884–9.
24. Brain KR, Walters KA, Green DM, et al. Percutaneous penetration of diethanolamine through human skin in vitro: application from cosmetic vehicles. Food Chem Toxicol 2005; 43:681–90.
25. Lalko J, Isola D, Api AM. Ethanol and diethyl phthalate: vehicle effects in the local lymph node assay. Int J Toxicol 2004; 23:171–7.
26. Politano VT, Isola DA, Lalko J, Api AM. The effects of vehicles on the human dermal irritation potentials of allyl esters. Int J Toxicol 2006; 25:183–93.
27. Nielsen JB. Natural oils affect the human skin integrity and the percutaneous penetration of benzoic acid dose-dependently. Basic Clin Pharmacol Toxicol 2006; 98:575–81.
28. Nielsen JB, Nielsen F. Topical use of tea tree oil reduces the dermal absorption of benzoic acid and methiocarb. Arch Dermatol Res 2006; 297:395–402.
29. RIFM (Research Institute for Fragrance Materials Inc.). In-vitro human skin penetration of methyl eugenol, estragole, acetyl cedrene and OTNE, Report Number 37084, 2001 (RIFM, Woodcliff Lake, NJ, U.S.A.).
30. Jimbo Y. Penetration of fragrance compounds through human epidermis. J Dermatol 1983; 10:229–39.
31. Ford RA, Hawkins DR, Schwaezenbach R, Api AM. The systemic exposure to the polycyclic musks, AHTN and HHCB, under conditions of use as fragrance ingredients: evidence of lack of complete absorption from a skin reservoir. Toxicol Lett 1999; 111:133–42.
32. RIFM (Research Institute for Fragrance Materials Inc.) In-vitro human skin penetration of radiolabelled fragrance material AHTN. Report Number 38099, 2001 (RIFM, Woodcliff Lake, NJ, U.S.A.).
33. RIFM (Research Institute for Fragrance Materials Inc.). Penetration studies in vitro on intact skin of naked rat with benzyl salicylate, Unpublished report from Givaudan. Report Number 33515, 1983 (RIFM, Woodcliff Lake, NJ, U.S.A.).
34. Hotchkiss SA, Miller JM, Caldwell J. Percutaneous absorption of benzyl acetate through rat skin in vitro. 2. Effect of vehicle and occlusion. Food Chem Toxicol 1992; 30:145–53.
35. Garnett A, Hotchkiss SA, Caldwell J. Percutaneous absorption of benzyl acetate through rat skin in vitro. 3. A comparison with human skin. Food Chem Toxicol 1994; 32:1061–5.
36. Bronaugh RL, Stewart RF, Wester RC, Bucks D, Mailbach HI, Anderson J. Comparison of percutaneous absorption of fragrances by humans and monkeys. Food Chem Toxicol 1985; 23:111–4.
37. Smith CK, Moore CA, Elahi EN, Smart AT, Hotchkiss SAM. Human skin absorption and metabolism of the contact allergens, cinnamic aldehyde and cinnamic alcohol. Toxicol Appl Pharmacol 2000; 168:189–99.
38. Weibel H, Hansen J. Penetration of the fragrance compounds, cinnamaldehyde and cinnamamyl alcohol, through human skin in vitro. Contact Dermatitis 1989; 20:167–72.
39. Yourick JJ, Bronaugh RL. Percutaneous absorption and metabolism of Coumarin in human and rat skin. J Appl Toxicol 1997; 17:153–8.
40. Ford RA, Hawkins DR, Mayo BC, Api AM. The in vivo dermal absorption and metabolism of [4-14C] coumarin by rats and by human volunteers under simulated conditions of use in fragrances. Food Chem Toxicol 2001; 39:153–62.

41. Hotchkiss SA. Absorption of fragrance ingredients using in vitro models with human skin. In: Frosch PJ, Johansen JD, White IR, eds. Fragrances: Beneficial and Adverse Effects. Berlin: Springer, 1998:125–35.

42. RIFM (Research Institute for Fragrance Materials Inc.) In-vitro human skin penetration of radiolabelled fragrance material HHCB. Report Number 38100, 2001 (RIFM, Woodcliff Lake, NJ, U.S.A.).

43. Jager W, Buchbauer G, Jirovetz L, Fritzer M. Percutaneous absorption of lavender oil from a massage oil. J Soc Cosmet Chem Japan 1992; 43(1):49–54.

44. RIFM (Research Institute for Fragrance Materials Inc.). In-vitro human skin penetration MMDHCA, methyl dehydrojasmonate and methyl atrarate, Report Number 37083, 2001 (RIFM, Woodcliff Lake, NJ, U.S.A.).

45. Hawkins DR, Ford RA. Dermal absorption and disposition of musk ambrette, musk ketone and musk xylene in rats. Toxicol Lett 1999; 111:95–103.

46. Hawkins DR, Elsom LF, Kirkpatrick D, Ford RA, Api AM. Dermal absorption and disposition of musk ambrette, musk ketone and musk xylene in human subjects. Toxicol Lett 2002; 131:147–51.

47. Hood HL, Wickett RR, Bronaugh RL. In vitro percutaneous absorption of the fragrance ingredient musk xylol. Food Chem Toxicol 1996; 34:483–8.

48. Reichling J, Landvatter U, Wagner H, Kostka KH, Schaefer UF. In vitro studies on release and human skin permeation of Australian tea tree oil (TTO) from topical formulations. Eur J Pharm Biopharm 2006; 64:222–8.

Index